HOSPITAL MANAGEMENT
A Guide to Departments

Edited by
Howard S. Rowland
and
Beatrice L. Rowland

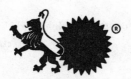

AN ASPEN PUBLICATION®
Aspen Systems Corporation
Rockville, Maryland
Royal Tunbridge Wells
1984

Library of Congress Cataloging in Publication Data
Main entry under title:

Hospital management.

"An Aspen publication."
Includes index.
1. Hospitals—Administration. I. Rowland, Howard S.
II. Rowland, Beatrice L. [DNLM: 1. Hospital Department—
Organization and Administration—Handbooks. WX 39 H828]
RA971.H5938   1984   362.1'1'068   84-324
ISBN: 0-89443-853-0

Publisher: John R.Marozsan
Associate Publisher: Jack W. Knowles, Jr.
Executive Managing Editor: Margot G. Raphael
Managing Editor: M. Eileen Higgins
Printing and Manufacturing: Debbie Collins

Library of Congress Catalog Card Number: 84-324
ISBN: 0-89443-853-0

Printed in the United States of America

1   2   3   4   5

To the men and women who, as hospital administrators,

have made the American system of health care delivery

a model and a standard for the entire world.

TABLE OF CONTENTS

INTRODUCTION

One of the festering problems of postindustrial society is society's failure to provide the individual with a sense of his or her unique importance in the work place. Even in the professions, the roles of individuals are often perceived as simply interchangeable components within increasingly complex and fragmented systems. It is the era of the specialized worker.

There may have been a time when a rare person like daVinci or Bacon or Jefferson could feel at home in any discipline, whether it be art or science or politics or philosophy. But those times are gone. The multiple explosions of knowledge in field after field have created vast reservoirs of fact, method, and skill that can be usefully explored only by the most dedicated and single-minded specialists. There seems no longer need or place for a "Renaissance man."

And yet there is one job today demanding a familiarity with a wide range of fields that would seem to suggest only a person of Renaissance dimensions need apply. The position requires a working knowledge of finance and accounting, industrial relations, systems analysis, mediation, public relations, marketing, social psychology, housekeeping, information management, high technology, law, computer science, education, and management . . . to name a few.

What is this job? It is that of the hospital administrator. Others within the hospital community may enjoy the glory, the professional recognition, the detailed knowledge, and the daily exercise of their special fields. But it is the administrator who brings all these distinct disciplines together and makes them work as an integral and effective whole. It is the administrator who often—when there is a hard decision to be made in one of these specialized departments—must take the final responsibility.

Indeed, the hospital administrator must be a person of remarkable parts, ready to meet whatever challenge comes along in a host of technical and professional fields. But no matter how quick this executive's mind or multifaceted the person's skills, the job is simply too broad, too deep, too complex for anyone to feel entirely comfortable in its performance.

That was the reason for undertaking this project—to make available to the hospital administrator, in a single handbook, the most current, pertinent, and authoritative information on managing the entire range of specialized functions within the hospital. Each chapter is designed to provide the administrator with not just a knowledge of a department's operation but with a detailed and practical guide for its management, improvement, and evaluation.

It is a "how-to" book, a definitive resource that a hospital administrator can consult with confidence whenever there is a need for informed guidance on the workings of a department or on methods for improving and bringing its services or procedures sharply up to date.

This book is not the work of one or two authors. The selections here are drawn from the most respected authorities and most significant literature in each of these specialized disciplines. That is why we call it a "state-of-the-art" library of information. Our intent was to create a "Renaissance" collection of rare intelligence, a treasure chest of knowledge, guidance, and practice in hospital management.

We trust you will find the result useful.

Howard S. Rowland
Beatrice L. Rowland
Peekskill, N.Y.
December 1983

Chapter 1—The Hospital Organization

THE ORGANIZATION CHART*

In a typical hospital organization chart, Figure 1-1, the governing body of the organization is generally referred to as the board of governors, board of trustees, or board of directors. The board delegates its authority to the administrator, chief executive officer, director, or president of the hospital. The administrator generally has associate administrators, or administrative assistants to handle the various operational aspects of the day-to-day functioning of the hospital. It is not unusual for an administrator to have support from assistant administrators, the number of whom will vary by hospital size. In very large institutions there may even be someone assigned as "Night Administrator." It is common for hospitals in the 200–300 bed range to have two assistant administrators.

Below the assistant administrator level in the hospital organization chart, there is a middle management group that becomes the departmental level of management. In the departmental or functional organization of the hospital there are generally at least four major types of functions to be carried out: (1) the nursing functions, (2) the business or fiscal functions, (3) the ancillary or professional services, and (4) the support services. It is not unusual for a hospital to have under the CEO at least four distinct ad-

ministrative or functional groupings responsible for these areas.

Overlapping Authority

The hospital has been termed a complex social system with conflict among the various participants, from patients to personnel. According to Rakich, Longest, and O'Connor (*Managing Health Care Organizations, 1977*):

The diversity of the institutional organization creates major problems. The governing board has the legal authority over, and responsibility for, the institution. The medical staff possesses the technical knowledge to make the decisions regarding questions of patient care and treatment. The administrative staff is responsible for the day-to-day operation of the hospital. These three elements, sometimes referred to as the organizational *triad*, share the same basic objectives. However, they interpret the means for meeting these objectives in terms of their own values and personalities. These values and personalities, unfortunately, are not the same for each element of the triad. This makes the hospital perhaps the most complex institution in American society.

For a prototype of the organizational structure in a medium size hospital see Figure 1-2. The complexity is apparent. The "dual pyramid" aspect is seen in the alignment of the medical staff portion of the organization with the administrative portion, including the

---

*Source: I. Donald Snook, Jr., *Hospitals: What They Are and How They Work,* Aspen Systems Corporation, 1981.

Figure 1-1 A typical hospital organization chart

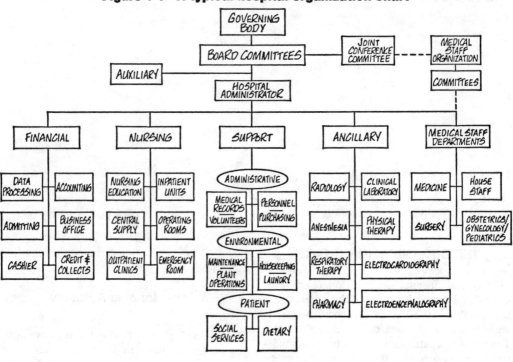

Figure 1-2 Overlapping authority in a voluntary general hospital

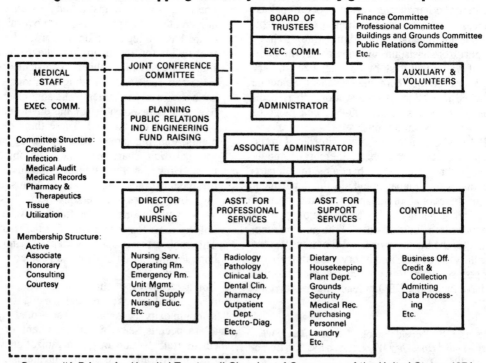

Source: "A Primer for Hospital Trustees," Chamber of Commerce of the United States, 1974.

administration, nursing division, professional services, support services, and controller. Note the position of the third element of the hospital's organizational triad, the Board of Trustees.

THE BOARD OF TRUSTEES*

Hospital trustees serve without pay; they are prohibited from profiting in any way from their membership on the board of trustees. Once appointed, the trustee has a responsibility to safeguard the hospital and its assets. The rewards for being a trustee are the satisfaction of having rendered a service to others in the community and the receipt of some measure of community status by being on the board. Because the trustees represent the ownership of the hospital, they have the ordinary liability of any owners of property. But they have the additional burden of protecting the patients from all foreseeable and preventable harm.

Trustees are frequently chosen from among the more prominent members of a community. Highly esteemed businessmen or professionals often serve on hospital boards. It is not uncommon to find representatives of well-established families with inherited wealth serving on boards. A more recent trend, however, has been one of providing community or consumer representation on boards. Yet, on balance, the traditional character of the board still holds. In a recent survey it was found that governing boards are dominated by business executives, members of the legal and accounting professions, and spokespersons for medicine and hospitals.

Profile of a Hospital Board

Just as hospitals vary considerably in size, purpose, and make-up, so do their boards. A recent survey by the American Hospital Association gives us a good overview of the make-up and structure of the typical hospital board. The average hospital board has 14 trustees, the smaller boards have 8 to 9 members, and the larger boards have around 25 members. Hospital boards typically meet between 10 and 12 times a year; the average is 10. This is reasonable considering a board may not meet during one of the

summer months or the Christmas season. Board membership likewise varies considerably. The average term of membership is slightly in excess of 3 years, with a majority of hospitals stipulating no limit on the number of consecutive terms a board member may serve. There is remarkable consistency throughout the nation's hospitals in board committee structure. Perhaps the reason for this consistency is the impetus toward review of hospital bylaws and suggestions from the JCAH. The most common committee is the Executive Committee, which is found in more than 70 percent of hospitals. With regard to the age of a typical board member, over 55 percent fall between the ages of 51 and 70, and 38 percent between the ages of 31 and 50. Over 80 percent of board members have at least a bachelor's degree in education, regardless of hospital size or ownership. Board membership is predominantly male. Across the United States, 83 percent of boards are made up of men, with women representing approximately 16 percent.

Functions

There are three primary functions or responsibilities of a board of trustees: (1) the formal and legal responsibility for controlling the hospital and assuring the community that the hospital works properly, (2) the responsibility to see that the hospital gains support from its community, and (3) the responsibility of ensuring that the board of trustees is accountable to the citizens and to the community it serves.

A review of the activities that hospital boards undertake across the country shows that the following functions can be attributed to them (see also Table 1-1):

● They establish hospital objectives.
● They organize themselves in order to perform their work; this is usually accomplished according to the hospital bylaws.
● They have important roles in reviewing and approving all major plans and programs of the hospital.
● They review all major administrative policies of the hospital.
● They appoint the administrator and evaluate the administrator's activities from year to year.
● They advise the administrator in the operational management of the hospital.

---

*Source: I. Donald Snook, Jr., *Hospitals: What They Are and How They Work,* Aspen Systems Corporation, 1981.

- They review and approve all major hospital decisions.
- They annually review the hospital's performance to see whether the hospital has reached its objectives.

The board's important role in the control of hospital funds should be noted. It is the board's responsibility to see that the hospital's finances be reviewed in some detail and approved by the trustees. Hopefully, most governing board members will be involved in obtaining endowments, grants, gifts, and other donation income. If the hospital is fortunate enough to have a significant amount of funds to be invested, it is the hospital board's responsibility to do this. Frequently, this is done at least once a year at the time the hospital budget is presented to the board of trustees by the hospital administrator.

One of the most important functions of a board of trustees is the investigation, review, and selection of the hospital administrator. Indeed, perhaps the most important thing a board of trustees does is to select an administrator. The board then delegates to the administrator the authority and responsibility to manage the day-to-day operations of the hospital. However, though the trustees must delegate enough authority so that the administrator can do this job well, the board still retains the ultimate responsibility for everything that happens in the hospital. The relationship between the administrator and the governing board is primarily that of employee-employer, but not in the usual sense of the term. Since the hospital is a very special type of organization, the relationship between the administrator and the governing board is in fact similar to a partnership. Just as it is the responsibility of the governing boards to hire administrators, it is also their responsibility to discharge them for cause at any time.

Relationship with the Medical Staff

The medical staff of the hospital operates within its own medical staff bylaws and regulations, but the physicians on the medical staff are accountable to the board of trustees for the professional care of their patients. The board of trustees is responsible for exercising due care in the selec-

Table 1-1   Hospital Trustees' Job Description

A comprehensive "job description" for hospital trustees was prepared by the Dallas County Hospital District to help hospital trustees assess the scope of their duties and functions:

- Attend board meetings regularly;
- Exercise general supervision over the corporation's affairs;
- Investigate and audit the corporation's decisions;
- Bring your "business experience" and "common sense" with you to decide corporate policies;
- Pursue the warning signs that come to your attention that something is wrong;
- Insist on regular and frequent board meetings;
- Insist on meaningful board meetings with full disclosure of operating results;

- Require the corporation to employ a CPA firm to audit the corporation's records;
- Require the corporation to engage competent legal counsel;
- Require the corporation to set up an executive committee to examine and carry out the policies of the board of directors;
- Require reports at the directors' meetings of all committees of the corporation;
- Evaluate officer performance and review officers' duties periodically;
- Select competent new executive officers;
- Authorize legitimate corporate indebtedness;
- Insist on a policy as to retirement of directors, officers, and employees at realistic standards of age and health condition;

- Know the trustees, officers, and corporate organization you are asked to serve;
- Adopt and follow sound business policies;
- Avoid self-serving policies;
- Avoid conflict of interest;
- Maintain a good credit standing for the corporation;
- Maintain reasonable capitalization;
- Observe the general corporation business laws;
- Review the adequacy of the corporation's insurance programs;
- Review the adequacy of your trustees' and officers' insurance programs;
- Review the fairness of the indemnification granted to trustees and officers of the corporation.

Source: Stephen M. Blaes, "Hospital Trusteeship: Corporate and Personal Liability," *Hospital Progress*, July 1982, pp. 78ff.

tion of physicians. A physician's application credentials and requested privileges are carefully examined by the medical staff, which in turn recommends the physician with requested privileges to the board. It is the responsibility of the trustees to act upon these recommendations, that is, to grant privileges, to request further clarification from the medical staff, or to reject the privileges on sound grounds.

The board of trustees has a legal and moral responsibility to control the quality of medical care in the hospital. Yet, though the governing body has the ultimate responsibility, quality control is a team effort. The CEO and the chief of the medical staff also have a part to play in the quality assurance program. Such a program has to be developed and implemented, and both the administrator and chief of the medical staff contribute greatly in these two areas. The board has the monitoring role in the program. Monitoring includes receiving monthly reports that display the medical staff's performance as measured against preestablished criteria, concurring with medical staff recommendations, or developing the board's own recommendations to improve medical staff performance and to ensure that it impacts positively on the quality of medical care.

The board's joint conference committee, which has representatives from the medical staff, serves as the main formal linkage between the medical arm of the hospital and the board and its administrator. It is through committees that the governing board usually gets its work accomplished. This committee structure is frequently established along special functional lines. Examples of typical board of trustee committees are an executive committee, a finance committee, a planning committee, and perhaps a committee for the building and its operations and grounds. Generally, recommendations through the separate committees affect the governance, management, and administration, as well as the medical staff in the hospital.

Selecting and Nurturing Board Members*

Boards are valuable assets for a health care organization—but they must be properly selected and nurtured. The right people must be selected.

Here, myth must be distinguished from reality. For every story about a board person who gave a building, there are a hundred other stories about someone whom "we thought would give a building, died, and gave nothing." Organizations should approach the selection of directors with considerable seriousness and select only those people who enhance the value of the organization because of their expertise, availability, and yes—in some cases, personal stature. Considered in this decision should be the question, If time and effort are invested in this person, will there be a return on that investment? A negative answer suggests that the search process should be continued.

Having selected the right people, the organization must then make an investment. This investment has several dimensions. First, the manager should learn as much as possible about the new director and that director's home organization, experience, or profession. This includes an assessment of areas of strength and weakness. Doing this diagnostic workup demonstrates an interest in the board member's professional and personal development, while simultaneously permitting an evaluation of how and where the new director can fit into the organizational scheme. Second, the board member must be educated in the major issues and problems faced in the health industry, in general, and the particular component, specifically. In doing this, it is not necessary to focus on detail as much as to look at issues and options. Finally, the board member has to keep informed.

Behavior of Directors*

Several types of behavior can be considered desirable in a director. A board member must be active and participate in the board meetings, as well as in the committee structure. The director who shows up occasionally and must always be "updated" wastes everyone's time and can be counterproductive. The director who wants to learn more and seeks additional expertise is respected by other directors and management. This interest should be construed as an indication that the director supports the organization, and such a person should be considered a major asset. Seeking additional responsibility is another important behavior, since it is a sign of

*Source: Seth B. Goldsmith, *Health Care Management*, Aspen Systems Corporation, 1981.

*Source: Seth B. Goldsmith, *Health Care Management*, Aspen Systems Corporation, 1981.

commitment. An individual who follows through is invaluable. Board members who offer suggestions and ideas but simply do not deliver are not nearly as helpful as those who develop their programs. In general then, the useful and effective director is one who is conscientious, thoughtful, articulate, concerned, and available—a tall order indeed.

Undesirable behaviors could, in many instances, lead to a managerial Armageddon or revolution. At the top of the undesirable list is the demanding board person who involves management with inconsequential work activities or focuses attention on trivial matters. The president of one hospital board had the assistant director trailing after her carrying a sample book of fabrics so that the manager could hold the samples against various couches throughout the hospital and the president could choose the new fabrics. A morning doing that is demeaning and demoralizing to a manager, as well as a waste of money.

Vying for the top of the list is the board member who has accepted the position for personal gain. This gain comes in various guises. At worst, there are board members who, despite conflict-of-interest laws, want to do business with the organization on whose board they serve. Sometimes being on a board works to their advantage in their own businesses; for example, one restaurateur who served as treasurer on the board of a large hospital insisted that the hospital use certain purveyors—the same ones he used. Subsequently, he received discounts from these purveyors for his own business. A less overt personal gain is seen when a person joins a board for the experience or "service" credits necessary to advance in the home organization.

The directors who may disturb managers most are those who like to end-run management. For example, they might make commitments without consulting management, or they might stir up enthusiasm for a new program without investigating it or discussing it with staff. When a policy is adopted that they object to, however, they respond by openly criticizing management and the board.

Small thinking is a characteristic of many board members. Along with this is a tendency to focus on a "hobbyhorse." For example, a board member whose pet project is the snack bar might insist on an overinvestment by manage-

ment in a program that should really have a lower priority.

The naive, uninformed, and lazy director is also a problem. Again, such a director expends energy, which is limited, for insignificant issues.

Trustees and Conflict of Interest: A Sample Memo to Trustees from CEO*

A conflict of interest may be considered to exist in those instances in which the action or activities of an individual on behalf of the hospital also involve (a) the obtaining of an improper personal gain or advantage; (b) an adverse effect on the hospital interests; or (c) the obtaining by a third party of an improper gain or advantage. Conflicts of interests can arise in other instances. Although it is impossible to list every circumstance giving rise to a possible conflict of interest, the following list will serve as a guide to the types of activities that might cause conflicts. For your protection and the protection of the corporation, such activities should be fully reported.

1. Interests
   a. Holding by a trustee, directly or indirectly, of a position or of a material financial interest in any outside concern (1) from which the hospital secures goods or services or (2) which provides services competitive with the hospital.
   b. Competition with the hospital by an individual, directly or indirectly, in the purchase or sale of property or property rights or interests.
2. Outside activities
   a. Rendition by an individual of directive, managerial, or consultative services to any outside concern that does business with, or is a competitor of, the hospital.
   b. (Applicable only to trustees who are employees.) Participation by an individual in any activity (whether for personal profit or incident to industry, civic, or charitable organization affairs) that is likely to involve significant use of the individual's time during normal business hours.
3. Gifts, gratuities, and entertainment
   Acceptance by an individual of gifts, ex-

*Source· Stephen M. Blaes, "Hospital Trusteeship: Corporate and Personal Liability," *Hospital Progress*, July 1982.

cessive entertainment, or other favors from an outside concern that does, or is seeking to do, business with, or is a competitor of, the hospital under circumstances from which it might be inferred that such action was intended to influence the individual in the performance of his duties. This does not include the acceptance of items of nominal or minor value that are of such a nature as to indicate that they are merely tokens of esteem or friendship and are not related to any particular transaction or hospital activity.

4. Inside information
   Disclosure or use of hospital information for the personal profit or advantage of the individual or anyone else.

Any situation in doubt should be fully disclosed so as to permit an impartial and objective determination. It should be particularly noted that this disclosure relates not only to your activities but also to those of your immediate family.

Distinctions between Governance and Management

The functions trustees perform pertain to most decision-making bodies in organizations. It is important to understand which functions constitute governance and which constitute management, since governance is the essence of trustees' responsibility. A challenge of governance and management is to distinguish who does what, since some areas overlap.

Robert Cunningham, Jr., described seven essential functions of hospital boards of trustees: ensure survival, set goals, make plans, organize resources, delegate authority, measure performance, and initiate change.[1]

One hospital's distinctions between governance and management responsibilities can be found in Table 1-2.

How to Appraise Board Performance*

Individual Performance

Inherently, performance appraisal at the board level must be treated differently than managerial appraisal. The purpose of an organizational structure is to pinpoint responsibility and ac-

---

[1]Sr. Mary M. Sengelaub, "Governance Sponsorship Management," *Hospital Progress,* July 1982.

*Source: Everett A. Johnson and Richard L. Johnson, *Hospitals in Transition,* Aspen Systems Corporation, 1982.

Table 1-2 Governance, Management: Complementary Responsibilities

Governance, a role which can be filled only by the legal owners themselves or by their appointed representatives, comprises the following responsibilities:

- To review and to act on philosophy, mission, role, and goals;
- To control and direct policymaking;
- To enhance the organization's total assets (financial, human, and material); and
- To appoint management and ensure that it is competent and carries out strategies that will meet the (hospital) corporation's goals and objectives.

Management may be described as complementing governance. Management functions include:

- Assisting the board in developing philosophy, mission, role, goals, and objectives;
- Defining strategies to achieve goals and objectives;
- Interpreting and communicating goals and objectives to those they affect;
- Ensuring that all organization activities are consonant with the philosophy, mission, role, goals, and objectives;

- Reporting to the governing board the organization's status in achieving its goals;
- Implementing governing board policy and ensuring that the implementation is achieved and reported to the board and providing input for developing and evaluating policies;
- Acquiring, conserving, preserving, and ensuring efficient and effective use of all resources; and
- Monitoring and controlling operations, evaluating performance, taking corrective actions, and affirming good outcomes.

Source: This material was adapted from "Integrated Governance and Management Process: Conceptual Design," Sisters of Mercy Health Corporation, Farmington Hills, Mich. 1980, pp. 76–77

countability for performance so that the individual manager can be measured. At the board level, the purpose of the structure is to provide a mechanism for deliberative group action in a way that minimizes the impact of individual performance. Yet, to measure the board only in a collective manner and not to discriminate between individual board member performance denies that any real differences can exist between levels of individual board performance.

Many boards still carry on with the charade of using a small group for making decisions and talking as if all the board members of a large board are effectively making contributions to the development of policy. The executive committee is really where the decisions are made. Large boards rarely exist without an executive committee that meets more frequently than the board and, in actual fact, operates as a *de facto* board.

As individuals charged with managing the hospital, administrators know the more time they spend on governance, the less time they will have available for operating matters. Because of this time factor, they tend to build personal relationships with this inner circle as a way of ensuring the adoption of their recommendations. Instinctively, chief executives recognize that if others are to become deeply involved in the real decision-making process, the demands on their own time for governance activities (on an individual basis) would increase, thereby leading to a further reduction in time for operational activities.

Two Types of Inquiry

In evaluating the performance of the governance level of a hospital with a board, two types of inquiry have to be made; the questions deal with the inputs to policy making and the outputs in terms of appropriateness of the policies reached.

Input Questions

The input questions include the following:

- Does the board carry out its responsibilities in the organizational framework outlined in its own bylaws?
- Have position descriptions been written and followed by board members, chairman, and chief executive officer?
- To what extent do all trustees exercise their responsibility for providing inputs into the decision-making process?

- What periodic and formal review is made of individual trustee performance?
- What periodic and formal review is made of the performance of the chief executive?

Output Questions

Output questions that should be studied include:

- From a careful review of board minutes, to what extent do they indicate the adoption of timely courses of action?
- To what extent does the regular reporting system provide trustees with a clear picture of the quality of care being given in the hospital?
- Do trustees receive appropriate financial information?
- Can it be demonstrated that the board acts appropriately on the reports it receives?
- Does the board periodically review the objectives and goals of the hospital and determine to what extent performance has met them?

Who Performs the Appraisal?

Since overall governing board performance is the collective result of individual trustee activities, evaluation of each one on an annual basis would seem to be in keeping with sound organizational practice. Because the nominating committee is charged with recommending trustees, as well as the slate of officers at the annual meeting of a hospital corporation, it is the most suitable for undertaking this task as an extension of its existing responsibilities. As the definition of the functions of a nominating committee is reviewed in hospital bylaws, it becomes obvious that a careful and thorough formal review of each trustee's performance annually would be an invaluable asset in determining whether or not to reappoint for another term. Written reviews by such a committee would be a first step in bringing about a minimum standard of performance for all trustees.

How Boards Measure Administrator Performance*

To assure accountability on a continuing basis, hospital management literature says the board

---

*Source: David G. Warren, *Problems in Hospital Law*, 3rd ed., Aspen Systems Corporation, 1978.

should set performance standards and mechanisms for measuring administrative performance. Some of the suggested indices by which they judge how well the administrative staff of a hospital is performing are these:

(a) budgets compare favorably with actual expenditures;
(b) costs per patient day compare favorably to those of similar hospitals;
(c) costs per case by department compare favorably to those of similar hospitals;
(d) cash on hand, payables, and receivables are judged to be in appropriate relationship with revenue;
(e) ratios of payroll to total expense, staff to numbers of patients, work performed to employee work-hours are appropriate;
(f) other fiscal reports are available and indicate measures of efficiency and effectiveness which can be compared internally with prior performance and externally with hospitals of similar size and setting.

THE HOSPITAL ADMINISTRATOR

The Hospital Administrator's Functions*

The responsibilities of a hospital administrator as described in an AHA Management Review Program are these:

(a) Submitting for approval a plan of organization for the conduct of hospital operation and recommending changes when necessary.
(b) Preparing a plan for the achievement of the hospital's specific objectives and periodically reviewing and evaluating it.
(c) Selecting, employing, controlling, and discharging all employees.
(d) Submitting for approval an annual budget showing expected receipts and expenditures.
(e) Recommending the rates to be charged for hospital services.
(f) Having charge and custody of and being responsible for all operating funds of the corporation.

(g) Representing the hospital in its relationships with other health agencies.
(h) Serving as liaison and channel of communications between the governing board or its committees and the medical staff.
(i) Assisting the medical staff with its organizational and medical-administrative problems and responsibilities.
(j) Submitting to the governing board reports showing the professional service and financial experience of the hospital, and submitting such special reports as may be requested by the governing board.
(k) Advising the governing board on matters of policy formulation.

In addition, the AHA says in a postscript to this catalog of responsibilities, the chief executive or his delegate is expected to attend all meetings of the governing board and its committees, and to advise and keep "the governing board currently informed on significant trends which enable it to carry out its function of policy formulation . . . [including] information [on] and explanation of (1) significant economic, legislative, and social factors which influence the hospital field in general and this hospital in particular; (2) activities of local, state, and national organizations which are related to the hospital's program of service; (3) conditions within the hospital which may require action by the governing board; [and] (4) technical and scientific advances in the health field."

The Chief Executive Officer's (CEO) Functions*

The chief executive officer

- Directs all activities of the institution within the framework of the established philosophy, objectives, and policies adopted by the board of trustees.
- Implements the policies established by the board of trustees.
- Acts as catalyst for establishing institutional goals, both short- and long-term, in support of the institution's philosophy and general objectives.

---

*Source: David G. Warren, *Problems in Hospital Law*, 3rd ed., Aspen Systems Corporation, 1978.

*Source: "Financial Career Opportunities," issue editor Richard C. Dolan, *Topics in Health Care Financing*, Fall 1980, Appendix.

- Educates and orients the board of trustees; works closely with the executive and nominating committees to plan for appropriate new members; assures that new members bring specific expertise needed by the board in areas such as finance, human resources, medicine, engineering and public relations; prepares meaningful board agendas; acts as catalyst to effectively persuade board to make important decisions.
- Consults with medical staff; remains fully informed regarding the views of the medical staff as to the quality of medical practice and patient care within the hospital.
- Involves medical staff leadership in evaluating and recommending the overall policies, objectives, and quality control of the institution; informs the professional staff regarding policies and objectives established or under consideration, including the availability of human, financial, and other resources to realize such objectives.
- Works outside the institution in planning and community relations, and with various regulatory bodies to ensure current feedback concerning the latest regulations, laws, and assorted encumbrances involved with managing a health care institution; attends association meetings especially at the state and regional levels; remains current on health care trends through extensive outside reading.
- Oversees the planning, control, and effective utilization of the physical, financial, and human resources of the institution.
- Strives to improve patient care by developing (in conjunction with the director of operations) a sound management organization that will provide maximum human resource, physical plant, and equipment support for professional and auxiliary staff.
- Reviews and approves the organization of internal function of the institution through appropriate departmentalization and delegation of duties; delegates management responsibilities to appropriate people; establishes formal means of accountability.
- Selects qualified personnel for management positions; approves objectives of each manager; follows up on objectives to assure compliance; takes responsibility for terminating ineffective managers without having

to consult the board of trustees or medical staff; approves individual managerial salary increases and other increases throughout the institution without consulting the board, provided they are within defined budgetary and management compensation plans.
- Directs the financial officer as appropriate to ensure the current and future viability of the institution.
- Remains aware of current and potential competitive forces in the marketplace; ensures that the institution has an active and continuous marketing plan that meets the objectives of the overall corporate plan.
- Ensures that all legal and statutory requirements are met for the operation of the institution; participates in all litigation for all institution activities; informs board of need to initiate litigation.
- Listens to the auxiliary, community, staff, volunteers, and other voluntary organizations interested in the institution; directs their overall activities to ensure they are in keeping with the institution's philosophy, objectives, and legal commitments.
- Establishes a system whereby the management staff develops contacts with groups within the community in order to ensure better community understanding and support for the institution's programs.
- Performs other duties as assigned by the board of trustees or as required to effectively meet the responsibilities for the position.

Qualifications

The CEO must have a proven record of successful leadership over line management functions in a large complex organization. He or she must have the ability to effectively select, motivate, and evaluate performance of key personnel. The person must have the mental skills to fully comprehend complex issues and problems, and analyze extensive reports, financial and statistical data. The person should have a mature management style and react with confidence and poise during times of stress. Tough-minded decision making occurs frequently, and the person should be able to tolerate considerable amounts of criticism on an infrequent basis and some amount of criticism on a frequent basis.

The Chief Operating Officer's Functions*

The chief operating officer manages the internal function of the institution under the overall direction of the CEO, directs all departments and nonfinancial functions connected with the day-to-day management of the institution, and performs routine duties of CEO in his or her absence.

Specifically, the chief operating officer:

- Manages virtually all areas of the institution; applies all of the modern management techniques of planning, organizing, and problem solving in managing virtually all facets of the day-to-day operations of the institution.
- Develops and motivates department managers and other key personnel to optimize their talents and meet the overall needs and goals of the organization; analyzes organizational needs and ensures that the institution has the effective personnel resources to accomplish its goals; recruits and orients key personnel.
- Provides for the development and implementation of managerial controls; oversees the proper use of systems, procedures, management engineering, data processing, and other methodology to ensure that up-to-date business management techniques are being utilized; stresses the importance of objective measurement in developing standards of performance.
- Performs a wide variety of organizational and human resource functions, including: performance evaluations of all department managers; recommendations for promotions, demotions, salary increases, discharges; participates in disciplinary actions involving department managers and assists department managers in the proper handling of disciplinary actions of their subordinates; assists department managers in developing their skills to better educate and motivate their personnel; acts as consulting resource for all departments regarding general management problems; makes final decisions regarding key problems as called for

in established management guidelines for the position; provides authoritative backup for department managers as part of their decision making; occasionally makes immediate decisions regarding emergencies affecting the institution's operations where no precedent exists.
- Assists the CEO in the development of general policies and in the formation of long-range programs and plans; implements specific policies and programs after approval by the CEO and the board of trustees.
- Works with the medical director, institution-based physicians and key members of the medical staff on day-to-day hospital operations problems; attends medical staff meetings that have a direct impact on hospital operations.
- Attends board of trustee meetings as a backup to the CEO and to serve on committees of the board as assigned.
- Works closely with the financial officer to ensure a sound financial position for the institution; acts as a liaison with department managers in matters pertaining to the institution's budget; participates in all important institutional budget meetings and determinations.
- Strives to improve patient care by developing a sound management organization that will provide maximum human resource allocations; assists CEO in management matters pertaining to physical plant and equipment that will benefit patient care.
- Oversees the efficient operations within the hospital; demands top-level performance from departmental managers and ensures that practical standards are set and met.
- Oversees the quality assurance program, including utilization review, medical audit, and administrative liaison with professional standards review organizations.
- Organizes and oversees the activities of hospital departments to ensure smooth management and compliance with Joint Commission on Accreditation of Hospitals standards, state health department rules and regulations, and other legislative directives.
- Performs other duties as required by the president and CEO or as required to effectively meet the responsibilities for the position.

---

*Source "Financial Career Opportunities," issue editor Richard C. Dolan, *Topics in Health Care Financing,* Fall 1980, Appendix.

Qualifications

This position is similar in kind to the "administrator" position of several years ago that reported to the board of trustees. It shares second place in overall importance with the CFO in many hospitals. The person must have a strong background in line management to qualify for this post. This position requires an individual with mature judgment and excellent people skills. The individual must have a proper balance between being analytical and decisive. Age and a specific educational background are not as important as the ability to work well with people and to make unpopular decisions with a minimum of unrest. Work involves a considerable amount of energy and the need to cater to the working hours of others, therefore the work schedule requires early morning arrivals and moderately late evening departures. The individual must be thick skinned and able to handle criticism because he/she will be looked upon by most managers and employees as the institution's disciplinarian.

The Administrator's Key Relationships*

An administrator must pay close attention to three important relationships: with the medical staff, with the governing body, and with hospital employees.

Medical Staff

For better or for worse, the administrator is a partner with the physicians in delivering health care in the modern hospital. The hospital provides the necessary facilities and personnel to aid the physician in the practice of medicine. The physician—and only the physician—can admit the patients to the hospital. Thus, a necessary partnership is forged.

The best circumstances between the administrator and the medical staff exist when there is a mutual understanding, respect, and trust between the two parties.

Administrators should keep their staff informed on organizational changes, board policies, and decisions that affect them and their patients. Physicians who understand the reasons for certain policies and decisions will tend to be more supportive. On the other hand, administrators should be sensitive to the medical staff's need for self-governance and support that need. There is a potential for conflicts and tensions between the administrator and the medical staff. Some of these tensions may be natural, since the physicians' interests tend to be directed primarily to the patient and the physicians' own economic survival. The administrators' interests tend to be broader in terms of the entire hospital, their relationships with all the employees, and the financial viability of the institution. These two objectives may in fact not necessarily be in concert.

Many of the tensions and frustrations that exist might be brought about by poor communications between the administrator and the medical staff. Misunderstandings flourish when effective communication is put in a secondary position. Administrators *must* communicate with their medical staffs—that is a key function of their role. They must be negotiators and integrators in their relationships with the medical staff. Although friction may exist, it is by no means the normal state of affairs in hospital administration and should be minimized. There should be no dividing lines between these two groups; there should be singleness of purpose, enabling the hospital to move ahead in its program effectively.

The medical staff views the administrator as a catalyst in management activities, as an implementer, one who is able to provide the physicians tools in the right place and at the right time to enable them to carry out their work in the hospital. They see the administrator as being accountable for the handling of these resources.

Board of Trustees

Boards of trustees give administrators their ultimate authority; boards hire them and can also fire them. The administrator is delegated the authority to administer the affairs of the hospital. Though this relationship is one of employee/employer, in actuality the two parties—the administrator and the board—function as partners. The administrator must turn the board's power into administrative action within the hospital. Just as with the medical staff, communication

---

*Source: I. Donald Snook, Jr., *Hospitals: What They Are and How They Work,* Aspen Systems Corporation, 1981.

with the board is critical to the administrator's proper functioning and to the future of the hospital.

Indeed, the partnership relationship between the board and the administrator has been solidified through the placement of the CEO as a voting member on many governing boards of hospitals. This is a common occurrence in industry, where the CEO is also a member of the board of directors and is an equal among equals, not just a hired employee. Typically, when administrators are members of boards, they have the title of president under the chairman of the board. CEOs can become active, with voting privileges, or as ex officio members on key board committees, including the nominating, bylaws, and planning committees.

Employees

Employees regard administrators as their work leaders, and they are expected to fill this role. Administrators have an image to uphold in the hospital; they are perceived as authority figures, as people of action who are supposed to make decisions with speed and wisdom. Employees respond best when they feel they are being brought into the communications link and that they are not being treated arbitrarily. One of the key roles of the administrator is to make the employees aware of the critical nature of their services in the mission of the hospital. This is easier with the nurses and others who deal directly with patients, but the administrator must continually inform all employees of their importance to the whole mission of the hospital. Again, as with the medical staff and the board of trustees, communication is a key to a successful relationship with the employees.

The administrator has the ultimate authority to employ, direct, discipline, and dismiss employees, though this is generally delegated to middle managers and department heads. Because of this, the administrator has a special relationship with department heads. Through the department heads, the administrator executes the rules and regulations concerning the employees' work duties. On the other hand, the administrator has the responsibility to provide the proper organization as well as a safe work environment within the hospital. The administrator must be sensitive to employee needs and see that the personnel are compensated adequately for their effort.

Chapter 2—Medical Staff

OVERVIEW

The medical staff has overall responsibility for the quality of all medical care provided to patients and for the ethical conduct and professional practices of individual physicians. It is accountable to the governing body, just as the administrator is. The medical staff can be on a line relationship to the governing body or may work on a line to the administrator. In many organizations the medical staff serves in a staff or advisory capacity to the administrator with line authority only to and from the governing body.

Staff Distinctions*

Active medical staff includes physicians who are responsible for the greatest amount of medical practice within the hospital and who perform all significant staff, organizational, and administrative functions.

Associate medical staff consists of physicians who are being considered for advancement to the medical staff. Included in this is a definition of the period of time to be served in associate medical staff as outlined in the bylaws. At the end of this period the member is considered for advancement through a mechanism established by staff bylaws.

Courtesy medical staff is a group of physicians who have privileges to admit and treat pa-

---

*Source: Kathleen A. Waters and Gretchen F. Murphy, *Medical Records in Health Information*, Aspen Systems Corporation, 1979.

tients only occasionally. The number of patients who may be admitted by these members is defined by medical staff bylaws along with any exceptions related to bed availability.

Consulting medical staff is a group established for those medical practitioners of recognized professional ability who, on an on-call or regularly scheduled basis, provide consulting services to other members of the staff.

Honorary staff are those individuals who are recognized for their noteworthy contributions to patient care, their outstanding professional reputation, and/or their long service to the hospital. If honorary status is to be established automatically at a certain age, this is defined in the medical staff bylaws.

Provisional staff includes all initial appointments to the medical staff except honorary and consulting. The initial provisional period should be the same for all new members of the medical staff. All characteristics of this group are defined in the bylaws. Each newly appointed medical staff member is usually assigned to a department or service where his or her performance and clinical competence are observed by a chairman, chief of the department, or some other physician assigned to perform the review function. If at the end of the provisional period individuals have not satisfied the requirements for staff eligibility, provisional status is usually automatically terminated and they are given written notice of such termination and of any rights that they have under the procedures specified in the medical staff bylaws to contest this decision.

Temporary staff are physicians who have been granted temporary privileges for a limited period of time by the chief medical staff officer or on the recommendation of the chief of a particular department. Temporary status is given to physicians who for some reason have a temporary need to provide patient care in a hospital where they do not usually work. Temporary privileges may be given for a stated period or for a period spanning the time needed for the specialized care of a specific patient.

Executive Committee*

To have an effective organization the medical staff must provide effective self-regulation. The duties, qualifications, and method of selecting officers of the medical staff should be defined in medical staff bylaws, rules, and regulations. Important to the administrator are such organization components of the medical staff as departments and committees. The executive committee of the medical staff is empowered to act for the staff in the intervals between medical staff meetings. This committee usually performs the following functions:

- Serves as a liaison between medical staff and hospital administration
- Receives and acts upon reports and recommendations from medical staff committees, departments, services, and assigned activity groups
- Implements the approved policies of the medical staff
- Recommends to the governing body all matters relating to appointments and reappointments, staff categorization, department service assignments, clinical privileges, and (except where there is such a function of the medical staff) corrective action
- Accounts to the governing body for the quality of the overall medical care rendered to the patient by the medical staff
- Initiates and pursues corrective action when warranted in accordance with medical staff bylaw provisions

---

*Source: Kathleen A. Waters and Gretchen F. Murphy, *Medical Records in Health Information*, Aspen Systems Corporation, 1979.

- Informs the medical staff of accrediting programs and the accreditation status of the hospital
- Assures that all medical staff members are actively involved in the accreditation process, including participation in any surveys or final critique session

Department Chairman*

In a hospital where duties and functions are too complex to be handled by the staff as a whole, the medical staff will be organized in departments. Usual duties of the department chairman should include:

- Accountability to the executive committee for all professional and medical staff administrative activities within departments
- Continuing surveillance of the professional performance of medical staff members who exercise privileges in the department, submitting regular reports on each member, at least at the time of reappointment/reappraisal
- Recommending to the medical staff the criteria for granting privileges in the department
- Conducting concurrent and retrospective patient care evaluation studies to determine the quality of care being given within the department
- Assuring participation of department members in continuing education programs and required meetings
- Appointing committees as needed to conduct department functions
- Participating in department budgetary planning and assisting in preparation of all required reports

Medical Staff Committees**

There are six other major medical staff committees that are traditionally found in hospitals. These committees are found in all accredited hospitals because they encompass functions recommended by the JCAH.

---

*Source: Kathleen A. Waters and Gretchen F. Murphy, *Medical Records in Health Information*, Aspen Systems Corporation, 1979.
**Source: Kathleen A. Waters and Gretchen F. Murphy, *Medical Records in Health Information*, Aspen Systems Corporation, 1979.

The Medical Record Committee

The primary purpose of the medical record committee is to see that accurate and complete medical records are developed and retained for every patient treated. Records are reviewed for their timely completion, clinical pertinence, and overall adequacy for use in patient care, patient care evaluation studies, and in some circumstances medico-legal documentation. The medical record committee review ensures that records reflect the condition and progress of the patient, including results of all tests and therapy given. Some other functions that may come under the consideration of the medical record committee are decisions on the format of the complete medical record, forms to be used in the record, and methods of retaining and retrieving medical data. Members of the medical record committee include members of the medical staff and the medical record administrator.

The Tissue Committee

Its prime responsibility is the review of surgical procedures, both those in which a specimen or human tissue was removed and those in which no specimen or human tissue was removed. The committee reviews documented indications for surgery and attempts to evaluate the relationship between the preoperative and the postoperative diagnoses. It is also concerned with the pathologic diagnoses of any specimens or tissue removed during surgery. Members of the tissue committee include members of the medical staff, the clinical laboratory, and the medical record administrator.

The Infection Committee

Its prime responsibility is distinguishing hospital from nonhospital-acquired infections, control of infection, and the coordination of all other activities regarding infection control, including the reporting, evaluating, and maintaining of records of infections among patients and personnel. This committee is responsible for written policies regarding specific requirements for isolation and for the prevention, surveillance, and control procedures regarding sterilization and disinfection practices in all departments of the hospital. Members of this committee include members of the medical staff, administration, the nursing staff, a microbiologist (if one is part

of the clinical laboratory) or other laboratory representative, and often the medical record administrator.

The Pharmacy Committee

Its primary responsibility is the development of policies and practices relating to the selection and distribution of drugs, including policies regarding safety and effective use of pharmaceuticals. This group also serves the medical staff in an advisory capacity on matters pertaining to drugs and develops and reviews periodically the formulary that is a drug list for the entire hospital. Members of this committee include a pharmacist, physicians, and nurses.

The Utilization Review Committee

Its primary purpose is the review of all aspects of care to assure high-quality patient care through the effective use of equipment, personnel, materials, and the facility as a whole. This committee utilizes medical records for most of its deliberations. The committee is always concerned that the need for care is well documented, including justification for admitting patients to the inpatient facility. The utilization review committee must have a written plan that describes the methods it will use for evaluating appropriateness and medical necessity of admissions, continued stays, supportive services, and the provision for discharge planning. This plan must specify the time frame in which the reviews will be conducted and outline the specifications for both concurrent and retrospective reviews. Concurrent review is an evaluation of individual patients during their hospitalization, and retrospective review is a review of patients after they have been discharged. Members of the utilization review committee include members of the medical staff, administration, and the medical record administrator or record technician.

The Medical Audit Committee

This committee, with its more contemporary title of Patient Care Evaluation Committee, has as its prime responsibility an evaluation of the quality of patient care provided to patients by the medical and other professional staffs. Criteria against which standards can be applied and care measured must be established or adapted by the medical and other professional staffs. The criteria must be explicit and measurable and must reflect components of care to enable verification that patients are receiving current technologic and professional services. Members of this committee include physicians, nursing personnel, and medical record professionals.

Other Committees*

Other committees include:

- Joint Conference Committee—Executive Committee and Hospital Board representation
- Department of Medicine
- Department of Surgery
- Department of Family Practice
- Department of Pediatrics
- Department of Obstetrics and Gynecology
- Department of Anesthesia
- Department of Outpatient Services and Emergency Room
- Department of Radiology
- Department of Pathology and Laboratory Services
- Credentials Committee
- Critical Care Committee
- Continuing Medical Education Committee
- Patient Care Services Committee
- Library Committee

These committees may require the administrator to serve on several of them throughout his tenure.

The advantage of multiple committee assignments is the opportunity to choose the most suitable location for expounding new proposals and ideas. The disadvantage is that if you are involved in more than one committee and you cannot be present at all of the meetings, you may be assured, by the principle of Murphy's law, that if something can go wrong, it will. It is in the one meeting you miss that something will be discussed in far greater detail than you might have wished. Of course, that can also happen on committees of which you are not a member. If you have an assistant, it is useful to make his availability known to all committee chairmen. Thus if questions arise and you are not available to answer them, the questioners have someone else to approach.

You may also request that the assistant be allowed to attend meetings when you are not available, not only to provide necessary input but also to receive feedback that might modify hospital activities. Unfortunately, physicians on the whole prefer not to have nonphysicians at their meetings, owing to the delicate matters that they sometimes discuss in a rather spontaneous fashion. It is increasingly common for administrative personnel to be at major committee meetings, but it would be political to get approval before you have your assistant stand in for you.

Who's in Charge?*

Despite his enhanced authority and status, the typical administrator has a trying and often anomalous job. The old tensions between the medical staff and administration, built into the structure of the voluntary hospital, remain. In the eyes of most physicians, the administrator is in charge only of the nonmedical aspects of the hospital's operations.

Medical responsibility is divided among individual doctors and the collective staff. The staff has collective responsibility for medical policies (or making recommendations to the trustees). Some hospitals have "open staff" privileges; its facilities are available to any doctor in the community. Others have a "closed staff;" only those doctors elected by the staff (or trustees) may use its facilities, although such hospitals may extend courtesy privileges to additional physicians who may use the hospital without becoming members of the active staff. In metropolitan areas, many doctors have staff appointments in two, three, or more hospitals and, of necessity, wear their staff duties lightly.

The medical staff also has collective responsibility for the conduct of its members. In practice, this is usually quite loose. The staff is primarily a professional fraternal order, not an organization. To some extent the activities of the staff will depend upon whether the hospital has full-time chiefs and whether the administrator is a physician. The staff's power is generally

---

*Source: S. H. Appelbaum and W. F. Rohrs, *Time Management for Health Care Professionals,* Aspen Systems Corporation, 1981.

*Source: H. M. Somers and A. R. Somers, *Medicare and the Hospitals,* The Brookings Institution, 1967.

pretty much what it wishes to make of it. The trustees are laymen, serving part-time without compensation, but the institution is there to render professional health services. The doctors make a special point that the hospital cannot practice medicine, that the patient is the doctor's, not the hospital's—a precious distinction that dilutes the unity and authority of the hospital.

The doctor's relationship to the hospital has become increasingly contradictory as its place in his professional life grows. Although the degree of his dependence varies with type of practice, probably at least 50 percent of the average physician's income is earned in the hospital. A surgeon or radiologist may earn up to 100 percent of his income there. In any case, even with staff duties, the physician who is the key and indispensable figure in the hospital, with wide authority and latitude, is not a real part of the administrative or financial organization. On the other hand, a united and aggressive medical staff can effectively take over an entire hospital and conduct its affairs almost independently without any of the financial risks or responsibilities that would otherwise be expected.

Hospital Privileges and Legal Considerations*

The Joint Commission on Accreditation of Hospitals' (JCAH's) Accreditation Manual sets forth procedures and criteria that hospitals should use in granting physicians staff privileges. According to the manual, "[T]he medical staff shall ensure that each [physician] is qualified for membership and shall strive to maintain the optimal level of professional performance of its members. . . ." Accordingly, JCAH requires a reasonably comprehensive delineation of each member's privileges and some evidence of demonstrated competence at the time of admission. Prospective members are obligated to complete an application form containing information required by the hospital's medical staff bylaws. They are also asked to disclose any successful or currently pending challenges against their license to practice medicine, any prior loss of medical society or hospital staff privileges, and any adverse malpractice action.

*Source: Marguerite R. Mancini and Alice T. Gale, *Emergency Care and the Law,* Aspen Systems Corporation, 1981.

Staff privileges, JCAH states, should not be granted to a physician merely because he or she is licensed in a state to practice medicine, is a member of a professional organization, or has staff privileges elsewhere. Specialty board certification is, however, an "excellent benchmark to serve as a basis for privilege delineation."

Physicians who have contracted to provide emergency room services for a hospital must, as must all applicants, satisfy medical staff requirements and be staff members. Finally, all physicians applying for hospital staff privileges are regarded by the JCAH as implicitly consenting, by virtue of the applications, to the hospital's inspection of all documents related to their qualifications.

Hospital governing boards and medical staff appoint various committees to carry out the business of governing and operating the hospital. The credentials or privileges committee is one of the committees that may collect confidential information in order to fulfill its responsibility to review physicians for appointment or reappointment to the medical staff. Commonly, the medical staff credentials committee will have gathered data about a physician and will make a recommendation to the governing board's committee. Sometimes these reports will contain information about the physician's treatment of particular patients.

These proceedings are subject to several kinds of legal problems. First, if a physician is denied privileges at the hospital she or he may choose to challenge that decision in court and seek to subpoena the committee records. Ordinarily the physician will succeed in obtaining those records for the purpose of the lawsuit.

Second, several states—including New York, Montana, and Georgia—have enacted statutes requiring that reports be made to the medical licensing board about information that appears to show that a physician is medically incompetent, mentally or physically unable to safely engage in the practice of medicine, or is guilty of unprofessional conduct. Failure to report is penalized by suspending or revoking the license of the physician, hospital, insurer, or medical association that does not report as required. Persons who make these reports in good faith are protected from civil and criminal liability. The New York statute specifically declares that this disclosure does not violate the physician-patient privilege.

Third, there has been a considerable amount of litigation over the question of whether the work of medical staff committees, particularly utilization review and other peer review committees, should remain confidential. In order to counter the trend of court decisions that granted patients and other plaintiffs access to these records by subpoena, legislatures have been enacting provisions that protect these committee proceedings from discovery.

Fourth, unauthorized disclosure of hospital or medical staff records that might tend to injure a physician's reputation in the community could invite a defamation suit by the affected physician. If the hospital acted out of malice, the doctor might recover for defamation in some states even if the charges were based in fact. Conceivably, public dissemination of the unfavorable information could constitute grounds for a lawsuit claiming invasion of privacy.

In order to avoid some problems that can accompany appointment or reappointment procedures, a physician could be required to sign a document authorizing the hospital and medical staff to release any information made in connection with the consideration of the appointment. This release could specify that the members of the medical staff, the hospital governing board, and the hospital administration are allowed to make statements affecting the consideration of the appointment, and that a record of the deliberations can be released to others with a legiti-

mate interest (such as another hospital where the physician is seeking employment).

This release would not bind any patient about whom information was disclosed in connection with the appointment process. Thus, the release does not prevent a patient (as it does the physician) from suing the hospital. Hospital boards and medical staffs should therefore act prudently in handling patients' information during the consideration of physician appointments as well as during peer review and inhouse disciplinary actions.

Physician Peer Review*

The peer review function can be performed in a number of ways but it is routinely accomplished by a series of medical staff committees that review different aspects of a physician's clinical performance.

The information that would be considered in a peer review can be drawn from a number of documents in addition to patient's medical records (Table 2-1).

The characteristics of peer review documents tend to militate against their being admitted into evidence. Documents generated by peer review

---

*Source: Lee J. Dunn, Jr., and Reid F. Holbrook, "Legal Issues Concerning Peer Review Documents," *Topics in Health Record Management,* September 1981.

Table 2-1   Documents Relevant to Peer Review

1. Clinical and related administrative records
   - unusual incident reports
   - operating room circulating slips
   - fetal monitoring tapes
   - operating room and other logs
   - respiratory records
   - apnea monitor records
2. Hospital corporate documents
   - hospital articles of incorporation, bylaws, and regulations
   - medical staff bylaws and regulations
   - JCAH survey results
   - auditor management letters
   - medical staff disciplinary documents
   - business office records
3. Quality assurance, safety, and health care delivery policy documents
   - quality assurance committee records (e.g., utilization review committee, medical audit committee, tissue committee)
   - nursing care and procedural manuals
   - standing orders
   - grand round presentations
   - resident evaluations
   - bioengineering and equipment guidelines
   - operating instructions for biomedical equipment

Source: Lee F. Dunn, Jr. and Reid F. Holbrook, "Legal Issues Concerning Review Documents," *Topics in Health Record Management,* September 1981.

activity often contain condensed opinions of perceptions by committee members taken from hearsay records, such as a patient's charts, which are made subsequent to the event being evaluated. Such opinions are basically second-level retrospective evaluations (except in the case of a credentials committee report, where the records would be prospective). Peer review committee records are not part of a patient's chart or record, and therefore not directly related to a patient's case. Arguably, they are not kept in the ordinary course of a hospital's routine business (considering the routine business is patient care). The records generally do not contain entries made by a person who was present during the administration of patient care and usually are not made by a person who is required to record the treatment. The records contain the opinions and conclusions of physicians not directly involved in the patient's treatment. All these points militate against admitting this information into evidence.

PROBLEM PHYSICIANS*

Because the medical staff is by nature *self-policing* (subject to the ultimate authority of the governing body), it has a responsibility to identify problem individuals and situations within its ranks. In addition to normal patient care evaluation activities conducted through committees, a medical staff is required to pass judgment on its individual members. Too often, the annual reappointment process results in a hurried, thoughtless recommendation for reappointment of all members with the same privileges, year after year.

In an effort to assist the medical staff and governing body in monitoring both staff privileges and annual reappointments, physician "profiles" are being developed in some hospitals. In institutions with data-processing capacity, such a program is easily handled, but basic information can also be maintained manually for this purpose.

Some of the data that may be included in the profile follows:

*Source: Bernard L. Brown, Jr., *Risk Management for Hospitals: A Practical Approach,* Aspen Systems Corporation, 1979.

- Physician's utilization of hospital facilities (including outpatient and emergency services)
- Physician's attendance of staff and committee meetings (including excused absences)
- Physician's continuing medical education credits earned
- Physician's participation in internal educational activities within the hospital (both as instructor and participant)
- Physician's specialty board eligibility or certification status
- Other basic information concerning such things as formal training, work experience, memberships on other staffs, liability insurance, and malpractice claim experience

If a medical staff is accurately to monitor and evaluate its members and then act appropriately in regard to them, such basic information needs to be available.

Professional Misconduct

There has been a reaction against the inability or unwillingness of licensing authorities to revoke licenses for demonstrated incompetence and a reluctance of medical societies to censure members, and this is reflected in some of the new laws as well as within the profession. Against considerable resistance, some doctors are demanding professional self-policing to deal with those who are disabled by drug addiction, alcoholism, mental illness, and the like, as well as those who refuse to retire long after advanced age has caused them to lose their effectiveness.

Refusal to testify for plaintiffs and failure to report the observed malfeasance of other physicians—the so-called "conspiracy of silence"—are diminishing and are no longer quietly accepted as appropriate professional conduct. Specialty boards are displaying increased sensitivity to their responsibilities for quality performance.

Also, about a dozen state medical societies have voted to require members to participate in continuing education or be removed from the society. Moreover, medical societies supported, or did not oppose, the state laws that permit boards of medical examiners to compel all doctors to continue their education or lose their licenses or have them suspended.

State boards of medical misconduct have been established in several states. For example, professional misconduct in New York includes:*

1. obtaining a license fraudulently;
2. practicing a profession fraudulently, beyond its authorized scope, with gross incompetence on a particular occasion or negligence or incompetence on more than one occasion;
3. practicing a profession while the ability to practice is impaired by alcohol, drugs, physical disability or mental disability;
4. refusing to provide professional service to a person because of such person's race, creed, color, or national origin; or
5. permitting, aiding, or abetting an unlicensed person to perform activities requiring a license.

Impaired Physicians**

The impaired physician, conservatively estimated by the American Medical Association to include one of every 10 physicians, has been defined by that group as "one who is unable to practice medicine with reasonable skill and safety to patients because of physical or mental illness, including deterioration through the aging process or loss of motor skill, or excessive use or abuse of drugs including alcohol." Studies show that physicians suffer from a greater incidence of impairment generally than do members of similarly educated groups, are more likely to abuse narcotics or alcohol than nonphysicians, and commit suicide with greater frequency and at an earlier age than members of the general population. Yet, most impaired physicians hesitate to seek help because they deny that a problem exists, don't comprehend the seriousness of the problem, or fear loss of license, income, or professional reputation.

Surprisingly few hospitals have established a committee that deals specifically with emotionally and behaviorally impaired physicians. One

California hospital that established a "physicians' health and well-being committee" to aid impaired physicians in a nondisciplinary manner may serve as a model to other health care facilities. Once the committee learns of aberrant physician behavior, the physician is contacted and advice and assistance is offered. If, however, help is refused, and the committee believes that patients may be in jeopardy, the case is referred to the medical care evaluation committee, which has the authority to recommend to the proper authorities that the suspect physician's staff privileges be immediately curtailed or suspended.

The AMA's Department of Mental Health has adopted general guidelines for establishing programs for impaired members of the medical staff. These guidelines, which should be reviewed carefully by all hospitals, suggest incorporating into the hospital's bylaws a formal policy regarding impairment; setting up a special committee to verify allegations of physician impairment; training hospital personnel in confrontation and intervention techniques; publicizing the existence of the hospital's policy on impairment; and initiating an educational program for

Table 2-2 Public Attitudes Toward Doctor's Honesty and Ethics [Ratings of Doctors and Other Professionals]

	Very high, high	Average	Low, very low	No opinion
	%	%	%	%
Clergymen	63	28	6	3
Druggists, pharmacists	59	33	5	3
Dentists	52	38	7	3
Medical doctors	50	38	10	2
Engineers	48	35	5	12
College teachers	45	36	8	11
Policemen	44	41	13	2
Bankers	39	47	10	4
TV reporters, commentators	36	45	15	4
Newspaper reporters	30	49	16	5
Funeral directors	30	41	19	10
Lawyers	25	41	27	7
Stockbrokers	21	46	7	26
Senators	20	50	25	5
Business executives	19	53	19	9
Building contractors	19	48	27	6
Congressmen	15	47	32	6
Local political officeholders	14	51	30	5
Realtors	14	48	30	8
Labor union leaders	14	29	48	9
State political officeholders	12	50	30	8
Insurance salesmen	11	49	36	4
Advertising practioners	9	41	38	12
Car salesmen	6	33	55	6

Source: The Gallup Poll, September 20, 1981.

*Source: George D. Pozgar, *Legal Aspects of Health Care Administration,* Aspen Systems Corporation, 1979.

**Source: Barbara L. Zelner, *Hospital Law Manual Newsletter #90,* Health Law Center, Aspen Systems Corporation, December 1981.

the medical staff and other hospital employees to increase their awareness of the impaired physician problem. The educational program would, among other things, provide information about the availability of community mental health services.

Hospitals should check with their respective state licensing boards when considering a physician's application for medical staff privileges to assure themselves that the applicant's privileges have not previously been revoked, suspended, or limited at other health care institutions in the state. To verify whether a physician has been disciplined in another state, a health care institution need only check with the Federation of State Medical Boards, which maintains a listing of physicians disciplined by state medical examining boards. [See Table 2-2 for a poll of the public's regard for the ethics of physicians.]

PHYSICIAN COMPENSATION

Types of Hospital-Based Physicians*

The term "hospital-based physicians" suggests that physicians conduct a majority of their practice within the physical confines of the hospital and are compensated through or by the hospital. There are two basic types of hospital-based physicians.

Specialist

The specialist is one whose medical practice is limited to a particular field or area of medicine. In a hospital environment, this specialty is usually associated with the various ancillary or service departments. Typical types of specialties include:

Radiology
EKG
CCU
Cardiorespiratory
Noninvasive cardiology
Medical education
Pathology
EEG
ICU
Physical therapy
Inhalation therapy
Catheterization lab

Emergency care
Isotopes
Cardiopulmonary
Anesthesiology
Medical director
Hemodialysis

A variation of the specialist category is the specialist who also is the administrative chief of a hospital service and therefore responsible for its operation. This specialist is considered a clinical department head within the hospital who not only provides a specialized medical service but also is the administrative liaison between that department and the hospital management.

House Staff Member

A house staff member contracts with the hospital to provide inhouse coverage of certain services. In most hospitals, this coverage consists of making general rounds in patient care areas as opposed to coverage of ancillary departments.

Setting Fees*

Most physician fee-setting arrangements address the following areas:

1. Cost of service rendered
   • Expenses incurred, office expenses, capital equipment, etc.
   • Time involved
2. Patient demand
   • Number of patients
   • Each patient's ability to pay
3. Value of service rendered
   • Success or failure
   • Importance of the disease to the survival of the patient
   • Complexity of the treatment
4. Customary fees in the community
5. Whether the client is the physician's regular patient
6. Limitations under the law or under the rules of professional associations

In recent years, and certainly since the advent of Medicare and Medicaid, customary fees in the community and limitations under the law have become especially important variables affecting physicians' fees.

---

*Source: E. Andrew Kaskiw, "Overview of Physician Compensation," *Topics in Health Care Financing,* Spring 1978.

*Source: E. Andrew Kaskiw, "Overview of Physician Compensation," *Topics in Health Care Financing,* Spring 1978.

Factors Influencing Contract Negotiations*

Effect of Supply of Physicians

If a community finds itself with an abundance of physicians in a particular specialty, then the hospitals in that community may find themselves in a "buyer's market." When this occurs, a hospital may be able to negotiate a lower remuneration than it would if there were a smaller number of specialists available. If a community has few specialists available to negotiate, the hospitals in the community may find themselves paying a premium in order to obtain physician services.

If the specialty is one of a new or superspecialty such as cardiac catheterization, the actual number of physicians available in the community or elsewhere may be minimal.

Determining a Benchmark for Negotiations

Hospitals, not surprisingly, have looked to other hospitals in determining a benchmark for negotiations with these physicians. This applies both to the types of agreement and to the amounts of remuneration. This "technique" can be used by both the hospital and the physician. This technique, however, is not an easy one to apply since there typically are considerable difficulties in trying to gather this information. Some information concerning hospital-based physician contracts is available for larger geographic areas through the state hospital associations. The knowledge of salary ranges and types of compensation typical in a state or area can be extremely helpful in preliminary negotiation sessions.

Other Factors

First, the ability of a hospital to pay may imply that either the hospital is financially sound or that a particular department is financially profitable.

A second factor is the standing or reputation of the hospital. A hospital which possesses an image of being a mecca for clinical management and medical research may find itself in a position of being able to negotiate a lower remuneration

in lieu of the status and professional growth involved.

In some areas, physician remuneration is directly related to the size (number of beds) of the hospital; up to a point, the dollar amount of physician reimbursement may increase as the size of the hospital increases. (See Table 2-3 for an administrator's review of the physician's contract.)

Trends in Compensation

Six different types of arrangements for physician compensation are listed in the *American Hospital Association Guidelines for Physician Compensation* discussed later in this chapter.

Considering all types of contract arrangements between hospital-based physicians and hospitals, the "percentage of gross" type has been and continues to be the most widely used, followed by fee for service. In some geographic areas such as the West Coast 90 percent of all contracts for radiologists and pathologists involved gross and net percentage.

The popularity of the percentage type contract is a function of the hospital-based physicians traditionally being in a better bargaining position than the hospital and the potential amount of income that can be generated by this method.[1]

Evaluating Physician Compensation Models*

An evaluation of the advantages and disadvantages of each of the compensation models requires the development of criteria for assessment. The hospital should select their criteria on the basis of their goals and objectives for selecting a desirable method of physician compensation. Some examples of possible goals and objectives for selecting a compensation model are:

● The hospital may desire to assess the impact the compensation model would have on its information and data management system. What are the accounting requirements of the compensation model, and

---

*Source: E. Andrew Kaskiw, "Overview of Physician Compensation," *Topics in Health Care Financing*, Spring 1978.

[1]E. Andrew Kaskiw, "Overview of Physician Compensation," *Topics in Health Care Financing*, Spring 1978.

*Source: James C. Morell and Peter G. Rogan, "Hospital-Based Physician Compensation Concepts," *Topics in Health Care Financing*, Spring 1978.

Table 2-3 Tax Status: Outline for Review of Physician's Contract

1. Consider first general items:
   - Does the doctor have a contract that defines specific duties?
   - Is the doctor's compensation fixed?
   These factors help lay the groundwork for further analysis.
2. Consider factors normally associated with employee status:
   - Does the doctor receive, or is he entitled to receive fringe benefits?
   If employee fringe benefits predominate, the physician probably should be classified as an employee.
3. If employee features are not present, consider whether any positive factors exist that would indicate independent contractor status.
   - Does the doctor have specific, segregative duties?
   - Does the doctor have a private practice?
   - Does the doctor hire employees?
   If *positive* independent contractor characteristics exist in the absence of employee features, the doctor should be classified as an independent contractor.

4. Inevitably, there are physicians whose relationship with a hospital cannot be clearly fixed as either employee-employer or independent contractor. Since the IRS will tend to resolve doubts in favor of employee status, carefully consider:
   a. Factors tending to show independent status:
      - variable compensation
      - direct hiring and supervision of employees by the physician
      - segregative duties
      - private practices
      - nonhospital billing
      - leased department
      - any factors tending to show that the physician bears business risk.
   b. Factors tending to show employee status:
      - fixed compensation
      - employee fringes
      - hospital-paid insurance, office space, supplies, expenses.

Source: Albert W. Herman, "Compensation of Hospital-Based Physicians," *Topics in Health Care Financing,* Winter 1980.

what does the hospital have to do to effectively implement the program?

- The hospital may be looking for a compensation model which would balance physician and hospital utilization levels. Cost-effective productivity on the part of both the physician and the hospital is desirable for maximizing the utilization of limited resources.
- If the hospital is a tax-exempt institution, consideration may be given to the impact the compensation model may have on their tax-exempt status. The cost of forfeiting one's tax-exempt status may outweigh the benefits received from adopting a particular compensation model.
- The hospital may be seeking a way to increase the physician's authority in the institution while providing for responsibility and accountability on the part of the physician. Selecting a compensation model that would outline physician authority, responsibility and accountability may be desirable.

- The hospital may be seeking a compensation model that would not change their relationship with the various third party reimbursement programs. In selecting a compensation model, the hospital would assess the impact their decision may have on their reimbursement status.
- The hospital may be concerned with the level of involvement the hospital-based physician may experience with the institution's employees and their work. Physician commitment to the hospital, its people, and the health care delivery process may be desired by the institution.
- Associated with the physician's involvement in the health care delivery process is the physician's participation in medical staff activities. The hospital may want the hospital-based physician to work on medical staff committees such as utilization review or quality assurance. Further, participation in medical staff activities could include being an officer of the staff. The hospital may be seeking continued physi-

cian commitment to the hospital and its programs through increased participation in the activities of the medical staff.

- The search for an acceptable compensation model may include a review of all applicable legislation to ensure the program is in compliance with all the appropriate laws. The cost of adopting a compensation model which is not in compliance with all applicable legislation may be greater than the benefits gained from the program.
- The hospital may be concerned with the impact the compensation model may have on their ability to retain their present hospital-based physicians as well as their ability to attract new hospital-based physicians. Physician recruitment is important to the hospital since the physician's practice contributes to the institution's utilization. The hospital may not want to limit its ability to recruit hospital-based physicians in the future due to the nature of the present compensation model.
- The hospital may desire a compensation model with a provision which provides for a renegotiation of the agreement at specified intervals or at the request of either party. The hospital should seek an arrangement which allows for such renegotiations.
- The hospital may seek to adopt a physician compensation model that provides for a good working relationship between the administration and the physician. This goal may be the most important in determining the acceptability and success of the selected compensation model.

Medicare Reimbursement and Physician Compensation*

The area of the Medicare law and regulations relating to cost paid for physician professional service is one of the most difficult to comprehend. The confusion and misunderstanding surrounding this topic is attributable primarily to the need to segregate payments for administrative and professional services between the Part A and Part B trust funds. The Medicare program is subsidized by two separate sources: the Part A trust fund (financed primarily by Social Security taxes), designed to cover reimbursement of the reasonable *cost* for services rendered by hospitals; and the Part B trust fund (financed primarily by patient premiums and deductible and coinsurance charges), designed to cover the reasonable *charge* for services rendered by a licensed physician. Since the hospital charge for ancillary services such as radiology, laboratory, EKG, and EEG normally includes an amount applicable to both an administrative and professional component, separate reimbursement under the two funds creates a problem.

Cost is the reimbursement basis for hospitals, while *charges* are the reimbursement basis for physicians. This is the case even when a physician is hospital based and bills through a hospital. Normally, the physician is under some type of contractual agreement with the hospital whereby he provides his professional service in the applicable department, and in turn, is paid by the hospital on a fee basis as a percentage of departmental revenue. That portion of the fee that represents payment for a professional service (i.e., the interpretation or reading of an x-ray or EKG) is recoverable under Part B of the program. That portion of the fee that represents payment for an administrative service rendered by the physician (i.e., general supervision of the particular department) is recoverable under Part A of the program.

In an attempt to simplify interim billing procedures, the program allows the provider to "combine bill" all radiology and laboratory charges under Part A of the program. (Note that this provision applies only to radiology and laboratory services.) At the end of the year, when the provider files its cost report, a separate computation is made that transfers reimbursement from Part A to Part B of the program. This is accomplished by excluding from Part A allowable costs—the professional component of all physician fees paid to the radiologist or pathologist—and by preparing a separate reimbursement computation based on the ratio of charges to charges in the applicable department to be reimbursed under Part B.

For those professional services that the provider is not allowed to combine bill under Part A during the interim period (EKG, EEG, and so forth), a separate claim form must be submitted to the program for the professional component of the hospital charge to be reimbursed by Part B of the program.

---

*Source: C.W. Frank, *Maximizing Hospital Cash Resources,* Aspen Systems Corporation, 1978.

Structuring the Physician Contract

To maximize payments effectively from *all* classes of payor, the actual structure of the physician contract deserves careful consideration. Financial arrangements that reimburse the physician on a percent of departmental revenue should be avoided. Contracts that provide for payment on a fee-for-service basis are more desirable, since a departmental price increase does not automatically provide for an adjustment of the physician's fee. Additionally, there should be some provision in the fee computation to recognize the bad debts that will result from physician-rendered services. Perhaps the best arrangement is to have the physician bill the patient directly for professional services. Professional fees then become an arrangement between patient and physician and the hospital does not become involved in the collection effort. In this way, the hospital shifts the administrative cost of billing, collection, and possible bad debt losses to the physician.

Because of the many types of physician arrangements, it is sometimes difficult to determine the exact treatment of the professional fee in the Medicare cost report. Table 2-4 reflects some of the factors to be considered in this process.

Tax Considerations for Hospital-Based Physicians*

Underlying all compensation arrangements with hospital-based physicians is the question of whether the IRS will view the arrangement as creating employee status or independent contractor status for the physician. Proper classification of a physician's status is extremely important to the hospital and physician.

From a hospital's standpoint, treating the physician as an independent contractor rather than an employee enables the hospital to exclude the physician from any of its benefit plans, eliminates the hospital's cost of Social Security, and eliminates any withholding tax requirements. From purely a tax standpoint, the hospital may prefer to have the physician treated as an independent contractor.

From a physician's point of view, employee status generally is not an attractive choice. Most physicians prefer independent contractor status for the relative autonomy it provides. With a properly structured professional corporation, a physician may be able to exceed the employee benefits available through a hospital, particularly in the amount of income that may be set aside in a qualified profit or pension plan.

Determining Physician's Employee Status

IRS rulings set forth four criteria for determining whether the requisite control and supervision exist to treat an individual as an employee:

1. the degree to which the physician is integrated in the operating organization of the hospital for which the services are performed;
2. the substantial nature, regularity, and continuity of the individual's work for such hospital;
3. the authority vested in or reserved by the hospital to require compliance with its general policies; and
4. the degree to which the physician is accorded the rights and privileges the hospital provides its employees.

The IRS provides that no one factor can be considered more important than others and points out that a strong indication of an independent contractor's status is the physician's employment and payment of associates. A restriction on the physician's outside practice or furnishing employee-type benefits is an indication of an employer-employee relationship. If a revenue agent finds an individual receiving employee fringe benefits, the agent usually concludes that the individual is an employee of the hospital.

Many contracts have been drafted without due consideration to the IRS criteria for classifying an individual as an employee or independent contractor. Many cases where the IRS has asserted that an individual was an employee have resulted from an improperly or poorly worded contract. (A basic outline which has been used for the review of physician's contracts appears in Table 2-3, above.)

Careful consideration of the tax implications of various compensation arrangements are necessary to provide the most attractive compensa-

---

*Source: Albert W. Herman, "Compensation of Hospital-Based Physicians," *Topics in Health Care Financing*, Winter 1980.

Table 2-4 Treatment of Physician Fees Under Various Compensation Arrangements

Description	Settlement Method	Comment
Group I, Fully Licensed Physicians		
a. Provider-based physician practicing in specialty areas (radiology, pathology, etc.)		
(1) Providing "administrative" services to the provider	SSA-2551/2552, Schedule E	Physician fee is an allowable Part A cost
(2) Providing identifiable professional services to patients	SSA-2551/2552, Schedule D-3 (1) SSA-1554 or 1490 (2)	Physician fee removed as Part B adjustment
b. Private practice physicians		
(1) Providing identifiable professional services to patients	SSA-1554 or 1490 (2)	Fee removed as Part B adjustment if paid
(2) "Guaranteed compensation" serving in emergency room	SSA-2551/2552, Schedule D-2	Fee is removed from Part A cost and is reimbursed under Part B
(3) Serving on provider's utilization review committee	SSA-2551/2552, Schedule E	Fee is an allowable Part A cost
(4) "Teaching" in association with approved intern/resident training program (excludes teaching in medical school facilities)	SSA-2551/2552, Schedule D-2	Fee is allowable Part A cost
(5) Serving on provider committees organized to improve overall medical care	SSA-2551/2552, Schedule E	Fee is allowable Part·A cost
(6) Serving as administrator	SSA-2551/2552 Schedule E	Fee is allowable Part A cost
(7) "House Physician"	SSA-1554 or 1490 (2)	Fee removed as Part B adjustment
(8) Provides *inpatient* medical services on a nightly or 24-hour basis	SSA-2551/2552, Schedule D-2	Fee is removed from Part A cost and is reimbursed under Part B
Group II, Interns-Residents		
a. Under approved training program	SSA-2551-2552, Schedule D-2	Fee is an allowable Part A cost
b. Under nonapproved training program	SSA-2551/2552, Schedule D-2	Fee is removed from Part A cost and is reimbursed under Part B
Group III, Licensure-restricted Physicians		
a. Resident of another provider "moonlighting" (even if under an approved training program in another provider facility)	SSA-2551/2552, Schedule D-2	Fee is removed from Part A cost and is reimbursed under Part B
b. Foreign resident limited to practice in the provider facility	SSA-2551/2552, Schedule D-2	
c. "House physician"/"Medical director"	SSA-2551/2552, Schedule D-2	Fee is removed from Part A cost and is reimbursed under Part B
d. Staff physicians	SSA-2551/2552, Schedule D-2	
(1) Applicable to combined billing under part A		
(2) Applicable to billing under Part B		

Source: C.W. Frank, *Maximizing Hospital Cash Resources,* Aspen Systems Corporation, 1978.

tion package to hospital-based physicians while avoiding undesired tax results.

American Hospital Association Guidelines on Contracts Between Hospital and Physicians*

Historically, hospitals have contracted with physicians in the traditional hospital-based specialties of anesthesiology, pathology, and radiology; however, a trend has developed to extend contractual arrangements to other hospital-based specialties, including cardiology, electrodiagnosis, and emergency medicine, and to hospital multispecialty practices in ambulatory care centers, satellite clinics, and surgical centers.

The AHA guidelines have been developed to assist hospitals that are considering entering into a contractual arrangement with a physician or group of physicians to provide professional and administrative services and to offer guidance to hospitals on entering into such contracts in light of current legal, regulatory, and economic trends. The guidelines are not intended as legal advice nor as an exhaustive treatment of the subject. They are not intended to apply to agreements with house staff.

An AHA Principle

A physician under contract is entitled to fair and equitable remuneration for services rendered. Factors to be considered include the physician's training and experience, the difficulty of the procedures to be performed and the degree of expertise required, the size and complexity of the department managed, the demands that will be made on the physician's time, the responsibilities for supervision, the levels of compensation prevailing locally and in comparable facilities for physicians with comparable qualifications, and the reasonable compensation equivalent (RCE) limits published pursuant to the Medicare provider-based physician regulations.

Key Elements of a Contract

The following list discusses certain key provisions that should be considered for inclusion in a

*Source: Reprinted, with permission, from *Guidelines on Contractual Relationships between Hospitals and Physicians,* published by the American Hospital Association, copyright 1983.

contract. The list is not intended to be all-inclusive. All of the parties should work with specialized legal counsel to ensure that the arrangement is equitable to all and complies with applicable state laws and other necessary legal requirements.

Legal characterization of the agreement. Whether the physician has independent contractor or employee status is critical in many areas of law. For a number of purposes, including workers' compensation, liability allocation, and tax liability, the hospital may wish to demonstrate that the physician is an independent contractor; if so, the contract should reflect an absence of hospital control or direction over the methods by which the physician performs services and functions. The contract also should state explicitly that the physician will not be treated as an employee for federal tax purposes.

Methods of compensation and other financial arrangements. Various compensation arrangements exist for physicians under contract. State statutes should be checked before a method of compensation is chosen because some states prohibit certain organizational and contractual arrangements.

The reimbursement implications of the proposed method of compensation also should be considered. Legal and financial advice should be obtained to ensure that the contractual arrangement does not unintentionally reduce reimbursement from third-party payers and that the hospital is compensated for its participation in the billing and collection of the physician's fees. The contract should contain a provision for renegotiation or termination on short notice if significant changes in the policies, criteria, or methods of public or private third-party payers or changes in applicable tax laws affect the amount of reimbursement received from third-party payers.

The contract also should address how the physician's schedule of charges will be established, how services will be billed, and how services will be reimbursed. Especially in the case of an exclusive contract, the hospital should give strong consideration to reviewing and approving or otherwise monitoring the physician's schedule of charges for professional services and increases in the physician's fees.

Substantial changes in hospital billing procedures may be required as a result of the 1982

Medicare provider-based physician regulations. The right of a nonteaching provider to profit from the professional component of physician services has been eliminated, and combined billing for the professional and administrative components of physician services has been proposed to be eliminated. The appropriate method of billing for each specialty depends on the contractual arrangement between the hospital and the physician.

Responsibilities of the contracting parties. When the physician is compensated by or through the hospital, the physician's administrative services, such as teaching, patient-care-related research, administration, supervision of technical and other personnel, service on hospital committees, and participation in quality assurance activities, must be distinguished from the physician's professional services, his or her direct personal services to individual patients. The former are considered provider component services and are included in the hospital's Medicare allowable cost.[1] The latter are considered professional component services and are reimbursable under Medicare on a reasonable charge basis. Compensation to physicians must be apportioned on the basis of the time spent in the various activities, and the allocation must be mutually agreed to by the hospital and the physician. To secure reimbursement, appropriate time records as well as a time allocation agreement must be maintained.

The administrative services of the contract physician who is head of a department include providing information on the budgetary and other needs of the department; maintaining the appropriate reports and records; complying with hospital and medical staff policies, rules, and regulations; and participating in the effective administration of the department and the hospital.

Noncompetition agreements (restrictive covenants). Any limitations on the outside activities of the physician during and after the term of the contract should be specified in the contract, and legal counsel should be consulted to determine the validity and enforceability of these limitations under state law. Such noncompetition agreements should be reasonable as to the activities restricted and to the duration and geographic scope of the restriction.

Term of the contract. The contract may terminate automatically after a stated period ("fixed-term") or may be renewed automatically for successive periods unless terminated by prior notice ("evergreen"). A one-year contract, by promoting competition among physicians vying to secure or retain the contract, may encourage continued enhancement and upgrading of the services provided. A multiyear contract, on the other hand, may prevent the turmoil that may accompany annual contract renewal and may be preferred by physicians.

Whatever its term, the contract should be reviewed annually by executive management and the physician to ensure that the terms of the agreement are being fulfilled and are still appropriate for current conditions. All contracts should be terminable on short notice in view of the rapidly changing legal, regulatory, and economic environment.

Termination procedures. The contract should specify the breaches for which the contract can be terminated and the physician's right, if any, to staff membership and due process on termination of the contract. The termination of a physician's right to clinical practice normally is governed by the medical staff bylaws. However, especially in exclusive-source contracts for ancillary services, the hospital may wish to consider such a provision. Any rights to due process to be accorded the associates, partners, or employees of the contract physician on termination of the contract should also be specified: the hospital should obtain individual waivers from each physician.

Liability insurance. The physician, whether an independent contractor or an employee, ordinarily should be required to obtain and maintain appropriate levels of professional and comprehensive general liability coverage with approved carriers during the term of the contract. Failure to carry insurance should be grounds for automatic termination of the contract.

Access to books and records. If the contract has an annual value of $10,000 or more for services that are to be claimed as allowable costs on the hospital's cost report, a clause should reflect the physician's agreement to comply with all obligations of Social Security Act section 1861 (v) (1) (I).

---

[1]The Medicare prospective pricing system established by the Social Security Amendments of 1983 changes the relationship between a hospital's costs and the amount of its Medicare payment.

Resolution of disputes. The orderly resolution of any disputes that may arise may be provided for through such mechanisms as an appropriate committee of the medical staff, a committee composed of governing board and medical staff representatives, or arbitration. Medical staff involvement is unnecessary unless patient care or clinical issues are at stake.

Physician Compensation Arrangements

[Fixed compensation and fee-for-service contracts are the most common financial arrangements between hospitals and physicians.]

1. *Fixed compensation:* May be associated with either employee or independent contractor status for the physician. A salary arrangement, a common type of fixed compensation arrangement, tends to be associated with employee status for the physician. Although a salary gives the hospital maximum control over the physician's compensation, the hospital should consider whether the physician is given sufficient incentive to increase departmental productivity.
2. *Percentage of departmental revenue:* Associated with independent contractor status for the physician. The predetermined percentage-of-*gross*-revenue arrangement gives the physician an incentive to increase departmental revenue but may offer less incentive to increase departmental productivity. Under a percentage-of-*net*-revenue arrangement, the physician receives a predetermined percentage of the department's net receipts. Such an arrangement gives the physician an incentive to improve departmental performance and cost-effectiveness. With the new provider-based physician regulations [Tax Equity and Fiscal Responsibility Act of 1982] and Medicare hospital payment policies [Social Security Amendments of 1983] hospitals that pay physicians on a percentage-of-departmental-revenue basis may find such arrangements increasingly unattractive because they may encourage unnecessary utilization and inadequate reimbursement, because the exact amount of compensation cannot be predicted in advance, and because hospitals cannot increase charges without increasing physician compensation or renegotiating the contract.
3. *Fee for service:* Under this arrangement, the physician is compensated on a predetermined fee schedule for the services provided. When the physician is an employee, the fees billed to patients are generally considered income of the hospital. When the physician is an independent contractor, the fees are generally considered income of the physician. However, ownership of fee income will be dependent on the reassignment provision in the contract. A fee-for-service arrangement generally gives the hospital little control over the physician's compensation.
4. *Departmental leasing:* With a lease arrangement, the physician assumes all or part of the costs of operating the department. Leasing gives the physician maximum autonomy and a clear incentive to improve departmental performance. The Medicare program, however, has always looked with disfavor on leased departments. Lease arrangements may be adversely affected by the new Medicare provider-based physician regulations. The Medicare program will make reasonable charge payments to physicians only for services provided to individual patients, not for technical component costs that the physician has assumed under an agreement with the hospital.

Source: Reprinted, with permission, from *Guidelines on Contractual Relationships between Hospitals and Physicians,* published by the American Hospital Association, copyright 1983.

Performance-Based Compensation Plan for Salaried Physicians*

Although employee performance evaluations have long been established as an essential management tool in assuring the efficient and effective operation of any complex organization, there has been a tacit exemption of physicians from such review processes. Yet a formal system of assessing performance can and should be applied to physicians. Such assessments should be a major determinant of compensation. [This example is derived from the plan in operation at the Jefferson Health Foundation (JHF), Birmingham, Ala.]

In order for a comprehensive physician compensation plan to be effective, it should:

1. attract and retain high-caliber physicians;
2. induce part-time staff to expand commitment;

---

*Source: Richard M. Cooper, "A Performance-Based Physician Compensation Plan," *The Journal of Ambulatory Care Management,* May 1980.

3. provide income levels competitive with those of comparable physicians in the local community;
4. minimize, within the constraints of the marketplace, the traditional inequities extant among various medical and surgical specialties;
5. include incentives for appropriate utilization and productivity;
6. recognize experience, professional stature, special skills or contributions, and medical/administrative responsibilities;
7. contain a substantial portion of total remuneration in the form of nontaxable, indirect compensation ("fringe benefits");
8. incorporate elements of risk sharing;
9. afford opportunities for personal and professional growth; and
10. reward individual merit.

Salaries and Salary Increments

Base salaries vary by specialty and may be augmented by additional remuneration provided for practice experience and for specialty board certification. New physicians are granted a longevity increase annually (in addition to regular budgeted salary increments) during their first three years of employment. Section chiefs and committee chairmen receive extra compensation (not computed in base salary) in recognition of their administrative duties.

Regular annual salary increments consist of two components (half fixed and half variable). All physicians receive the fixed portion as a percentage-of-base salary increase. The remaining variable portion is allocated to each specialty section, and is distributed to individual physicians according to merit.

Incentive Bonuses and Fringe Benefits

Incentive Bonuses

Incentive bonuses are granted subject to approval of, and in an amount determined by, the board of trustees based on overall financial condition of the organization and attainment of projections and assumptions. The bonus pool is allocated to each specialty section based on its percentage of total full-time equivalent physicians, rather than on its percentage of aggregate base salaries, thus providing parity among various specialists in terms of absolute potential bonus dollars. Amounts awarded to individual physicians within each section are based on performance, as described in the criteria for annual salary increments. Only those physicians with two or more years of continuous employment are eligible to receive incentive bonuses and such bonuses are not included in base salaries for computation of other benefits.

Fringe Benefits

Fringe benefits vary widely, their diversity seemingly limited only by the resources and ingenuity of each medical group.

Elements to consider in developing a fringe-benefit package might include:

- educational leave (graduated with longevity? reimbursement for travel/tuition?);
- sabbaticals (frequency and duration? percentage of full salary?);
- retirement plan (formula? vesting schedule? defined contribution versus defined benefit?);
- deferred compensation plan (tax-deferred annuity?)
- professional liability insurance (limits? occurrence versus claims made?);
- long-term disability insurance (percentage of base salary? maximum?);
- life insurance (percentage of base salary? maximum?);
- health insurance (major medical? dental?);
- hospital staff dues (which? how many?);
- professional fees, organizations (which? how many?);
- recruiting fees, relocation allowance (limits? prorated payback if terminated?);
- books, journals (which? how many?); and
- car allowance (purposes? amount?).

Evaluation Checklist for Salary-Based Physicians

A weighting system, assigning variable "points" to different items, is used to indicate relative importance of items assessed (there are 200 total attainable points—105 related to clinical performance, 75 for nonclinical performance and 20 for special accomplishments or achievements) (Tables 2-5 and 2-6).

Table 2-5   Supervisor's or Medical Director's Assessment of Salary-Based Physicians

Professional (Clinical) Performance	Point Rating	Nonclinical Performance	Point Rating
Medical Record Keeping: Adherence to problem-oriented system, thoroughness and reliability of documentation	____	Attitude ("Sense of group" enthusiasm, interest, commitment)	____
Outpatient Services: Panel size, number and types of visits, appropriateness of return intervals	____	Adherence to oral and written directives	____
Inpatient Services: Necessity and appropriateness of hospital admissions, number of hospital days, LOS	____	Flexibility in adapting to changing work situations and demands	____
Diagnostic Services: Appropriateness of acquisition and utilization of lab, x-ray, etc. in clinical decision making	____	Ability to train, develop, and motivate others	____
Referral Services: Soundness of logic and judgment in acquisition and utilization of consultations in management of patient problems, coordination and control of follow-up	____	Ability to communicate effectively with others	____
		Degree of leadership potential	____
Therapeutics: Appropriateness of prescribing habits (agents, volume, refills), use of nonapproved drugs, consideration of cost-benefit	____	Special accomplishments or achievements [rate from 1 (lowest) or 5 (highest) to indicate significance of contribution (if none, indicate "NA")]	____
Patient Satisfaction: Transfers, compliments/complaints received	____	Total Points	

Nonclinical Performance

Professional (Clinical) Performance	Point Rating
Understanding of facility's organization and policies (and own role and relationship to other staff)	____
Willingness and ability to consistently and accurately complete assignments in a timely fashion	____
Interpersonal relationships	____
Willingness to accept constructive criticism	____
Initiative in providing thoughtful comments	____

Specific strengths of physician

_____

_____

Specific weaknesses of physician or areas which require improvement

_____

_____

Special skills or areas of interest physician has displayed

_____

_____

Source: Richard M. Cooper, "A Performance-Based Physician Compensation Plan," *The Journal of Ambulatory Care Management,* May 1980.

Table 2-6 Physician's Self-Assessment

	Degree
A. Indicate your degree of satisfaction; mark the degree (1) Very Satisfied (2) Somewhat Satisfied (3) Somewhat Dissatisfied (4) Very Dissatisfied.

1. Volume and nature of clinical duties _____
2. Volume and nature of nonclinical and administrative duties _____
3. Patient care resources available to you (professional and ancillary staffing, facility, diagnostic and consultative services, ER, hospital, etc.) _____
4. Extent and nature of your input in medical and administrative policy decision-making process _____
5. Your relationships with patients _____
6. Your relationships with other staff _____
7. Opportunities to improve your professional knowledge and skills _____
8. Pay, fringe benefits, general working conditions _____
9. Your acceptance and stature in the hospital and medical community _____
10. Quantity and quality of direction and/or supervision you receive _____
11. Quantity and quality of your direction and/or supervision of others _____

B. What are your personal and professional goals for: (a) next year, (b) five years from now?

_____

_____

C. What changes would you suggest to improve your practice or your role here?

_____

_____

D. How would you rate your own overall performance?

☐ average
☐ well above average
☐ somewhat below average
☐ somewhat above average
☐ well below average

E. List any additional comments or other items you would like to discuss.

_____

_____

Source: Richard M. Cooper, "A Performance-Based Physician Compensation Plan," *The Journal of Ambulatory Care Management,* May 1980.

Chapter 3—Admissions, Billing, and Collections

OVERVIEW*

Reporting Structures

The most common organizational reporting structures found in admissions are: (1) through the hospital's financial organization; (2) through a hospital operation other than financial; (3) through a patient service representative organization; (4) through a modified patient service representative organization; and (5) through various combinations of structures 1 through 4 above. Each of these structures has its advantages and disadvantages.

Reporting Through the Financial Organization

The advantage of this organizational form (see Figure 3-1) is that admissions, billing and credit/collections are part of the same organization, facilitating accurate gathering of billing and financial information. In addition, the implementation and coordination of effective admissions, billing and credit collection policies and procedures are made easier. The major disadvantage of this organizational form is that the financial organization sometimes emphasizes the billing/collecting segment to the detriment of the patient service aspects.

---

*Source: John F. Clarkin and Sheldon D. Chizever, "Inpatient Front Office Functions," *Topics in Health Care Financing,* Spring 1982.

Reporting Through an Organization Other Than Financial

Admissions reporting through an organization other than financial is shown in Figure 3-2. This organization provides the atmosphere for patient service emphasis and can be an effective organizational structure if the director of hospital services and the director of fiscal affairs have a good working relationship. One major disadvantage of this structure is that the patient must now deal with two organizational entries (operations and finance). In addition, the implementation of important billing and credit and collection policies is sometimes overlooked.

Reporting Through a Patient Service Representative Organization (PSR)

The PSR in effect performs the functions of the admissions, billing, and credit and collection clerk found in traditional patient accounting organizational structures.

The PSR organization can be an effective one because the patient deals with only one individual throughout the hospital stay and often after discharge. One major disadvantage with this type of organization, however, is that it is difficult to find and maintain the quality of staff required, who must possess the diverse skills of administration, social service, billing, and credit and collection; when they can be found, their salary requirements are often high.

Figure 3-1 Admissions reports through the financial organization

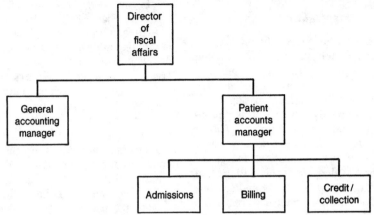

Source: John F. Clarkin and Sheldon D. Chizever, "Inpatient Front Office Functions," *Topics in Health Care Financing*, Spring 1982.

Reporting Through a Modified Patient Service Representative Organization

The modified patient service representative concept is defined as one in which the functions of admissions, patient services, and insurance verification are performed by the PSR with the functions of billing and collections being performed by patient accounts.

The major advantage of the modified patient service representative concept is that it combines the best aspects of the total patient service representative concept (one patient advocate) and the organizational structure where admissions reports through the financial organization (billing and collecting are performed by a separate entity under supervision). The major disadvantage is that more staff could be required under this organizational form, especially if the PSR continues patient contact after discharge.

Reporting Through Various Combinations

Under this organizational structure, admissions reports to the director of hospital services and patient accounts, and credit/collections reports to the director of fiscal affairs. The admissions reporting segment carries the same advantages and disadvantages as the admissions reporting through an organization other than financial model. However, on the financial side, the separation of the patient accounts function from the credit/collection function carries the potential disadvantage of overlapping duties and respon-

sibilities between patient accounts and credit/collections. In addition, the lack of integration of the credit function into patient accounts could result in the credit department becoming involved in the patient accounting cycle much too late to be effective.

Figure 3-2 Admissions reports through organization other than financial

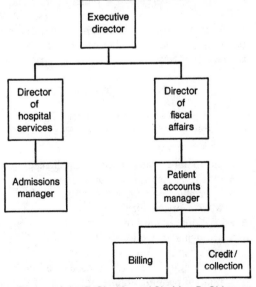

Source: John F. Clarkin and Sheldon D. Chizever, "Inpatient Front Office Functions," *Topics in Health Care Financing*, Spring 1982.

Financial Considerations

Patient Financial Counseling

The absence in some hospitals of financial counseling may inadvertently create a situation where the patient may neglect his or her personal obligations or where third parties may not pay the hospital bill because of missing or incomplete information. The end result is a problem for both the patient and hospital. This is why financial counseling should be performed. It provides a service to the patient and at the same time improves the patient accounting function by decreasing delays in billing and accelerating cash flow. Effective financial counselors are trained in all aspects of credit including Hill-Burton, Medicaid, free care, and state, county, and local welfare programs. In addition, effective financial counselors are familiar with state and federal regulations such as the Truth-in-Lending Act and the Fair Credit Reporting Act.

Definite policies are needed, as well as procedures to be followed, when the patient either is unable to pay for current or prior services or is able but unwilling to pay for these services.

One example of such policies is deposit requirements. Deposits should be required based on the patient's projected length of stay, with the patient's liability portion calculated according to the deductible co-insurance or other amounts not covered by the patient's insurance. Patients without third party coverage (self-pay) should be required to make a minimum deposit based on the average daily charge multiplied by the length of stay.

Preadmission Procedures

From the patient accounting viewpoint, the following functions could be performed prior to admissions:

- informing patient of hospital policies;
- obtaining insurance information;
- informing patient of financial liabilities where applicable;
- verifying method of payment;
- arranging admissions date;
- verifying insurance coverage;
- notifying business office/credit and collections of pending admission;
- mailing preadmission form.

The implementation of the preadmission process begins with the design of a preadmission form (see Figure 3-3).

A preadmission form generally contains the identifying information required for billing, such as the patient's name, address, third party coverage, and insurance numbers.

Once the preadmission form is received, the hospital will have more time to verify the insurance coverage and inform the patient of any financial liabilities prior to admission.

Problems concerning third party payments are greatly reduced, eliminating billing delays, decreasing the number of days' revenue in accounts receivable, and improving cash flow.

With the use of a preadmission system, the admissions routine becomes a more efficient process since most of the required information has already been gathered and verified. Patients are normally pleased with the preadmission process because long waiting periods during the day of admission are avoided.

Of course the preadmission process cannot be used 100 percent of the time, because of emergency or nonscheduled admissions.

Monitoring Performance

Some hospitals have implemented management reporting systems designed to monitor, control and report on the effectiveness of their admissions functions. For example, Figure 3-4 shows one hospital's admitting performance indicator chart. This hospital established staffing for the admissions department by formulating estimated man-hours and associated dollar costs per admission. The chart also monitors and reports on the success of the preadmission system in relationship to the total nonemergency admissions.

Using Figure 3-4, this hospital constructed an admitting department performance analysis (see Figure 3-5.) This chart indicates the direct relationship of the increase in hours per admission to the cost of admission. Many types of performance indicators could be established to monitor, control, and report on the performance of the admissions department. The importance of the management reporting system lies in assuring hospital management that the critical elements of the systems are working effectively.

Figure 3-3 Sample hospital preadmission form

Patient name _____

Address _____ County _____ Township _____

Place of birth _____ Date of birth _____ Age _____

Marital status _____ Religion _____ Telephone _____ S.S.# _____

Have you ever stayed overnight at _____ Hospital? _____

Patient's employer _____ Occupation _____

Employer's address _____ Telephone no. _____

Spouse's name _____ Occupation _____

Spouse's employer _____ Address _____

Patient's father's name (if minor) _____ Mother's maiden name _____

Person responsible for bill _____

Address _____ _____

Employer name and address _____

Physician name _____ Expected date of hospitalization _____

Reason for hospitalization _____

Hospital bill will be paid by the following (check one):

_____ Blue Cross—Name of subscriber _____ Name of Blue Cross plan _____

Contract number _____ Code number _____

_____ Other group insurance—Name of company _____

Address _____

Policy number _____

_____ Medicare—Medicare number _____

_____ Patient

_____ Other— _____

_____

Signature _____

Unless other arrangements are made with the hospital, the hospital bill is payable in full upon discharge.

Please complete this form and return at once to:

_____

_____

Source: John F. Clarkin and Sheldon D. Chizever, "Inpatient Front Office Functions," *Topics in Health Care Financing*, Spring 1982.

Figure 3-4 Sample form for monitoring effectiveness of admissions functions

No.	Period From	Dates To	1 Total Admissions	2 Total Non-Emergency Admissions	3 Total Dept. Man-Hours	4 Total Dept. Dollars	5 Total Pre-Admitted Patients	6 Man-Hours Per Admission	7 Dollars Per Admission	8 Pre-Admission Ratio
1										
2										
3										
4										
5										
6										
7										
8										
9										
0										
1										
2										
3										
4										
5										
6										
7										
8										
9										
0										
1										
2										
3										
4										
5										
6										

Column 1: From Daily Admission Book
Column 2: From Daily Admission Book
Column 3: From Departmental Personnel Budget Report
Column 4: From Departmental Personnel Budget Report
Column 5: From Daily Admission Book
Column 6: Divide Column 3 by Column 1
Column 7: Divide Column 4 by Column 1
Column 8: Divide Column 5 by Column 2

Source: John F. Clarkin and Sheldon D. Chizever, "Inpatient Front Office Functions," *Topics in Health Care Financing*, Spring 1982.

Figure 3-5 Sample admitting department performance analysis

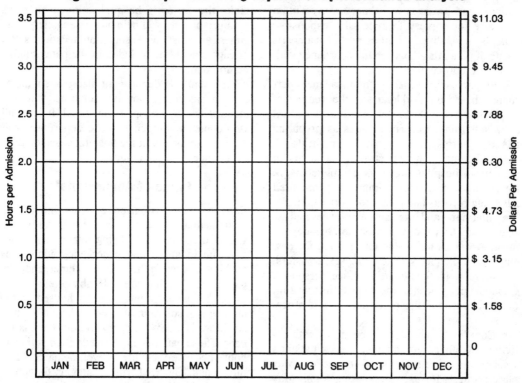

Source: John F. Clarkin and Sheldon D. Chizever, "Inpatient Front Office Functions," *Topics in Health Care Financing,* Spring 1982.

ADMITTING DEPARTMENT

Director of Admissions—Job Duties*

• Makes future reservations for patients, arranges for admission of patients to hospital, and directs and coordinates activities of hospital admitting office personnel.

• Determines hospital privileges of physician who is making reservations by checking against a staff list. Records information that identifies physician and patient, type of accommodation desired, insurance coverage, date of admission, and type and date of operation if case is surgical. Reviews list of unoccupied beds and makes pre-admission reservations according to type of case

---

*Source: *Job Descriptions and Organizational Analysis for Hospitals and Related Health Services,* U.S. Training and Employment Service, Department of Labor, 1971.

and accommodation desired. Frequently forwards admission form to patients to be filled out in advance of hospitalization.

• Interviews patient, his relatives, or other responsible individual to obtain identifying and biographical information. Interprets hospital regulations to patient concerning visitors, visiting hours, and disposition of clothing and valuables. Explains rates, charges, services, discounts, and hospital policy regarding payment of bills. May request partial payment in advance. Notifies particular hospital division to expect patient and arranges for escort of patient to room or ward station. If patient is brought into emergency room, secures necessary information from patient, or from relative or person accompanying patient. Assigns bed or, if patient is to be sent home, explains emergency room charges and arranges for payment. Enters information on record book and forwards cash to business office. Explains differences in rates and charges to patients desiring change of accommodations, and arranges for change. May obtain signature for surgery from legally responsible patients or relatives. Notifies pertinent departments of patient's admission in accordance with established procedures.

• Prepares work schedule for department personnel, based on workload and the number of employees available to perform the tasks. Directs subordinates in such duties as preparing admitting forms, room transfers, admitting reports, and maintaining a current bed index of patients in hospital. Reviews completed work for accuracy and returns improperly prepared admitting records and forms for correction.

• Interviews and hires new employees and assigns them to various sections of the department. Arranges for on-the-job training for new employees. Requests wage increases, transfers, and promotions for admitting office personnel. Conducts periodic staff meetings to inform staff of changes in admitting office policies and procedures.

• Coordinates admitting procedures with activities of other departments. Places patient's valuables in office safe and issues receipt. May place requests for use of operating room. May answer inquiries concerning condition of patient in accordance with regulations governing such information. May notify family when patient is placed on critical list. May contact police in connection with admission of patients classed within police or medicolegal area. In smaller hospitals the duties usually assigned to the credit department are frequently assigned to this job.

• Usually 3 months' on-the-job training is required to become familiar with admitting office policies and procedures.

The Patient's First Impression*

A patient's impression of the hospital begins at the admitting office. A positive image can be generated through patient information booklets or brochures that are either distributed before or at the admission of the patient; frequently these are given to the patient's family and to visitors as well. A booklet for patients outlining the "do's" and "don'ts" of the hospital stay will make the patient's hospitalization a bit more comfortable and will help alleviate anxiety. The American Hospital Association's Patient's Bill of Rights could be included in the patient information booklet.

The admitting department also plays a major role in sustaining positive relations with the medical staff and hospital personnel. Indeed, all who come in contact with the department will form a reaction about the hospital based on their experience with the admitting staff.

Types of Admissions*

Emergency admissions are patients who have to be immediately admitted to the hospital for the sake of their life or well-being. When there is not a vacant inpatient bed, emergency admissions could be housed in the hospital's emergency department's holding area. If absolutely necessary, the patient could also be housed in the nursing unit solarium or even in the patient unit corridor. The next category of admission is *urgent*. These patients must be admitted within 48 hours because their life or well-being could be threatened. The least critical category for admissions is *elective*. These patients' lives are not endangered if their admission is delayed. Under crowded conditions, elective patients generally go on a waiting list. It is common for the hospital's medical staff to be asked to review or to modify these admission definitions. Also the hospital's medical staff has an obligation to review the categories of admission and define them based on local community conditions, for example, by considering the age of the population and the services available in the hospital.

Preadmission Testing**

Prior to the patient's admission, certain clinical preadmission testing is conducted on many elective patients. Third party payers concerned with the high cost of medical care encourage this preadmission testing process. The process of pread-

---

*Source: I. Donald Snook, Jr., *Hospitals: What They Are and How They Work*, Aspen Systems Corporation, 1981.

*Source: I. Donald Snook, Jr., *Hospitals: What They Are and How They Work*, Aspen Systems Corporation, 1981.

**Source: I. Donald Snook, Jr., *Hospitals: What They Are and How They Work*, Aspen Systems Corporation, 1981.

mission clinical testing involves the patient coming to the hospital for ancillary studies, including laboratory tests, x-ray examinations, or electrocardiograms. Testing generally is done on an outpatient basis prior to the day of admission.

Preadmission testing has four recognized benefits for the patient, the physician, and the hospital:

1. It frequently reduces the need to postpone or cancel surgery by discovering unusual test results prior to admission.
2. It allows the hospital's busy ancillary areas (x-ray and laboratory) to distribute the workload more evenly.
3. It provides information to the physician prior to the admission and makes the physician's preoperative patient workup much easier.
4. Since the testing is done on an outpatient basis, it frequently shortens the length of the patient's hospital stay; it thereby reduces the cost to the patient and to the insurance company and also frees beds for other patients.

Preadmission testing does have some drawbacks. Sometimes the patient is too ill to go to the hospital for diagnostic studies. Obviously, preadmission will not work on emergency admissions. Some patients are unwilling or unable to leave work or to go to the hospital a day or two prior to admission. Some patients find it inconvenient to travel long distances to the hospital.

Bed Assignments*

Establishment of the specific policies and procedures is up to the individual hospital in concert with its medical staff. However, some criteria that are used include: (1) maximizing occupancy; (2) clinical segregation of patients (more often done in teaching or university hospitals), which allows the medical department, the surgical department, and other specialty areas to receive a reasonable balance of patients in the hospital; (3) minimizing the bad debts or maximizing revenue or income; and (4) allotting certain hospital beds for teaching cases (fre-

quently seen in medical teaching centers where it is used to maximize the teaching cases for residents and medical students).

Indigent Patients*

The Hill-Burton Act regulations create two categories of persons unable to pay for care. Category A includes those persons whose individual or family income for the preceding 12 months is at or below the poverty income guideline of the Community Services Administration. For such persons a facility must provide services without charge. Category B includes those persons whose individual or family income for the preceding 12 months is greater than the poverty income guideline established by the Community Services Administration, but no more than twice the guideline amount. The provision of uncompensated services to individuals in this category is at the facility's option. Should a hospital provide uncompensated services to individuals in this group, it may exercise flexibility, providing its services at no charge or in accordance with a schedule of charges established in its allocation plan. The facility should maintain separate accounts for uncompensated services. In addition, provision is made for public inspection and HHS review, consistent with personal privacy, of certain information.

Under the new regulations, a facility may provide uncompensated services in accordance with an allocation plan that describes the method by which it will distribute such care. The allocation plan must be published prior to the beginning of the fiscal year. Should a facility not adopt an allocation plan, it will be presumed to have adopted a first-come, first-served method of distributing uncompensated services to persons eligible for such care.

The current Hill-Burton regulations require that facilities provide notice of the availability of uncompensated services. This is accomplished by notices published in newspapers with a general circulation; notices posted in such places as the admissions area, emergency department and business office of the hospital; notices given to individuals; and notice given to the Health Systems Agency (HSA) for the area.

*Source: I. Donald Snook, Jr., *Hospitals: What They Are and How They Work,* Aspen Systems Corporation, 1981.

*Source: Health Law Center, *Hospital Law Manual,* Vol. 1, Aspen Systems Corporation, December 1981.

The newspaper notices must be published at least 60 days prior to the beginning of the hospital's fiscal year. The contents of the notice must include the hospital's allocation plan, the amount of uncompensated care available during the ensuing fiscal year, and where applicable, a statement explaining why the hospital does not anticipate meeting its annual compliance level. The fact that a facility met its uncompensated care obligation during the previous year or will do so in the next fiscal year should be stated.

The regulations also include "community service" provisions requiring that services be furnished without discrimination as to creed, race, color, national origin, or other bases unrelated to the person's need for or availability of care. Moreover, the regulations prohibit a facility from denying a person emergency care if that person resides in the area (or works in the area according to Title XVI) because of an inability to pay for care rendered. However, a patient accepted for care under this provision may be discharged or transferred to another facility when doing so would not carry a substantial risk of deterioration in the patient's medical condition.

There are also community service regulations that are designed to eliminate exclusionary admission policies. The regulations set forth three types of policies that constitute noncompliance with the community service obligation. First, if a hospital has a policy of admitting only those individuals who are referred by physicians with staff privileges and this has the effect of excluding persons in the community because they do not have a personal physician with staff privileges, the hospital would be deemed in noncompliance with the regulation. To correct such a situation, the hospital must take steps to assist individuals in the service area who would otherwise be unable to receive care at the facility. For example, a hospital would establish a primary care clinic through which such patients could be hospitalized, or alternatively, it could hire or contract with qualified doctors to treat those who do not have a personal physician.

Second, if the hospital participates in the Medicaid program, but few physicians with staff privileges treat Medicaid patients and this has the effect of denying such patients care at the facility, this too, would be seen as noncompliance. While a hospital need not require all staff physicians to treat Medicaid patients, it must initiate measures to ensure Medicaid beneficiaries full access to services available at the facility. This could be accomplished by a voluntary arrangement with staff physicians willing to accept Medicaid beneficiaries or by hiring or contracting with doctors to treat Medicaid patients. If an insufficient number of staff physicians agree to participate in a referral arrangement, then the facility may require acceptance of referrals as a condition of renewing or obtaining staff privileges. Another step that may be taken includes establishing a clinic through which Medicaid beneficiaries needing hospitalization may be admitted.

If a hospital requires preadmission deposits and this has the effect of denying hospitalization or care or creates substantial delays in gaining admission or care because the individual cannot pay the deposit, this would be seen as noncompliance with the community service obligation. In correcting this third type of noncompliant policy, the facility need not eliminate the deposit requirement in all cases. Rather, the hospital must establish alternative arrangements so that individuals who do not have the necessary cash when the services are requested, but are likely to be able to pay at a later date, are not denied care.

To deny a person treatment or admission solely because he or she has no demonstrable way of paying for such services has been seen by some courts as an unlawful, arbitrary action by an institution charged with the responsibility of serving the community in which the facility is located. A court may draw upon a facility's charter, incorporation papers, licensure application, or the state indigency laws in carving out a hospital's duty to look beyond a person's ability to pay in deciding whether to treat or admit that individual.

The extent of a hospital's duty to provide either treatment or admission for care is not without limit. Several states still follow the traditional principle that a hospital does not have a responsibility to admit or treat a person in a nonemergency situation. Yet, differentiating emergency from nonemergency matters is not a simple task. Denial of care based on such a distinction can result in civil litigation charging wrongful denial of care. Given the developing trend extending the duty of a hospital in a nonemergency situation, it is necessary for institutions to develop guidelines that require emergency department personnel to evaluate the seriousness of a person's complaint of injury or illness without first assessing ability to pay for care. A hospital and its employees are charged with the responsibility of exercising reasonable care under the circumstances. If treatment or admission is warranted, steps could then be taken to determine whether the person has any means of paying for care. Deposits may be requested at this point, or transfer to another facility may be warranted. In this way, the hospital would be acting reasonably in meeting its duty of care to nonemergency patients.

Hospitals' Liability*

. . . For Wrongful Discharge or Transfer of Patients

Although a hospital may be held liable for the wrongful detention of a patient, it bears a responsibility to prevent the escape or elopement of a patient in need of further care when the patient's leaving creates an unreasonable risk of harm. Reasonable restraint may be used with patients who are mentally unbalanced or who are afflicted with a communicable disease. Detaining such patients is legally sound if it can be demonstrated that they require further medical care and that their release would endanger their personal well-being or the health and safety of persons in the community.

Hospitals may also be held liable for the wrongful discharge or transfer of patients who injure themselves or others as a result of their inappropriate release from the facility. Similarly, hospitals will be held responsible for the death of patients or others who die as the result of a patient's inappropriate release. Liability will attach in either instance if the hospital knew or should have known that the patients posed a substantial risk of harm or danger to themselves or others. Thus, government hospitals have been found negligent for the wrongful discharge of persons who went on to commit homicide.

. . . In Retention and Detaining of Patients

In most of the reported cases based on allegations of false imprisonment, the patients argued

that they were detained against their will for failure to pay their hospital bills. It is fundamental that no one should be detained for such a reason. An action for false imprisonment will also be entertained for the detention of a voluntarily committed patient beyond a statutory period without benefit of a court proceeding.

Internal Audit Checkpoints*

Admitting and Discharge Policies

An internal audit must evaluate the adequacy of written policies for admitting and discharging patients, how they were generated, who is responsible for keeping them up to date, the method used, and whether employees are aware of them. Following are starting points for auditors to design custom tailored audits for their hospitals.

General

1. Are there any particular types of illnesses that will not be admitted?
2. What is the policy for emergency admissions? What priority do they have over other admissions and how is the procedure protected from abuses of the privilege?
3. What liability release forms are required?
4. What patient classification system exists and does it describe the various patient groups adequately?
5. Are patients routinely segregated by type of admitting diagnosis?

Financial

1. What policy is used to admit charity patients and how does the hospital control its charity load?
2. What is the policy on requiring advance deposits from patients without third-party payor coverage?
3. What is the screening process for determining patient ability to pay, for acquiring financial information, and for verifying insurance coverage?
4. How are patients handled for readmission when they have outstanding balances?
5. What is the policy for discounts on hospital bills?

---

*Source: Health Law Center, *Hospital Law Manual,* Vol. 1, Aspen Systems Corporation, December 1981.

---

*Source: Seth Allcorn, *Internal Auditing for Hospitals,* Aspen Systems Corporation, 1979.

Organization of Admissions

1. Is the admitting office located in one area under one supervisor or decentralized to other buildings and areas under several supervisors? Is the form of organization effective?
2. To whom do the supervisors of admissions report?
3. What authority and responsibilities do the supervisors have?
4. Is the organizational pattern documented and do all employees know and understand it?
5. What provision is there for coordinating other hospital operations with admissions?

Staffing Admissions

1. Do adequate job descriptions exist for all employee positions and do they complement the existing organization? Do employees know their jobs?
2. What provision is there for monitoring employee turnover, absenteeism, and overtime? How are staff shortages dealt with? Are temporary employees used or do persons from other departments fill in temporarily in admissions?
3. What provisions exist for orientation of new employees, training, performance evaluation, wage and salary administration, and staff benefits?
4. Do employees appear motivated, do they identify with the hospital's goals, and are they loyal?
5. What provisions exist for employee feedback?

Physical Facilities for Admissions

1. Where is the admissions office located in relation to the lobby, main entrances, emergency room, medical records, the business and cashier offices, and patient and physician traffic patterns?
2. Is there sufficient space to provide for patient privacy during interviews and has adequate space been assigned for waiting areas, toilets, equipment, records storage, and personnel?
3. Are operating conditions safe and comfortable and do they encourage good employee performance? Is the area clean, climate controlled, nicely decorated and furnished, and well lighted, and are there enough clearly marked exits and sufficient aisle space?
4. Is admissions equipped properly with business machines, copy machines, and telephones?
5. Is the area laid out to facilitate a normal flow of operation?

Admitting Procedures

1. Is there a system of preregistering elective admission patients and, if so, do the forms and instructions sent to patients provide enough information for the hospital and the individuals?
2. Is the current census known at all times and are available beds well controlled?
3. Do admitting forms provide complete information for all hospital business systems? What is the distribution of the forms?
4. How are patient clothes and valuables handled? How are advance payments handled?
5. Is there an effort to control workload by staggering patient arrival times?
6. Are patients received with warmth and courtesy? What provisions exist for patient and family feedback regarding treatment by staff?
7. How are patients escorted to the wards and what forms and records accompany them?
8. What care related activities come under admissions' responsibility? What routine tests are part of the admitting process, does admissions request the medical record, and is admissions responsible for notifying the attending physician of the patient's arrival?
9. Are physicians kept informed of bed occupancy levels?
10. Does admissions compile daily and weekly statistics on all activities?

Discharge Procedures

1. Who has the authority to discharge or transfer a patient and how is admissions informed?
2. What is the procedure for returning clothes and valuables?

3. Are relatives informed as early as possible and is transportation arranged for the patient? Who is responsible for being certain the patient can make the trip safely?
4. Who is responsible that the patient has received proper health care instructions and drugs if needed? What is the procedure for follow-up appointments as an outpatient?
5. What control procedures exist for the patient's medical record and other records and reports?

BILLING DEPARTMENT

In many instances the billing process is viewed narrowly as the system that produces only bills, dunning messages, and aged trial balance listings and applies cash. It is essential to broaden this perspective to include all the related billing functions from the process of admissions or outpatient registration to the ultimate collection of the patient's bill. The interactions and dependencies of these functions are shown in Figure 3-6.

Functions of Accounts Receivable Management*

It is also important to distinguish between front and back office functions of accounts receivable management. Front office functions may be defined as those surrounding both the initial contact with the patient and the gathering of the proper identifying and charge information required for billing. These include inpatient admissions, appointments, registration, master patient index, charge capture and financial counseling. Back office functions may be defined as those involving the patient after discharge, including

---

*Source: John F. Clarkin and Sheldon D. Chizever, "Accounts Receivable Management—an Overview," *Topics in Health Care Financing,* Spring 1982. The authors are health care consultants with Coopers & Lybrand, Philadelphia.

Figure 3-6 Accounts receivable management system: interactions and dependencies of billing functions

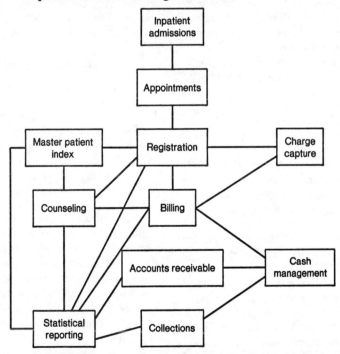

Source: John F. Clarkin and Sheldon D. Chizever, "Accounts Receivable Management—An Overview," *Topics in Health Care Financing,* Spring 1982, chart © 1981 by Coopers & Lybrand, Philadelphia, reprinted with permission.

billing, accounts receivable, cash management, collections and statistical reporting. Back office functions normally take place during the "discharge routine" for both inpatients and outpatients and involve billing and collecting for hospital services.

Inpatient and Outpatient

It is important to analyze accounts receivable management in terms of both inpatient and outpatient services because the two services are quite different.

In the case of inpatient service, bills are normally of higher dollar value and fewer in number than those of outpatient. In addition, there are many opportunities to gather the information required for billing and collect the patient liability portion of the hospital bill. For example, cash collection can be accomplished at preadmission, on the day of admission, during the hospital stay, on the day of discharge or after the patient has been discharged.

The outpatient service, on the other hand, creates an entirely different set of circumstances. For instance, the outpatient is examined, treated and discharged on the same day; for this reason, the collection of cash and the gathering of the proper financial information on the day of service are important. The hospital may have only a few minutes or hours to execute these tasks. This is why it is important to have documented policies and procedures that outline, in advance, at what point in the outpatient process cash collection will be performed and what steps are to be taken if the patient is unwilling or unable to pay for the service. Cash collection on the day of service is particularly important for outpatients because the bills are normally of lower dollar amounts and higher volumes than those of inpatients. This difference causes a higher cost for billing and collection to the point that the cost for sending out the bill sometimes exceeds the value of the charge itself.

Many hospitals are expanding their outpatient facilities, yet some do so without revising existing EDP systems designed to process much smaller volumes. As a result of these expanded facilities, volume of patient visits increases and existing systems collapse under the increased volume. Furthermore, there is a general lack of EDP systems designed to handle the specific problems associated with outpatient registration, financial counseling, billing, credit and collections.

This scarcity has evolved because many systems on the market today were primarily designed as inpatient systems, and outpatient processing was not or could not be given adequate consideration because of hardware or software limitations and costs. This situation is changing now with the technological advances being made in mini- and microcomputers and associated software. These mini- and microprocessors are enabling automated outpatient processing and billing to be performed in a cost-effective manner.

One of the most important aspects of the relationship between inpatient and outpatient services is that more and more examinations and treatments previously requiring an inpatient stay are now able to be performed, due to an increase in technology, on an outpatient basis. Insurance coverage for these services, however, has not kept pace with the types of examinations and tests now able to be performed safely on an outpatient basis. The outpatient upward trend can be expected to grow in the future, and third party payers are now reviewing and evaluating this condition, although few corrective measures have yet been implemented.

Monitoring Billing*

Problems in billing and accounts receivable and in cash management are not difficult to uncover because they are readily identifiable in the hospital's financial reports. For example, a significant increase in the days of revenue in accounts receivable, a negative variance in the expected cash from accounts receivable, and an increase in the dollar value of the accounts in the 90-days-and-older category on the aged trial balance are all warning signals of problems in the billing process. However, in many cases by the time these reports have been published, the damage is already done.

To avoid these problems, some hospitals have instituted systems and management reports that identify when and where problems occur in the billing/accounts receivable and cash management functions.

---

*Source: John F. Clarkin and Sheldon D. Chizever, "Back Office Functions of the Billing Process," *Topics in Health Care Financing,* Spring 1982.

One report that has been used effectively by hospitals is the Billing Process Report (see Table 3-1). This report provides the manager with an inventory and status report of the total billing process in billed and unbilled accounts. It also establishes targets (or goals) for billed and unbilled accounts broken down by all payers. In using a target system that establishes goals, billing clerks will normally work toward meeting the established target bills first and work on problem accounts as a group later on or will sometimes pass these accounts to their immediate supervisor for resolution. The Billing Process Report also includes measurement criteria for unapplied payments.

Another report that hospitals have used effectively is the Third Party Follow-Up Report (see Table 3-2). This report is used in much the same way as the Billing Process Report with inventories and targets being established for follow-up to third parties. The report is submitted daily and summarized weekly with comments on any variances and the action taken. The status of follow-up on rejected or otherwise unpaid insurance claims is a statistic that is frequently not accurately known or reported. Once again, the patient accounts manager or controller might not be aware of the problem until it subsequently surfaces as a cash flow difficulty.

Table 3-1   Billing Process Report

Category	Total / Target / Comments
Billed	By Payer class:
Current	Medicaid
Prior	Blue Cross
Unbilled	Medicare
Current	Commercial
Prior	Workmens comp.
Unapplied payments	Self-pay
Current	Others
Prior	
Unanswered	
correspondence	
Current	
Prior	
Comments/action taken:	

Source: John F. Clarkin and Sheldon D. Chizever, "Back Office Functions of the Billing Process," *Topics in Health Care Financing,* Spring 1982, table © 1981 by Coopers & Lybrand, Philadelphia, reprinted with permission.

Table 3-2   Third Party Follow-Up Report

Inventory / Target / Comments
Beginning inventory
New claims
Reviewed this week
Ending inventory
Target balance
Variance
Comments
By:
Commercial
Workmen's comp.
Champus
Medicare
Blue Cross
Self-pay
Comments/action taken:

Source: John F. Clarkin and Sheldon D. Chizever, "Back Office Functions of the Billing Process," *Topics in Health Care Financing,* Spring 1982, table © 1981 by Coopers & Lybrand, Philadelphia, reprinted with permission.

One particular report that hospital financial managers have found very helpful in controlling the entire back office function is the Controller's Weekly Status Report (see Table 3-3). The purpose of this report is to provide the manager with a snapshot of the status of the entire patient accounting process. Contained in this report are (1) performance measures for the current week compared to the prior week, and (2) targets for billing and collection activities. Targets are established for each component of the processing/control functions within the billing process, including total patient receipts, billings, credit, receivables/cash applications and collections. Each week the various units report on their performance and comment on the reasons for any variances and, more importantly, the action taken.

Staffing*

Guidelines can be used to establish staffing requirements in credit and collection departments. One guideline involves the maintenance of logs and management reports where the number of

*Source: John F. Clarkin and Sheldon D. Chizever, "Back Office Functions of the Billing Process," *Topics in Health Care Financing,* Spring 1982.

Table 3-3   Controller's Weekly Status Report

Performance measure	Week of	Prior week	Target
Cash			
Total patient receipts			
Blue Cross			
Insurance			
Medicare			
Medicaid			
Self-pay			
Other			
Billing			
Total dollars billed			
Unbilled inpatient accounts			
Unbilled outpatient accounts			
Unbillable inpatient accounts			
Bills on system over 3 days			
Credit			
Total billed, unpaid $			
Blue Cross			
Insurance			
Medicare			
Medicaid			
Self-pay			
Credit interviews			
Dollars collected			
Unanswered correspondence			
Receivables & cash application			
Total active A/R accounts			
Total receivables			
Days of revenue			
Unapplied cash			
Collections			
Amount sent to agencies			
Amount sent to date			
Amount recovered to date			
Percent recovered			
In-house collections			
In-house collections to date			
Percent recovered			
Dunning calls			
Comments/action taken:			

Source: John F. Clarkin and Sheldon D. Chizever, "Back Office Functions of the Billing Process," *Topics in Health Care Financing,* Spring 1982, table © 1981 by Coopers & Lybrand, Philadelphia, reprinted with permission.

items in each category that can realistically be processed by departmental personnel is maintained over a 30- to 60-day period. Specifically, for each category of staffing, these logs would contain the following:

- collectors (number of telephone calls and dollar value; number of letters answered and dollar value);
- financial counselors (number of patients interviewed and dollar value);

- paralegal (number of accounts requiring appearance in court and dollar value; number of attorney referrals and dollar value).

The totals in each category would then be divided into the total inventory in each category to arrive at the number of employees required. The hospital should ascertain what backlogs would be acceptable in each category and consider these totals when deciding on the number of employees required. Performance measures and targets should then be established for each category and reported upon.

Theft in Billing and Collection*

The billing and collection process in hospitals and other health care institutions has become so complex that it is a favorite topic of discussion among journalists, the media and hospital consultants. All the advance admitting preparations, the automated charge methods, and the computerization have done little to reduce the monstrous proportion of errors and the staggering load of patient complaints and claims adjustments.

Collection

The potential for fraud in the collection process may be small in comparison to other areas in the hospital, but when such fraud is successfully perpetrated over a period of time, it can substantially drain the hospital's assets.

There have been cases of massive collusion between collection personnel within the hospital and collection agencies. Perfectly collectable accounts are sometimes declared uncollectable. They are then handed over to an agency and collected in full. A portion may be deposited with the hospital with the remainder being divided between the collection clerical and the collection agency.

Billing

With ever-increasing coverage by third party carriers, the opportunities for theft in the billing and collection process may gradually diminish. However, the opportunity for theft will always be great when the entire billing process is suffering from a staggering load of unresolved receivable balances. The less up-to-date the legitimate billing and collection processes are, the easier the defalcations will be.

Preventing theft in this area is difficult. Billing systems vary, as do the loopholes and the opportunities for fraud. Suffice it to say that eager attention to legitimate billing and collection processes is not enough. Alertness to potential fraud is essential. The total system of checks and balances, internal audit methods and investigative techniques has to be geared to the problem.

Theft in Ancillary Charges*

Though some hospitals have an all-inclusive rate for patient care, Medicare, Medicaid or other third party plans usually require a separate listing of ancillary charges. Also, certain services such as x-ray, cardiac and respiratory may be excluded from the all-inclusive rate. In some hospitals these types of departments are established as private corporations (PCs) and process their own charges. Depending on the data processing facilities at the hospital and arrangements made with these departments, charges to patients can be processed through the hospital's computer, an outside service organization or manually by the department itself. Therefore, whether the hospital charges for each item separately or operates on a full-inclusive or partial-inclusive rate, ancillary charges usually have to be billed to the proper patient or processed through the internal accounting system.

Patient Accounts

Most hospitals today have some type of computer system for patient accounts. The older systems use a charge card type of patient identification, which includes the patient's name and number (sequential city or state number, as required), the name of the physician and other pertinent information. Ancillary charges are processed by impairing the patient identification onto an ancillary charge form. The forms are then key punched and entered into the computer. The more sophisticated systems employ CRTs at the nursing stations for entering patient information. In other cases, charges for special items are "precharged" and retained in computer memory until the second entry at the nursing station removes the precharge and transfers the amount with coding to the patient's account. In most cases, services are charged to patients when administered.

*Source: Walter Nagel, "Health Care Industry's Vulnerability to Theft," *Topics in Health Care Financing,* Winter 1978.

*Source: Walter Nagel, "Health Care Industry's Vulnerability to Theft," *Topics in Health Care Financing,* Winter 1978.

CRTs

Administration should not assume that they will capture all ancillary charges by the use of CRTs. The medical staff may accidentally forget to charge a patient, or a nurse purposely fail to enter a charge for a patient who is a friend or relative.

Administrators tend to assume incorrectly that in the newer systems using CRTs the patient identification number (with a check digit) ensures that the proper patient is charged and that if departmental charge codes and dollar amounts are programmed correctly the right charge is billed. The CRT can not ensure that certain charges, such as those for monitors and defibrillators, go to the appropriate patient. Equipment such as monitors and defibrillators are moved from patient to patient, and often the wrong patient is charged for these services. The cardiology or biomedical engineering departments must be responsible for issuance and control of equipment.

CREDIT AND COLLECTION DEPARTMENT*

Hospitals have been effective in resolving problems with their collection departments by first reviewing organization and hospital policies and procedures. In many hospitals, the collection department does not become involved until an account is 120 to 150 days old. This is generally too late in the billing cycle to be helpful; somewhere between 60 and 90 days would be desirable. When the collection department enters the billing cycle as early as possible, a hospital's cash flow is normally accelerated, and the bad-debt write-off figures are decreased.

The next step to be taken is to review the support being provided to the department by electronic data processing. Weekly aged trial balance reports, broken down by third party payers, are proven documents that can be used effectively. When collectors receive a weekly trial balance, the account is more current because payments by third parties have been applied.

---

*Source: John F. Clarkin and Sheldon D. Chizever, "Back Office Functions of the Billing Process," *Topics in Health Care Financing,* Spring 1982.

This step should be followed by a review of the dunning messages that appear on the patient's bill to ensure that they are worded in the most effective manner.

Problems often occur in the credit and collection department because of the absence of a good collection manual. A good manual will specifically outline the duties and responsibilities of each individual within the unit. The manual should also contain the hospital's policies, including: free care, delinquent accounts, outside collectors, budget payments and bad-debt write-offs.

Finally, an absence of performance goals and measurement standards can be a problem to a credit and collection department. Hospitals have successfully instituted targets for the credit and collection department. One is a measure of the amount of dollars sent to outside collectors as well as their percentage of collections. This statistic can be important because if an outside collector's performance is too good, perhaps the hospital's collection department is not spending enough time on these accounts. Another measure used by hospitals is the number of dunning calls made and the effectiveness of these calls. These and other performance measures, along with established weekly targets, can be found on the Controller's Weekly Status Report (Table 3-3, above).

Functions

Functions typically found in hospital credit and collection departments are:

- delinquent account follow-up (collectors): telephone dunning, collection letters, interviews;
- correspondence: telephone inquiry, mail;
- financial counseling;
- policy and procedure development;
- knowledge of federal and state regulations;
- paralegal expertise: liens, Small Claims Court, bankruptcies, legal aspects of federal and state regulations, attorney referral;
- outside collection agency selection and control;
- insurance billing, follow-up (sometimes found in billing); and
- systems development, including electronic data processing interface and interaction with other departments.

Table 3-4 aligns those functions typically found in hospital credit and collection departments with each position.

Policies and Procedures

Preadmission

All completed preadmission forms should be delivered to the credit section for review. The credit section or its designee should have documented policies and procedures which instruct personnel to:

- check all patients against the bad-debt and self-pay open account file;
- verify coverage for all third party payers; and
- estimate, based on the projected length of stay, the patient liability portion of the bill. This computation should include amounts not covered by insurance, deductible and coinsurance amounts, room differentials and telephone fees.

In addition, a deposit should be required by admissions from all patients for the estimated self-pay responsibility for noninsurance-covered items. Patients without third party coverage (self-pay) should be required to make a minimum deposit based on the per diem charge for the estimated length of stay. Patients on the bad-debt or open account list should be required to make settlement arrangements prior to admission. Deposit requirements would then be communicated by telephone, and patients with limited financial resources would be interviewed and assisted in applying for Medicaid or other charitable organizations. Admissions are sometimes postponed in those cases where suitable financial arrangements cannot be made.

Admission

Emergency admissions for the most part are processed without regard for financial adequacy. If the patient does not have adequate third party coverage or means to pay, the credit department would assist the patient or his or her representative in obtaining financial assistance from Medicare, Medicaid or some other governmental or charitable organization.

Elective and other nonemergency admissions who arrive without having the preadmission review should be admitted if there is evidence of adequate third party coverage and the required deposit is paid, or the patient is self-pay and pays the required deposit, and the assignment of benefits form is signed.

In cases where the patient has third party coverage but cannot pay his or her estimated self-pay liability, the patient should be referred to the credit department. During the credit interview, the patient should agree to meet the self-pay obligation before discharge. Admissions are sometimes postponed in cases where suitable financial arrangements cannot be made. In all cases, the physician should be notified when admissions are postponed.

Discharge

Policies and procedures should be established whereby all patient liability portions of bills must be paid at the time of discharge, or credit arrangements must be made with the hospital's credit and collection department. Once billing has taken place, effective policies and procedures must be in place for timely follow-up of patient and third party bills to ensure prompt receipt of payment.

In cases where the patient does not pay in a timely fashion, policies and procedures should be in place for either sending the patient bill to a collection agency, settlement, bad-debt write-off or free care. Settlement authorizations should contain guidelines similar in format, but not necessarily in content, to these: 3 to 6 months past due, 60 percent settlement; 6 to 12 months past due, 50 percent settlement; and over 12 months past due, 30 percent settlement.

Outpatients

The rationale for written credit and collection policies and procedures for outpatients is the same as that for inpatients. The type of policies differs somewhat because of the larger number of encounters at a lower charge per encounter. The outpatient system of credit and collection procedures needs to encompass:

- controlled registration of patients for each outpatient visit, including positive identification of the patient;
- treatment of patients only when properly registered prior to service, and complete recording of all services provided;

Table 3-4   Functional Organization of Credit and Collection Department

Manager

Reviews activity logs and management control reports daily to monitor performance and resolve problems.

Recommends policies to hospital administration.

Trains new personnel on credit and collection procedures.

Directs and is responsible for the successful performance of all components of credit and collection.

Correspondence clerk

Receives patient inquiries via the telephone and resolves:
- incorrect balances
- unapplied payments
- balances not covered by patient insurance
- incorrect insurance numbers and addresses
- etc.

Receives mail from patients commenting on whether:
- payment has been made in full to hospital
- patient has insurance coverage which is not reflected on bill
- patient never received a bill

Resolves mail correspondence problems and answers by return mail.

Maintains daily activity logs on inquiries and answered and unanswered correspondence.

Collection clerk

Performs telephone dunning of delinquent patient accounts and makes arrangements for payment.

Records all calls, correspondence, interviews and activities relating to collection efforts to an activity log.

Interviews patients referred by financial counselors who are able but unwilling to pay.

Interviews patients with large delinquent accounts where telephone resolution is not practical:
- determines settlement on accounts in accordance with hospital policy
- arranges for budget payment plans where applicable

Uses collection letters and mailgrams as necessary.

Forwards to the paralegal supervisor accounts that cannot be resolved or that threaten legal action against the hospital.

Forwards and monitors accounts sent to the outside collection agency in accordance with hospital policies.

Monitors prelist for bad-debt write-off.

Financial counselor

Interviews patients referred from admissions or outpatient department without full insurance coverage and/or who have delinquent accounts to:
- inform patients of hospital policies
- arrange suitable financial coverage for self-pay patients
- assist patients in obtaining medical assistance cards if qualified
- arrange contractual payments for patients able to meet financial liabilities
- recommend patients for free care, according to hospital policy

Paralegal clerk

Works closely with the hospital's attorney regarding:
- Small Claims Court
- legal suits
- other legal actions

Interviews patients, with the approval of the hospital's attorney, who are threatening to sue but who have not taken legal action.

Keeps abreast of the legal aspects of federal and state regulations.

Prepares and maintains an activity log on interviews, cases for Small Claims Court, correspondence, cases ready for legal action, etc.

Source: John F. Clarkin and Sheldon D. Chizever, "Back Office Functions of the Billing Process," *Topics in Health Care Financing*, Spring 1982.

- strict accountability of documents authorizing and recording services; and
- accurate and timely billing for services.

Proof of identification should be required at the time of registration, including driver's license or third party cards as appropriate. Cash should be required for all self-pay amounts, and Master Card and VISA cards should be evaluated. The remainder of the credit and collection policies for inpatients can be applied to outpatients.

Management Reporting

The purpose of management reporting is to enable the credit and collection department to measure its employees' job effectiveness as well as the effectiveness of the department as a whole. Several logs and management reports that have been used successfully by hospitals are:

- *Financial Counselor's Log.* The purpose of this log is to maintain a record of patient referrals for financial counseling—the reasons, the amount of the bill and the terms arranged. At the end of the day and each week, both the financial counselors and the credit and collection manager will have a document to communicate progress achieved and areas for improvement.
- *Correspondence Log—Telephone.* The purpose of this log is to enable the correspondence clerks to analyze the effectiveness of their daily activities. The log lists the patient's name, reason for the call, disposition, payment arrangements made and remarks which might include, for example, the fact that the patient was billed as self-pay but really has third party insurance. The telephone correspondence log is also a good barometer of how well the other functions of accounts receivable management are performing. For example, a great many calls stating that the patient has third party coverage might indicate that admissions is not performing the functions of preadmission or insurance verification effectively.
- *Correspondence Log—Mail.* This log serves the same purpose as the telephone correspondence log in providing a mechanism for the correspondence clerks to measure the effectiveness of their daily activi-

ties. Mail correspondence can also point out problems that may be occurring at various stages of the accounts receivable management process. For example, many complaints from patients who insist that payments have been made in full to the hospital might suggest that there may be a misapplied cash problem somewhere in the billing process.

- *Collection Activity Log.* This log is an important document for the collectors. It enables the collectors to record and analyze their telephone performance on a daily basis. The log provides for the name, balance and age of the account, whether contact was made and with whom, and information regarding payment arrangements. The log should be used in conjunction with the telephone interviewing technique discussed on pages 54 and 56.
- *Paralegal Log.* This log enables the effectiveness of the paralegal section to be measured. The supervisor and paralegal clerk can review and discuss workloads on a daily and weekly basis and decide on areas for concentration.
- *Daily and Weekly Collection Activity Summary Reports.* The daily summary report summarizes the contact, payments arranged, accounts turned over to a collection agency or attorney, and free care on a daily basis. This information is garnered from the financial counselor's daily logs, correspondence logs, (telephone and mail) collection activity logs and paralegal logs. The weekly summary report is a compilation of the daily summary reports.

Slow and Nonpayers

A major problem found in many hospitals is aged trial balance listings (ATB). Hospitals that have cost-effective credit and collection efforts often use for different purposes a variety of ATB reports. These include ATBs by:

- *Financial class, aging category, largest balances first*—This ATB allows specific collectors to work on certain financial classes beginning with the largest balances. For example, one collector could be following up on Medicare accounts while another is following up on Blue Cross accounts that have not been paid.

- *Bad-debt write-off accounts*—This ATB provides quick access to accounts that have been written off and proves useful when these patients again visit the hospital and request admission or treatment.
- *Collector accounts*—This ATB permits close monitoring of those accounts sent to an outside collection agency.
- *Self-pay alpha*—This ATB allows follow-up and special handling by a designated collector for self-pay delinquent accounts.

Other support can be provided to credit and collection departments by electronic data processing in the form of procedures for automatic balance write-off. Once accounts have been approved for write-off, these account balances can be written off automatically by the computer and adjustments made to accounts receivable without voluminous and time-consuming manual entries being performed.

The Outside Collection Agency

Hospitals ask many questions concerning the use of and basis for selection of an outside collection agency. One such question is whether a local, regional or national collection agency should be used. The answer given most frequently by hospitals that have experience with all three is that a local firm is satisfactory if it has access to or affiliation with a regional or national firm.

Regardless of the type of agency, it is important to examine the credentials of the agency before selection. Always ask for references and make sure you check on those references before any decision is made. Ensure that the collection agency under consideration has experience with dealing with a hospital of your size and in your type of community. If your institution is a 1,200-bed medical center located in the inner city, make sure the agency is accustomed to dealing with large institutions with significant volumes. If your hospital is in the affluent suburbs, select an agency with appropriate experience. The manner in which you deal with the patient in each location may be somewhat different.

The agency selected should be bonded and licensed and have viable financing. It should have a proven track record for professionalism to avoid potential public relations problems between the hospital and the community. Finally, since fees charged by outside agencies vary

from approximately a 30 to 40 percent flat rate to a sliding scale based on age of the account and dollar value, the competition should always be checked and comparisons made as to effectiveness and rates.

Hospitals turn accounts over to outside collection agencies on different bases. Most frequently, the decisions to turn over accounts are based on the degree of internal effort expended, the age of the account and the account's dollar value. However, the hospital may decide in some cases that the ratio of collection fees to amounts collected is simply too high to warrant retaining the agency's services. Excessive patient complaints may indicate that the outside agency is not exercising the degree of professionalism desired by the hospital.

Key Tools for Credit and Collection

Two key tools for credit and collection which are not always used or used effectively by hospitals are telephone interviewing and follow-up letters.

The purpose of telephone interviewing is to obtain information from patients as to why they have not paid their hospital bills. The responses for nonpayment of bills often include incorrect insurance information, wrong account balances and inability of the patient to pay the outstanding balance. The manner in which the telephone call is handled, regardless of the telephone situation, will determine the success or failure of the call. Follow-up letters are sometimes required when messages on bills and telephone collecting are not appropriate methods of communicating with patients or do not produce the desired results.

Telephone Interviewing

General guidelines should be established for all telephone interviewing (see Tables 3-5 and 3-6). Prior to making a call, the collector should become familiar with both the debtor and the account, including: debtor's name, spouse's name, amount owed, age of account, date and amount of last payment, last collection attempt and promises made, and other pertinent information.

During the call, the collector should always identify himself or herself and the name of the hospital. Payment in full by a specified date should always be requested, and if this is not practical, a series of specified payment dates

Table 3-5　General Telephone Situations (Slow and Nonpayers)

General Telephone Situations

Telephone situation	Guidelines
Responsible party is ill	Identify yourself. Identify the person with whom you are talking. Who is ill (patient, spouse, children)? Why didn't the debtor let us know? Is debtor really affected by the illness? Is this really the cause of delinquency or a stall? Impress debtor that he or she must keep us advised. Try to get promise of payment.
Motivating the responsible party to pay the bill	**Good credit rating**—Isn't a good credit rating worth \$_____? Good credit is your most valuable asset. **Peace of mind**—You could relieve your mind and avoid our taking further action by paying now. **Avoid trouble**—If you do not make payment, we will have no other alternative but to turn your account over to a professional collection agency, and you know the trouble this could cause you. **Honesty**—We believe you are honest and will pay us. **Urgency**—If you can't send the \$_____ today, perhaps you can send it tomorrow.
"I can't pay"	Source of money for payment in full: Loan (credit union, employer, bank, advance on paycheck, loan company, increase in existing loan, relatives, mortgage of home). Sources of money for monthly payments: (paycheck, spouse's payroll check, pension, roomer, hobby, second job, unemployment check, military reserve pay, support and/or alimony checks), assets (checking account, savings account, savings bonds, tax refund). Establish assistance (other): working children, relatives.
Responsible party is out of work	Identify yourself. Be sure you are speaking with the responsible party. Where off work and why? How long off work? What are prospects for employment? Why didn't responsible party let us know? Can relatives or friends assist? Unemployment compensation? Supplemental unemployment?
Responsible party is separated or divorced	Identify yourself. Be sure you are talking to the right person. Establish if divorced or separated. Date of legal separation or divorce? Employer of responsible party? Address and telephone number of responsible party? Contact other responsible party. Tell debtor that he or she is responsible for the bill.
Responsible party is deceased	Identify yourself. Identify the person you are talking with. Date and place of death? Name and address of administrator of estate, if any? If not established, when will this party be named? Name and address of attorney? Is spouse responsible for payment?

Source: John F. Clarkin and Sheldon D. Chizever, "Back Office Functions of the Billing Process," *Topics in Health Care Financing,* Spring 1982.

Table 3-6 Specific Telephone Situations (Slow and Nonpayers)

Specific Telephone Situations

Telephone situation	Guidelines
First collection	Make sure you are talking to debtor. Identify yourself. Ask for payment in full today. If debtor says he or she can't, find out reason and offer solutions to problem. On what day will payment reach us? Mail or personal delivery? Check, money order or cash? Re-verify employer, spouse's employer, resident address. Ask debtor to write down your name, amount and date payment will reach us.
Responsible party or spouse not at home	Identify yourself. Establish to whom you are talking. If not the guarantor or the guarantor's spouse: When will guarantor be home? Leave name and telephone number, stress urgency of call.
Payment is in the mail	When was it sent? How (check, money order or cash)? Amount? If not the amount arranged for, why not and when will balance of payment be made? Re-verify employer, spouse's employer, resident address. Reconfirm figure arrangements.
Partial payment by responsible party	Identify yourself. Be sure you are talking to the responsible party. Thank debtor for payment. Ask for payment in full today. If debtor says he or she cannot, determine the problem and offer solutions. If necessary, make and accept best arrangements possible. Re-verify employer, spouse's employer address. Repeat arrangements and have debtor write them down.
Responsible party has broken payment promise	Make sure you are talking to the debtor. Identify yourself. Why didn't debtor let us know he or she couldn't keep the promise? The arrangements were made as favor. It is hospital policy that bills be paid in full when received. Ask for payment in full today. On what date will payment reach us? Mail or personal delivery? Check, money order or cash? Before agreeing to another promise, make sure that the debtor understands that this will be the last promise accepted, no more favors. Re-verify employer, spouse's employer, resident address. Ask debtor to write down your name, amount and date payment will reach us. Reconfirm future arrangements.

Source: John F. Clarkin and Sheldon D. Chizever, "Back Office Functions of the Billing Process," *Topics in Health Care Financing*, Spring 1982.

Figure 3-7   Sample letter to insurance carrier

Date:

Re: Policy #, Insurance Co.

To Whom It May Concern:

Our records indicate that on _____ our hospital submitted completed assignment forms and billing for _____ inpatient _____ outpatient treatment rendered to _____ of _____ Your insured is _____ and the employer is _____. The period of treatment is _____ to _____ .

In view of the length of time that has elapsed, we must assume that since no payment or correspondence has been received from you in response to our billing, you are denying payment of this claim. Before we seek payment directly from the patient/insured, we are allowing you fifteen (15) days from receipt of this investigation to remit payment of the claim to us or to explain why payment has been delayed.

If payment/information is not received, the hospital will seek payment for services rendered directly from the patient/insured. If necessary, other credit alternatives available to us will be utilized. It will then be the responsibility of the patient/insured to bill you directly for reimbursement as the hospital will process no further filing for this claim.

Your prompt attention to this matter will be appreciated.

Sincerely,

(TO BE SENT AT 45 DAYS TO THE CARRIER)

Source: John F. Clarkin and Sheldon D. Chizever, "Back Office Functions of the Billing Process," *Topics in Health Care Financing*, Spring 1982.

Figure 3-8   Sample letter to patient

Date:

Dear _____ :

Your hospital bill for (inpatient/outpatient) treatment _____ was submitted to your insurance carrier _____ on _____ .

To date your insurance carrier has not remitted payment on your claim. I must inform you that if I do not receive payment from your insurance company within the next thirty (30) days, I shall have to look to you for payment in full on your account.

Any assistance you can provide in obtaining immediate payment from your insurance carrier will be greatly appreciated and will provide mutual benefits to both of us.

Sincerely,

(TO BE SENT AT 60 DAYS TO THE PATIENT)

Source: John F. Clarkin and Sheldon D. Chizever, "Back Office Functions of the Billing Process," *Topics in Health Care Financing*, Spring 1982.

Follow-Up Letters

Letters are sometimes required when messages and telephone collecting do not produce the desired results. Letters may be required for insurance follow-up when insurance companies do not pay claims within 45 days after submission by the hospital (see Figure 3-7 for a sample insurance follow-up letter). If the insurance carrier does not pay within 15 days, a letter could be sent informing the patient that if payment is not received from his or her insurance company within 30 days, the hospital will look to payment in full from the patient (see Figure 3-8). In cases where the patient has expired and a balance is outstanding to the hospital, a patient estate letter is sometimes required. Letters are also required when, after payment arrangements have been agreed upon between the hospital and the patient, the patient defaults.

should be arranged. A sense of urgency for payment should be created, but tempers should always be kept under control since angry remarks do not motivate payment. Tables 3-5 and 3-6 show common situations in which collectors normally become involved during telephone conversations with debtors as well as response guidelines for those situations.

Chapter 4—Medical Records

OVERVIEW*

Organization of the Department

The organization and staffing of the medical record department reflect in a very straightforward manner the tasks and functions of the department. The department is staffed to handle (1) release of information, (2) admission and discharge analyses, (3) medical transcriptions, (4) coding and abstracting (generally this involves diagnostic and procedural coding), and (5) storage and retrieval.

In the area of statistics and recordkeeping, the statistical section of the medical records department provides the input to many of the computerized data services that hospitals use to generate computerized patient data profiles. The primary source of these data is the patient's discharge abstract that is submitted to computerized agencies, such as the Hospital Utilization Program (HUP) or the Commission on Professional Hospital Activities (CPHA). These data are summarized in computer language and sent to a computer with large memory banks. The hospitals can then receive the information in a readable and quickly retrievable fashion.

Typically, a medical record is hard copy; that is, it is bound in paper. However, as bulk storage becomes a problem and space becomes more scarce, the microfilming of medical rec-

ords has become quite common. In recent years, microfilm formats have improved greatly. Earlier, rolls of film were put into cartridges and could be indexed. Today, motor viewers used for high speed retrieval have been replaced in some areas by microfiche, which is a more efficient, cost effective means of storage and retrieval.

The transcription section of the medical record department is an area in which medical typists transcribe the summaries and reports dictated by physicians onto paper for filing in the medical record. At one time, many hospitals employed medical transcribers; today, it is common to use outside transcription services. With these outside systems, the transcription is dictated over the telephone, typed, and then sent by messenger or mail to the hospital. This system offers the hospital the advantage of not having to deal with various hospital employees. Also, the hospital is paying exactly for what it receives in typing, and the outside service relieves the hospital from the task of maintaining a bank of technical transcription equipment.

The Medical Record Administrator

Part of the medical record administrator's job is to organize and manage the medical record system and to provide efficient medical record services to the hospital. Generally this person's duties include: (1) planning, designing, and technically evaluating patient information; (2) planning, directing, and controlling the administration of the medical record department and its

*Source: I. Donald Snook, Jr., *Hospitals: What They Are & How They Work,"* Aspen Systems Corporation, 1981.

services; (3) aiding the medical staff in its work on medical records; (4) developing statistical reports for management and the medical staff; and (5) analyzing technical evaluations of health records and indices.

More specifically:

Functions. Develop, retain, and retrieve patient/client records in accordance with established policies that include retention, protection, and disposition of reports, forms, correspondence, and other records.

Organizational relationships. Reports to assistant administrator or administrator—administrative services; supervises assistant records manager, retention/retrieval supervisor, records center supervisor, central records clerks, microfilm technicians, forms clerks, keypunch, and CRT operators.

Interdepartmental relationships. Systems and procedures department, legal counsel, business and accounting office, all department heads, medical staff, patients, and clients.

Extradepartmental relationships. Third party payers, health planning agencies, patients/clients, legal counsels, biostatisticians, data collection representatives, physicians, hospitals, and other direct and indirect health care providers.

Responsibility for the institution. (1) Establish procedures for retention and destruction of all types of records on a departmental and facility-wide basis; (2) design and revise forms and procedures pertaining to the use of health information; and (3) coordinate problems concerning the flow of information, retention/retrieval of records, files, delivery of medical reports, and medical records.

Departmental. (1) Plan, develop, implement, and modernize record availability and departmental services; (2) maintain and control all records, including files, index cards, registers, policy manuals, microfilm or microfiche, magnetic tape, or other media used in the preparation and retention of records; (3) delegate authority through supervisors or directly to personnel for specific projects; and (4) prepare departmental and institutional manual regarding retention and retrieval of health information.[1]

---

[1]Kathleen A. Waters and Gretchen F. Murphy, *Medical Records in Health Information,* Aspen Systems Corporation, 1979.

The Medical Records Committee

The medical staff's medical records committee is the liaison between the medical record department and the physicians in the hospital. This committee is charged with the responsibility of reviewing and evaluating the medical records function. These tasks should be performed not less than quarterly. Generally, based on random sampling and recommendations from a variety of medical sources, the committee will review certain records on a regular basis for appropriateness. However, the principal responsibility for quality of peer review rests with the medical staff's audit and utilization review committees.

The medical records committee's principal responsibility is to supervise the organization of the record. The committee must review and approve all new medical record forms. In view of the fact that the traditional record is a potpourri of medical forms, this can be, at certain hospitals, a very time-consuming task. The committee should evaluate the accuracy of certain record notations relating to management and administrative matters of the record. For example, if physicians are not writing the discharge diagnosis on the medical record at the proper time or in the proper place, the medical records committee should take directive action. It is the committee's responsibility to police the traditional and chronic problem of physicians' delinquency in completing medical records.

The medical records committee does not generally get involved in making recommendations on management issues in the medical records department. For example, filing procedures, coding of medical records, storage, microfilming potentials, and preservation of certain sections of the record are matters usually left to the medical records administrator in conjunction with the hospital management. However, if the hospital were to change from a traditional medical record system to a problem-oriented medical record system, this committee would play a key role in analyzing the pro's and con's of switching.

The Medical Record

Historically, medical records have been a chronological assembly of notes, forms, reports, and summaries. The traditional or classical record, used in most hospitals today, is a combination of these forms, reports, and notes. The forms are the vehicle for the physician and health practitioners to record the patient's illness and course of recovery. Reports (based on studies such as laboratory tests, x-ray examinations, and operating room procedures) are also included in the medical record. Usually, the record contains written notations, clinical analyses, and handwritten or typed consultation summaries. All of these forms and reports are usually contained in a folder called a chart. Most often the record is maintained in chronological order; that is, the first events regarding the patient in the hospital are noted first in the medical record, followed by subsequent occurrences.

Thus, the traditional record is a package of forms and reports, including the patient's admission form, medical history, physical examination form, and laboratory, x-ray and special report forms. If the patient undergoes surgery, there will usually be authorization and consent forms (including a signed authorization or informed consent) obtained prior to surgery. The patient's anesthesia record will usually be attached to the surgeon's operative report, which is usually dictated and typed. Frequently, physicians' orders will follow the admission form. These orders are on forms, maintained in chronological fashion, by which the physician communicates to the nurses and other health care professionals instructions for carrying out the patient's diagnosis and therapy. Usually near the physician's order sheets are progress note sheets. The progress note sheets are often the largest part of any patient's medical record. The nurses' notes or nursing records are really progress notes from a nursing standpoint. The nursing notes contain the nurses' around-the-clock observations of the patient. Finally, in the record there will be a discharge order written on the physician's order blank, indicating that the patient can be discharged. Following the discharge of the patient, it is required that the physician dictate a narrative summary; this is usually typed and placed into the medical record after the patient has left the hospital. Although this is the last document recorded by the physician, it is generally placed in first position when the record is finally stored so that reviewers can quickly see the course of the patient's hospital stay.

The arrangement and dictating of all these separate forms in chronological order is the traditional or classical method of maintaining hospital patient medical records. More recently, the traditional record has become known as the source-oriented medical record. Prior to the permanent filing of the medical record in storage, the traditional record is somewhat rearranged as follows: The demographic data and identification data come first, followed by the patient's historical medical information and base line medical data; finally nursing data and nursing notes are stored in the record.

The Problem-Oriented Medical Record

The problem-oriented medical record or POMR highlights the patient's problems rather than buries them chronologically as the classical medical record does. The POMR is supposed to aid the physician by identifying the patient's problems and then outlining the plan for a course of treatment for the specified problems. The emphasis in the POMR is to coordinate the various health skills, and is not limited to only those of the physician. The emphasis is on solving the patient's whole problem, not just episodic situations. The POMR has been reported to be a better organized, more rational, and more consistent way of gathering medical facts about the patient's clinical problems. It provides an organized way of planning the therapy and following the patient's progress. Compared with the traditional record, the advantages of POMR become evident. Apart from the fact that the POMR tends to be easier for medical students and for health professionals to use, it has these additional advantages:

- It is easier to use as an educational tool.
- It is a more logical system for PSRO and other agencies to review.
- It lends itself better to a rational review of medical progress and care rendered.
- It allows for improved continuity of care, since the professionals all use the same set of recording rules (the patient's problems are thereby not lost or as easily confused).
- It is more adaptable to computerization.
- It is easier for the nonmedical personnel to read.

In the traditional medical record, chronological events, specific forms, and reports are the basis of the record. The POMR system uses specific elements, namely, data base information that is gathered together and clearly recorded, and a numbered list of specific patient problems. In the POMR system, a problem-oriented plan is agreed upon and as in the traditional system, progress notes made. But, in the POMR, these notes refer specifically to the numbered patient problems. In recording POMR progress notes, a definite system called "SOAP" is used, incorporating (1) *s*ubjective data, (2) *o*bjective data, (3) *a*ssessment or interpretation of impressions, and (4) an ongoing clinical *p*lan for the patient.

Delinquent Medical Records

Hospital medical records are highly visible instruments used in the evaluation of patient care. This being the case, it is very common for third parties, and especially the JCAH, during their annual or biannual surveys to study and review carefully the patients' medical records.

One of the traditional areas that is almost always reviewed is the timely completion of the medical record. Outside reviewers can be expected to inspect the matter of delinquent medical records at any given point in time during the survey. In fact, if the delinquent record problems are serious, they could jeopardize the hospital's accreditation by the JCAH.

Many physicians do not complete their medical records in a timely and accurate manner. This tends to be a chronic problem faced by medical record administrators across the country. In the final analysis, the most potent weapon against these delinquencies is suspension of privileges of physicians until they complete their records.

Computerized Medical Records

Medical records administrators are constantly attempting to make the processing of medical records and information more efficient (see Figure 4-1). One area that shows promise for increased efficiency in the storage and handling of information is the word processing computer. Usually this type of computer hardware is used in conjunction with a centralized medical typing pool. With the ease and speed permitted by the word processing computer, handwritten records can be replaced by typed reports, including pa-

Figure 4-1 Complexity of data flow within a hospital

① Business Office ⑤ Medical Administration ⑨ Pharmacy
② Nursing Services ⑥ Diagnostic Services ⑩ Dietary
③ Medical Services ⑦ Admitting/Discharge ⑪ Medical Research
④ Administration ⑧ Outpatient & Education

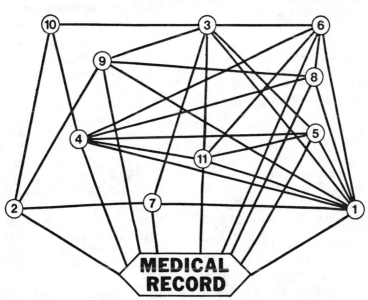

Source: Gerald S. Langan and Kenneth J. Dickie, *The Practice-Oriented Method,* Aspen Systems Corporation, 1978, p. 26.

tient histories, results of physical examinations, and consultant reports.

Computer applications have been developed for both the traditional and problem-oriented medical record. One such system that has been in operation for several years in the Massachusetts General Hospital in Boston is called MUMPS (Massachusetts General Hospital Utility-Programing System). Applications of MUMPS have been developed in the following areas: laboratory test reporting, automated patient histories, patient summary reports, critical patient care planning, medical education, medical examination, automated medication systems, physician-generated narrative notes, statistical packages, and medical care utilization statistics. Given the kinds of material that have to be computerized, medical information systems are very complex to develop and to maintain, since it is necessary to allow multiple inputs and inquiries and to have a large capacity of peripheral storage. One of the most important aspects of developing information systems is getting user acceptance, that is, making it comfortable for nurses, physicians, and other health care professionals to use sophisticated computerized systems.

The implementation of computerized medical information systems is in its infancy. It is clear, however, that when such systems become more widely available and used, they will be a powerful force for change in the traditional hospital environment.

Many hospitals even now participate in a shared computer medical record system called the Professional Activity Study (PAS). The PAS is purchased from the Commission on Professional Hospital Activities (CPHA), a nonprofit computer center, located in Ann Arbor, Michigan. With this system, the hospital's medical records technicians complete a discharge abstract for every discharged patient. The information on the abstract is then displayed and returned to the hospital in the form of a series of monthly and semiannual reports showing such data as the patient's average length of stay by disease categories and the number of clinical tests and studies performed during the period. An extension of the PAS that displays hospital clinical data quarterly is called the Medical Audit Program (MAP). MAP reports are used in continuous, comprehensive medical audits and retrospective utilization reviews.

Legal Concerns

The medical records administrator is the custodian of the medical records and must be alert to certain legal requirements with regard to the handling and release of medical information and medical records. (See pp. 73–77 for a full discussion.)

PROCEDURES AND SERVICES

Users of Medical Records

Medical record department personnel are responsible to design and implement a system to provide for evaluation, retention and future utilization of patient information. Patient information is used to plan patient care, perform medical research, evaluate patient care and provide information to authorized users.

Current users of medical information and the purposes for which the information is used may be classified as in Table 4-1.

Retention/Retrieval*

The Retention/Retrieval Manual

This manual is prepared to provide a means of sharing information about the many elements in the record retention/retrieval process.

Some of the important elements that must be addressed in the written manual are:

1. Designate the individual who has authority for the centralized control of the record management function.
2. Identify the relationship between the records retention/retrieval function and user departments or individuals.
3. Establish uniform procedures in the origination, processing, retention, and destruction of records for the whole facility.
4. Publish instructions and guidelines for all personnel who develop, use, or retrieve the facility's records.
5. Develop an attitude among all facility employees that there is a basic principle of good records management that necessitates control of data flow.

---

*Source: Kathleen A. Waters and Gretchen F. Murphy, *Medical Records in Health Information*, Aspen Systems Corporation, 1979.

6. Encourage employees to provide constructive suggestions concerning the retention/retrieval program.
7. Communicate change in policies and procedures.
8. Coordinate similar records management functions and activities throughout the organization.
9. Serve as a training center or source of information for all new or transferred employees.

Contents

Contents of the manual should include:

- Retention and retrieval schedules for particular types of data
- Policies regarding the time that data may be allowed out of the central file area
- Policies regarding information available for particular users of the data
- Sample forms, such as release-of-information forms, consent forms, and summaries that are used for preparing information for external users of data
- Policies regarding the use of photocopies and the charges for those copies
- Policies regarding photocopies vs. summarizations of records

- Policies regarding release of information to patients/clients
- Policies regarding audit of the record retention function

The manual should also include as many current samples of forms, flow charts, and *retention schedules* as possible, as well as other salient information that would point out the current directions of the department.

Policies

The retention/retrieval program should include a policy regarding the release of information. Other policies considered in a retention/retrieval program are those governing retention of various types of information. There must be a policy that describes how long secondary records, indexes, and medical records will be retained. These policies will be based on the objectives of the administration and medical staff under the professional direction of a medical record administrator working closely with legal counsel for the facility. A destruction schedule will probably be controlled by a policy for any facility that prepares and uses health information.

Table 4-1 Uses and Users of Medical Records

Users of Medical Records	Uses of Information in Medical Records
A. Health Care Providers, Institutional and Individual (Primary Users)	1. as a medium of communication among health care providers during the current episode of illness 2. as a reference for treatment of future illnesses 3. for training of physicians and other personnel—to assist students to relate theory with medical practice 4. for prospective and retrospective evaluation of the quality of patient care through review and analysis of patterns of care as documented in the medical record 5. for promotion of effective and efficient use of facilities, equipment, services, personnel and financial resources through statistical analysis of information abstracted from the medical record 6. for documentation of voluntary compliance with standards for accreditation of the institution 7. for research aimed at the improvement of treatment, assessment of disease detection methods, assessment of the effectiveness of medication and other treatments through study of appropriate cases 8. for documentation which demonstrates conformity to government regulations 9. follow-up care of patients with long-term illnesses and assessment of the efficacy of the care given

Table 4-1 continued

Users of Medical Records	Uses of Information in Medical Records
B. Payors for Services, private insurance plans, government insurance plans and programs (Secondary Users)	1. for substantiation of patient claims for payment of health care services 2. for audits of claims for health care services and professional fees 3. to monitor the quality and equity of care and services rendered to those insured 4. to assess and control the cost of health care services to those insured
C. Social Users 1. Public Health Agencies	1. in surveillance of diseases of epidemiologic significance through statistical analysis of information abstracted from medical records
2. Medical and Social Researchers, institutional and extra-institutional	1. for investigations of disease patterns, effects of disease on functions of daily living, including occupational health and safety
3. Rehabilitation and Social Welfare Programs	1. in determination of need for specific types of rehabilitation programs through analysis of incidence data 2. in development of individual rehabilitation and training plans for participants in programs for the handicapped, retarded and drug and alcohol abusers
4. Employers	*1. for administration of employer-provided health insurance plans *2. for determination of employment suitability 3. in treatment and analysis of job related injuries and correction of occupational hazards 4. to determine disability
5. Insurance Companies	*1. in determination of risks in writing insurance 2. in determination of liability for claims
6. Government Agencies: federal, state and local	1. for allocation of government resources for schools, health care facilities, education institutions, etc. based on vital statistics submitted from medical records
7. Education Institutions	*1. for assessment of suitability for admission to selected education programs 2. for maintenance of student and employee health programs
8. Judicial process	1. in adjudication of civil and criminal matters through use of the medical record as evidence through the legal process 2. in judicial process for involuntary admission of mentally ill
9. Law enforcement and investigation	*1. in criminal investigation *2. for security clearance programs
10. Credit investigation agencies	*1. for determination of credit eligibility
11. Accrediting, Licensing and Certifying Agencies	1. for demonstration of individual fulfillment of criteria for professional licensing by a state government agency 2. to ascertain competence of practitioners 3. for determination of compliance with criteria for hospital based education programs 4. as documentation of compliance with standards for institutional accreditation
12. Media: press, radio, TV	1. for announcements of developments in medical research 2. for reporting of health hazards, diseases affecting the public health and newsworthy events

*May in some instances be improper use.

Source: *Confidentiality of Patient Health Information: A Position Statement of the American Medical Record Association,* © 1981 by the American Medical Record Association.

The Register

An important accessory of the manual is a register or log that records all requests for information. It lists the names of all the requesters, dates reports were requested, dates reports were sent out, and the name of the patient or client identified in the report.

The register can be divided into two sections: one regarding records pulled for research purposes for physicians or other users or health care providers; the other to list reports that are provided to direct and indirect patient care providers or users for patient care or purposes other than research.

Materials and Equipment

In developing a system of retention/retrieval, health information management also identifies and selects appropriate materials and storage equipment. Table 4-2 outlines what takes place.

Medical Data in Medical Records*

During a patient's hospitalization, the transactions that comprise the overall medical record are of daily interest to the physician in charge of the case, the ward nursing staff, interns and residents. At times, an occasional interest in the total medical record is expressed by others, such as medical consultants, anesthesiologists, dieticians, business office personnel, licensure and audit groups, accreditation organizations, and statistical support personnel. Amidst these needs are transitory information situations, e.g. a radiologist wants to know what patient problems are being explored, or when a pathology report deviates from his/her findings, or a laboratory clinician deems an ordered test inconsistent with the patient's problems or inappropriate because the patient's medication records reveal use of a certain drug which will affect the values of the parameter being tested.

These examples typify the class of practitioners whose work is chronicled in the medical record. As a result, the medical record becomes a medium of open discussion or "forum" for the hospital staff; but because of the physical problems of storing and displaying data, it has evolved into a segmented and disjointed data repository (e.g., a physician may have to view two different parts of the medical record to find a patient's blood pressure as measured by cuff to compare it with the pressure measured by the intra-arterial line; similarly, the blood gases and blood glucose may be in separate sections.

To illustrate the data repository function of the medical record, refer to Table 4-3 for a list of independent inputs.

Patient Census Service*

Two major components of quantitative analysis in hospitals are the daily census and the discharge analysis carried out by the medical record service.

Statistical information and standard reports commence when the patient is admitted. At the point of admission, the patient is listed on the census report. The census is the number of inpatients present at any one time. Some patients may be admitted, treated, and discharged between the census-taking hours of the same day. The daily inpatient census must account for this to accurately reflect the activity. Daily inpatient census taking, therefore, is the number of inpatients present at the census-taking time each day, plus any patients who were *both* admitted and discharged after the census-taking time the previous day.

Census data are initiated at the point of patient care. This means that the nursing station is the place where the census is taken in hospitals. In most hospitals, however, the medical record department is responsible for compiling and using the census data. The medical record administrator makes sure that census taking is carried out consistently. This means that the census must be taken at a consistent time each day. If one consistently takes the census at the same time during any given 24-hour period or calendar day, the census data will be standard and useful. If not, errors may arise. For instance, if one counts patients at 9 A.M. one day and at 2 P.M. the next day, there is a reasonable chance that some admissions or discharges will be miscounted or missed altogether.

---

*Source: Gerald S. Langan and Kenneth J. Dickie, *The Practice-Oriented Method,* Aspen Systems Corporation, 1978.

---

*Source: Kathleen A. Waters and Gretchen F. Murphy, *Medical Records in Health Information,* Aspen Systems Corporation, 1979.

Table 4-2   Comparison of Retention/Retrieval Methods and Their Impact on Equipment Selection

Data Entries in a Paper Record System	Data Entries in a Computerized Record System	Mechanical Data Processing Methods	Subsystems Operations Within Medical Record Department
Data entries entered on forms	Data entries entered through CRT terminals	Data are condensed through keypunch	These activities will also require selection of materials and equipment for retention/retrieval
Forms grouped together in a logical format to make up a record	Stored on computer direct access storage device	Master patient index is placed on computer output microfilm	
Record is housed in a folder	Transferred to magnetic tape for permanent storage;	Physician's index keypunched	Operations of the department
Folders are housed in files	or	Disease index keypunched	Indexing
Drawer/open shelf/ electrical	Processed into microfiche via	Special index indexes keypunched	Medical reporting activities
Can be condensed through microfilm	computer output microfilm techniques	Key sorted on an as-needed basis	Maintenance of reports
Destroyed through organizational plans according to legal statutes	Retained in paper record folders as part of original document;	Printed out on tabulating machine for hard copy retrieval	Special purpose files
	or		Storage of printouts
	Filed in microfilm filing and storage units		Microfilm operations
			Materials and supplies handling

Source: Kathleen A. Waters and Gretchen F. Murphy, *Medical Records in Health Information,* Aspen Systems Corporation, 1979.

The location of the patient is tracked from day to day on the census. The census report provides specific daily counts of patients in the hospital as well as average daily counts and percentage of occupancy for the hospital. Census information is critical to daily management and future planning as well. The census is intended to reflect current hospital activity. It can be calculated for the entire hospital population or broken down into special populations. For example, the average daily census can be calculated for a single fiscal source such as Medicare or an individual age group of patients. Activity of each care unit or category of service, such as medical, surgical, pediatrics, and others, can also be counted. The census taking is the use of descriptive statistics in hospitals.

Administrative Uses of the Census

First, it depicts the volume of care or the service rendered in any one period. Second, information on the census can be used by accrediting agencies and health agencies for planning. Third, census information is directly related to staffing

and supply needs for the hospital. Fourth, cost accounting can be calculated according to average patient load in individual care units and for overall hospital services. Fifth, census portrays the activity of hospitals for administrative decision making. Sixth, the census affords the basis for analysis of service costs for patients.

The average daily census can also be designed to count various types of patient subgroupings. For instance, it would be quite simple with a computerized census system to routinely count Medicare patients, or male patients, and so on. A computerized census also would allow count of patients by zip code, health problem, or initial treatment plan broken down into elements, such as lab work to be performed, drugs to be taken, or diet to be started. Such sophisticated census counts might be used to track down persons involved in a natural disaster. Suspected leaking of poisonous gas in a given neighborhood or city, new information contraindicating use of a commonly ordered drug, or research interest in patients being treated currently are instances in which the lab work, drugs, or diet census counts might be helpful.

Table 4-3 Sections Maintained within the Medical Record

Hospital Summary
Patient's Problem List
Administrative Data
Allergies and Sensitivities
History

Physical Examination
Medical Certificate and History
Doctor's Orders
Doctor's Progress Notes
Consultation Sheet (may be multiple)
Social Services—Reports and Summaries

Tumor Board Report, Neuropsychiatric (NP) Staff Conference, Neurology Conference
Laboratory Report Display Forms (may be several types and multiple)
Flow Charts
Radio-Active Iodine Uptake (RAI) or Radioisotope Sheet
Radiographic Reports

Oral Examination and Treatment Record (Dental)
Anesthesia
Operation Report
Tissue Examination
Report of Special Procedures

Physical Medicine and Rehabilitation Reports (may be multiple)
Inhalation Therapy
Blood Transfusion
Radiation Therapy
Radiation Therapy Summary
Radium Therapy
CAT Scan Report
Diet History
Continuing Medication and Treatment

Diabetic Record
Temperature-Pulse-Respiration
Weight Chart
Nursing Notes
Nursing Procedure Record (Cardex)

Electrocardiographic (ECG) Record
Electroencephalogram (EEG) Record
Scans
Neurological Examination
Diagnostic Skin Test (Mycobacteria and Fungi)

Manual Muscle Evaluation
Eye Test Forms
Joint Motion Measurements

Table 4-3 continued

Muscle and/or Nerve Evaluation-Manual and Electrical: (EMG)
Pulmonary Function Report

Alcoholics and Narcotics Record Trunks
Anatomical Figure
Plotting Chart (may have several)
Authorization for Administration of Anesthesia and Performance of Operations and Other Procedures
Authorization for Use of Drugs and/or Procedures for Investigational Purposes

Seizure Report
Summary of Special Incidents
Miscellaneous Material and Admitting Office Consults
Photographs
Special Laboratory Reports

The medical record also contains all medical reports and summaries received from other hospitals, physicians, etc., during this admission.

Source: Gerald S. Langan and Kenneth J. Dickie, *The Practice-Oriented Method,* Aspen Systems Corporation, 1978.

The more consistently health information professionals elect to use standard hospital terms, the more reliable the reporting will be. Some hospital statistical terms, definitions, and formulas are shown in Table 4-4.

Uniform Hospital Discharge Data: Minimum Data Set*

1. *Person identification.* Each patient is to have a unique number within the hospital, to distinguish that patient from all other patients. The patient's name need not be recorded.
2. *Date of birth.* The month, day, and year of birth.
3. *Sex.* Male or female.
4. *Race and Ethnicity.* American Indian or Alaskan native, Asian or Pacific islander, black, Hispanic, white, other.
5. *Residence.* Record zip code.

*Source: *Uniform Hospital Discharge Data: Minimum Data Set,* National Center for Health Statistics, April 1980, Pub. No. (PHS) 80-1157.

Table 4-4   Statistical Terms and Formulas

Terms	Formulas

ADMISSION

Hospital patient
An individual receiving, in person, hospital-based or coordinated medical services for which the hospital is responsible.

Inpatient admission
The formal acceptance by a hospital of a patient who is to be provided with room, board, and continuous nursing service in an area of the hospital where patients generally stay at least overnight.

Number of patients in the hospital at
midnight April 29   535

Plus . . . . . Number of patients admitted April 30 .   + 30

565

Hospital inpatient
A hospital patient who is provided with room, board, and continuous general nursing service in an area of the hospital where patients generally stay at least overnight.

Minus . . . . Patients discharged (including deaths)
April 30 . . . .   − 18

Patients in hospital at 12 p.m. (midnight) April 30.   547

Inpatient census
The number of inpatients present at any one time.

Plus . . . . . Patients both admitted and discharged (including deaths) on April 30 . . . . .   + 3

Daily inpatient census
The number of inpatients present at the census-taking time each day, plus any inpatients who were both admitted and discharged after the census-taking time the previous day.

Inpatient census (inpatient service days) April 30   550

Example of Care Unit Breakdown:

Intensive Care Unit
Inpatient Service Days
(Inpatient Census)

Inpatient service day (also called Census day)
A unit of measure denoting the services received by one inpatient in one 24-hour period.

Patients remaining midnight April 29 .   8

Plus . . . . . Patients admitted April 30. . . . .   + 1

Plus . . . . . Patients transferred on unit from
another unit in hospital . . . .   + 1

Minus . . . . Patients discharged . . . .   − 0

Minus . . . . Patients died . . . .   − 2

Minus . . . . Patients transferred off unit to another
unit in hospital . . . .   − 1

Midnight census April 30.   7

Plus . . . . . Patients both admitted and discharged
on April 30 . . . .   + 1

(These patients have already been counted as admission and discharges or deaths. However, since their patient days have been canceled out by adding them as admissions and subtracting them as discharges, they must be added again to determine the inpatient service days on this unit.)

Table 4-4 continued

Terms	Formulas

Total inpatient service days (also called Census days)
The sum of all inpatient service days for each of the days in the period under consideration. Notice it is the numerator in the formula.

The formula to obtain the average daily inpatient census for a whole hospital is:

$$\frac{\text{Total inpatient service days for a period}}{\text{Total number of days in the period}}$$

Average daily inpatient census
Average number of inpatients present each day for a given period of time. This is always calculated by a formula as indicated in the example.

The average daily inpatient census (average daily census) for newborn inpatients is generally reported separately. When it is, the following formula is used to determine the average daily inpatient census excluding newborn:

Inpatient bed occupancy ratio
The proportion of inpatient beds occupied, defined as the ratio of inpatient service days to inpatient bed count days in the period under consideration.

$$\frac{\text{Total inpatient service days (excluding newborn)}}{\text{Total number of days in the period}}$$

Synonymous terms: percent occupancy, occupancy percent, percentage of occupancy, occupancy ratio

$$\frac{\text{Total inpatient service days for a period} \times 100}{\text{Total inpatient bed count days} \times \text{number of days in the period}}$$

Example: A hospital has an inpatient bed count (bed complement) of 150 (excluding the newborn bassinet count of 15). During April, the hospital rendered 3,650 inpatient service days to adults and children. April has 30 days. According to the formula, this is $3,650 \times 100 \div 150 \times 30 = 365,000 \div 4,500 = 81.11\%$. Therefore, the inpatient bed occupancy percentage for April was 81.1%, or 81%.

EVENTS DURING HOSPITAL STAY

Transfer (intrahospital)
A change in medical care unit, medical staff unit, or responsible physician of an inpatient during hospitalization.

Not applicable

Adjunct diagnostic or therapeutic unit (ancillary unit)
An organized unit of a hospital, other than an operating room, delivery room, or medical care unit, with facilities and personnel to aid physicians in the diagnosis and treatment of patients through the performance of diagnostic or therapeutic procedures.

Not applicable

Consultations may be viewed from two perspectives.

Medical consultation
The response by one member of the medical staff to a request for consultation by another member of the medical staff, characterized by review of the patient's history, examination of the patient, and completion of a consultation report giving recommendations and/or opinions.

1. Total consultations rendered. This may be used to show specialty activity, such as the total number of psychiatric consultations rendered by the psychiatric service.
2. The percentage of consultations rendered per patients treated in the hospital. The formula for this would be:

$$\frac{\text{Total number of patients receiving consultations} \times 100}{\text{Total number of patients discharged and died for the period}}$$

Table 4-4 continued

Terms	Formulas

Surgical operation
One or more surgical procedures performed at one time for one patient via a common approach or for a common purpose.

The formula approved by the Joint Commission on Accreditation of Hospitals for computing the postoperative infection rate is:

Complication
An additional diagnosis that describes a condition arising after the beginning of hospital observation and treatment and modifying the course of the patient's illness or the medical care required.

$$\frac{\text{Number of infections in clean surgical cases for a period} \times 100}{\text{Number of surgical operations for the period}}$$

Usually calculated in a rate only in infection cases, since the formula above clearly assigns the source of the complication.

Hospital live birth
The complete expulsion or extraction from the mother, in a hospital facility, of a product of conception, irrespective of the duration of pregnancy, which after such separation, breathes or shows any other evidence of life such as beating of the heart, pulsation of the umbilical cord, or definite movement of voluntary muscles, whether or not the umbilical cord has been cut or the placenta is attached; each product of such a birth is considered live born.

Live births may be classified according to the birth weight:

1,000 grams (2 pounds, 3 ounces) or less;
1,001 grams to 2,500 grams (5 pounds, 8 ounces);
over 2,500 grams.

Hospital cesarean section rate
Hospital cesarean section rate is the ratio of cesarean sections performed to deliveries. For statistical purposes, when a delivery results in a multiple birth, it is counted as one delivery.

Formula:

$$\frac{\text{Total number of cesarean sections performed in a period} \times 100}{\text{Total number of deliveries in the period}}$$

Inpatient discharge
The termination of a period of inpatient hospitalization through the formal release of the inpatient by the hospital.

Discharge transfer
The disposition of an inpatient to another health care institution at the time of discharge.

Length of stay (for one inpatient)
The number of calendar days from admission to discharge.

Admit Jan 20   Calculation:
Disch Jan 24

	24
	− 20
Disch days	= 4

or

Admit Jan 20   Total days in
Disch Feb 14   Jan

	31
	− 20
days in Jan	= 11
days in Feb	+ 14
Disch days	= 25

The length of an inpatient's hospitalization is considered to be one day if he is admitted and discharged the same day and also if he is admitted one day and discharged the next day.

Table 4-4 continued

Terms	Formulas

Total length of stay (for all inpatients) ⟶ Total duration (discharge days)
The sum-of-the-days stay of any group of inpatients discharged during a specified period of time.

$$\frac{\text{Total duration (discharge days) of inpatient hospitalization (including deaths; excluding newborn)}}{\text{Total discharges (including deaths; excluding newborn)}}$$

Average length of stay
The average length of hospitalization of inpatients discharged during the period under consideration.

Gross death rate

$$\frac{\text{Total number of deaths (including newborn) for a period} \times 100}{\text{Total number of discharges (including deaths and newborn deaths) for the period}}$$

Net death rate (also called Institutional death rate)

$$\frac{\text{Total number of deaths (including newborn) minus those under 48 hours for a period} \times 100}{\text{Total number of discharges (including deaths and newborn) minus deaths under 48 hours for the period}}$$

Postoperative death rate

$$\frac{\text{Total number of deaths within 10 days postoperative for a period} \times 100}{\text{Total number of patients operated on for the period}}$$

Maternal death rate

$$\frac{\text{Total number of maternal deaths for a period} \times 100}{\text{Total number of maternal (obstetrical) discharges (including deaths) for the period}}$$

Anesthesia death rate

$$\frac{\text{Total number of deaths caused by anesthetic agents for a period} \times 100}{\text{Total number of anesthetics administered for the period}}$$

Hospital fetal death
Death prior to the complete expulsion or extraction from its mother, in a hospital facility, of a product of conception, irrespective of the duration of pregnancy; death is indicated by the fact that after such separation, the fetus does not breathe or show any other evidence of life such as beating of the heart, pulsation of the umbilical cord, or definite movement of voluntary muscles.

Early: Less than 20 complete weeks of gestation (500 grams or less)

Intermediate: 20 completed weeks of gestation, but less than 28 (501 to 1,000 grams)

Late: 28 completed weeks of gestation and over (1,001 grams and over)

Abortion
Abortion is the expulsion or extraction of all (complete) or any part (incomplete) of the placenta or membranes, without an identifiable fetus or with a live-born infant or a stillborn infant weighing less than 500 gm. In the absence of known weight, an estimated length of gestation of less than 20 completed weeks (139 days) is calculated from the first day of the last normal menstrual period.

Usually only intermediate and late fetal deaths are included.

Formula:

$$\frac{\text{Total number of intermediate and/or late fetal deaths for a period} \times 100}{\text{Total number of births (including intermediate and late fetal deaths) for the period}}$$

Table 4-4   continued

Terms	Formulas
Gross autopsy rate —— The ratio during any given period of time of all inpatient autopsies of all inpatient deaths.	$$\frac{\text{Total inpatient autopsies for a given period} \times 100}{\text{Total inpatient deaths for the period}}$$
Net autopsy rate —— The ratio during any given period of time of all inpatient autopsies to all inpatient deaths minus unautopsied coroner's or medical examiner's cases.	$$\frac{\text{Total inpatient autopsies for a given period} \times 100}{\text{Total inpatient deaths minus unautopsied coroner's or medical examiner's cases}}$$
Hospital autopsy rate (adjusted) —— The proportion of deaths of hospital patients following which the bodies of the deceased persons are available for autopsy and hospital autopsies are performed.	$$\frac{\text{Total hospital autopsies} \times 100}{\text{Number of deaths of hospital patients whose bodies are available for hospital autopsy}}$$

SPECIAL NEEDS

Psychiatric survival rates
The monthly statistics provided to staff gave no information as to how long a patient was able to function independently.

Admission date — Discharge date of last visit = Survival time

This formula was created when it became evident that staff was being discouraged by the high reported readmission rate, in spite of additions to staff and improved therapy programs.

The use of survival time statistics demonstrated two factors to administration that were then used to revise procedures:

$$\frac{\text{Cumulative survival time for all patients for the period utilizing outpatient clinics}}{\text{Total number of admissions for the period}} = \text{Average survival rate of patients utilizing clinics}$$

- The survival time for which patients were functioning without support was increased with each discharge.

- There was no evidence that outpatient visits increased the survival time between hospitalizations. (Patients were returning due to attachments to staff.)

$$\frac{\text{Cumulative survival time for all patients for the period not utilizing outpatient clinics}}{\text{Total number of admissions for the period}} = \text{Average survival rate of patients } not \text{ utilizing clinics}$$

A program was developed to introduce outpatient clinic staff to patients and create attachments to the appropriate staff prior to discharge to reduce dependency on the patient facility.

Source: Kathleen A. Waters and Gretchen F. Murphy, *Medical Records in Health Information,* Aspen Systems Corporation, 1979. The information has been adapted from Edna K. Huffman, *Medical Records Management,* Physicians Record Company Publisher, 1972; *Glossary of Medical Terms,* American Medical Record Association, 1974; and Candace Dillman, RRA, who designed the section on "Psychiatric Survival Rates" for use in the Alaska Psychiatric Institute.

6. *Hospital identification.* Each hospital must have a unique number within the abstracting system.
7. *Admission and discharge dates.*
   a. Admission Date includes month, day, year, and hour (1–24) of admission.
   b. Discharge Date includes month, day, and year of discharge.
8. *Physician identification.* Each physician is to have a unique number within the hospital. The attending physician and operating physician are to be identified.
   a. Attending Physician. This is the physician who was primarily responsible for the care of the patient at the beginning of each hospital episode.
   b. Operating Physician. This is the physician who performed the principal procedure.
9. *Diagnoses.* All diagnoses that affect the current stay. Old diagnoses that relate to an earlier episode and have no bearing on this hospital stay are excluded.
   a. Principal Diagnosis is listed first and is defined as the condition established after study to be chiefly responsible for occasioning the admission of the patient to the hospital for care.
   b. Other Diagnoses to be listed are all conditions that coexist at the time of admission or develop subsequently and affect the treatment received and/or the length of stay.
10. *Procedures and Dates.*
    a. In addition to surgical procedures, all other significant procedures are to be recorded together with the dates. A significant procedure is one that carries an operative or anesthetic risk or requires highly trained personnel or special facilities or equipment. The identity code of the person performing the surgical procedure is required.
    b. The principal procedure is to be listed first. If only one procedure was performed, it is considered the principal procedure.
       In determining which of multiple procedures is the principal procedure, the following criteria are to be applied.
       1) The principal procedure is one that was performed for definitive treatment rather than diagnostic or exploratory purposes, or a procedure that was necessary to take care of a complication.
       2) The principal procedure is that procedure most related to the principal diagnosis.
11. *Disposition of patient.*
    a. Discharged to home (routine discharge)
    b. Discharged or transferred to another short-term hospital
    c. Discharged or transferred to a long-term institution
    d. Died
    e. Left against medical advice
12. *Principal source of payment.*
    a. Self-pay
    b. Worker's compensation
    c. Medicare
    d. Medicaid
    e. Maternal and Child Health
    f. Other government payments
    g. Blue Cross
    h. Insurance companies
    i. No charge (free, special research, or teaching)
    j. Other

HOSPITAL POLICIES FOR ACCESS TO MEDICAL RECORDS*

Hospitals must have well-defined policies on the use and disclosure of medical information, encompassing all patient-identifiable record systems maintained within the institution. There should be no patient-identifiable record system within the institution whose existence is unknown to the chief executive officer or the chief executive officer's designee.

It may be necessary to conduct a survey to determine the record systems currently being maintained in various ancillary and clinical departments. Such a survey should include the type of information being kept in patient-identifiable form and the rules and procedures pres-

*Source: Mary E. Converse, "Privacy Protection of Medical Records," *Topics in Health Record Management,* June 1981.

ently followed for granting access to the record system and disclosing information to sources outside the institution.

The definition of medical records used in legal parlance often includes departmental records if they contain information on diagnostic findings, treatment, or care given to the patient. The same is true of record systems containing information abstracted from medical records and maintained in patient-identifiable form, such as tumor file records, research study records, and automated discharge abstract records. Hospital policy and procedures for access and disclosure of medical record information should include all these patient-identifiable record systems. Criteria should be developed for use in determining the need for maintaining such systems.

Internal policies should be established to provide for proper use of patient-identifiable records as necessary to carry out functions within the hospitals. These include identifying when access by hospital and medical staff does and does not require the written consent of the patient, as well as provisions for security of patient-identifiable records.

The authority and responsibility of the hospital or medical staff or the duly appointed committee or panel requesting access, the reason for the request, and the kind of information requested are determining points in granting access without written consent of the patient. Requesters who would be permitted access to the medical record without written authorization of the patient include:

- the governing board for purposes of ensuring quality of patient care;
- the chief executive officer in carrying out management duties;
- physicians and health care personnel involved in the care of a patient and the integration of previous episodes of illness and care with the current episode;
- chiefs of clinical services and departmental directors in evaluating the performance of their staff or the quality of services in providing patient care;
- duly appointed committees of the medical staff and hospital in determining whether the quality of care provided to all patients is consistent with medical staff bylaws, provisions of clinical privileges, hospital poli-

cies, .and requisites for hospital accreditation;
- medical record personnel as necessary to carry out departmental functions; and
- designees of the chief executive officer only on a need-to-know basis in the conduct of hospital affairs, such as in conducting a risk-management program, receiving legal counsel, and planning health services. In this respect, staff access should be commensurate with the individual's responsibility and authority for conducting hospital business.

Security Measures

Security measures should be taken to reasonably safeguard medical records and departmental patient records, whether in hard copy, on film, or in computerized form, against loss, defacement, tampering, unauthorized disclosure, and use by unauthorized persons. Policies and procedures are needed for governing who can make corrections or amendments in the medical record and under what conditions. Staff must be aware of procedures to follow in not obliterating corrected material and in authenticating corrections. Precautions should be taken to prevent removal of content material by third parties authorized to read the record.

There should be means of identifying staff authorized to use the records. Conditions under which students of hospital-approved programs may use the record for classroom assignments may include written permission requisite and exclude removal of the record from the medical record department, either in hard copy or tape-recorded form.

Finally, a clear statement is needed establishing who in the hospital has responsibility for processing all requests for disclosure to sources outside the hospital.

Rules of the hospital should be reviewed for any further delineation of the extent to which physicians and other staff professionals in good standing are privileged to use hospital records for bona fide study and research. Circumstances that would require patient authorization should be identified. Responsibility for protecting confidentiality should be included in the rules established for use of medical records in hospital-approved education programs.

Sign-Out Procedures

Procedures for requisitioning and signing out records from medical record and ancillary departmental files should be reviewed for appropriateness. The sign-out system should contain the name of the person requesting the record, the name of the person who will be using the record if different from that of the requester, the name of the clinic or unit in the event of visits or admissions, date requested, date retrieved from the files, and identification of person who retrieved the record from the file. The latter provision may not be feasible when large numbers of records are retrieved for clinic visits.

The purpose of this sign-out procedure is to provide record clerks with sufficient information for determining if certain requests should be referred to a supervisor for security decisions or follow through.

Outside Requests

Policies and procedures for external disclosure of medical record information should be designed to handle the various requests received from outside sources. Factors to be identified and considered are: the type of requests received; the kind of information requested; the persons, agencies, or organizations authorized to receive information without written consent of the patient; the type of permission needed for disclosure by the hospital; the necessity to conform to laws, regulations, and other measures in the public interest; and reasonable charges to be made for furnishing copies of records. Provision should be made for handling unusual requests that may merit establishing additional policies or important modifications of existing policies.

External Record Disclosure

The policy generally agreed upon is that no hospital should disclose, or be required to disclose, medical record information in patient-identifiable form to a third party without the patient's authorization, *unless* such disclosure is: pursuant to law or statutory regulations requiring the hospital to report certain information; in accordance with compelling circumstances affecting the health or safety of the patient or of another person; permitted under certain circumstances by the hospital in the conduct of biomedical, epidemiologic, or health services research.

Information on patients currently hospitalized should be limited to name, date of admission, and general condition, except in those instances when the patient or an authorized representative requests that even this limited information not be released. Laws or regulations (for example, alcohol and drug abuse treatment) forbid disclosure of this information.

Other exceptions to requirements for patient's authorization may be necessary. The hospital's agreement with a government agency or other third-party payer for payment of hospital service charges to authorized beneficiaries may provide for inspection of certain portions of a medical record in the performance of claims processing or financial audit. Such inspection is conducted to determine necessity for admission, validate the physician's order with hospital charges, and confirm benefits entitlement.

There are also instances where the hospital must act on behalf of a patient to determine benefits entitlement when the patient is unable to communicate an authorization for disclosure and no authorized representative is presently available. This occurs at the time of admission and often with elderly patients.

Privacy Review Group

A number of privacy protection proposals provide for an institutional review board. The board would be charged with the responsibility of reviewing requests from outside parties for use of hospital medical records in the conduct of a study or research project. The outside party would be asked to justify the necessity for access to medical records and to cite the precautions for safeguarding the confidentiality and integrity of medical record information. Such a hospital-based review group could provide recommendations to the hospital's chief executive officer on whether or not to permit medical records to be used for proposed study and research projects.

Authorization Format

Hospitals on an individual, local, or statewide basis may wish to develop and promote the use of a more specific patient consent form authorizing the hospital to disclose information. It would specify why subject matter is being authorized for disclosure by period of time to be covered, specified information, or type of treatment. It would also require the name of the person or organization to receive the information and any applicable time limit for valid authorization.

Another item that could be incorporated is the purpose of the request. However, this item would be completed as required by the patient and not the hospital. There will be instances when the patient or the patient's lawyer may not want the purpose identified.

It is recommended that authorizations contain a statement to the effect that any disclosure of medical record information by the recipient(s) is prohibited except when implicit in the purpose of this disclosure.

Patient Access

Statutory or judicial laws in many states recognize a reasonable right of access to medical record information by the patient. If the objective of privacy protection is to provide fairness to the patient, consideration should be given to allowing access by the patient except in those instances where information may be detrimental to the physical or mental health of the patient, as determined by the physician. In the latter instance, information should be released in a manner that will minimize any adverse effects on the patient, such as having a physician communicate the appropriate information.

Minors

Access to the medical record by a minor may be permitted under general state law or a state law permitting a minor to seek on his or her own behalf, without the knowledge or consent of the parents, treatment for certain conditions. These conditions are usually venereal disease, alcohol or drug abuse, or pregnancy. Access may also be permitted for minors seeking family planning or abortion services. In privacy protection proposals for minors, the suggested minimum age for permitting minors to decide what disclosure can be made from their medical records and to whom have ranged from 13 to 16 years. Hospital counsel should be consulted regarding the legal rights of minors in making such decisions.

Hospital counsel, in cooperation with the medical staff, should develop procedures for handling those instances where access to psychiatric or other sensitive information in the record of a minor by the minor's parent(s) or guardian may prove detrimental to the child. Information should be disclosed in a manner that minimizes any adverse effects on the child. This may be accomplished by the attending or another physician.

Fairness Protection

Fairness protection in the hospital's record-keeping relationship with patients should include policies and procedures to cover the following:

- A person has the right to verify whether or not the hospital has created and is maintaining a medical record pertaining to care or services provided to that person (not all inquiries will represent former patients).
- A patient has the right to find out if a disclosure of his or her medical record has been made by the hospital and to whom it was made, if such information is available on older records.
- A patient may look at the record of medical care provided and may request a copy on payment of reasonable charges for the service, unless access is believed by the attending physician to be medically contraindicated.
- A patient may request correction or amendment of information in his or her medical record.
- A patient's personal representative(s) or duly authorized nominee(s), on good cause shown by such person(s), may be granted reasonable access to information contained in the patient's medical record.

Reasonable access refers to a time and location procedure that allows the hospital to arrange for access in an orderly manner. As part of the hospital's objectives for fairness, the attending physician should be notified of the patient's request for access to the medical record.

Patient Corrections or Amendments

Any request by patients for changes to be made in their medical records should be made in writing and should specify the entry or entries in dispute. The hospital and the attending physician will decide whether or not the correction or amendment is to be made. If the decision is made to correct or amend the record, the patient should be so advised. In making any changes in the medical record, care must be exercised not to obliterate the material corrected or amended.

If the request for change is not granted, the patient should be so informed and advised that a statement of his or her disagreement can be filed with the hospital.

Methods of Infiltrating Computerized Records*

Among the activities that an infiltrator might wish to undertake are the following:

- Gaining access to desired information in the files, or discovering the information interests of a particular user.
- Changing information in the files (including destruction of entire files).
- Obtaining free computer time or the unauthorized use of proprietary programs.

For active infiltration, an appropriate terminal and entry into the communication link are essential. In fact, considerable equipment and know-how are required to launch sophisticated infiltration attempts. The methods for gaining access through normal access procedures include:

- Using legitimate access to a part of the system to ask unauthorized questions (e.g., requesting payroll information or trying to associate an individual with certain data), or to "browse" in unauthorized files.
- "Masquerading" as a legitimate user after having obtained proper identifications through wiretapping or other means.
- Having access to the system by virtue of a position with the information center or the communication network but without a "need to know" (e.g., system programmer, operator, maintenance, and management personnel).

An infiltrator may also attempt to enter the system covertly (i.e., avoiding the control and protection programs) by:

- Using entry points planted in the system by unscrupulous programmers or maintenance engineers, or probing for and discovering "trap doors" which may exist by virtue of

the combinatorial aspects of the many system control variables.
- Employing special terminals tapped into communication channels to effect:

—"piggy back" entry into the system by selective interception of communications between a user and the processor, and then releasing these with modifications or substituting entirely new messages while returning an "error" message;

—"between lines" entry to the system when a legitimate user is inactive but still holds the communication channel;

—cancellation of the user's sign-off signals, so as to continue operating in his name.

In all of these variations the legitimate user provides procedures for the infiltrator to obtain proper access. The infiltrator is limited, however, to the legitimate user's authorized files.

AUDIT CHECKLISTS*

Evaluating the Overall Records Management Program

No hospital can afford to be without a sound records management program that provides clear guidelines for what types of information must be kept and where, with what security and safeguards, and for how long. Below are ten sets of checkpoints on which to begin an audit program design.

1. Do all records have definite retention and destruction schedules? Who developed the policies and were they approved by the governing board? Is there a continuing program of records management, with personnel assigned to carry it out?
2. Do retention schedules meet applicable federal and state regulations? Do the schedules meet the hospital's needs for records while not keeping an excessive volume of material on hand?
3. Has adequate consideration been given to the types of records and their retention schedules? The issue here is one of eco-

---

*Source: Eric W. Springer, *Automated Medical Records*, Aspen Systems Corporation, 1971.

*Source: Seth Allcorn, *Internal Auditing for Hospitals*, Aspen Systems Corporation, 1979.

nomics. A policy may require records to be retained for a specific period to document a transaction with a patient or employee. Experience may indicate the records seldom are used after a year and that the risk of loss from disposing of them is less than the cost of storing them. The auditor should recommend the retention schedule be reexamined and adjusted to bring the storage costs more in line with the risks involved.

4. Are there enough types of records? Are they organized in such a way as to minimize paper processing needs and provide maximum documentation and information? Is there much duplication of records in part or in full? Do departments routinely retain documentation of charges that also are kept by the business office?

5. Are the records retained in a manner that facilitates quick retrieval and accurate filing? There are many proved methods for organizing all types of records, including using various types of equipment. Auditors must be alert for requests for records that require an extended amount of work to locate.

6. What use is made of a central records storage facility? Is it properly equipped and staffed? Is its service well known throughout the hospital? Is it properly utilized?

7. What use has been made of microfilm in the business record area? If data processing is used, for business purposes, have applications of computer output microfilm been explored?

8. How are important records safeguarded from loss or destruction? Are storage areas clean and well organized? Are the policies and procedures for record access and removal adequate and are they followed?

9. How are records destroyed? Do the hospital's procedures for disposing of records and trash ensure maximum confidentiality?

10. Is the generating of new reports and forms monitored by an administrator? Is the staff generally informed of what records are available? Is there an index of all of the hospital's records?

Evaluating the Patient Medical Records System

Hospitals have found the management of medical records to be a difficult task. Two types of problems have been encountered. First, systems that provide for positive control of patient medical records often prove to be restrictive and inconvenient for physicians and staff while those that provide easy access often fail to keep accurate information on where the records can be located. Second, it is extremely important that the medical record be kept accurate.

There are two reasons for this. The obvious one is for patient care. The patient's medical history must be available for review at all times and must provide an accurate and complete record of all tests and therapy results. The second reason is less important for patient care but directly affects the hospital's receiving payments from government health insurance programs. The medical record must support all charges to patients. Failure to provide this documentation can result in considerable loss of payments from the government. Internal auditors must evaluate the hospital's management and control of medical records. Below are important points to audit.

1. What procedures are there for ensuring that medical records are complete and support the patient billings? Does the system get the job done effectively and with a minimum of delays? How is this monitored?

2. What group is responsible for the management of the medical records department? Are the group members qualified to supervise the department and do they actively manage medical records systems and procedures?

3. Are medical records personnel qualified for their jobs? Are there training programs for staff?

4. Does medical records have an operating manual? Is it up to date and complete? Are the procedures adequate?

5. Are the physical facilities of the medical records department adequate? Is there sufficient equipment? Is comfortable space provided for department personnel and for physicians who come to review or complete patient records?

6. How are medical records filed? Do proce-

dures facilitate accurate filing and quick retrieval?

7. Who is allowed access to the records and how is this enforced? Are there specific standing orders on the release of information on patients?

8. How are medical records protected from loss and destruction?

9. What reports are compiled routinely by medical records? Are there enough or too many and do the right people receive them?

10. In general, do the physicians and ward personnel believe medical records management and control procedures get the job done?

CONTROLLING FORMS

A forms control program can be beneficial in several areas:

1. establishment of logical buying patterns;
2. reduction of obsolescence; and
3. reduction of dollar investment in forms.

By developing good inventory control, purchasing through groups and systems contracting, all forms can be ordered at preset intervals. Obsolescence can be reduced with a well-organized print shop and an administratively supported forms control committee. A forms exchange system will not only aid in this obsolescence reduction; it will also result in a reduced inventory, lower dollar investment, increased cash flow and reduction in inventory holding costs in the storeroom.

The first step necessary to controlling forms is to catalog each one used in the hospital. This effort should include both internally and externally produced forms.

Once the file has been completed, the development of a numbering system will both help to keep it accurate and allow a degree of control. But the control of an expanding forms system should not be the responsibility of one individual: It is best handled through a committee approach.*

The following explains the role of the forms control committee and the procedures for obtaining approval of the purchase or printing of forms.

The Forms Control Committee*

A. Objectives

1. to achieve maximum economy and administrative efficiency with a minimum of paper;
2. to make optimum use of available resources; and
3. to use well-designed forms effectively as a means of presenting information concisely to conserve time and effort.

B. Definitions

1. Form—Forms or form letters are administrative aids, predesigned and printed or typed with space provided for the insertion of information. Work sheets—which are reproduced in any manner or stocked for future use—and items such as labels, tags and coversheets—which may not require insertion of information—are included in this definition.

2. One-Time Form—This is a form or form letter designed for accomplishment of a specific once-only purpose.

3. Temporary Form—This is a form or form letter designed to accomplish a specific purpose within a short period of time—normally from 30 to 90 days.

4. Permanent Form—This is a form or form letter used within the hospital either by one area or more than one area in sufficient quantity to warrant reproduction and storage either in materiel management or the using department(s).

C. Forms Are Categorized in the Following Groups

1. Medical Record—used to record patient's medical data (this may or may not be an actual part of the patient's medical record).

2. Charge and Requisition—used to request service and initiate service charges to the patients;

3. Payroll and Personnel—used to maintain necessary payroll and personnel information by appropriate departments;

---

*Source: Michael J. Brzezicki, "Forms Control: Is It Possible?" *Hospital Materiel Management Quarterly,* May 1980.

4. Business Records—used to maintain patient business accounts as necessary;
5. General and Administrative—used for communication and documentation;
6. Budget and Financial Control—used to prepare and control the budget; and
7. Information System—used with the computer information system.

D. Forms Committee

1. Function:
   a. to review *all* forms presently being used within the hospital;
   b. to determine, with appropriate communication with using areas, if the present forms are consistent with the objectives of the forms management system;
   c. to review all requests for new forms with an annual usage of more than 15 copies to be printed within the hospital or to be purchased from an outside source;
   d. to determine, with appropriate communications with using areas, if the new forms are consistent with the objectives of the forms management system; and
   e. to approve or disapprove requests for new forms or revisions and to inform the administrative council of its actions.
2. Membership:
   a. director of materiel management,
   b. representative of hospital education;
   c. representative of business office;
   d. representative of medical records;
   e. representative of data processing;
   f. purchasing agent; and
   g. printer.

E. Procedures

1. Present forms. The committee will be responsible for the—
   a. review of *all* forms presently being utilized within the hospital and their placement into one of the forms categories.
   b. establishment of a complete catalog index file of all hospital forms, based on the forms categories and specific forms used by each department.
   c. review, with appropriate communication with the using areas, of all forms, and the determination of whether the

forms are consistent with the objectives of the forms management system.
2. Requests for new forms or revisions of present forms (including inventory forms and forms that are maintained in specific departments):
   a. presentation to the forms committee for approval of all requests for new forms or revisions of present forms that have an annual usage of more than 15 copies;
   b. review by the committee of the request to determine if it is consistent with the objectives of the forms management system;
   c. review and approval by the medical records committee, after presentation to the forms control committee, of all requests for printing or revisions of forms that pertain to the patient's medical record (the forms control committee will forward the form to the records committee after approval);
   d. review by the committee of the request (the committee will inform the administrative council of its action);
   e. inclusion in the committee's review of a decision on whether the form is to be printed by the hospital or purchased from an outside source;
   f. placement by the committee of new forms or revisions, after approval, in the forms catalog index and file; and
   g. notification by the materiel management department of all using departments one month prior to requisition a reorder of an outside-purchased form to allow for review of the form prior to ordering (to be done in writing and requiring the using department to submit any requested changes through the forms control committee in the same manner as other requested changes).
3. One-time forms (management engineering worksheets, forms for evaluation purposes only, form letter questionnaires, etc.) and emergency requests for forms:
   a. may be approved for printing and use by the director of materiel management. These forms must meet the definition of a one-time form and must be for short-term use only (usually less than 30 days).
   b. Temporary forms must follow the same

procedure for review and approval as permanent forms. The forms control committee will be responsible to ensure that temporary forms are not allowed to be used on a permanent basis.

c. The printing department or purchasing department will not print or authorize the purchase of forms that have not been approved by the forms control committee. The print shop will maintain a file of forms authorized to be printed for each department.

Common Hospital Forms*

The following list provides a brief descriptive overview of the titles and contents of common hospital forms.

1. Identification Data and Consent Forms
2. Provisional Diagnosis. There should be an admitting problem identified on every patient at the time of admission. If a patient requires hospitalization, the hospital staff needs this information to proceed intelligently.
3. History: Chief Complaint, Present Illness, Past History, Present History, and Family History
4. Physical Examination.
5. Consultations. Consultations imply an examination of the patient and the patient's record. The consultation note should be recorded and either signed or authenticated by the consultant.
6. Clinical Laboratory Reports. The original signed laboratory report is entered in the patient's record. Duplicates are filed in the laboratory.
7. X-ray Reports. The original signed radiological report is entered in the patient's record. Duplicates are filed in the x-ray department.
8. Tissue (Pathological Specimen) Report. Since all tissues removed in surgery are sent to the laboratory, acknowledgment that the tissue has been received and a gross description should be entered in the record. If a microscopic examination is

done, a description of the findings should be made a part of the record. The decision to do a microscopic examination is determined by the medical staff and the pathologist according to the rules and regulations of the hospital.

9. Physician's Diagnostic and Therapeutic Orders
10. Treatment: Medical and Surgical. All treatment procedures are in the medical record. Except in cases of grave emergency, the patient should receive a complete diagnostic workup before surgery. Operative notes should be dictated immediately after surgery and should contain both a description of the findings and a detailed account of the technique used and tissue removed.
11. Progress Notes. Provide a chronological picture and analysis of the clinical course of the patient. The frequency with which they are made is determined by the condition of the patient, the complexity of the treatment, and the need for information exchange among the medical team providers.
12. Nurses' Notes. Provide a description of daily objective and subjective findings.
13. Final Diagnosis. A definitive final diagnosis or a complete problem list is entered on each record.
14. Summary. A summary of the patient's condition on discharge and course in the hospital is valuable as a recapitulation of the patient's hospitalization.
15. Autopsy Findings. When an autopsy is performed, a complete protocol of the findings should be made a part of the record.

Guidelines for Designing Forms*

One of the most important things in designing forms is considering a design that will facilitate ease in data collection, data completeness, and error control. Data can be collected several ways. They can be entered on a form through handwriting or dictated and transcribed on reports for inclusion in patient records. They can

---

*Source: Kathleen A. Waters and Gretchen F. Murphy, *Medical Records in Health Information,* Aspen Systems Corporation, 1979.

*Source: Kathleen A. Waters and Gretchen F. Murphy, *Medical Records in Health Information,* Aspen Systems Corporation, 1979.

be collected for computer processing by key-punching cards, by being keyed directly to magnetic tape, and by being entered directly into CRT terminals.

Table 4-5 lists guidelines that are helpful in

Table 4-5   Guidelines for Designing Forms

1. Assess each form individually to
   a. insure its necessity.
   b. avoid duplicate recording.
   c. insure it integrates with the existing records system.
2. Determine the purpose of the form, which will determine information to be included.
3. Identify benefits that will be derived from introduction of the form into the record.
4. Design forms as simply as possible; do not clutter them with headings, captions, or instructions.
5. Consider use of unstructured, multipurpose flow sheets. They will eliminate the need for several special forms to monitor special care factors and reduce chart bulk.
6. Plan all forms in the record to be a uniform size.
7. Place form titles and patient identification consistently on every form.
8. Include space for at least
   a. full patient name.
   b. medical, health, or client record file number.
9. Consider printing headings and captions in bold print.
10. Line up headings to provide an uncluttered appearance and to promote ease in locating desired information.
11. Consider logical sequence of subject headings.
12. Use white paper with color-coded borders for quick identification of different forms; colored paper may be difficult to read or photocopy.
13. Select captions that clearly state what information is to be entered.
14. Use a box arrangement to save time in checklists.
15. Plan spacing according to the specific method of documentation.
    a. Typewritten entries: set lines according to number of lines per inch on a typewriter and to accommodate vertical spacing.
    b. Handwritten entries: set lines far enough apart to insure readability.
    c. CRT or computer printout format: set margin, spacing, and punctuation clearly.
    d. Consider the period of time each side of the form covers.

Table 4-5   continued

16. Identify certain portions that are restricted for use by designated staff or groups (for example, medical record service, infection control committee, utilization review committee); those areas should be surrounded with bold lines.
17. Consider printing on both sides of the sheet to maximize paper use and reduce chart bulk.
18. Consider printing on reverse side to facilitate reference when form is in chart holder and/or fastened at top as a closed record.
19. When possible, eliminate the need for a special form by utilizing a rubber stamp on an existing form.
20. Allow sufficient space for signatures of those making entries.
21. Because newly designed forms often need revisions, mimeograph or photocopy a small supply for trial use.
22. Use good quality paper stock in final printing to avoid dog-earring and tearing, and to insure permanence; 20-pound weight paper stock is recommended for long-term use.
23. Card stock should be avoided since it creates bulk, is difficult to handle, and may complicate photocopy technique.
24. Stock only a six-month supply of the form to prevent waste in the event of a revision or change in documentation procedures.
25. Always introduce a proposed new form before implementation and preferably during initial design phases; this promotes input by those making entries and using the data.
26. Complete final review and approval of the draft form prior to implementation; this is accomplished by a multidisciplinary forms committee that includes the medical record administrator.
27. Simple printed instructions will insure uniformity, if a form is to be used by various departments.
28. If instructions are detailed, prepare separate directions regarding
    a. purpose.
    b. use.
    c. instructions for completion.
    d. staff responsibilities.
    e. references, if any.
29. Include the name, address, and city of the facility on forms that are likely to be sent elsewhere.
30. Identify all forms by
    a. a descriptive and simple title.
    b. a stock control number.
    c. the month and year of first, revised, or last printing.

Source: Kathleen A. Waters and Gretchen F. Murphy, *Medical Records in Health Information*, Aspen Systems Corporation, 1979.

knowing where to begin and what steps to take in designing a form.

The more opportunities there are for copying and reentering information, the greater the chance of error. It is important to design forms that will capture data at the most propitious time. That is, data should be recorded during or immediately after an encounter and collected on an instrument that provides permanence. This will reduce the possibility of transposing and making other errors when the data are copied.

Another important consideration is grouping similar types of data on one form. Identification data, for instance, can be grouped in one section of a form, as can patient provider entries. Other ways of identifying data are through the use of shaded coloring, boldface print, or underscoring particular items. Information managers should review various forms to illustrate these characteristics and others when developing forms design programs.

The following list suggests a few policies necessary in controlling forms design.

- There should be a forms inventory that outlines the most recent revision dates.
- There should be policies established by a forms review committee that clearly delineate parameters for entry.
- There should be procedures specifying the steps necessary to redesign a form, enter a new form, or revise or remove a current form from the inventory.

These policies are necessary to prevent individual departments or providers from proliferating forms in the system and causing unnecessary bulk for the total document. In some organizations, forms design is so controlled that physicians and other health care providers are not allowed to work or maintain staff privileges in a facility unless they agree to utilize and comply with policies established by the organization and monitored by the records manager or forms control committee. Another method of controlling forms is to purchase preprinted, packaged forms from commercial printers who specialize in health and medical records. This illustrates a method of standardizing and fostering control of forms and formats. Any form that is not preprinted is not allowed in the record and can be discarded.

Providing Direction

The design of the form can facilitate or obstruct the ease of data entry as well as the understanding of the data entered on that form. It is difficult to prepare a summary or an abstract or even to read a medical record if data entries are scattered and not standardized. If a medical record contains mixed forms of entry, it is difficult to read and understand. For instance, if the record contains some forms that are handwritten, others that are typewritten, and still others of various sizes and colors, it is most difficult to try to abstract or summarize information from that record.

The following questions summarize the targets used in creating effective documents through forms design.

- Where does the form originate; that is, what department originally enters data onto the form or enters the form into the system to be used by others?
- What individual enters data on the form?
- What information should be on the form?
- What information is currently being entered on the form?
- Who ascertains the completeness of the data entries?
- Where will the form finally be filed?
- Who will use the information on the form?
- Who will receive copies of the form?
- How long should the form be retained?

MEDICAL RECORDS GLOSSARY*

Abortion—the expulsion or extraction of all (complete) or any part (incomplete) of the placenta or membranes without an identifiable fetus, with a live born infant or a stillborn infant weighing less than 500 gm, or after an estimated length of gestation of less than 20 completed weeks (139 days) calculated from the first day of the last normal menstrual period.

Abscissa side—the horizontal side of a graph, used for values.

Accession number—the number given each order as it occurs.

---

*Source: Kathleen A. Waters and Gretchen F. Murphy, *Medical Records in Health Information*, Aspen Systems Corporation, 1979.

Accreditation—a process of evaluation of the physical, medical, and administrative as well as social and rehabilitative services provided by a health care facility.

ACS—American College of Surgeons.

Active medical staff—physicians and dentists who are responsible for the greatest amount of medical practice within the hospital and who perform all significant staff, organizational, and administrative functions.

Adjunct diagnostic or therapeutic unit (ancillary unit)—an organized unit of a hospital, other than an operating room, delivery room, or medical care unit, with facilities and personnel to aid physicians in the diagnosis and treatment of patients through the performance of diagnostic or therapeutic procedures.

Administrator—an individual who works at the direction of the Board of Trustees to carry out the specific functional activity of the organization.

Admission certification—a set of medical elements that are used to determine justification for hospital admission.

Agencies, associations, societies—extensions of the individuals who deliver or participate in the delivery of health care; organized groups.

AHA—American Hospital Association.

AHR—Association for Health Records; a multidisciplinary forum for the exchange of information among all persons in the field of medical and health information.

AMRA—American Medical Record Association.

Aperture card—punch card with film attached.

ART—Accredited Record Technician; an individual who has achieved a specified educational level and successfully completed a national qualifying examination.

Associate medical staff—physicians or dentists who are new to the staff and are being considered for advancement to the medical staff.

Audit measurement—comparison of actual practice to preestablished criteria.

Audit trial report—a report of an audit or check on the accuracy of a computer application. These reports can be computer generated as a part of a data security program.

Auxiliary computer storage—supplements to the main storage which are usually of higher capacity and lower speed or longer access time. Because central memory is limited and expensive relative to the size of programs and the data sets requiring processing, most computers have devices, usually disks, attached to them which store large amounts of data (millions or billions of characters). Data are then transferred in blocks between auxiliary storage and central memory as the data in central memory are exhausted. Transfer of data between auxiliary storage and central memory is slower than the rate at which data may be moved between the CPU and memory. Secondary storage can also include magnetic tape, magnetic drum, and card readers.

Average daily inpatient census—the average number of inpatients present each day for a given period of time.

Average length of stay—the average length of hospitalization of inpatients discharged during the period under consideration.

Bar charts—the depiction of relationships among elements. The rectangle is the essential representation of the area of the bar.

Batch processing method—the processing of the data that has been accumulated in advance such that each accumulation of data or batch thus formed is processed during the computer run. An in-house computer system could use batch processing to prepare a discharge analysis of services each month.

Board of Directors of AMRA—a ten member board elected by the active membership of the American Medical Record Association.

Board of trustees—governing body; the highest level of organization administration, it bears full legal and moral responsibility for professional services provided by the facility.

Bureau of Quality Assurance (BQA)—agency which reports to the Health Services Administration and is responsible for the administration of the Professional Standards Review Organization (PSRO).

Business records as evidence—a record of an act, condition, or event which, insofar as it is relevant, shall be competent evidence if the custodian or other qualified witness testifies to its identity and the mode of its preparation, if it was made in the regular course of business at time near the time of the act, condition, or event, and if in the opinion of the court the source of information, method, and time of preparation were such as to justify its admission. This refers to admitting the medical record to the court as evidence and the testimony by the medical record administrator or a designee that this is in fact a record kept in the regular course of business.

CARE—Computerized Audit and Record Evaluation System.

Cathode Ray Tube Terminals (CRTs)—common instruments for transmitting data to a computer, retrieving data from the computer and displaying them in a visual manner so that anyone can read them. Cathode ray terminals may have typewriter keyboards for communication and display data on a TV-like screen.

Census—the number of inpatients present in a health care facility at any one time.

Central Processing Unit (CPU)—the part of a computer system that contains the circuits which control the interpretation and execution of instructions, including the arithmetic, logic, and control functions.

Centralized filing system—a system in which all information is filed in one central location.

Charge-out devices—simple cardboard ledgers in a file that a user or a clerk fills out, noting date and destination of chart.

Chart analysis—careful review of the entire record; identification of specific areas that are incomplete.

Chart-out guide—a file ledger that records the date and name of the person removing the record and the reason for removing it.

Clinic—a physical site that provides office space for several physicians who are organized to serve patients through their cooperative efforts.

Clinical algorithm—application of algorithms which are procedures consisting of a finite number of steps for solving a problem in medicine. Algorithms may contain a number of branch points where the next step depends on the outcome of the preceding step.

Cluster sampling—a sampling procedure that selects population elements in groups or clusters. Medical record administrators may use sampling when ascertaining particular growth patterns of cards in a master patient index file, for example.

CMT—current medical terminology; a dictionary of preferred terms in medicine.

Coding—a numerical assignment that provides an organized approach to data retrieval. Codes are symbolic abbreviations that allow information to be categorized into succinct forms for ease of storage and use.

COM—computer output microfilm system; the process of translating computer-generated information into a miniature image on film.

Complication—a detrimental condition arising after the beginning of hospital observation and treatment and modifying the course of the patient's illness or the medical care required.

Computer conversion plan—a formal plan for converting to a new computer system.

Computer interactive processing (mode, conversational)—an operation of data processing systems such that the user, at an input-output terminal, carries on a conversation with the system. Since a prompt response is obtained from the system as each unit of input is entered, a sequence of runs can take place between the user and the system typical of a conversation.

Computer primary or main storage (also referred to as main memory)—a device in a computer in which the binary bit representations of program instructions and data are stored. The memory device is very closely linked with the CPU so that individual program instructions and data elements may be obtained from memory very rapidly.

Computer program—a set of instructions stored in the computer which directs it to perform a specific process.

Computer system design and resource allocation phase—the process of formulating a plan which describes the specifications determined in the study phase. It includes allocation of staff time, determination of required software, identification of required documentation for computer operations programs and user applications, and determination of required hardware functions.

Computer system development and conversion planning phase—time period or phase in which the actual computer programs are written, hardware purchased, and conversion plan formally prepared for a specific computer application.

Computer system operation phase—the phase in which the computer system becomes operational and its performance is reviewed and measured against original objectives.

Computer system study phase—a fundamental examination of an operation that needs to be improved or evaluated. It includes problem identification and can include all the steps of a feasibility analysis. It may be used synonymously with feasibility analysis.

Computer user manual—a procedure manual for computer applications usually prepared in the computer system design process as part of the documentation of the system.

Computerized word processing system—a system, based on microprocessor technology, in which medical stenographers type dictation directly into computer terminals. Errors can be easily corrected by inserting items or lines when appropriate. This information, once it is proofread, is then printed out on an impact printer.

Concurrent review—a form of medical care review that occurs during the patient's hospitalization. It consists of a review of the patient's need for a hospital or skilled nursing facility's level of care and may include an assessment of the quality of care being provided.

Confidential information—a statement made to a lawyer, physician, or clergyman in confidence with the implicit understanding that it should remain a secret.

Confidentiality—status accorded to data or information which is sensitive for some reason and therefore must be protected against theft or improper use and disseminated only to individuals or organizations authorized to have it.

Consent—concurrence of wills; voluntary yielding of one's will to the proposition of another; acquiescence or compliance.

Consulting medical staff—staff members who provide consulting services to other members of the staff on an on-call or regularly scheduled basis.

Contestant—one contesting a decision.

Continued stay review—the review carried on during a patient's hospitalization to determine the medical necessity and appropriateness of continuation of care at that level.

Control selection—a technique of sampling developed to increase the likelihood (over that of random sampling) of choosing a preferred combination of sampling units while maintaining probability methods.

Controlled-decentralized system—a system in which all forms, requisitions, filing procedures, methods, and processes are standardized so that records in the various areas are maintained identically.

Courtesy medical staff—physicians or dentists who have privileges to admit patients only occasionally.

CPT—current procedural terminology; a coding method for diagnostic and therapeutic procedures in surgery, medicine, and the specialties.

Criteria—predetermined elements against which aspects of the quality of medical service may be measured; for instance, two criteria for care of a urinary tract infection might be a urinalysis and urine culture.

Critical management—the minimal preventive and responsive procedures concerning a complication that must be documented in the record to convince the audit committee that everything necessary was done to prevent the complication or that the complication was promptly recognized and appropriately treated.

Daily inpatient census—the number of inpatients present at the census-taking time each day, plus any inpatients who were both admitted and discharged after the census-taking time the previous day.

Data Collection Network (DCN)—a computer-coordinated system that collects, stores, and disseminates information from a computer center. The information is collected initially from several health care institutions or agencies, which also have access to a central computer or group of linked computers.

Data entries—all the items of information that are entered into a health record.

Data entry—inputting information into a computer for processing.

Data security—the policies and procedures established by an organization to protect its information from unauthorized or accidental modification, destruction, and disclosure.

Data Security Administrator—a specially trained medical record administrator who is proficient in information science, medical information handling, and data security systems maintenance and supervision. The person must be trained and/or certified by a recognized authority verifying the individual's level of expertise.

Debug—to detect, identify the source, and fix errors in a computer program.

Decentralized filing system—a system in which files are usually located close to the source of their active use.

Defendant—a person required to make answer in an action or suit; a person to whom an action is brought. In malpractice this could be the physician and the hospital.

Deficiency—a nonjustifiable variation from expected standards.

Delegation of review—method of performing peer review whereby the PSRO delegates to the health care facility responsibility for performing actual review functions.

Denial—disapproval of continued payment by the fiscal intermediary. In Medicare a patient may be disallowed benefits if the length of stay exceeds the norm or standard without appropriate justification.

Denominator—number that represents a large group of related conditions, individuals, or events counted; the part of the fraction below the line.

Deposition—the written testimony of a sworn witness in response to interrogation, testimony taken on oath in writing outside of the courtroom to be used as evidence.

Descriptive statistics—numerically described events, services, patients, charges, and other agency activity to demonstrate and quantify the operations of the agency.

Direct patient data—facts that the patient actually states or displays to another person.

Discharge analysis—the tabulation of data on discharged hospital patient to reflect the professional services provided in the hospital.

Discharge transfer—the disposition of an inpatient to another health care institution at the time of discharge.

Disease and operation index—a numerical index of patient problems, diagnoses, and procedures by individual categories.

Dividers—heavy-weight fabric forms of pressboard, used to designate alphabetical breaks in the folders or highlight numerical divisions within the filing system.

DSM—Diagnostic and Statistical Manual of Mental Disorders.

ECF—extended care facility. This term preceded SNF (Skilled Nursing Facility) to designate nursing homes which had been certified to care for Medicare patients.

Elements—specific services, tests, and/or parameters of care which are grouped together and considered the identifiable parts that make up a criterion. For instance, a reviewer may look at three individual elements to see if a particular criterion was met.

Emergency—any condition which could result in serious permanent harm to a patient or aggravation of injury or disease, or in which the life of a patient is in immediate danger and any delay in administering treatment could add to that danger.

Evidence (primary)—that evidence that suffices for the proof of a particular fact until contradicted or overcome by other evidence.

Exception—identified case to which specified standards do not apply. For instance, complications may warrant an extension of the patient's stay in the hospital.

Executive committee of the medical staff—group of staff members empowered to act for the staff in intervals between medical staff meetings.

Expert witness—a person testifying to facts within his or her own knowledge, who may give opinions upon assumed facts.

Family numbering—a system in which the family is assigned one number and the individual family members are assigned subnumbers.

Feasibility analysis—the process that examines, identifies, and ranks alternative solutions to a problem. It evaluates the probable soundness of such elements as hardware, software, cost analysis, and staffing against performance specifications required in a given application.

Federal Register—a publication that makes regulations and legal notices issued by federal agencies available to the public.

File folders—solid, two-sided binders of Kraft, manila, pressboard, or patented composition used to store paper records.

Fiscal intermediary—an organization acting in an intermediate role for dispersing funds from the federal government. Blue Cross, for example, acts as a fiscal intermediary in the Medicare program.

Focused review—a review of target areas or cases identified through analysis of the data system as questionable in effective utilization of resources. This allows a utilization review program to bypass repetitive activities on well-defined topic areas that have exhibited consistent effective utilization of services.

Format—the arrangement of a form, or an organization of forms in a permanent file folder, which directs the type of entries, the way entries are made, and the future use of those entries.

Frequency distribution—a number of predetermined classes with counts of the number of cases or observations that fall within the interval for each class.

GANTT chart—a program management chart that tracks the progress of a project against a predetermined schedule.

Glossary of hospital terms—hospital statistical terms, definitions, and formulas.

Grants—projects funded through federal appropriations approved by the U.S. Congress and provided through the direction of federal agencies and programs for ongoing and new health care programs.

Gross autopsy rate—the ratio during any given period of time of all inpatient autopsies to all inpatient deaths.

Group practice—care provided by a group of physicians who usually represent a fairly broad spectrum of medical specialties.

Hardware—the physical machinery and equipment that comprise a computer system.

Health—the state of complete physical, mental, and social well-being.

Health care—the restoration or preservation of health; the providing of relief, comfort, and healing to the sick.

Health care delivery—a set of separate, related, but essentially nonunified health care activities not all working toward a single purpose.

Health care practitioners—other than physicians, those health professionals who (a) do not hold a doctor of medicine or doctor of osteopathy degree, (b) meet all applicable state or federal requirements for practice of their profession, and (c) are actively involved in the delivery of patient care or services that may be paid for, directly or indirectly, under Titles V, XVIII, and/or XIX of the Social Security Act.

Health information—any data pertaining to the physical, mental, or social well-being of an individual or group of individuals.

Health record—documentation of direct or indirect health care services to patients/clients by providers and users of the data in any type of health-related institution.

Hearsay—statements not made under oath by someone who is not a party in interest, nor a party to the action.

HEW—Department of Health, Education and Welfare.

HMO—health maintenance organization.

Honorary staff—those individuals recognized for their noteworthy contributions to patient care, outstanding professional reputation, and/or their long service to the hospital.

Hospital autopsy rate (adjusted)—ratio of autopsies actually performed to the number of bodies of deceased persons available for autopsy.

Hospital cesarean section rate—the ratio of cesarean sections performed in a hospital to deliveries. For statistical purposes, a delivery resulting in a multiple birth is counted as one delivery.

Hospital computer system—a hospital electronic data processing and communications system which provides on-line processing with interactive responses for patient data within the hospital and its outpatient department, including ancillary services such as clinical, laboratory, x-ray, pharmacy, etc.

Hospital fetal death—a death prior to the complete expulsion or extraction from the mother, in a hospital facility, of a product of conception, irrespective of the duration of pregnancy. Death is indicated by the fact that, after such separation, the fetus does not breathe or show any other evidence of life such as beating of the heart, pulsation of the umbilical cord, or definite movement of voluntary muscles.

Hospital inpatient—a hospital patient who is provided with room, board, and continuous general nursing service in an area of the hospital where patients generally stay at least overnight.

Hospital inpatient autopsy—a postmortem examination performed in a hospital facility, by a hospital pathologist or by a physician of the medical staff to whom the responsibility has been delegated, on the body of a patient who died during inpatient hospitalization.

Hospital live birth—the complete expulsion or extraction from the mother, in a hospital facility, of a product of conception which, after such separation, breathes or shows any other evidence of life such as beating of the heart, pulsation of the umbilical cord, or definite movement of voluntary muscles, whether or not the umbilical cord has been cut or the placenta is attached; each product of such a birth is considered live born.

Hospital patient—an individual receiving, in person, hospital-based or coordinated medical services for which the hospital is responsible.

Hospital record—a written account of all the services provided the patient from the time of admission until discharge. It identifies the dates and ward or room where the patient was physically located, names of the physicians, nurses, and other health professionals who provided care, and the results of the care.

House of Delegates of the AMRA—the official legislative body of the American Medical Record Association.

ICD—international classification of diseases; a basic three-digit code with four- and five-digit categories in some areas.

ICF—intermediate care facility.

ICHPPC—international classification of health problems in primary care; a method of classification for use by physicians in general and family practice throughout the world.

IMR—institution for the mentally retarded.

In loco parentis—in the relationship of a parent.

Independent contractor—one who exercises an independent calling and is subject to the control of no one in his or her work.

Index—an organized, condensed list of data that reflects more extensive data pertaining to one subject or source of information.

Indirect patient data—information which comes from the patient but requires an interpretation before it is usable.

Individual plan of care—document established to view the patient from the aspect of each health care provider. It pulls all portions of the available information together to develop a coordinated, individual plan for use by health care providers or family in further treatment programs.

Infection committee—committee responsible for substantiation of hospital v. nonhospital acquired infections, control of infection, and coordination of all other activities regarding infection control, including the reporting, evaluating, and maintaining of records of infections among patients and personnel.

Inference statistics—an analysis of population samples, services, or treatment results which is used to make an inferred judgment or assessment on the whole. Medical research, patient care appraisal, utilization review, length of stay by selected diagnosis, projected effects of new therapy, and studies on effects of nutrition on underprivileged children are all examples of inference statistics.

Information—knowledge or intelligence; facts, data.

Information activity list—a detailed record that provides information about the usage of patient information, i.e., how often it is requested.

Inpatient admission—the formal acceptance by a hospital of a patient who is to be provided with room, board, and continuous nursing service in an area of the hospital where patients generally stay at least overnight.

Inpatient bed count—the designated number of available hospital inpatient beds, both occupied and vacant, on any given day.

Inpatient bed occupancy ratio—the proportion of inpatient beds occupied defined as the ratio of inpatient service days to the inpatient bed count days in the period under consideration; percent occupancy; occupancy percent; percentage of occupancy, occupancy ratio.

Inpatient census—the number of inpatients present at any one time.

Inpatient discharge—the termination of a period of inpatient hospitalization through the formal release of the inpatient by the hospital.

Inpatient service day—a unit of measure denoting the services received by one inpatient in one 24-hour period.

Interim patient record—a paper record made up primarily of computer printouts in those settings where patient information is maintained on the computer until discharge or cessation of treatment.

Intervention—peer review criteria that are applied during the process of medical care of an individual patient which may directly influence the action of the attending physician during care.

JCAH—Joint Commission on Accreditation of Hospitals.

Job description—a document containing information about a position such as required education or training, experience, lines of authority and designation of supervisor, as well as a general description of the job and major job objectives.

Judicial contest—any controversy that must be decided upon evidence.

Length of stay—the number of calendar days from admission to discharge of one inpatient.

Length of stay certification (also called recertification)—a statement in writing by the attending physician assuring that continued hospitalization is medically necessary. It must include diagnosis, complications, plan for care, and anticipated length of stay. It justifies a length of stay beyond the norm.

Letter distribution classification—a list prepared by the Department of the Navy and the Social Security Administration which shows how certain letters of the alphabet expand in a filing system. The expansion of each letter is described in percentages.

Level of care—the degree of services and health care available. The degree may be extensive or minimal depending on the health care needs of an individual patient.

Level of care criteria—standards used to determine the appropriate level of care—hospital, skilled nursing facility, intermediate care—for a given patient based on the types of service that can only be provided at that level.

Liability—state or quality of being liable; that which is under obligation to pay. Hospitals, nursing homes, and health care providers can all be considered liable for services they render.

Liability insurance—insurance to cover answerable claims, such as malpractice insurance.

Line chart—a graph which depicts movement and generally aids the reader in comprehending the material.

Litigation—the act of carrying on a suit in a law court.

Longitudinal health record—a patient record that includes medical information collected over an extended time, such as a family practice record that includes all medical data on an individual from birth to the present.

Majority—that age which qualifies an individual as legally responsible for his or her own acts; 21 years of age in most states.

Malpractice—improper, careless, or ignorant treatment.

Management data—data used by those who support the development, retention, and retrieval of patient data through their professional direction; information used by providers and users as well as patients, such as policy and procedure manuals, memos, bylaws, budgets, correspondence, and individual or specialized worksheets developed for individual departmental needs.

Master patient index—a condensed listing of data that provides identification and location information regarding medical or health records.

Mean—the arithmetic average of the value of a sample.

Median—the point at which half of the values of a sample fall above and half below.

Medicaid—the federal health program designed for the recipients of categorical aid programs, i.e., the medically indigent.

Medical audit—an evaluation system in which established standards are used to measure performance. Once corrective action has been taken on problems identified through a review process, performance is remeasured after an appropriate time period.

Medical audit committee—committee responsible for evaluation of the quality of patient care provided to patients by the medical and other professional staff who are directly responsible for patient care.

Medical audit follow-up—action taken as a result of medical audit committee recommendations. Action must be immediate if problems are life-threatening and must be documented to show improvement in patient care.

Medical care appraisal programs—program components which include utilization review of services, assessment of the patient's treatment, and examination of the end result of patient care.

Medical care evaluation—a structured program to measure the quality of care given to patients. It is a global term that encompasses methods used to carry out such measurement functions as audit, appraisal, peer review, quality assurance, and assessment in various specific forms.

Medical care evaluation studies (MCEs)—a retrospective medical care review in which an in-depth assessment is made of the quality and nature of the use of identified health services.

Medical care outcome—the end result of a patient's state of illness during an episode of treatment or a period of care during chronic illness.

Medical consultation—the response by one member of the medical staff to a request for consultation by another member of the medical staff, characterized by review of the patient's history, examination of the patient, and completion of a consultation report giving recommendations and/or opinions.

Medical Record Administrator—the individual responsible for developing and directing the objectives and activities that comprise an information system to compile and distribute patient/client data.

Medical record committee—committee which sees that accurate and complete medical records are developed and retained for every patient treated.

Medical staff—qualified medical personnel responsible for the quality of all medical care provided to patients and for the ethical conduct and professional practices of individual physicians.

Medical staff bylaws—rules and regulations which define duties, qualifications, and method of selection of officers of the medical staff.

Medicare—the federal health care program designed for persons over 65 years of age.

MEDLARS—Medical Literature Analysis and Retrieval System: a computer-based system derived from journals indexed for *Index Medicus, Index to Dental Literature,* and the *International Nursing Index.*

MEDLINE—MEDLARS on-line; a shortened form of the MEDLAR system.

Memorandum of understanding—a signed statement outlining the responsibilities of each party involved. Memoranda of understanding are between hospitals and PSROs and between fiscal intermediaries and PSROs.

Microfilming—a process of photographing and reducing a given report to a miniature of the original on film.

Mode—the one value in a sample that occurs with most frequency.

Monitor—to watch, observe, and check, especially to track, a particular item of information.

Morbidity—the incidence of disease or the proportion of diseases in a given population; statistical data that represents rates or ratios of disease.

Mortality—the incidence of deaths or the proportion of deaths in a given population; statistical data that represents rates or ratios of deaths.

MRP—medical record practitioner; an individual who works with medical records but has not successfully completed a national qualifying examination.

MSIS—Multi-State Information System, an automated information system for mental patients' records.

NAMCS—National Ambulatory Care Survey.

Negligence—failure to exercise the reasonable prudent care that the circumstances justly demand.

Net autopsy rate—the ratio during any given period of time of all inpatient autopsies to all inpatient deaths minus unautopsied coroners' or medical examiners' cases.

Nominal scales—the enumeration of attribute data, i.e., survival status. The summary measure is the proportion of cases that exhibit the attribute.

Non compos mentis—of unsound mind, including all forms of mental unsoundness.

Nonphysician health care providers—those health professionals who do not hold a doctor of medicine or osteopathy degree but are qualified by education or licensure to practice a profession and are involved in direct patient care services.

Nonprobability samples—samples which at some stage of sampling permit arbitrary choice of sampling units by the sampler.

Norm—a numerical or statistical measure of usually observed performance. Norms are identified by analyzing statistical data that record particular activities and results of a defined problem, diagnosis, or treatment.

Normal distribution—the bell-shaped curve which is a method of mathematically explaining the frequency of occurrences.

Notary public—public officer whose function is to administer oaths and to attest and certify by his or her hand or official seal certain classes of documents to give them authenticity in foreign jurisdictions.

Notary subpoena—an order issued by a notary public for the medical record to be taken to an attorney's office instead of to court. Used as part of a pretrial discovery procedure, this type of subpoena is intended to expedite the trial of cases.

Number index—a chronological listing of all numbers issued with cross references to the names of the patients to which the numbers have been assigned.

Numbering system—an identifying method that utilizes assigned numbers to label each record for filing in a systematic manner for easy retention and retrieval.

Numerator—that number representing the actual number of conditions, individuals, and events counted; the part of the fraction above the line.

Numerical continuum scale—the continuum along which clinical measurements such as blood pressure, height, and weight fall.

Objectives—a determination and a description of activities, stated in measurable terms, that lead toward a unified goal. They must be formulated in such a manner that all participants in the system understand what is to be achieved. The objective should have specific activities identified to describe what is to be done between the date of establishing the plan and the target date for reaching the goal.

Office of Professional Standards Review (OPSR)—agency which reports to the Assistant Secretary of the Department of Health, Education and Welfare (DHEW) and is responsible for staff activities for PSRO.

On-line—a device that currently is an operating part of the computer system. A terminal is on-line if it is logged into the system. An idle service is on-line if it may be activated by the computer.

On-line patient records—computerized patient records stored on a storage device which permits direct, immediate access through terminals.

Ordinate axis—the vertical side of a graph, usually used to designate the frequency.

Output descriptions—a detailed explanation of what will result from a computer action in a specific application. For example, a new form, format, or other combination of documents that produces data previously unavailable, such as a printout produced in the main file room that automatically prints all chart requests in two-part labels. The labels include patient number, name, requesting party, authorization code .number (which tells the staff the requestor is authorized to access the chart), date, and time of request. One label is placed on the outguide and one on the chart. Another example is an activity summary produced at the end of the day that lists the number of charts requested, distribution of request frequency, and a list of all charts not returned for that day.

Parameters—values which vary according to the circumstances of their application. Each health problem has a unique set of parameters, that is, plans, tests, and treatments that are individually adapted to that problem.

Patient care audit—an objective, systematic evaluation of the quality of patient care based on two principles: (1) it is neither necessary nor efficient to examine every aspect of the patient care process; and (2) the results of careful comparison of actual practice against certain predetermined, objective measurable criteria accurately reflect the quality of patient care.

Patient carried personal health record—the written information which people keep about their personal health care and actually are responsible for physically storing and transporting.

Patient data—information gathered during a patient encounter with a professional care provider.

Pattern analysis—a program to evaluate the effectiveness of medical care evaluation by comparing similar data over time. It is generally directed at the comparison of data regarding particular topics or characteristics.

PEP—performance evaluation procedure for auditing and approving patient care. Originated by the Joint Commission on Accreditation of Hospitals, this procedure originally focused on patient care outcomes.

Percentile—a value on a scale of 100 that indicates the percent of a distribution that is equal to or below it. For instance, 50th percentile for a group of hospitalized patients may be five days, which means that 50 percent of the patients stayed five days or less.

Performance testing—a dry run of the particular computer application to see if the results produced matched the specifications laid out in the study phase.

PERT—Program Evaluation Review Technique.

Pharmacy committee—committee responsible for development of policies and practices relating to the selection and distribution of drugs.

Pharmacy profile record system—a system which provides immediate retrieval of information necessary for the pharmacist to identify previously dispensed medication at the time a prescription is presented. One profile card may be maintained for all members of a family living at the same address and possessing the same family name.

Pie charts—graphic presentation of relationships as percentages.

Plaintiff—one who commences personal action or suit to obtain a remedy for injury to his or her rights; the complaining party in any litigation. A patient suing a physician for malpractice would be the plaintiff.

Plan (POMR)—notation in the problem oriented medical record consisting of three parts:

the plan for (1) collecting further data; (2) for initial treatment; and (3) for patient education. It explains what the patient must do, the results of the patient's own activities in the management of that problem, the results of the tests, and any prognosis that is available; it educates the patient regarding changes that may have to come about in life style in order to recover fully or live comfortably with a particular problem.

Playscript procedure—a procedure written in two columns in which the source or person carrying out the step is listed in the left-hand column and the steps to be carried out are listed in the right-hand column in exact chronological sequence.

Policy—a basic guide to action that prescribes the boundaries within which activities are to take place.

POMR (Problem Oriented Medical Record)—a system of organizing data entries in a patient record by titled and numbered problems that are determined by the clinician in reviewing the patient's direct data and the data base. The data base includes medical history, physical findings, and patient life-style information. Plans for investigation, treatment, and patient education as well as progress recording are all keyed to the problem numbers and titles.

Preadmission certification—a preadmission process that provides for formal certification of necessity for hospitalization prior to a patient occupying a bed in the hospital.

Prefix with the year—a system in which a number including the year of current treatment is assigned.

Prepaid care—health program which offers the patient the opportunity to pay for health care regularly whether it is needed or not, in exchange for which no charge is made when care is provided.

Prima facie—evidence sufficient to establish the fact and, if not rebutted, conclusive of the fact.

Printout—the printed data document from a computer operation. An on-line patient admission system in a hospital may create a printout of the admission information to be used as an identification and summary sheet in the hospital patient record.

Privacy—a right. To declare information confidential is to recognize formally the patient's inherent right to privacy.

Privileged communication—any information acquired by a physician or surgeon in attending a patient which was necessary to enable him or her to prescribe or act for the patient and which cannot be revealed in a civil action without the consent of the patient.

Problem—an aspect of the patient that disturbs or endangers the patient's health and that requires further attention for diagnosis, treatment, or observation.

Process—components of the total health care activity that are evaluated to determine adequacy of care. For instance, process components might include contraindicated drugs, excessive exposure to radiation, surgical intervention without documented workup, misfiled lab work, denied admission, adjustments in the care plan to accommodate changes in a patient's condition, routine physical exams, follow-up of abnormal lab or x-ray findings, etc. Process can be performed concurrent with care, addresses all direct and indirect providers, can directly interface and depend on patient's actions, and can relate directly to administrative and fiscal controls. The process of care also refers to effective documentation of the details of the patient's history and physical examination, other diagnostic measures, and specific treatment procedures. The Problem Oriented Medical Record is particularly geared to in-depth, effective operation of process audits.

Processing cycle—*see* Batch processing method, Computer interactive processing, Real time processing.

Professional—one who renders a personal service, possesses a specialized body of knowledge, observes ethical principles, maintains high standards, and participates in continuing education.

Profile analysis—a mechanism to judge the effectiveness of a PSRO or a hospital's review program by comparing similar data over time. It is generally directed at the comparison of data regarding a particular physician or health care provider.

PROMIS program—hospital-based computerized problem oriented medical record program that uses specific computer applications to aid health providers in recalling the memory elements of the patient record via CRT terminals.

Prospective review—a procedure for conducting the review process prior to the receipt of care. The purpose is to review the patient's condition and assure that the planned admission and the level of care are appropriate.

Provisional staff—individuals who have only recently been appointed to the medical staff. All initial appointments to the medical staff, except honorary and consulting, are provisional.

PSRO—Professional Standards Review Organization.

Punch cards—80- or 96-column cards widely used for computer input. The hole combinations punched into cards are converted with electronic pulses by the card readers and sent to the CPU for processing.

QAP—Quality Assurance Program.

Quality assurance—activities performed to determine the extent to which a phenomenon fulfills certain values and standards, and to assure changes in practice that will fulfill the highest or a predetermined level of values.

Quality assurance mechanism—retrospective review program by the organized medical staff. It assesses the quality of care as compared to locally or internally developed standards and verifies that the standards or exceptions are met, that deficiencies are corrected, and that the original problem is reassessed on a planned program basis.

Quantitative analysis—descriptive statistics; a basic means of describing and understanding the population served by the health care system. There are three basic types: (1) numbers and demographic information; (2) health status, commonly referred to as morbidity (sickness) and mortality (death) information; and (3) utilization of goods and services.

Rate—a numerical expression that describes a relationship per time interval.

Ratio—a numerical expression that describes a relationship per number of total relationships.

Real time processing—a form of interactive processing in which the computer system records each change immediately and updates all the necessary files, etc. immediately. In health information a computerized on-line appointment system could be real time; intensive care computers that monitor patient heart functions, breathing, etc. are real time systems.

Rebuttal—defeat or removal of the effect of something; testimony intended to deny or contradict.

Recommended medical audit action—specific steps determined by the medical audit committee as a result of a completed audit. It must be specific to the problems identified and effective in accomplishing change.

Record control—that part of record retention and retrieval that provides (1) procedural elements that assure a permanent location for data to be maintained, (2) defined limits on retrieval of the data by particular users, and (3) methods to communicate continually the current location of a record.

Record destruction program—a plan that includes a time schedule and facility for routinely eliminating selected records from the files.

Record linkage—the process of connecting one individual's records, even though they were developed at different times and in different places, and combining them into one file by means of a common identifier.

Recorded instruments—certified copies of any deconveyance, bond, mortgage, or other writing that has been recorded, which can be accepted as evidence.

Refutation—the act of proving the falsity or error in a statement, a proposition, or an argument.

Register—a log that records all requests for information.

Registry—a synopsized listing of data that categorizes a larger group of data.

Release—a written instrument by which some claim or interest is surrendered to another person.

Reliable data—information obtained by means of a well-defined objective method for measurement which involves all or a representative sample of patients and practitioners.

Reported—acknowledged by executive committee, chief of the medical staff, chief executive officer, and governing body (for medical studies); acknowledged by chief executive officer, governing body, and chief of medical staff (for nursing service and other health care professionals' studies).

Res ipsa loquiter—"The occurrence speaks for itself" (the proof that an accident took place).

Research Grants Index—annual publication which is a source of information on health research currently supported by the health agencies of DHEW.

Research sampling techniques—alternative methods used to select appropriate representation of a given population; to use analysis of that representation to draw conclusions on the population.

Respondeat superior principle—principle that states "Let the master answer." Two factors must exist: employee-employer relationship, that is, the person must be employed by a facility, and the employee must act within the scope of his or her employment. This doctrine says the employer is responsible for the act of his or her agent or servant. A patient who sues a nurse also sues the hospital because the nurse is employed by the hospital.

Retention/retrieval—keeping information so that it may be used in the future; planning, implementation, and control of a system that safeguards the physical and information characteristics of medical or health data for future use.

Retention/retrieval manual—a written manual that describes what is to be completed, the method to be used, and the productivity level expected.

Retroactive denial—disapproval of payment based on retrospective review of the case. When this occurs, an appeals process is usually initiated in which further documentation from the patient's record is submitted and an additional review requested.

Retrospective review—an in-depth assessment of the quality or nature of the utilization of health services performed after the patient has been discharged.

Review—examination of a medical record by a physician to determine if continued hospitalization is medically necessary.

Review coordinator—a person responsible for the smooth functioning of the review program and the communication of information among patient, attending physician, hospital, and PSRO.

RFP—request for proposal.

RFVC—reason for visit classification.

RRA—Registered Record Administrator; one who has achieved a specified educational level and has successfully completed a national qualifying examination.

Rules of exclusion—rules that evidence offered will be excluded from the record of proceedings or from being received in evidence if it is not properly qualified or not properly identi-

fied. For this reason, medical record administrators direct staff to take medical records to court and testify to their identity as medical records from the institution in which they originated.

Satellite record system—a system in which the majority of records are filed in one major location but some records needed in other areas may be moved and may be kept in those areas for a certain period of time, being returned to the central file room only for permanent filing.

SCM—Society for Computer Medicine; an association which promotes the use of computers in medicine.

Screen—to compare documentation recorded in the medical record against preestablished criteria.

Screening—a process in which norms, criteria, and standards are used to analyze large numbers of cases in order to select cases not meeting these norms, criteria, and standards for study in greater depth.

Serial numbering—a system of numbering in which the patient is assigned a new number each time treatment is received.

Serial unit numbering—a system in which patients are assigned a new number each time they enter the system. All previous records are brought forward and reassigned the new number.

Service or care unit—a group of patients who have related diagnoses and/or kinds of treatment; a group of inpatient beds designated for a single specialty of the medical staff.

Shared Computer Systems—a commercial program that collects, processes, and reports statistics on patient services and needs assessments, based on analysis of abstracts of hospital discharges. Studies comparing individual hospital performance with similar facilities are available to client hospitals.

Shop book rule—a rule of evidence allowing the admission in evidence of a party's account books of original entry, that is, the business record of the facility. The medical record is in this category.

Simple random sampling—method of sampling in which every unit in the population is assured an equal and independent chance of selection. A table of random numbers applied to sequential accession numbers assigned to clinic patients is an example of this.

SNF—skilled nursing facility.

SNODO—standard nomenclature of disease and operations.

SNOMED—systematized nomenclature of medicine.

SNOP—systematized nomenclature of pathology.

SOAP (POMR)—subjective objective assessment plan. **S** subjective; notation of items, as symptomatic complaints of the patient, that cannot necessarily be measured or strictly defined and are considered subjective. **O** objective; notation of items that are observable and measurable, such as laboratory findings, color of skin, results of tests, blood pressure, pulse rate, and any other activity that can be observed by one of the health care providers. **A** assessment; a statement of what is currently happening to the patient, the severity of the illness, any changes or conclusions to be drawn about diagnoses, prognosis, or change in the patient's statement. **P** plan; short-range, diagnostic, patient educational, or long-range treatment, according to the assessment.

Social Security numbering—a system of numbering in which records are identified by the individual patient's Social Security number.

Software—the programs (and associated documentation) produced to operate the computer system.

Soundex system—a phonetic filing system that uses a combination of letter and code numbers to designate names.

Source document—document on which data are originally recorded (handwritten or typed) and from which data elements are extracted for input into a computerized data system.

Source oriented record—a record that maintains all reports and data from a given department in one section and keeps them in chronological sequence within each subsection.

Standard—generally, a measure set by competent authority as the rule for measuring quantity or quality. Conformity with standards is usually a condition of licensure, accreditation, or payment of services.

Standardization—the establishment of a baseline guide as to the minimum acceptable level of performance.

State statutory law—written law that is created and enacted by the state legislature. It is also referred to as administrative code.

Statistical display—a graphic arrangement of statistical information; for example, tables, charts, graphic illustrations, and computer plots.

Statute of limitations—a law limiting the period of time during which an action must be brought; the legal requirement regarding retention time periods for various business and medical documents.

Step chart—illustration of patterns of motion often used in place of a line chart.

Straight numerical filing—a method of filing in which documents are filed according to chronological sequence of assigned number.

Stratified sampling—dividing the patient population into homogeneous groups according to some characteristic such as the type of service (surgical or cardiology) or source of payment (such as Medicare) and selecting a separate sample within each of those categories.

Subpoena duces tecum—a notice compelling the attendance of a person in court and ordering them to bring the books, documents, or other evidence described in the writ. It is signed by a clerk of the court or a deputy and directs a record administrator or employee of a medical record department to bring a particular record to court.

Suit—an action or process in a court for the recovery of a right or claim.

Summons—a process (document) served on a defendant in civil court action to secure his or her appearance in the action.

Surgical operation—one or more surgical procedures performed at one time for one patient via a common approach or for a common purpose.

System—related elements that are coordinated to form a unified result, specifically people, activities, equipment, materials, plans, and controls, working together to achieve a unified objective or whole; an array of components that interact to achieve some objective through a network of procedures that are integrated and designed to carry out a major activity.

Systematic sampling—the selection of every x number of individuals from a list or card file of patients, i.e., every fifth entry on a register or index, or all patients admitted on a certain day or intervals of days during a month.

Systems analysis—a problem-solving method for an overall, thorough analysis of an activity to determine the most appropriate method for accomplishing it. It is directed, but not limited to, knowledge and processes required for planning and implementing computer-based systems in health and patient information handling.

Tabs—the identifying extensions of folders.

Teleprocessing—data processing through the use of a combination of data processors, or computers, and telecommunications facilities.

Temporary staff—physicians or dentists who have been granted privileges for a limited period of time by the chief medical staff officer on the recommendation of the chief of a particular department.

Terminal digit filing—a method of filing by the last digits of a number instead of by the first digits. The entire number is broken into groups of twos or threes, with the last group being filed first.

Third party payment—that type of payment utilized by those who spend a regular part of their income or work benefits on health care insurance and, in turn, receive full or partial payment for their health care.

Time sharing operation—a system in which a number of users buy time and share resources of a central computer.

Tissue committee—committee responsible for the review of surgical procedures in the facility.

Title V—a federal health program for maternal and child health and crippled children's services.

Title XIX, Medicaid—a federal program designed to meet the health needs of persons who receive aid through the program for families with dependent children or who have only marginal income.

Title XVIII, Medicare—a federal health insurance program for people 65 years of age and older, and some people under 65 years who are disabled.

Tort—an injury or wrong committed with or without force to the person or property of another. Tort claims deal with civil or federal wrongs.

Total inpatient service days—the sum of all inpatient service days for each of the days in the period under consideration.

Total length of stay—the sum of the days stay of any group of inpatients discharged during a specified period of time.

Transfer (intrahospital)—a change in medical care unit, medical staff unit, or responsible physician of an inpatient during hospitalization.

Transfer data—an abstract or summary of an individual patient care plan to accompany the patient to another care facility.

Trial court—the formal examination of the matter in issue in a case before a competent tribunal for the purpose of determining such issues; the court before which issues of fact and law are first determined.

Type of care—the facilities and personnel available for health care and, more importantly, the objective of the care.

Unit numbering—a system in which only one number is assigned to the patient's record and is retained permanently.

Unit record system—a method that compiles all information on a single patient or subject and records it in one document and file folder.

Utilization review—the evaluation of the necessity, appropriateness, and efficiency of the use of medical services, procedures, and facilities. In a hospital this includes review of the appropriateness of admissions, services ordered and provided, length of stay, and discharge practices on the concurrent and retrospective basis. This can be done by a utilization review committee, PSRO peer review, or public agency.

Utilization review committee—committee which reviews all aspects of care in order to assure high-quality patient care through the effective use of equipment, personnel, materials, and the facility as a whole.

Valid criteria—standards stated in measurable rather than descriptive terms, precise enough to permit accurate evaluation; statements of optimal achievable care; measures of quality, which are (1) validation of diagnosis, (2) justification for admission, surgery, and/or special hazardous procedures, (3) statement of expected patient outcomes, and (4) processes of care or patient management, under appropriate circumstances.

Variation—finding or element not in agreement with the norm or standard.

Variation analysis—identification of conformance to and variations from the audit criteria. It requires explicit justification for all variations that are clinically acceptable, identification of problems in the provision of patient care (variations that are not clinically acceptable), and attribution of the problems to their source.

Variation justification—an acceptable reason why a given finding or element is not in agreement with the norm or standard.

Verdict—the finding or decision of a jury on the matter submitted in trial; decision or judgment; opinion pronounced.

Waiver—the voluntary relinquishing of a known right.

Witness—one who testifies to facts within his or her own knowledge.

WONCA—World Organization of National Colleges, Academies, and Academic Associations of General Practitioners/Family Physicians.

Written authorization—a written statement to clothe with legal power; to empower.

Chapter 5—Nursing Service

OVERVIEW*

Nursing is the largest department in the hospital. At its head is the nursing service administrator who is variously called director of nursing, head of the department of nursing, chief of nursing, chief of nursing practice. It is customary for her to have at least one assistant for each period of the day, since the nursing department is staffed for 24 hours. The department of nursing also has clinical specialists to administer at least some of its services, such as pediatrics, maternity, and operating room. Every service has two or more divisions, each of which has a head nurse in charge. The head nurse, in turn, has helpers who have varying types and degrees of preparation. All these individuals are part of the line organization. The nurse administrator may also have assistants in staff positions such as the director of inservice education. Although this organizational pattern is the most common today, other designs are being used in some hospitals which are not satisfied with traditional arrangements.

Special Nursing Units

The special nursing units in the Nursing Service Department usually include medical, surgical, pediatric, obstetric, and psychiatric. In addition

---

*Source: *Job Descriptions & Organizational Analysis for Hospitals and Related Health Services,* U.S. Training and Employment Service, U.S. Department of Labor, 1971.

to the overall responsibilities and functions of nursing service, the units also carry more specific responsibilities and functions of patient care, varying with each nursing unit. The establishment and execution of educational programs for staff and student nurses may also be functions of these special nursing units.

Medical and Surgical

Nursing care is provided in medical and surgical units in accordance with physician's instructions and recognized techniques and procedures. While medical conditions are not easily divided into distinct categories, medical nursing is considered a specialty in that normal and abnormal reactions or symptoms of diagnosed disease must be recognized and reported. The patient with a stroke or a cardiac condition requires a much different type of nursing from that given the patient with an ulcer or diabetes. Surgical patients also require special preoperative and postoperative care.

Pediatrics

This service embraces the care of children. Care of the newborn is usually in a separate unit located in the obstetric unit. The activities of the pediatric unit require understanding of the unique needs, fears, and behavior of children, which is reflected in the type and degree of nursing care given. Where illnesses require protracted convalescence, educational and occupational therapy become concerns of the nursing service. Relationships with parents pose further important responsibilities.

Obstetrics

Prenatal care, observation, and comfort of patients in labor, delivery room assistance, and care of mother after delivery, as well as nursing care of newborn, are important responsibilities of this unit. Obstetric nurses assist in instructing new mothers in postnatal care and care of the newborn. Care of the newborn, particularly the premature, requires special nursing skills dictated by their unique requirements.

Psychiatric

While most emotionally disturbed patients are treated in specialized hospitals, the general hospital also recognizes a responsibility and provides facilities for the mentally ill. Nursing care of the mentally ill requires a knowledge of their various behavior patterns and how to cope with them. Techniques must be learned for dealing with all types of problem behavior, so that skilled, therapeutic care is given to such patients.

Other Units

Operating Room

This unit has primary responsibility for comforting patients in the O.R.; maintaining aseptic techniques; scheduling all operations in cooperation with surgeons; and determining that adequate personnel, space, and equipment are available. Nursing personnel assist the surgeon during operations and are part of the surgical team. Preparation for operations includes sterilization of instruments and equipment; cleaning up after operations is also part of the unit's responsibility.

Recovery Room

In many hospitals, the Recovery Room unit is an adjunct responsibility of the Operating Room unit. Special nursing attention must be given patients after an operation until they have completely recovered from the effects of anesthesia.

Emergency Room

This unit is responsible for emergency care, and for arrangements to admit the patient to the hospital, if necessary. The unit completes required records; makes reports to police and safety and health agencies; handles matters of payment, and notification of relatives; and refers patients to other services within the hospital or community, as needed.

Intensive Care

Many hospitals have an Intensive Care unit; some hospitals have several. These units usually accommodate a limited number of patients whose conditions are very critical or require specialized care and equipment such as electronic instruments for observation, signaling, recording, and measuring physiological functions. In addition to providing continuous recording of cardiac function, bedside systems may monitor temperature, blood pressure, respiration rate, and other measurements. More nurses are assigned per number of patients and they are continuously in the room or within sight of the patient under care. This makes it possible to give close attention to the critically ill or postoperative patient requiring intensive care and to concentrate special equipment where it is most likely to be needed. An increasing number of specialized "teams" consists of one or more physicians and other medical specialists, nurses, and ancillary personnel who respond to emergency situations. They are known by the specialized function they perform such as "cardiac team" or "kidney failure team."

NURSING MANAGEMENT POSITIONS

In the United States, there are approximately 160,000 registered nurses in administrative positions in hospitals and about 35,000 in nursing homes. These nurses have many titles, among which the most frequently used are director of nursing or chief nurse (top management); associate or assistant director of nursing and/or staff development or assistant chief nurse (middle management); day, evening, or night supervisor (middle management); and head nurse (first-line management). Other newer titles designated for the top nursing management person, particularly in the large health care institutions, are vice-president for nursing, vice-president for patient care, or assistant administrator for nursing.

Following are brief descriptions of the nursing management jobs within the hospital, followed by descriptions of the staff jobs within the nursing service.

Director of Nursing

Job Duties

Organizes and administers the department of nursing:

Establishes objectives for the department of nursing and the organizational structure for achieving these objectives. Interprets and puts into effect administrative policies established by the governing authority. Assists in preparing and administering budget for the department. Selects and recommends appointment of nursing staff.

Directs and delegates management of professional and ancillary nursing personnel. Plans and conducts conferences and discussions with administrative and professional nursing staff to encourage participation in formulating departmental policies and procedures, promote initiative, solve problems, and interpret new policies and procedures. Coordinates activities of various nursing units, promoting and maintaining harmonious relationships among nursing personnel and with medical staff, patients, and public. Plans and directs orientation and inservice training programs for professional and nonprofessional nursing staff. Analyzes and evaluates nursing and related services rendered to improve quality of patient care and plan better utilization of staff time and activities. Participates in community educational health programs.

Education, Training, and Experience

A baccalaureate degree in nursing is a minimum requirement, with a master's degree preferable. Current licensure by State Board of Nursing is a necessity. Five years administrative experience as a director, assistant director, or supervisor of nursing services required.

Specific Qualifications*

What follows are the qualifications which were defined as important for the administrator of

---

*Source: *The Role of the Director of Nursing Service*, National League for Nursing, Publ. No. 20-1646, 1977.

nursing in a recent NLN publication under three categories: an experienced nurse, a management colleague and an educator.

Experienced Nurse

The administrator of nursing must be a nurse who:

- Understands both patient care and nurses; has demonstrated stature in the nursing profession; has had some influence in the nursing field, has kept abreast of changes in the profession.
- Plans for the department; establishes goals and directions for that department and helps the hospital establish its own goals; assures that nursing has proper influence on the total institutional goals and that nursing goals and directions complement and support the total.
- Has integrity and can be relied on to speak frankly and not waste time playing games; one whose voice is respected.
- Is a leader who can measure, evaluate, act, motivate and deal with people; can calculate trouble in advance and steady the organization; excludes unnecessary interference in the internal operations of the department by being a strong and effective manager.
- Is an interpreter for nursing and the hospital, both intramurally and extramurally; speaks for quality and can motivate people in general; understands elements of human behavior.
- Thinks independently; is knowledgeable in the field and willing to draw upon that knowledge to establish a position; can say no and then find a productive alternative. Policies and procedures, organizational charts and regulations are not substitutes for thinking. The nursing administrator must properly proportion rules, hardware and talent to gain the most effective means of achieving the best in total patient care.
- Is a member of the management team with a business mind and attitude; is able to delegate responsibility so that available resources are utilized; keeps decision making close to the patient, thus, responds to patient needs and not professional resentment; demonstrates warmth and concern for people as individuals and has an interest

in total patient care; above all, has a sense of humor and is able to supply a light touch when the going gets rough.

Management Colleague

The position of nursing director is a top administrative one and an extension of the administrator or chief executive officer. It would not be enough for a potential candidate to be simply interested in nursing management. This management colleague should be able to meet certain considerations, such as:

- Being qualified through having some management training and preferably a masters degree plus a demonstrable ability to cope with management responsibilities seemed to be legitimate criteria for such an important position.
- Having the ability to perform as a management representative. This colleague must represent management, which means having direct access to the administrator, the medical staff, and the trustees; being able to sit down with the doctors and plan problem-solving techniques with them; being multidepartment-oriented and a constructive change agent to move ideas forward in the organization.
- Having knowledge of volunteers and their respect to help them channel their energies in the most effective, productive way possible to the benefit of the hospital and patients.
- Having knowledge of community health needs. A person who would become a working member of the community and help plan community health.
- Being an organizer; a planner of strategies; one who keeps an eye on the objectives and functions of the organization and develops resources to achieve such goals through planning, idea development and clear perspectives.
- Having knowledge of budgets. A person in a management capacity must use all the tools for management, and one of the tasks of the nurse executive is to understand and participate in the budget process. This person must recognize that the budget is a tool used to get things done; it is not just something that interferes with nursing opportunities. One who can put budget pieces together correctly and stand accountable for personal actions as well as for the actions of others under her jurisdiction; one who understands the control mechanism and has the attitude and the ability to apply it; one who understands economics in the field (the key to survival of the hospital department), who understands that competition does not necessarily reduce the price of care. In fact, it is just the opposite. The oversupply of facilities, underutilization, increases the cost of care. Perhaps one of the most important considerations in the process of budgeting is to be able to relate dollars to quality.
- Having knowledge of the role the government plays in health care and its effect on that care. Regulatory processes, in a large measure, are aimed directly at doctors. The government has learned that the best strategy is to use the hospitals to apply restraints and restrictions on the medical profession, a devious and divisive process. Top level management must be able to cope with the regulatory process, sometimes anticipating problems and planning defenses in advance.
- Being knowledgeable about labor relations; someone who understands labor relations and the techniques of dealing with people; one who can handle professional pressures when conflicts develop. For example, when union activity is presented under the umbrella of professional organization, there is a problem when the organization says one thing and the employer another. This creates a tremendous pressure within the hospital and situations will occur that must be handled diplomatically but firmly.

Educator

- Someone able to understand the balance between education and practice; to know what is necessary in the area of personnel education as required by the employer to ensure the best possible patient care, and to be able to correlate hospital needs with educational requirements.
- Someone to provide input into educational programs for the hospital and bring new ideas into the organization concerning education.

- Someone with adequate information on educational laws and who knows how they apply in the state as well as nationally.
- Someone able to demonstrate self-improvement and have the ability to motivate others to higher levels of performance through better educational opportunities.

Profile of the Director of Nursing

The most recent comprehensive study of nurse administrators is the 1968 National League for Nursing survey on organizational patterns of nursing service in hospitals. Among the findings were: The ages of the directors ranged from 21 to 77 years, with the median age 48. Eighty-eight percent graduated from diploma schools, 9% were basic baccalaureate graduates. While most had sought education beyond their basic program, slightly less than one-third had earned no academic credential beyond the diploma. Of the 1,172 directors surveyed, 2 had doctorates, 467 (39.8%) had master's, and 310 (26.5%) had bachelor's degrees. About 38% of the directors with master's degrees had majored in nursing service administration, about 34% in nursing education; and about 29% in other fields.

Assistant Director, Nursing Service*

Job Duties

Assists in organizing and administering the department of nursing; assumes responsibilities delegated by the nursing service director.

Conducts conferences and discussions with personnel to encourage participation in formulating departmental policies, promote initiative, solve problems, and present new policies and procedures.

Analyzes nursing and auxiliary services to improve quality of patient care and to obtain maximum utilization of staff time and abilities. Coordinates activities of the nursing service units to achieve and maintain efficient and competent nursing service and to promote and maintain harmonious relationships among personnel

---

*Source: Descriptions for these supervisory positions are adapted from *Job Descriptions & Organizational Analysis for Hospitals and Related Health Services*, U.S. Training and Employment Service, Department of Labor, 1971.

supervised, medical staff, patients, and others. Assists in establishing lines of authority and responsibility, and defining the duties of nursing service personnel, consistent with good administrative techniques, to assure that department objectives are accomplished.

Assists in review and evaluation of budget requests against current and projected needs of nursing service.

Interviews applicants and recommends appointment of staff personnel, outlining their duties, scope of authority, and responsibilities. Participates in establishing and administering orientation and inservice training programs for both professional and nonprofessional personnel. Insures proper and economical use of equipment, supplies, and facilities for maintaining patient care. Maintains personnel and other records, and directs maintenance of patient care records.

Cooperates with medical staff performing research projects or studies as they affect nursing. Works with other agencies and groups in the community to promote the growth and broaden knowledge and skills of professional staff, and improve quality of hospital services.

Education, Training, and Experience

Graduation from an accredited school of nursing with bachelor's degree preferred, and master's degree desirable. Current licensure by State Board of Nursing required, and demonstrated administrative ability.

Experience in a supervisory capacity with demonstrated executive ability and leadership.

Qualifications

The role of an assistant director of nursing is filled with numerous administrative and clinical responsibilities. To be prepared, an assistant director might well hold an MSN degree and be backed up by one year of experience in management and two years in clinical service. Additional workshops or courses in management topics should provide support in handling labor relations, problem solving and planning. On the personal level, the assistant director should be purposeful but not rigid, assertive but not overly aggressive, articulate in her own views but not deaf to the opinions of others.

Skills and Responsibilities

Leadership skills in decision-making, problem-solving and interpersonal relations are involved in the daily contacts of working with head nurses on the unit. Assistance is given, on an individual or group level, for setting objectives, structuring plans, handling complaints and finding solutions. Administrative skills are called for in the performance of several functions. The assistant director is concerned with budgeting, helping the head nurse to document, justify and submit requests for positions, and evaluating head nurse performance. She is concerned with staff development, identifying staff instructional requirements to the inservice department and suggesting or teaching new programs. She is also concerned with committee participation, serving on the nursing service administration council and in a representational capacity on her clinical units' committees, specialty interest committees, department-wide committees, such as the committee on quality assurance, and inter-departmental committees.

The maintenance of quality patient care in the units under her supervision is a major responsibility of the assistant director. For some assistant directors the objective is demonstrated practically, by periodically working the unit floor to become acquainted with staff members as working partners and to act as models in the giving of proper care. Others increase communication contacts during the normal course of duties; they show a heightened involvement in short-term crises and long-term projects. Still others concern themselves with technical improvements, streamlining systems, altering forms, clarifying procedures and implementing standards.

Supervisor Nurse

Job Duties

Supervises and coordinates activities of nursing personnel engaged in specific nursing services, such as obstetrics, pediatrics, or surgery, or for two or more patient care units; also assigned to such areas as the operating room, the outpatient department, the recovery room, and special or intensive care units.

Participates with the director of nursing in the development and implementation of the philosophy and objectives for nursing service.

Supervises Head Nurses in carrying out their responsibilities in the management of nursing care. Evaluates performance of Head Nurse and nursing care as a whole and suggests modifications. Inspects unit areas to verify that patient needs are met.

Participates in planning work of own units and coordinates activities with other patient care units and with those of related departments.

Consults with the Head Nurse on specific nursing problems and interpretation of hospital policies. Supervises maintenance of personnel and nursing records.

Plans and organizes orientation and inservice training for unit staff members and participates in guidance and educational programs. Interviews prescreened applicants and makes recommendations for employing or for terminating personnel. Assists the Director of Nursing Service in formulating unit budget. Engages in studies and investigations related to improving nursing care.

The Supervisor Nurse is usually known by name of nursing section to which assigned or in which she has specialized, such as Supervisor Nurse, Medical and Surgical or Supervisor Nurse, Pediatrics. Specialized duties will be required by the specialized section.

Supervisor Nurse, Evening or Night Assistant Director of Nursing, Evening or Night

Job Duties

Supervises and coordinates activities of nursing personnel on evening or night tour to maintain continuity for around-the-clock nursing care:

Visits nursing units to oversee nursing care and to ascertain condition of patients. Advises and assists nurses in administering new or unusual treatments. Gives advice for treatments, medications, and narcotics, in accordance with medical staff policies, in absence of physician. Arranges for emergency operations and reallocates personnel during emergencies. Admits or delegates admissions of new patients. Arranges for services of private-duty nurses. Determines necessity of calling physician. May perform some bedside nursing services.

Delegates preparation of reports covering such items as critically ill patients, new admissions, discharges or deaths, emergency situations encountered, and private-duty nurses employed. Informs supervisory personnel on ensuing tour of duty of patients' condition and hospital services rendered during work period.

Education, Training, and Experience

Graduation from an accredited school of nursing and current licensure by State Board of Nursing. Advanced education desirable. Experience as a Head Nurse in which administrative, supervisory, and teaching abilities have been demonstrated.

Specific Qualifications

The beginning supervisor should:

- Have at least five years experience as a head nurse;
- Be intelligent, capable of learning readily and of retaining the knowledge;
- Be able to convey knowledge to others in an understanding and interesting way;
- Be tolerant and understanding;
- Be objective;
- Be able, when necessary, to show authority without being too demanding and without losing the respect of subordinates;
- Have self confidence and be able to gain the confidence of others;
- Have good physical and mental health;
- Be able to promote good public relations;
- Keep up with new trends in nursing and be able to convey this information to others;
- Be able to do new procedures and to use new equipment (as well as older methods) and to instruct others with clarity;
- Maintain interest in good nursing care;
- Know administrative regulations of the general hospital and how they apply to her and her coworkers;
- Give support where needed and a helping hand at times;
- Set the climate for cooperation between coworkers and shifts for a smooth-running institution.[1]

Director of Staff Development (Inservice-Education Coordinator)
Job Duties

Plans, develops, and directs program of education for all hospital nursing service personnel,

---

[1]Betty J. Robinson, "Supervision As I See It," *Supervisor Nurse*, October 1974.

and coordinates staff development with nursing service program:

Develops, schedules, and directs orientation program for professional and auxiliary nursing service personnel. Develops instructional materials to assist new personnel in becoming oriented to hospital operational techniques. If not scheduled by Personnel Department, schedules hospital tours and addresses by administrative staff to acquaint new personnel with overall operation and interrelationship of hospital services. Determines effectiveness of orientation materials and procedures through practice sessions. Sets up demonstrations of nursing service equipment to acquaint hospital staff with new equipment and make them more familiar with established equipment.

Plans, coordinates, and conducts regular and special inservice training sessions for hospital nursing staff to acquaint them with new procedures and policies and new trends and developments in patient care techniques; and to provide opportunity for individual members to develop to their full potential.

Keeps current on latest developments by attending professional seminars, institutes, and reading professional journals. Assists Supervisors and Head Nurses in planning and implementing staff development programs in their units. Keeps bulletin boards current by listing information on seminars and institutes and promotes appropriate staff attendance at these professional meetings. Plans training sessions for supervisory staff members.

May participate with committees in writing and maintaining policies and procedures manuals and nursing service forms. Reviews suggestions submitted by nursing service staff for changes or clarification in policies and procedures.

Writes annual reports on activities and prepares plans for future activities. Prepares budget requests.

Education, Training, and Experience

Graduation from an accredited school of nursing and current licensure by State Board of Nursing; graduation from a recognized college or university with specialization in education; bachelor's degree required. Experience as Head Nurse, Supervisor Nurse or Nurse Educator.

It would be a positive advantage for her to have had professional experiences that would encompass clinical, teaching, and supervisory practice within a large active nursing service organization. It is important that she be "service minded" and familiar with the needs and problems of service personnel. She should have a broad and thorough knowledge of nursing skills that would enable her to appraise the quality of nursing care being given as well as to assess the abilities enabling an individual nursing practitioner to meet the expectations of a specific job.

Head Nurse

Job Duties

Directs nursing service activities including the preparation of nursing care plans, and instructs nurses in an organized hospital patient care unit:

Usually responsible for the direct and indirect nursing care of patients within an organized unit of a clinical area, such as surgery, medicine, or pediatrics, or a specialized unit, such as the nursery, tumor clinic in the outpatient department, coronary care unit, or the emergency room.

May also be responsible for ward 24 hours a day in the sense that evening and night nurses report to her and she is responsible for assigning duties on other shifts.

Assigns duties to professional and ancillary nursing personnel based on patients' needs, available staff, and unit needs. Supervises and evaluates work performance in terms of patient care, staff relations, and efficiency of service. Provides for nursing care in unit and cooperates with other members of medical care team in coordinating patients' total needs. Identifies and studies nursing service problems and assists in their solution. Observes nursing care and visits patients to insure that nursing care is carried out as directed and treatment is administered in accordance with physicians' instructions and to ascertain need for additional or modified services. Maintains a safe environment for patients. Operates or supervises operation of specialized equipment assigned to unit and provides assistance and guidance to nursing team as required.

Accompanies physician on rounds to answer questions, receive instructions, and note patients' care requirements. Reports to replacement on next tour on condition of patients or of any unusual actions taken. May render professional nursing care and instruct patients and members of their families in techniques and methods of home care after discharge.

Directs preparation and maintenance of patients' clinical records, including nursing and medical treatments and related services provided by staff nurse. Compiles daily reports on staff hours worked and care and condition of patients. Investigates and adjusts complaints or refers them to supervisor.

Insures established inventory standards for medicines, solutions, supplies, and equipment. Accounts for narcotics. Provides orientation for new personnel to job requirements, equipment, and unit personnel. Instructs unit personnel in new nursing care techniques, procedures, and equipment. Presides over unit personnel meetings to discuss patient care needs. Evaluates individual work performance through observation, spot-checking work completed, and conferences. Promotes individual staff development.

Attends meetings of supervisory and administrative staff to discuss unit operation and staff training needs and to formulate programs to improve these areas. May assist in developing and administering budget for nursing unit to which assigned. Assists with studies related to improvement of nursing care.

The Head Nurse is usually known by the nursing unit to which assigned or in which she has specialized, such as Head Nurse, Medical and Surgical; or Head Nurse, Pediatrics. Specialized duties will be required by the specialized unit.

Education, Training, and Experience

Graduation from an accredited school of nursing and current licensure by State Board of Nursing. Advanced preparation in the clinical specialty, ward management, principles of supervision, and teaching is preferred.

Experience as a professional nurse in which potential administrative and supervisory competence has been demonstrated.

Nurse Specialists*

1. Clinical Coordinator, Nursing Service

The major responsibilities of this position are directly to the director of the department of nursing.

---

*Source: Russell C. Swansburg, *Management of Patient Care Services,* St. Louis: The C. V. Mosby Co., 1976.

- Coordinates activities with all hospital services and families in providing for the patients' total needs. She directly supervises charge nurses of inpatient units.
- Makes walk-through rounds and observes all patients—visits all seriously ill, very seriously ill, and other patients reported on the 24-hour report.
- Assists in providing adequate staffing for all inpatient units.
- Serves as advisor and resource person for nursing personnel on duty as needed.
- Advises committees as designated by the chairman of the department of nursing.
- Performs weekly rounds using checklist:
  a. Sees that medications are secure and that pouring of medications is done at time due.
  b. Checks ward alcoholic and narcotic register book.
  c. Reviews list of nurses proficient in intravenous medication administration.
  d. Checks biologicals:
    —Checks documentation of temperature of refrigeration unit.
    —Checks to see that thermometer is present.
    —Checks discarding of outdated drugs.
    —Checks dating of open vials.
- Performs PRN checklist:
  a. Checks admission schedules; coordinates with admissions and discharges clerk on bed availability.
  b. Reviews time schedules every 2 weeks as submitted.
  c. Coordinates scheduling of personnel for courses and programs such as race relations.
  d. Reviews nursing licenses: registration number, state, expiration date.

2. Clinical Nursing Specialist

Public Health Nurse

- Is in charge of the organization, management, and supervision of visiting nurse service. She makes nursing diagnosis and prescription and provides guidance, counseling, and teaching to patients and families in the home.
- Performs public health nursing consultant role to the nursing staff so that nursing activities include the social, environmental, and community aspects of care.

Rehabilitation Clinical Nurse Specialist

- Plans, organizes, directs, coordinates, and evaluates the practice of rehabilitative nursing, both inpatient and outpatient.
- Performs expert clinical nursing care as a member of the health care team.
- Practices nursing independently within the scope of legal parameters and educational preparation.

Pediatric Clinical Nurse Specialist

- Plans, organizes, directs, coordinates, and evaluates the practice of nursing, both inpatient and outpatient, of all pediatric patients.
- Examines and treats children with uncomplicated problems.
- Evaluates growth and development and administers screening tests on all high-risk infants and other children with problems in this area.
- Provides well-baby follow-up and parent counseling in hygiene, nutrition, discipline, and behavior.
- Establishes programs for follow-up care of children with chronic illnesses and handicaps.

Cobalt and Chemotherapy Nurse

- Provides nursing care, chemotherapy, and radiation therapy treatments to cancer patients, working closely with the physician oncologist.
- Operates therapeutic radiological equipment including Maxitron 250 U, cobalt 60, and other related types of supervoltage radiation equipment.
- Assists radiologists in handling radium, radon, gold grains, and other radioactive substances.

3. Charge Nurse—Clinics

General Therapy Clinic

- Assesses and identifies patients' health problems and needs.
- Assists with or initiates emergency lifesaving procedures.
- Provides health teaching for patients and families.
- Assists with research related to the improvement of the delivery of health care services.

Surgical Clinic

- Plans, organizes, directs, coordinates, and evaluates all nursing functions in the surgical specialty clinics.
- Screens patients and refers them to appropriate physicians, clinical specialists, or hospital department.
- Identifies patients' nursing care needs and problems and practices nursing to meet established goals.
- Maintains accurate records of nursing assessments, plans, and care.
- Is self-directing in practice; makes professional judgments, counsels and teaches patients, families, and co-workers.

Obstetrical-Gynecological Clinic

- Directs and coordinates all nursing activities in the obstetrical-gynecological clinic.
- Provides health services, which include health education, maintenance, prevention, and early case finding.
- Plays an important role in interpretation of treatment, making diagnostic reports, giving emergency care, taking patients' histories, and initiating charts.

4. Supervisor—Operating Room

The supervisor of the operating room is in charge of nursing personnel in the operating room, recovery room, and central sterile supply. The major responsibilities of this position are directly to the chairman.

- Plans, directs, and controls the staffing assignments to ensure 24-hour daily coverage and effective utilization of personnel.
- Directs and controls the flow and operational efficiency of equipment and supplies needed in the treatment of patients.
- Maintains a bacteria-free, safe physical environment for patients and personnel in accordance with established standards.
- Coordinates nursing services with those related services performed by other group members.

5. Charge Nurse—Central Sterile Supply

- Manages central nursing sterile supply service, including the management of personnel over a 24-hour period.

- Plans, directs, and coordinates all activities relating to the procurement, processing, storage, and distribution of supplies and equipment needed to give patient care efficiently and safely.

6. Charge Nurse—Anesthesia

- Supervises, directs, and controls the staffing assignments of nurse anesthetists to ensure 24-hour daily coverage.
- Maintains adequate levels of drugs, anesthetic agents, and supplies used in the treatment of patients.
- Assists in the anesthesia training of dental and surgical interns and residents.
- Is supervised directly by the chief of the anesthesiology service.

7. Superintendent of the Department of Nursing—Inpatient Units

The major responsibilities of this position are to the chairman of the department of nursing.

- Assigns technical nursing personnel and provides adequate staffing of all the inpatient units.
- Assists with supervising all nursing technicians assigned to the inpatient units.
- Inspects wards daily; identifies the necessity for rotation of technician personnel, for training, and for adjusting schedules to provide for competent patient care at all times.
- Interviews and counsels the assigned technicians and keeps pertinent information such as projected or actual gains or losses.
- Keeps supervisors informed of special abilities of technician personnel or other pertinent items of special interest.
- Performs rounds checklist of week:
  a. Ensures that management and control of needles and syringes are adequate.
  b. Checks safety measures:
     i. Fire regulations enforced.
     ii. Oxygen cylinders stored properly.
  c. Checks supplies to see that levels are realistic with no overstocking.
  d. Checks bedside units:
     i. Pillows protected with plastic covers.
     ii. Urinal covers used.
     iii. Bedside lamps available for all inpatients.

- Makes monthly checklist:
  a. Checks to see that there are locator cards on all patients.
  b. Checks signs; they should be professionally made.
  c. Checks bulletin boards and patient identification boards.
- Manages the unit manager, ward clerk activities.

8. Superintendent of the Department of Nursing—Outpatient Clinics

The major responsibilities of this position are to the chairman of the department of nursing.

- Assigns nursing technician personnel and provides adequate staffing of all outpatient clinics.
- Supervises all nursing technicians assigned to the outpatient clinics where there are no charge nurses.
- Inspects clinics daily and identifies the necessity for rotation of personnel in general therapy clinic and emergency room, for training, and for adjusting schedules to provide for competent patient care at all times.
- Keeps supervisors informed of special abilities of technicians or other pertinent items of special interest.

9. Evening and Weekend Nurse Clinicians

- Organizes, manages, and supervises all nursing activities within the general therapy clinic and the emergency treatment room during the evening (4 PM to midnight) tour of duty and the department of nursing during the day (8 AM to 4 PM) tour of duty on weekends.
- Screens patients, performs nursing procedures and treatments as required, and teaches nursing technicians in the clinical area.
- Coordinates activities within nursing service as senior nurse on duty.
- Provides adequate staffing for all inpatient units for the evening and weekend tours of duty as emergency situations arise.
- Serves as advisor and resource person for nursing personnel on duty as needed.

10. Night Technician of Nursing Services

To fulfill major responsibilities, the night technician of nursing services—

- Provides adequate staffing for inpatient care for the night tour of duty as emergency situations arise, conferring with senior nurse on call as needed.
- Procures supplies and equipment from central nursing sterile supply and other departments as needed by the wards and emergency treatment room.
- Assists with patient care on any inpatient care unit when the situation warrants it.
- Coordinates with admissions and discharges clerk to assure complete data is available for morning report.
- Accounts for administrative activities of nursing service to the chairman of the department of nursing, conferring with senior nurse on call, reporting any unusual problem as situation deems necessary.

Nursing Instructors*

1. Nursing Instructor: Ancillary Nursing Personnel

Job Duties

Plans, coordinates, and carries out educational programs (theoretical and practical aspects of nursing) to train ancillary nursing personnel:

Prepares and issues trainee manuals (which describe duties and responsibilities of nursing assistants) to be used as training guides. Familiarizes new employees with physical layout of hospital and hospital policies and procedures, organizational structure, hospital etiquette, and employee benefits. Plans educational program and schedules classes in basic patient care procedures, such as bedmaking, blood-pressure and temperature taking, and feeding of patients. Teaches Nursing Aides and Orderlies nursing procedures by demonstration in classrooms and clinical units and by lectures in classrooms, using such aids as motion pictures, charts, and slides. Observes trainees in practical application

---

*Source: *Job Descriptions & Organizational Analysis for Hospitals and Related Health Services*, U.S. Training and Employment Service, Department of Labor, 1971.

of procedures. Secures cooperation of Supervisors and Head Nurses to assist in teaching their specialty; coordinates training with all nursing service units to maintain consistency in practice and establish relationships, to give scope to program, and to point out variations of duties required by different units and on different shifts.

Prepares, administers, and scores examinations to determine trainees' suitability for the job. Makes recommendations to nursing service regarding placement of trainees according to test scores and practical application performance. Evaluates trainees' progress following training period and submits report to nursing service for further processing. Conducts meetings with trainees and with supervisors to discuss problems and ideas for improving nursing service training program.

Education, Training, and Experience

Graduation from an accredited school of nursing and current licensure by State Board of Nursing; advanced training in teaching methods and supervision.

One year's experience as Head Nurse or Supervisor Nurse.

2. Nursing Instructor: Inservice

Job Duties

Plans, directs, and coordinates inservice orientation and educational program for professional nursing personnel:

Assists Director of Staff Development in planning and carrying out program of staff development. Confers with Director of Staff Development to schedule training programs for professional nurses already on the staff, according to departmental work requirements. Lectures to nurses and demonstrates improved methods of nursing service. Lectures and demonstrates procedures, using motion pictures, charts, and slides.

Orients new staff members and provides inservice refresher training for professional nurses returning to hospital nursing service.

Instructs volunteer workers in routine procedures such as aseptic practices and blood-pressure and temperature taking.

Education, Training, and Experience

Graduation from an accredited school of nursing and current licensure by State Board of Nursing;

advanced training in teaching methods and supervision.

One year's experience as Head Nurse or Supervisor Nurse.

STAFF POSITIONS*

Unit Manager
(Ward Supervisor)

Job Duties

Supervises and coordinates administrative management functions for one or more patient care units:

Supervises clerical staff and assures accomplishment of administrative functions on a 24-hour basis by scheduling working hours and arranging for coverage of nursing care unit by nonnursing personnel. Performs personnel-management tasks by orienting and training new personnel. Evaluates performance of assigned workers by checking for quality and quantity.

Inventories and stores patients' personal effects either within the unit or in the hospital vault.

Establishes and maintains an adequate inventory of drugs and supplies for the unit.

Coordinates with other departments such as housekeeping and maintenance to maintain a unit that is hygienically safe and functional. Checks for cleanliness of the units and reports discrepancies to the appropriate supervisor. Performs daily maintenance inspection, and through proper channels initiates minor facility improvement projects.

Maintains close contact with medical and surgical reservations in regard to admissions, transfers, discharges, and other services. Serves as liaison between the specific patient care unit and other departments. Reviews special tests at the end of shift.

Insures that the medical record is completed in accordance with the standards of the Joint Commission on Accreditation of Hospitals. Insures hospital compliance with Medicare requirements insofar as certification and related administrative matters are concerned. Checks charts of patients scheduled for surgery or other

*Source: *Job Descriptions & Organizational Analysis for Hospitals and Related Health Services*, U.S. Training and Employment Service, Department of Labor, 1971.

special procedures to verify completeness of orders of consents, preparation of orders, and lab results, and for necessary signatures.

Greets, directs, and gives nonprofessional factual information to patients, visitors, and personnel from other departments.

Participates in projects, surveys, and other information-gathering activities approved by hospital management.

Education, Training, and Experience

One year of college or equivalent.

A minimum of 1 year's supervisory experience.

On-the-job training in coordinating nonnursing services for the assigned nursing units.

Staff Nurse

Job Duties

Renders professional nursing care to patients within an assigned unit of a hospital, in support of medical care as directed by medical staff and pursuant to objectives and policies of the hospital:

Performs nursing techniques for the comfort and well-being of the patient. Prepares equipment and assists physician during treatments and examinations of patients. Administers prescribed medications, orally and by injections; provides treatments using therapeutic equipment; observes patients' reactions to medications and treatments; observes progress of intravenous infusions and subcutaneous infiltrations; changes or assists physician in changing dressings and cleaning wounds or incisions; takes temperature, pulse, respiration rate, blood pressure, and heart beat to detect deviations from normal and gauge progress of patient, following physician's orders and approved nursing care plan. Observes, records, and reports to supervisor or physician patients' condition and reaction to drugs, treatments, and significant incidents.

Maintains patients' medical records on nursing observations and actions taken such as medications and treatments given, reactions, tests, intake and emission of liquids and solids, temperature, pulse, and respiration rate. Records nursing needs of patients on nursing care plan to assure continuity of care.

Observes emotional stability of patients, expresses interest in their progress, and prepares them for continuing care after discharge. Explains procedures and treatments ordered to gain patients' cooperation and allay apprehension.

Rotates on day, evening, and night tours of duty and may be asked to rotate among various clinical and nursing services of institution. Each service will have specialized duties and Staff Nurse may be known by the section to which assigned such as Staff Nurse, Obstetrics or Staff Nurse, Pediatrics. May serve as a team leader for a group of personnel rendering nursing care to a number of patients.

Assists in planning, supervising, and instructing Licensed Practical Nurses, Nursing Aides, Orderlies, and students. Demonstrates nursing techniques and procedures, and assists nonprofessional nursing care personnel in rendering nursing care in unit.

May assist with operations and deliveries by preparing rooms; sterilizing instruments, equipment, and supplies; and handing them, in order of use, to surgeon or other medical specialist.

Education, Training, and Experience

Graduation from an accredited school of nursing and current licensure by State Board of Nursing.

Orientation training in specific unit only; no experience required beyond that obtained in school of nursing.

Ward Clerk
(Floor Clerk, Nursing Station Assistant)

Job Duties

Performs general clerical duties by preparing, compiling, and maintaining records in a hospital nursing unit:

Records name of patient, address, and name of attending physician on medical record forms. Copies information, such as patients' temperature, pulse rate, and blood pressure, from nurses' records. Writes requisitions for laboratory tests and procedures such as basal metabolism, X-ray, EKG, blood examinations, and urinalysis. Under supervision, plots temperature, pulse rate, and other data on appropriate graph charts. Copies and computes other data, as directed, and enters on patients' charts. May record diet instructions. Keeps file of medical records on patients in unit. Routes charts when patients are transferred or dismissed, following specified procedures. May compile census of patients.

Keeps record of absences and hours worked by unit personnel. Types various records, schedules, and reports and delivers them to appropriate office. May maintain records of special monetary charges to patient and forward them to the business office. May verify stock supplies on unit and prepare requisitions to maintain established inventories. Dispatches messages to other departments or to persons in other departments and makes appointments for patients' services in other departments as requested by nursing staff. Makes posthospitalization appointments with patients' physicians. Delivers mail, newspapers, and flowers to patients.

Education, Training, and Experience

High school graduation or equivalent, including courses in English, typing, spelling, and arithmetic, or high school graduation supplemented by commercial school course in subjects indicated.

No previous experience is required.

On-the-job training in practices and procedures of the hospital and certain medical terminology.

Licensed Practical Nurse
(Licensed Vocational Nurse)

Job Duties

Performs a wide variety of patient care activities and accommodative services for assigned hospital patients, as directed by the Head Nurse and/or team leader:

Performs assigned nursing procedures for the comfort and well-being of patients such as assisting in admission of new patients, bathing and feeding patients, making beds, helping patients into and out of bed. Takes patients' temperature, blood pressure, pulse, and respiration, and records results on patients' charts. Collects specimens, such as sputum and urine, in containers, labels containers, and sends to laboratory for analysis. Dresses wounds, administers prescribed procedures, such as enemas, douches, alcohol rubs, and massages. Applies compresses, ice bags, and hot water bottles. Observes patients for reaction to drugs, treatment, cyanosis, weak pulse, excessive respiratory rate, or any other unusual condition, and reports adverse reactions to Head Nurse or Staff Nurse. Administers specified medication, and notes time and amount on patients' charts. Assembles and uses such equipment as catheters, tracheotomy tubes, and oxygen supplies. Drapes or gowns patients for various types of examinations. Assists patients to walk about unit as permitted, or transports patient by wheelchair to various departments. Records food and fluid intake and emission. Sterilizes equipment and supplies, using germicides, sterilizer, or autoclave. Answers patients' call signals, and assists staff nurse or physician in advanced medical treatments. Assists in the care of deceased persons.

May specialize in work of a particular patient care unit and be known by the name of that unit, such as Licensed Practical Nurse, Recovery Room or Licensed Practical Nurse, Psychiatrics.

May be required to work rotating shifts.

Education, Training, and Experience

High school graduation plus graduation from a recognized 1-year practical nurse program. Must pass State Board of Nursing licensing examination.

Nursing Aide
(Nurse Aide, Nursing Assistant)

Job Duties

Performs various patient care activities and related nonprofessional services necessary in caring for the personal needs and comfort of patients:

Answers signal lights and bells to determine patients' needs. Bathes, dresses, and undresses patients and assists with personal hygiene to increase their comfort and well-being. May serve and collect food trays, feed patients requiring help, and provide between-meal nourishment and fresh drinking water, when indicated. Transports patients to treatment units, using wheelchair or wheeled carriage, or assists them to walk. Drapes patients for examinations and treatments; remains with patients, performing such duties as holding instruments and adjusting lights. Takes and records temperatures, pulse, respiration rates, and food intake and output, as directed. May apply ice bags and hot water bottles. Gives alcohol rubs. Reports all unusual conditions or reactions to nurse in charge. May assemble equipment and supplies in preparation for various diagnostic or treatment procedures performed by physicians or nurses.

Tidies patients' rooms and cares for flowers. Changes bed linen, runs errands, directs visitors, and answers telephone. Collects charts, records, and reports, delivers them to authorized personnel. Collects and bags soiled linen and stores clean linen. May clean, sterilize, store, and prepare treatment trays and other supplies used in the unit. May be known by unit or section of hospital to which assigned, such as Nursing Aide, Psychiatric or Nursing Aide, Nursery, where special duties required by patients are performed.

May be required to work rotating shifts.

Education, Training, and Experience

High school graduation preferred.

Hospital-conducted on-the-job training programs. To work in some departments, additional training is given.

Orderly
(Nursing Assistant, Male)

Job Duties

Assists nursing service personnel by performing a variety of duties for patients (usually male) and certain heavy duties in the care of the physically or mentally ill and the mentally retarded:

Performs same job duties as Nursing Aide.

Education, Training, and Experience

High school graduation preferred.

Hospital-conducted on-the-job training programs. For work in some departments, additional training is given.

Surgical Technician
(Scrub Technician)

Job Duties

Performs a variety of duties in an operating room to assist the surgical team:

Assists surgical team during operative procedure. Changes into operative clothing, scrubs hands and arms, puts on sterile gown and gloves. Arranges sterile setup for operation. Passes instruments, sponges, and sutures to surgeon and surgical assistants. Assists circulating nurse to prepare patient for surgery. May assist in positioning patient in prescribed position for

type of surgery to be performed. May assist in preparation of operative area of patient. May assist the Anesthesiologist during administration of anesthetic. Adjusts lights and other equipment as directed. Assists other team members, upon completion of surgery, in moving patient onto wheeled stretcher for delivery to the recovery room. Assists in cleanup of operating theater following operation including disposal of used linen, gloves, instruments, utensils, equipment, and waste.

May count sponges, needles, and instruments used during operation. May prepare operative specimens, place in preservative solution, and deliver to laboratory for analysis. May record data on patients' record data sheets.

May be required to work rotating shifts.

Education, Training, and Experience

High school graduation or equivalent. Some employers prefer graduation from a recognized 1-year practical nurse program.

Hospital-conducted on-the-job training in operating room techniques.

NEED FOR NURSING MANAGEMENT TRAINING*

All too often, nurses are promoted into the ranks of management as a reward and as recognition of the nurse's technical skills. These nurses may be highly skilled and professionally competent, but they may be unprepared theoretically and practically for management responsibilities.

Such managers manage primarily on the basis of previous work experience—doing things correctly, following the right rules, acting the way traditional managers said they should act.

A study of head nurses in general hospitals showed that, prior to becoming head nurses, most had worked as assistant head nurses or charge nurses, but they had not been in programs designed for developmental purposes. The head nurses further stated that their learning process consisted of their own observations and evaluations rather than a planned exchange of information or a development program.

*Source: Juliana Manez, "The Untraditional Manager: Agent of Change and the Change Agent." Adapted, with permission, from an article originally published in *Hospitals, Journal of American Hospital Association*, vol. 52, no. 1, Jan. 1, 1978, © copyright 1978, American Hospital Association.

Nurses in top management positions are equally, if not acutely, affected by inadequate management development programs. A recent study to develop a group profile of contemporary nurse administrators underlines the seriousness of the problem. "Lack of management training" was the most frequently cited deficit in the nursing administrators' analysis.

One survey of directors of nursing in comprehensive health centers gave clear indication of the content and/or experiential areas that would have or had helped these nurses to function in their positions in these new health care delivery settings. The areas indicated were personnel management and human resources development; nursing administration; community organization; political science, termed by some as "practical politics"; program planning and evaluation; teaching methods; nursing care of the family; education and supervision of paraprofessionals; collaboration with consumers; interdisciplinary and interagency communications, cooperation, and flexibility; and orientation toward prevention of illness and promotion of health, rather than toward treatment of illness and meeting crises.

Survey of Supervisors and Head Nurses*

In still another survey supervisors and head nurses revealed that approximately 70 percent felt an urgent need or use for instruction in a full array of management skills techniques. Top priority was given to learning about methods for handling grievances, problem-solving, counseling-guidance and employee-relations. Other subjects deemed necessary, in descending order of importance, were concerned with techniques in motivation, leadership, interviewing, human relations, supervision and communications. Lesser need was expressed for some subjects such as performance evaluation and accident prevention, where a proportion of supervisors had already received training; but even so, over half the supervisors required the subject knowledge. In only two areas was there any significant indication (25 percent) that training really

wasn't necessary: 1. job-evaluation and salary control and 2. personnel interview, recruitment, and selection methods. This may well reflect respectively the lower-management level of the subjects or the organizational system of the individual hospital where personnel selection is centralized.

Despite the issues surrounding the advanced training of nurse leaders, there is a growing consensus that the acquisition of management skills must play a more central role in the education of nurse administrators.

New training programs in nursing administration are now being offered which will ensure that graduates will be able to:

1. employ top level management skills
2. apply management methods to the supervision of nursing personnel and nursing systems
3. utilize systematic techniques to meet professional nursing objectives
4. communicate authoritatively with other managers and professionals in the institution and within the health care field
5. advance the nursing profession by functioning as a knowledgeable leader, an explicator of its services and a supporter of newly researched developments

NURSING SERVICE POLICIES
Policy Development*

There are three general areas in nursing that require policy formulation: (1) areas in which confusion about the locus of responsibility might result in neglect or malperformance of an act necessary to a patient's welfare; (2) areas pertaining to the protection of patients' and families' rights, e.g., right to privacy, property rights; and (3) areas involving matters of personnel management and welfare.

The criteria by which one can judge the appropriateness of departmental policies have to do with the degree to which they facilitate the achievement of the goals of the department. Policies that do this will probably show the following characteristics:

---

*Source: *The Nursing Administration Handbook,* ed. Howard S. Rowland and Beatrice L. Rowland, Aspen Systems Corporation, 1980.

---

*Source: M.M. Cantor, "Policies . . . Guidelines for Action," *JONA,* May–June 1972.

1. The purposes of the policies can be stated in terms of the effects to be achieved as a result of their formulation and implementation.
2. The expected consequences of the policies can be shown to be instrumental toward achieving the objectives of the department.
3. The content of the policies is directly related to their stated purposes and reflects the due consideration given to relevant factors in their formulation.
4. The amount of direction included is based on the level characterizing the position in which the implementation must occur.

Objectives*

Objectives are the fundamental strategy of nursing, since they are the end product of all nursing activities. They must be capable of being converted into specific targets and specific assignments so that nurse persons will know what they have to do to accomplish them. Objectives become the basis and motivation for the nursing work necessary to accomplish them and for measuring nursing achievement.

Management must balance objectives. Some will be short range with their accomplishment in easy view or reach. Others will be long range, and some may even be in the "hope to be accomplished" target date timetable. The budget is the mechanical expression of setting and balancing objectives.

In nursing all objectives should be performance objectives. They should provide for existing nursing services for existing patient groups. They should provide for abandonment of unneeded and outmoded nursing services and health care products. They should provide for new nursing services and health care products for existing patients. They should provide for new groups of patients, for the distributive organization, and for standards of nursing service and performance.

Objectives are the basis for work and assignments. They determine the organizational structure, the key activities, and the allocation of people to tasks. Objectives make the work of nursing such that it is clear and unambiguous, the results are measurable, there are deadlines to be met, and there is a specific assignment of accountability. They give direction and make commitments that mobilize the resources and energies of nursing for the making of the future. Objectives are needed for the department and all wards or units. They should be changed as necessary, particularly when there is a change in mission or purpose or when they are no longer functional.

Operational Plan for Objectives

Objectives must be converted into action: activities, assignments, deadlines, and clear accountability. This is where nurse managers get rid of the old and plan for the new. It is where time dimensions are put into perspective and new and different methods can be tried. It is where nurse managers answer these questions over and over again: What is it? What will it be? What should it be?

An operational plan is the written blueprint for achieving objectives. It tells the activities and procedures that will be used to achieve them. It sets timetables for their achievement. It tells who the responsible persons are for each and every activity and procedure. It describes ways of preparing people for jobs and procedures for evaluating care of patients. It specifies the records that will be kept and the policies needed. It gives the individual manager freedom to accomplish her own objectives as well as those of the institution, department, ward, or unit. It is sometimes called a management plan.

An Example of a Nursing Service's Mission, Philosophy and Objectives*

Purpose or Mission

The mission of the department of nursing is to provide comprehensive nursing care for all patients admitted to the hospital or treated on an outpatient status.

High ethical conduct, loyalty, professionalism, efficiency, and personalized services are expected of each person assigned to the department of nursing. Proficiency must be maintained by continuous inservice programs and individual self-improvement efforts.

---

*Source: Russell C. Swansburg, *Management of Patient Care Services,* St. Louis: The C.V. Mosby Co., 1976, pp. 6–10, 13–19.

The department of nursing has a stated philosophy and objectives. Personnel of each unit within the department will have their own objectives. The objectives will be continuously evaluated, and a written statement as to progress will be sent to the chairman's office each August and February.

Philosophy

1. We believe that the department of nursing possesses the primary responsibility of providing comprehensive, individualized nursing care to the assigned patients, which will aid them in attaining and maintaining a healthy and independent state of mind and body.

2. We believe that the primary function of department of nursing personnel is the welfare of patients and their families. Therefore the whole patient must be considered, and his or her nursing needs must be identified and met—physical, emotional, personal, cultural, social, and rehabilitational. Nursing personnel must seek cooperation of and work with all agencies within the medical center and community in planning for and providing total patient care.

3. We believe that patients' health care needs will best be met by having nursing personnel focus on the primary functions of clinical nursing, that professional nurses will make assessments, nursing diagnosis, and nursing prescription, and will direct and participate in improvement of patient care programs including teaching of them and their families, and that safety factors and patients' rights will at all times be considered.

4. We believe that all nursing personnel should be effectively utilized commensurate with their education, level of training, abilities, and potential, and that their efforts and all nursing service activities will be directed toward the improvement of nursing care.

5. We believe that a continuous program of inservice education for all department of nursing personnel must be provided if the quality of nursing is to be improved and kept current with developments in the medical and nursing fields. All nursing personnel must be encouraged to continue their education.

6. We believe that a continuous evaluation of the activities of the department of nursing is necessary to assess how effectively the needs of the patients are being met and to take action to improve nursing service when indicated. Research must be performed, and the results must be analyzed, adapted, and implemented to modify nursing procedures and practices for the attainment of more effective patient care.

Objectives

1. The patient receives individualized care in a safe environment to meet the total therapeutic nursing needs—physical, emotional, spiritual, environmental, social, economic, and rehabilitative—as diagnosed through nursing assessments.

2. The patient is provided with an effective patient and patient-family teaching program, which will include guidance and assistance in the use of medical center resources and community agencies that can contribute support to his or her total needs.

3. The patient benefits from effective communication, cooperation, and coordination with all professional and administrative services involved in the planning of total patient care.

4. The patient benefits from a continuous, flexible program of inservice education for all department of nursing personnel, adapted to orientation, skill training, continuing education, and leadership development.

5. The patient benefits from supervised on-the-job training programs that will assist nonprofessional personnel in attaining the required proficiency in their designated jobs and in developing their skills for optimum effectiveness.

6. The patient benefits from close nursing supervision of all nonprofessional personnel who give patient care and from continuous evaluation of the nursing care given and of the performances of all nursing service personnel based on professional and medical center standards.

7. The patient benefits from research directed toward the best possible care of the patient and from adaptation and implementation of the results of the research to nursing practices and procedures to attain better care.

8. The patient benefits from the procurement, maintenance, and utilization of supplies and equipment required for activities of the department of nursing to the end that all resources are effectively utilized to achieve high-quality care.

9. The patient benefits from creation of a stimulating work atmosphere in which job satis-

faction is attained, high morale is maintained, and all department of nursing personnel have an opportunity to develop their potential leadership, personal, and professional abilities.

10. The patient benefits from a close association between department of nursing personnel and community nursing organizations and groups to keep abreast of current trends and advancements in nursing.

11. The patient benefits from the direct nursing care hours of all department of nursing personnel by relieving them of nonnursing duties.

12. The patient or his family gives consent to all nursing actions.

Checklist for a General Nursing Service Policy Manual*

The suggested checklist (Table 5-1) is intended as a guide in developing nursing service policies. Though it can scarcely be all-inclusive, it is an indication of the type of material that should be included in a policy manual.

A similar manual should be prepared for each clinical unit which would include those items pertinent to that area.

JCAH Standards for Nursing Services**

Standard I

The nursing department/service shall be directed by a qualified nurse administrator and shall be appropriately integrated with the medical staff and with other hospital staffs that provide and contribute to patient care.

Interpretation

The administrator of the nursing department/service shall be a qualified, registered nurse with appropriate education, experience, and licensure, and demonstrated ability in nursing practice and administration. It is desirable, but not required, that the nurse administrator have at least a baccalaureate in nursing. The nurse ad-

ministrator shall be employed on a full-time basis and shall have authority and responsibility for taking all reasonable steps to assure that the optimal achievable quality of nursing care is provided. When a hospital nursing department/service is decentralized and each clinical department/service has a director of nursing, there shall be one administrator to whom the directors shall be accountable for providing a uniformly optimal level of nursing care throughout the hospital.

A qualified registered nurse shall be designated and authorized to act in the nurse administrator's absence. The organizational structure of the nursing department/service shall provide for appropriate administration of nursing services on all shifts.

The nurse administrator shall have authority and responsibility for assuring that nursing care objectives are established and met, and, in accordance with delegated authority, shall assure that the policies, procedures, and practices of the nursing department/service are consistent with the hospital's goals and with the policies and procedures of the hospital and the medical staff. The development, allocation, and administration of the nursing department/service budget is necessary for the accomplishment of objectives and programs.

The nurse administrator, or an individual designated by the nurse administrator, should represent the nursing department/service in institutional planning and, when requested, should provide periodic reports on the status of nursing care. The nurse administrator should provide any formal liaison required between the medical staff and nursing department/service. Qualified registered nurses shall participate in other patient care activities, including, but not limited to, the infection control committee, the pharmacy and therapeutics function, the medical record function, the hospital safety committee, and, when such exist, the professional library committee, special care unit committee, and emergency care committee. The role of the nursing department/service in the hospital's internal and external disaster plans shall be defined.

When the hospital provides clinical facilities for the education of nursing students, there shall be a written agreement that defines the respective roles and responsibilities of the hospital nursing department/service and of the educational program.

---

*Source: Sr. Jean Marie Braun, S.C.S.C., "A Checklist for Nursing Service Policy Manual," The Catholic Health Association.

**Source: Joint Commission on Accreditation of Hospitals, *Accreditation Manual for Hospitals, 1983*, Reprinted by permission.

Table 5-1 Checklist for a General Nursing Service Policy Manual

1. *Accidents*
   A. Care
      1. Who
         a. Patients
         b. Personnel
         c. Visitors
      2. Where
      3. Whose responsibility
   B. Reporting
      1. Forms
         a. Number of copies
         b. Who fills out
         c. Who receives
      2. Oral
         a. Who
         b. What office
         c. Telephone number
   C. Precautions to prevent
II. *Admissions*
   A. Receiving patients
      1. Information obtained
      2. Instructions given
   B. Notifying
      1. Intern
      2. Doctor
      3. Other departments
III. *Autopsies*
   A. Obtaining permission
      1. By whom
      2. From whom—relationship
      3. Witness
   B. Arrangement
      1. By whom
      2. Use of morgue
IV. *Breakage*
   A. Classification
   B. Responsibility
   C. Reporting
V. *Bulletin Boards*
   A. Location
   B. Posting of information
      1. What
      2. Who
   C. Removing information
VI. *Communicable Diseases*
   A. Types accepted
   B. Where placed
   C. Cared for by whom
   D. Reporting
   E. Immunization of personnel
   F. Isolation techniques
      1. Concurrent disinfection
      2. Terminal disinfection
      3. Gowning and masking

   4. Disposal
      a. Food
      b. Linen
      c. Waste
   G. Visiting
VII. *Complaints*
   A. How handled
      1. Type
         a. Patient
         b. Personnel
         c. Visitors
      2. Kind
         a. Routine
         b. Emergency
   B. Action taken
      1. By whom
      2. When
VIII. *Consents*
   A. Obtaining
      1. By whom
      2. From whom
         a. Husband and wife
         b. Parents
         c. Emancipated minors
      3. For what
         a. Legal responsibility
         b. State regulations
      4. Witness
   B. Filing
IX. *Consultations*
   A. List of required
   B. List of appropriate
X. *Deaths*
   A. Notifying
      1. Who
         a. Doctor
         b. Family
      2. By whom
   B. Care and identification of body
   C. Care of personal belongings
   D. Death certificate
      1. Making out
      2. Signing
XI. *Discharge*
   A. Time
   B. Notifications
   C. Checking of clothes and valuables
   D. Accompaniment of patient
XII. *Doctors*
   A. Relationship with
   B. What to do if they cannot be contacted

XIII. *Doctor's Orders*
   A. Automatic stop orders
   B. Cancellations—surgery cancels all previous orders
   C. Telephone
   D. Verbal
XIV. *Documents, Legal*
   A. Types
   B. Notary Public
      1. When necessary
      2. Where obtained
   C. Who may witness
XV. *Emergency*
   A. Definition
   B. Use of available beds
   C. No available beds
XVI. *Elevator service*
   A. Where
   B. Who
XVII. *Equipment and supplies*
   A. List
      1. Expendable
      2. Non-expendable
   B. Care
   C. Lending
   D. Repairing
   E. Requesting
XVIII. *Fire Regulations; Evacuation; Disaster*
   A. Drills
      1. Frequency
      2. Plan
         a. Who in charge
         b. Departmental instructions
   B. Prevention
      1. Hazards
      2. Extinguishers
         a. Location
         b. Use
XIX. *Funeral Directors*
   A. Notification
      1. By whom
      2. How selected
   B. Release of body
XX. *Flowers*
   A. Delivery
      1. To hospital
         a. When
         b. Where
      2. To patient
XXI. *Interns and residents*
   A. Relationship with
   B. Notification of
      1. When
      2. Where

Table 5-1 continued

XXII. *Information*
A. Nature of hospital information
B. Publication
  1. When
  2. What
  3. By whom
  4. To whom
    a. Press
      1) Name
      2) Telephone number
    b. Police
      1) Station
      2) Telephone number
    c. Relatives

XXIII. *Linen*
A. Distribution
B. Requesting
C. Damaged

XXIV. *Lost and Found*
A. Where kept
B. How long
C. Whose
  1. Patients
  2. Personnel
  3. Visitors
D. Whose responsibility

XXV. *Meetings*
A. Frequency
B. Purpose
C. Types
D. Members
E. Minutes

XXVI. *Mentally Ill*
A. Admission
B. Notification
C. Restraints
D. Supervision
E. Transfer

XXVII. *Messenger Service*
A. Who served
B. By whom
C. Where
D. When

XXVIII. *Night Watchman*
A. Services
B. How contacted

XXIX. *Nursing Care*
A. Borderline functions
  1. Administration and preparation
    a. Intravenous fluids
    b. Blood transfusions
    c. Removing sutures
    d. Applying traction

    e. Acute cardiac care
    f. Other
B. Charting
  1. Forms used
  2. Red and blue ink
  3. Things to note
C. Daily Assignments
  1. By whom
  2. Where
  3. When
D. Dentures
  1. Identification
  2. Responsibility
E. Emergency drug supply
  1. Contents
  2. Responsibility
  3. Location
F. Ice Water
  1. Where obtained
  2. Who allowed
G. Kardex
  1. Use
  2. Sample form
H. Lights out regulations
I. Medications
  1. Card system
    a. Color
    b. Responsibility
    c. Checking
  2. Errors
    a. Correction
    b. Reporting
J. Oxygen
  1. When given without an order
  2. Storage of equipment
  3. Care of equipment
K. Property of patient
  1. Responsibility
  2. Placement

XXX. *Patients*
A. Relationship to
B. Booklet of privileges
  1. Activity
  2. Postal service
  3. Questionnaires
  4. Radios and Televisions
    a. Renting
    b. Time limit
    c. Use in wards
  5. Smoking
  6. Telephones
  7. Tipping
  8. Visiting

XXXI. *Photography*
A. Requesting
B. Consent
C. Ownership

XXXII. *Private Duty Nurses*
A. Cancellation
B. Engaging
C. Obligations to hospital
  1. Reporting
  2. Following regulations
D. Supervision
E. Evaluation
F. Remuneration

XXXIII. *Reasonable and Due Care*
A. Definition
B. Explanation
C. Legal implications

XXXIV. *Release from Responsibility*
A. Abortions
B. Discharges without order
C. Use of electric pads
D. Valuables

XXXV. *Reports*
A. Forms
  1. Number
  2. Where kept
  3. Where sent
  4. Types
B. Responsibility

XXXVI. *Reporting*
A. On and off duty
  1. Information given
  2. Who present
B. Leaving unit
  1. When
  2. To whom

XXXVII. *Restraints*
A. When applied
B. Whose order

XXXVIII. *Safety*
A. Dangerous materials
  1. Drugs
  2. Poisons
  3. Radioactive substances
B. Proper labeling
C. Control
  1. Equipment and appliances
  2. Temperatures
  3. Infections
D. Siderails
  1. Age range
  2. Conditions
  3. Type of patient

(continued)

Table 5-1　continued

4. Where obtained
5. By whom
E. Explosions
F. Smoking
 1. When
 2. Where
 3. Who
G. Disposal
 1. Broken objects
 2. Closed cans
H. Electric cords
XXXIX. *Soliciting and Vending*
A. Tips and gifts
 1. When accepted
 2. By whom
B. Vending
 1. When
 2. Who
XL. *Suicide*
A. Reporting
 1. To whom
 2. By whom
B. Forms necessary
XLI. *Suspicious Persons*
A. Who to notify
B. Telephone number
XLII. *Telephone*
A. Use
 1. Personal
 2. Patients
 3. Visitors
B. Handling of incoming and outgoing calls
XLIII. *Taxi or Ambulance Service*
A. Service
B. How obtained
XLIV. *Transfer of Patients*
A. Within the hospital
 1. Clearing house
 2. Reasons
 3. Special care units
B. From hospital
 1. Who contacted
 2. Responsibility
XLV. *Unusual occurrences*
A. Report
 1. To whom
  a. Day
  b. Evening
  c. Night
 2. Number of copies
  a. Where send
  b. By whom
B. Emergency action

XLVI. *Visitors*
A. Hours
B. Number
C. Children
D. Special requests
XLVII. *Wills*
A. Drawing up
B. Witnessing
 1. Who
 2. When

Interdepartmental

Interdepartmental policies are in keeping with overall hospital policies, thus ensuring unity and harmonious relationships among departments. The nursing unit will endeavor to make good use of the professional and technical services which render help to the patient. This requires a clear understanding of how these services can be carried out smoothly to the betterment of all concerned. Coordination of all their activities in obtaining the same final goal may be reached by the use of written policies.

I. *Admitting Office*
A. Admissions
 1. Type of patients
 2. Time
  a. Elective surgery
  b. Medical care
 3. Reservations
  a. When made
  b. How long
 4. Identification of patient
  a. How
  b. When
 5. Signing of consents
 6. Accompanying patient to unit
B. Transfers
 1. Requests
 2. Departments to be notified
C. Discharges
 1. Notification
 2. Request for transportation
II. *Barber and Beautician Service*
A. Arrangements
 1. How contacted

2. Time
  a. Bed patients
  b. Ambulatory patients
B. Remuneration
 1. Paying patients
 2. Service patients
III. *Blood Bank*
A. Obtaining
 1. Written requisition
  a. What information
  b. Number of copies
 2. Issuance
  a. By whom
   1) Day
   2) Evening
   3) Night
  b. Re-checking information
B. Reactions
 1. Who notified
 2. Records filed
C. Replacement
 1. Time
 2. Who
 3. Where
IV. *Cafeteria*
A. Hours
B. Late meals
C. Who may use
D. Removal of food
V. *Cashier's Office*
A. Notification of discharge
B. Check-out time
C. Information given
D. Valuables
 1. Safe-keeping
 2. Receipt
VI. *Dietary*
A. Requisitions
 1. New diets
  a. Therapeutic
  b. House
 2. Extra nourishments
 3. Discharge diets
 4. Change in diet
 5. Late meals
B. Tray service
C. Dish room
VII. *Electrocardiograms*
A. Requisition
 1. Routine
 2. Emergency
B. Bed or ambulatory patients
VIII. *Health Service*
A. Hours

Table 5-1   continued

B. Types of service
  1. Routine
  2. Emergency
C. Who may use

IX. *Housekeeping*
  A. Assignments
  B. Inspections
  C. Responsibility
  D. Cleaning of patients' rooms
    1. How notified
      a. Daily
      b. After discharge
    2. Precautions to be taken

X. *Laboratory*
  A. Requisition
    1. Routine orders
    2. Emergency orders
      a. Who to call
      b. Where
  B. Charting
    1. Hours
    2. By whom
  C. Manual for nurse's responsibilities

XI. *Laundry*
  A. Issuance
    1. Routine
    2. Emergency
  B. Disposal of soiled linen
  C. Special items
    1. Uniforms
    2. Patient's clothes
  D. Safeguards

XII. *Maintenance*
  A. Requisitions
    1. Routine
    2. Emergency
  B. Inspection of units
  C. Movable articles, care of

XIII. *Medical Library*
  A. Hours
  B. Who may use
  C. Overdues

XIV. *Medical Record Library*
  A. Medical Record
    1. How compiled

  2. Whose property
  3. Return of completed record
  4. Previous admissions
  5. Nurse's responsibility
  B. Late reports
  C. Release of information

XV. *Occupational Therapy*
  A. Hours of service
  B. Requisitions
  C. Kinds of activities
    1. Ambulatory patients
    2. Bed patients

XVI. *Patient's Library*
  A. Hours
  B. Time limits
  C. Service
    1. Ambulatory
    2. Bed patients
  D. Overdue books
  E. Damage or loss of books

XVII. *Personnel Department*
  A. Requisition for personnel
    1. Replacement
    2. New employee
  B. Interviewing
    1. Pre-employment
    2. Post-employment
  C. Record keeping
  D. Assistance given personnel
    1. Counseling
    2. Grievances
    3. Health and Welfare program
    4. Training
  E. Job analysis and specifications
  F. Personnel policies
  G. General orientation

XVIII. *Pharmacy*
  A. Hours of service
    1. Day
    2. Evening
    3. Night

B. Ordering of drugs
  1. Unit supply
  2. Prescription orders
C. Narcotic and barbiturate regulations
D. Label changing
E. Inspection of stock drugs and solutions on units
  1. How often
  2. By whom
F. Safety precautions

XIX. *Physical Therapy*
  A. Hours of service
  B. Requisitions
  C. Types of treatments

XX. *Purchasing Department*
  A. Hours of service
  B. Requisitions
    1. Routine
    2. Emergency
    3. Types
    4. Number of copies
  C. Back orders

XXI. *Social Service*
  A. Hours of service
  B. Referrals
    1. By whom
    2. Who
  C. (Contact) agencies contacted

XXII. *X-Ray*
  A. Requisition
    1. Information necessary
    2. Time
      a. Routine
      b. Emergency
        1) Who contacted
        2) Where
  B. Preparation of patient
    1. Details in procedure manual
      a. Prepared by x-ray
      b. Kept on nursing units
  C. Notification of unit
    1. Before and after x-ray
      a. Who
      b. When
    2. Cancellation of x-ray

Source: Sr. Jean Marie Braun, S.C.S.C., "A Checklist for Nursing Service Policy Manual," The Catholic Health Association.

Standard II

The nursing department/service shall be organized to meet the nursing care needs of patients and to maintain established standards of nursing practice.

Interpretation

The nursing department/service shall have a written organizational plan that delineates lines of authority, accountability, and communication. The manner in which the nursing department/service is organized shall be consistent with the variety of patient services offered and the scope of nursing care activities.

The nursing department/service shall be organized to assure that nursing management functions are effectively fulfilled. Nursing management functions shall include at least the following:

- Reviewing and approving policies and procedures that relate to the qualifications and employment of nursing department/service members.
- Establishing standards of nursing care and mechanisms for evaluating such care. This shall include the conduct of nursing monitoring functions and any review and evaluation performed to assess the quality and appropriateness of nursing care provided.
- Accounting for professional and administrative nursing staff activities. This includes receiving and, as necessary, acting upon the reports and recommendations of nursing department/service committees and other committees concerned with patient care.
- Implementing the approved policies of the nursing department/service.
- Appointing committees, as needed, to conduct nursing department/service functions. The purpose and function of each standing committee shall be defined and a record of its activities shall be maintained.
- Encouraging nursing staff personnel to participate in staff education programs and attend required meetings.

Appropriate nursing department/service personnel should meet as often as necessary, but not less than six times a year, to identify problems in the provision of nursing care and propose solutions, taking into consideration the findings from relevant nursing care monitoring and evaluation activities. This function may be performed on a department/service/unit level and should be carried out in a manner suitable to the hospital. A record shall be maintained that documents any resultant recommendations or proposed actions.

The nursing staff shall be involved in the accreditation process, including participation in the hospital survey and the summation conference.

All individuals, including graduates of foreign nursing schools and nursing personnel from outside sources, utilized in a registered nurse capacity shall be fully licensed by the state or shall have a current temporary license with a stated expiration date. There shall be a method for follow-up on temporary licenses.

Performance Appraisal A written evaluation of the performance of registered nurses and ancillary nursing personnel shall be made at the end of the probationary period and at a defined interval thereafter. An annual evaluation is recommended. The evaluation must be criteria-based and shall relate to the standards of performance specified in the individual's job description. Job descriptions for each position classification shall also delineate the functions, responsibilities, and specific qualifications of each classification, and shall be made available to nursing personnel at the time they are hired and when requested. Job descriptions shall be reviewed periodically and revised as needed to reflect current job requirements.

Outside Sources When outside agencies, registries, or other sources of temporary nursing personnel are used by the nursing department/service to meet nurse staffing needs, the registered nurses and ancillary nursing personnel from such outside sources ordinarily shall be evaluated by the hospital nursing department/service through its designated mechanism. If evaluation is performed by the outside source, the mechanism for evaluation and verification of its use must be available and acceptable to the hospital. When an appropriate evaluation has not been accomplished prior to the individual's working in the hospital, the assignment of such nurses shall be limited to units that are supervised by an experienced registered nurse from the hospital nursing staff on duty at the time.

Standard III

Nursing department/service assignments in the provision of nursing care shall be commensurate with the qualifications of nursing personnel and shall be designed to meet the nursing care needs of patients.

Interpretation

A sufficient number of qualified registered nurses shall be on duty at all times to give patients the nursing care that requires the judgment and specialized skills of a registered nurse. Nursing personnel staffing shall also be sufficient to assure prompt recognition of an untoward change in a patient's condition and to facilitate appropriate intervention by the nursing, medical, or hospital staffs. In striving to assure optimal achievable quality nursing care and a safe patient environment, nursing personnel staffing and assignment shall be based at least on the following:

- A registered nurse plans, supervises, and evaluates the nursing care of each patient;
- To the extent possible, a registered nurse makes a patient assessment before delegating appropriate aspects of nursing care to ancillary nursing personnel;
- The patient care assignment minimizes the risk of the transfer of infection and accidental contamination;
- The patient care assignment is commensurate with the qualifications of each nursing staff member, the identified nursing needs of the patient, and the prescribed medical regimen;
- Responsibility for nursing care and related duties is retained by the hospital nursing department/service when nursing students and nursing personnel from outside sources are providing care within a patient care unit.

The nursing department/service shall define, implement, and maintain a system for determining patient requirements for nursing care on the basis of demonstrated patient needs, appropriate nursing intervention, and priority for care. Specific nursing personnel staffing for each nursing care unit, including, as appropriate, the surgical suite, obstetrical suite, ambulatory care department/service, and emergency department/ service, shall be commensurate with the patient care requirements, staff expertise, unit geography, availability of support services, and method of patient care delivery. The hospital admissions system should allow for input from the nursing department/service in coordinating patient requirements for nursing care with available nursing resources.

Only qualified registered nurses shall be assigned to head nurse/supervisor and circulating nurse positions in the surgical and obstetrical suites. An operating-room technician may assist in circulating duties under the direct supervision of a qualified registered nurse.

Standard IV

Individualized, goal-directed nursing care shall be provided to patients through the use of the nursing process.

Interpretation

The nursing process (assessment, planning, intervention, evaluation) shall be documented for each hospitalized patient from admission through discharge. Each patient's nursing needs shall be assessed by a registered nurse at the time of admission or within the period established by nursing department/service policy. These assessment data shall be consistent with the medical plan of care and shall be available to all nursing personnel involved in the care of the patient.

A registered nurse must plan each patient's nursing care and, whenever possible, nursing goals should be mutually set with the patient and/or family. Goals shall be based on the nursing assessment and shall be realistic, measurable, and consistent with the therapy prescribed by the responsible medical practitioner. Patient education and patient/family knowledge of self-care shall be given special consideration in the nursing plan. The instructions and counseling given to the patient must be consistent with that of the responsible medical practitioner. The plan of care must be documented and should reflect current standards of nursing practice. The plan shall include nursing measures that will facilitate the medical care prescribed and that will restore, maintain, or promote the patient's well-being. As appropriate, such measures should include physiological, psychosocial, and environmental factors; patient/family education; and patient discharge planning. The scope

of the plan shall be determined by the anticipated needs of the patient and shall be revised as
the needs of the patient change. Exceptions to
the requirement for a care plan shall be defined
in writing.

Documentation of nursing care shall be pertinent and concise, and shall reflect the patient's
status. Nursing documentation should address
the patient's needs, problems, capabilities, and
limitations. Nursing intervention and patient response must be noted. When a patient is transferred within or discharged from the hospital, a
nurse shall note the patient's status in the medical record. As appropriate, patients who are discharged from the hospital requiring nursing care
should receive instructions and individualized
counseling prior to discharge, and evidence of
the instructions and the patient's or family's understanding of these instructions should be
noted in the medical record. Such instructions
and counseling must be consistent with the responsible medical practitioner's instructions.

The nursing department/service is encouraged to standardize documentation of routine elements of care and repeated monitoring of, for
example, personal hygiene, administration of
medication, and physiological parameters.

Standard V

Nursing department/service personnel shall be
prepared through appropriate education and
training programs for their responsibilities in the
provision of nursing care.

Interpretation

Education/training programs for nursing depart-
ment/service personnel shall be ongoing and designed to augment their knowledge of pertinent
new developments in patient care and to maintain current competence. The scope and complexity of the program shall be based on the documented educational needs of nursing staff
personnel and the resources available to meet
those needs. The needs shall be identified, at
least in part, through the findings of the review
and evaluation of nursing care and nursing de-
partment/service monitoring activities. The extent of participation of each nursing staff member shall be documented.

The individual responsible for developing and
coordinating nursing educational/training programs should be knowledgeable in educational

methods and current nursing practice. Registered nurses who provide direct patient care
shall contribute to such programs. An evaluation of the educational activities should be performed periodically. The educational programs
shall include instruction in safety and infection
control requirements.

Cardiopulmonary resuscitation training shall
be conducted as often as necessary, but not less
than annually, for appropriate nursing staff
members who cannot otherwise document their
competence.

Nursing department/service personnel, at
least on the supervisory level, should also participate in outside meetings that are relevant to
their patient care responsibilities, and such participation should be documented. Nursing staff
members should be encouraged to participate in
any available pertinent self-assessment programs.

New nursing department/service personnel
shall receive an orientation of sufficient duration
and content to prepare them for their specific
duties and responsibilities in the hospital. The
orientation shall be based on the educational
needs identified by assessment of the individual's ability, knowledge, and skills. Any necessary instruction shall be provided nursing service personnel before they administer direct
patient care. Prior to their performing nursing
functions within a patient care area, nursing personnel who are not hospital employees must be
provided any required orientation by the nursing
department/service.

Pertinent professional books and current
nursing periodicals should be made available to
nursing personnel. Appropriate reference material should be made available to each patient
care unit.

Standard VI

Written policies and procedures that reflect optimal standards of nursing practice shall guide the
provision of nursing care.

Interpretation

Written standards of nursing practice and related policies and procedures shall define and
describe the scope and conduct of patient care
provided by the nursing staff. These standards,
policies, and procedures shall be reviewed at
least annually, revised as necessary, dated to

indicate the time of the last review, signed by the responsible reviewing authority, and implemented. Nursing department/service policies and procedures shall relate at least to:

- assignment of nursing care consistent with patient needs, as determined by the nursing process;
- acknowledgement, coordination, and implementation of the diagnostic and therapeutic orders of medical staff members;
- medication administration;
- confidentiality of information;
- the role of the nursing staff in discharge planning;
- the role of the nursing staff in patient and family education;
- maintenance of required records, reports, and statistical information;
- cardiopulmonary resuscitation;
- patient, employee, and visitor safety; and
- the scope of activity of volunteers or paid attendants.

Additional policies and procedures are usually required for units in which special care is provided. Current hospital and medical staff policies and procedures that affect the nursing staff's provision of care shall also be available in each patient care area.

Standard VII

The nursing department/service shall provide mechanisms for the regular review and evaluation of the quality and appropriateness of nursing department/service practice and functions. Such mechanisms shall be designed to attain optimal achievable standards of nursing care.

Interpretation

The nurse administrator shall be responsible for assuring that a review and evaluation of the quality and appropriateness of nursing care is accomplished in a timely manner. The review and evaluation may be performed by the nursing department/service as a whole, by a designated representative committee, or by the professional nursing staff assigned to clinical departments, services, or units. When possible, nursing quality assurance efforts should be integrated with similar activities in the hospital. The review and evaluation shall be based upon written criteria, shall be performed at least quarterly, and should

examine the provision of nursing care and its effect on patients. Methods of review and evaluation may include, but are not necessarily limited to, patient observation or interview, specific monitoring functions, or use of the patient medical record. Nursing staff personnel who provide patient care shall participate in the review. When possible, the medical record department should help the nursing department/service perform medical record functions related to the nursing department's/service's review of nursing care. The quality and appropriateness of nursing care provided by personnel who are not hospital employees, that is, those obtained through agencies, registries, or other outside sources, shall be included in the regular review and evaluation of nursing care.

A mechanism shall be designed to assure that pertinent findings from the evaluation of nursing care are disseminated within the nursing department/service, and that appropriate action is taken.

Nurse Licensure*

Licensing Boards

The common organizational pattern of nurse licensing authority in each state establishes a separate board, organized and operated within the guidelines of specific legislation, to license all professional and practical nurses. Each board is in turn responsible for the determination of eligibility for initial licensing and relicensing; for the enforcement of licensing statutes, including suspension, revocation, and restoration of licenses; and for the approval and supervision of training institutions.

The governor of the state generally appoints the members of the nurse licensing board. Although many state nurse licensing boards still adhere to their own standards for accreditation, an increasing number of boards now accept standards established by professional nursing associations and national accrediting agencies. This trend toward application of a national standard has tended to standardize the program of instruction at nursing schools.

Many nurse licensing acts permit the substitution of actual work experience for certain educational requirements.

---

*Source: George D. Pozgar, *Legal Aspects of Health Care Administration,* Aspen Systems Corporation, 1979.

For nurse licensure, each state requires that the applicant pass an examination—usually written, although it may be oral, practical, or a combination—generally administered twice a year. The examinations may be formulated completely by the nurse licensing board, or they may consist in whole, or part, of material prepared by professional examination services or national examining boards. Some states will waive their written examination for applicants who present a certificate from a national nursing examination board.

Suspension and Revocation

All nurse licensing boards have the authority to suspend or revoke the license of a nurse who is found violating specified norms of conduct. Such violations may include procurement of a license by fraud; unprofessional, dishonorable, immoral, or illegal conduct; performance of specific actions prohibited by the act; and malpractice. Minimum due process standards must be maintained. These include: (1) notifying the nurse of the charges, with enough certainty and definiteness so the nurse is able to prepare a defense, and (2) holding a hearing at which the nurse is permitted to present evidence. The hearing does not have to conform to full judicial hearings, but the final order must spell out the grounds for any action taken.

Several states have a great number and variety of grounds for revoking a nurse's license to practice. For example, revocation of license has been warranted when a nurse removed drugs from the employer's supply without authorization or for an unauthorized use, and when a nurse's interference in matters concerning the treatment of patients tended to promote friction between physicians and their patients.

Scope of Practice Issues

A matter of considerable concern to many professional nurses is whether some of their patient care activities infringe upon the area of practice reserved by state licensing legislation for physicians only. The question can arise in almost any patient care setting, but it has been raised most frequently in regard to the emergency room and special care units such as the coronary care unit. A nurse may believe that the assigned duties and functions imply that the nurse is being called upon to make medical diagnoses and select ther-

apeutic measures, which are basic elements of medical practice. However, a nurse who engages in activities beyond the legally recognized scope of practice runs the risk of prosecution for violating the state medical practice act; the hospital that employs the nurse could also be held criminally responsible for aiding and abetting the illegal practice of medicine.

In addition to the risk of criminal prosecution, the risk of civil liability for harm suffered by a patient may be enhanced in a suit alleging negligence if the nurse has exceeded the legal scope of nursing. However, the nurse who follows medically established guidelines applicable to factual situations and is qualified to recognize these situations is not engaging in the illegal practice of medicine. A nurse carrying out medical standing orders, in a situation where the nurse is allowed to determine the existence of specified conditions indicating the need to execute the orders, is generally recognized as functioning within the scope of professional nursing practice.

The trend is clearly toward greater flexibility in assigning responsibilities to nurses. The focus is on the individual nurse's competence, in light of education and experience, to fulfill the responsibilities without increased risk to patients. Interpreting the definitions of practice in licensing legislation has become less important. The role of the nurse is rapidly expanding due to a shortage of primary physicians in certain rural and inner city areas, ever-increasing specialization (i.e. Intensive Care Unit and Coronary Care Unit), improved technology and public demand.

ORGANIZATION

Decentralized Organization Models

1. Staff Assistant Method*

At The New York Hospital supervisor (line) positions were eliminated and a new set of staff positions were created. These staff assistants were to function in an advisory and auditing capacity. They would report to the Nursing Department Head and maintain a staff relationship

*Source: Nursing Staff, New York Hospital, "Patient Care Management," *Nursing Clinics of North America,* June 1973.

with the head nurses. An organizational chart was drawn up (see Figure 5-1) and the supervisors were evaluated and given a chance to choose their area of preference with the requirement that they substantiate their choice. (In contrast, see the Traditional Centralized Nursing Service organizational chart in Figure 5-2.) The following staff positions were created:

● *Staff Assistant for Personnel*

The Staff Assistant for Personnel is a resource person to the head nurse in matters of time planning and the most effective use of personnel. She is responsible for selecting slates of applicants from which the head nurses make the final selection, and for variable staffing procedures suitable to census-imposed cost-control needs.

● *Staff Assistant for Logistics*

The Staff Assistant for Logistics and Equipment functions as a resource person in all departmental matters of equipment and supplies. She plans with the other assistants for the most efficient method for installing and implementing department-wide standardization and improvement

programs. The Staff Assistant is responsible for keeping abreast of the best current practices in her field and making recommendations accordingly.

● *Staff Assistant for Education*

The Staff Assistant for Education is responsible for developing programs and materials for orientation, training, and development of both professional and nonprofessional staff in the department. She is available to guide and counsel the head nurse in the training of her staff. She coordinates affiliating educational programs in the department and participates in hospital-wide educational programs.

● *Staff Assistant for Nursing Practices*

The Staff Assistant for Nursing Practices is responsible for counseling, education, and guidance of head nurses in the use of standard nursing practices. These practices include both hospital and departmental policies and procedures. The development of methods and procedures of patient care involving physical as well as conceptual techniques is equally as important

Figure 5-1 Organization of a nursing department: Staff assistant method

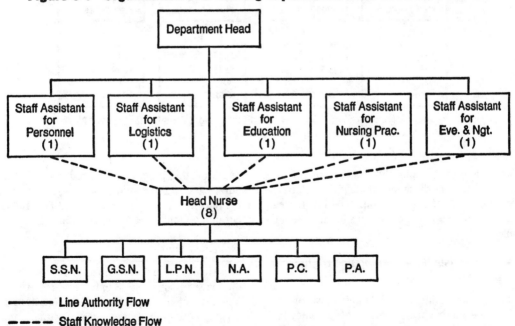

Source: Nursing Staff, New York Hospital, "Patient Care Management," *Nursing Clinics of North America,* June 1973.

Figure 5-2 Traditional centralized nursing service

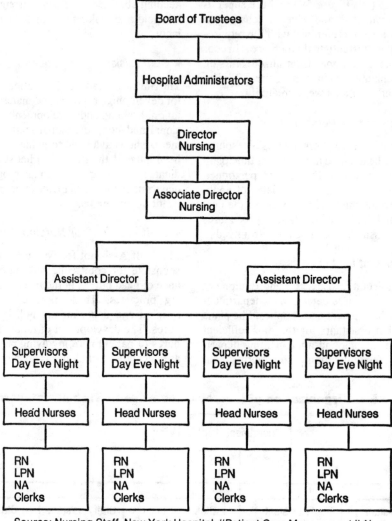

Source: Nursing Staff, New York Hospital, "Patient Care Management," *Nursing Clinics of North America,* June 1973.

as the advisory responsibilities. Essential to the development of these techniques is close collaboration with the other staff assistants, head nurses, and resource colleagues in other departments.

• *Staff Assistant for Evening and Night Operations*

The responsibilities of the Staff Assistant for Evening and Night Operations differ somewhat. She functions as the representative of the Department Head. She is responsible for the conti-

nuity of the programs planned by the head nurses and staff assistants. She also functions as the liaison person who ensures that fast and accurate communications are maintained.

Implementation

The Head Nurse is now directly responsible to the Department Head. She has control over the functions of her unit. She makes decisions regarding both patient care and staff situations as required on the unit. This meant that all staff members on all tours of duty would truly be responsible to their head nurse. The next higher level of authority was the Department Head.

Then introduced were the positions of the staff assistants, who were to be available for guidance and consultation to the line organization and to each other. Each staff assistant individually met with the head nurse group, presenting her job responsibilities with short- and long-range goals. This dialogue gave an opportunity for questions and answers, for the line to express its needs, for mutual expression of expectations, and for discussion of the staff assistants' proposed methods for the accomplishment of these expressed needs. The head nurse then shared this information with her professional and nonprofessional staff, interpreting for them her new role as well as that of the staff assistants.

Another area of responsibility came with the budgetary management of the unit. In the past the head nurse knew the budget existed but not how it was formulated. The Department Head reviewed the head nurse's total budget. Items included were medications, supplies, equipment, and personnel quotas and salaries. As all managers soon learn, she had to live within allotted figures. Here the Staff Assistant for Logistics was available when guidance was needed.

Evaluations of her staff were now the head nurse's responsibility. The head nurse writes the evaluation and holds conferences with each of her staff members. Promotions are initiated by the head nurse and recommended to the Department Head.

The head nurse had the opportunity to be selective when a new staff member is to be added to her unit. She interviews the new applicant and discusses her impressions with the Staff Assistant for Personnel. Together they make a decision.

The head nurse is responsible for orientation and development of her staff. She works in conjunction with the Staff Assistant for Education.

2. Clinical Supervisor Method*

Allegheny General is a 700 bed private voluntary hospital in the metropolitan setting of Pitts-

---

*Source: Doris M. Stitely, "The Role of the Division Head in a Decentralized Nursing Service System," *Nursing Clinics of North America,* June 1973.

burgh. Under its decentralized nursing service system (Figure 5-3) each major clinical nursing specialty has become a division, for example, Division of Medical-Surgical Nursing, Division of Obstetric-Pediatric Nursing, Emergency-Ambulatory Services, Operating-Recovery Room Services, and Inservice Education. The individual divisions function with a high degree of autonomy under the direction of a division head, and with the coordinated efforts of clinical coordinators and clinical supervisors.

Just as each major clinical specialty becomes a division, each patient care area becomes a unit under the direction of a clinical supervisor. The units may vary in patient census and patient care complexity. Therefore, the management aspects will differ from unit to unit in material as well as personnel needs. The clinical supervisor, as the first-level management person, must establish and maintain quotas for supplies and equipment through the Department of Materials Management for automatic delivery service. Other duties are the preparation of personnel time schedules, evaluation of personnel work performance, and the initiation of personnel disciplinary action. The clinical supervisor is expected to make the day-by-day operational decisions that are specific to the individual unit. However, a most important element of these administrative duties is the sharing of information related to the management and operation of each and every unit with the division head. Thus, the lines of administrative responsibility are clinical supervisor to division head to the Department Head.

Clinical Responsibilities

The clinical advantage of a decentralized system is that the key figures in each division are clinically proficient. For example, the division head of medical-surgical nursing must be prepared educationally and with experience in the care of adult patients, while a maternal-child health background is essential for the division head of obstetrics and pediatrics. Another advantage of this system is the ability to utilize a clinical expert who has no administrative responsibilities, that is, the clinical coordinator. This person has the responsibility and the authority to make nursing decisions related to direct patient care. The clinical coordinator may function as a specialist with direct relationships to the patients and families, as a consultant to all staff members

Figure 5-3   Decentralized nursing service

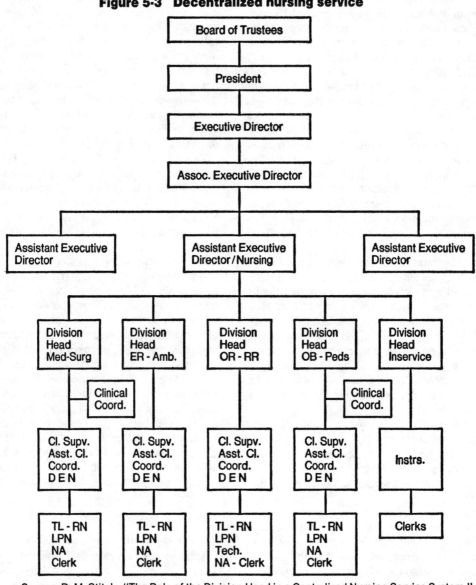

Source: D. M. Stitely, "The Role of the Division Head in a Centralized Nursing Service System," *Nursing Clinics of North America*, June 1973.

for improving nursing arts and skills, and as an evaluator of clinical nursing practice. Thus, the clinical lines of the organizational chart will follow from the clinical supervisor on each patient care unit, to the clinical coordinator in an area of expertise, to the division head, and to the Department Head.

The Division Head

Since the division head has the responsibility and authority for both the management operations and the clinical practice within the specific division, methods must be established to receive unit input, refer information through proper hospital channels, take appropriate action, and respond to personnel. The division head is in the thick of a communication system which must connect all levels of nursing personnel with top hospital management and top management with all nursing personnel. How does one individual meet these obligations? The first step is to establish a means of communicating within the individual division.

Intradivisional Communication

Of course, daily one-to-one contact between people is the most direct method of sharing information. However, this is impossible where patients and personnel are numbered in the hundreds. Daily reports and weekly rounds will permit the average unit problems to be solved. Each morning and afternoon the division head meets with the clinical coordinators and the off-tour assistant clinical coordinators at the divisional intershift reports. During these times the off-tour patient and operational needs are discussed. Following the morning and prior to the afternoon report a brief planning session between the clinical coordinators and the division head will allow for immediate clinical problems to be reviewed and extra supportive staff to be placed where the patient needs are greatest. General management problems may also be processed through the various hospital departments.

The division head schedules rounds with the clinical supervisors of each unit weekly. Other members of the unit staff, R.N.'s, L.P.N.'s, and clinical coordinators, are encouraged to join the rounds. At this time the unit operations are discussed and patients are reviewed.

Although reports and rounds are important for receiving information and establishing a close working relationship between individuals at the unit level, the *monthly operational council* is the most effective tool for intradivisional communication. The council consists of clinical coordinators, clinical supervisors, and representatives from the off-tour assistant clinical coordinators, and the registered nurse and licensed practical nurse staff. It is chaired by the division head. It is through this council that the division head is able to activate problem-solving techniques in a democratic atmosphere.

Interdivisional Communication

The second step in the decentralized nursing service communication system is a mechanism through which all division heads and the Department Head can effectively utilize the divisional input for planning patient care and operational management programs. Many nursing practice procedures and allied health care services are shared by all divisions. Therefore, a close interdivisional relationship must be developed. The Executive Council of Nursing is the method most often used for communication. The participating members are the division heads and the clinical coordinators, and the council is chaired by the Department Head. This group is charged with the responsibility of identifying the strengths and weaknesses of the care delivered to patients. The information from the division's operational council meetings is pooled and more formalized fact-finding programs are generated.

In this decentralized system, the division head becomes the primary participant on the planning committees involving a specific clinical specialty area. Since the lines of communication within the divisions are so direct, the nursing input is realistic from a functional aspect. The division head is also in the advantageous position of promoting nursing to a peer relationship with the medical and administrative committee members rather than the subservient relationship that so frequently exists in a hospital environment. This is sometimes a slow process, but eventually, the clinical knowledge and managerial skills required of the division head in a decentralized nursing service system are recognized and accepted.

Budgetary Responsibilities

The Department Head rather than the division head is the representative to the executive finance committee. However, each division head is delegated the responsibility to prepare a projected yearly budget for her division. Fortunately, the inter- and intradivisional programs can provide necessary facts to justify certain budget requests. Since nursing personnel is the largest item in the hospital budget, the division head will use the information from the activity study to develop a staffing pattern.

The division head also meets with each clinical coordinator and clinical supervisor to determine the major equipment needs. A written justification for additional hypothermia units, pacemakers, or other major items must accompany the request. The routine operational items are also adjusted. The division head makes an estimate of the operational costs by reviewing the expenditures for two previous years.

The final step in the budgetary procedure is to submit the total projected divisional costs with the justifications to the Department Head.

Nursing Service Facilities Design*

Activities and Objectives

Within the Nursing Services Department, activities can be analyzed as to three functions:

Administration. This supports the activity of a department. It consists of offices, files and reception areas.

Functioning Area. This is the prime reason for the department's existence. It occupies the greatest amount of space within a department.

Ancillary. The people who operate the department require convenience space, such as rest area, personal hygiene facilities and a place to eat. Lockers and showers may also be necessary.

As rooms can be collected into departments, so can departments be combined into facilities that have broad common objectives: administrative (management) facilities, diagnostic facilities, treatment facilities, materials management facilities (processing), general service facilities and nursing facilities.

These support areas outnumber the inpatient area and may occupy as much as 70 or 80 percent of the total structure. In the hotel, physically the most similar institution to the hospital, the reverse is true; guest space takes 75 to 80 percent of the whole.

Facilities specifically assigned for use by the Nursing Services Department consist of office space for the director and assistant director of nursing services, nursing stations on each of the patients areas and units that enable the nursing personnel and the medical staff to conduct activities associated with patient care, utility rooms which are in most cases adjacent to the nursing stations and used for storage of needed supplies and portable equipment, linen closets for storage of laundry items, and on two floors small conference rooms seating four to six people and used for medical consultations. Equipment and furnishings are much the same in each of the nursing stations and consist basically of charting desks, patient charts, medicine preparation tables and cabinets, and a minimum of paging and communication equipment. There is some portable equipment such as resuscitators, chest respirators, and irrigation apparatus charged to the department.

The Nursing Unit*

The nursing care of the hospital is organized in a decentralized fashion into patient care units or nursing units. The size of nursing units varies. They can be very small, with 8- to 10-bed units for specialized care, or they can be large, with 60- to 70-bed units. Perhaps the most common size is between 20 and 40 beds per unit. Nursing units operate on three shifts to cover the 24-hour period. They generally operate as a day shift between 7:00 A.M. and 3:00 P.M. The evening shift, called the evening tour, runs from 3:00 P.M. to 11:00 P.M., and the night shift from 11:00 P.M. to 7:00 A.M.

There are disagreements over the most effective way to organize the distribution of patient rooms on a nursing unit. Most rooms are semi-private or multibed accommodations, with two, three, four, or even up to six beds in one room. More recently, there has been a trend toward the private or single-bed accommodation. Studies on efficiency and effectiveness, comparing the private room to the multipatient accommodation, are still being evaluated.

The size of the nursing unit and the distribution of single and multibed rooms are considered before a unit is built. Consideration is given to the cost of construction of the unit, the duplication of equipment, and how much nursing service time will be required to staff the unit. If the unit is spacious and rooms are distributed a distance from the central nursing point, the staff

---

*Source: DHEW.

*Source: I. Donald Snook, Jr., *Hospitals: What They Are and How They Work,* Aspen Systems Corporation, 1981.

must continually travel to reach a patient and supplies. Although the unit may look pleasing, it may not be efficient to work in. There are a variety of designs and configurations for nursing units. Some of the more common nursing unit layouts are shown in Figure 5-4.

Patient Rooms

Whether the patient rooms are private or multi-accommodations, they will vary in size. It has been suggested that the minimum size for a private room should be not less than 125 square

Figure 5-4 Schematic designs for nursing units

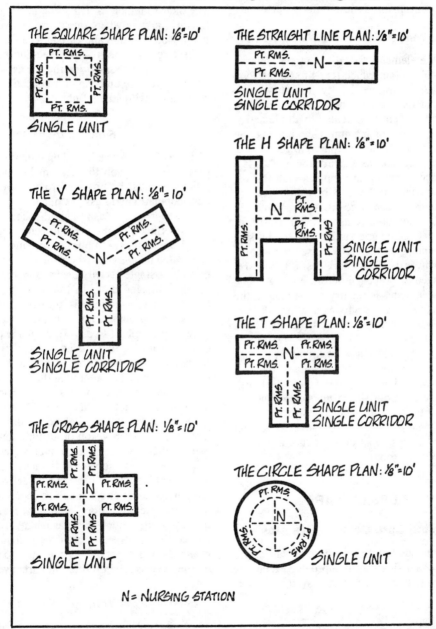

Source: I. Donald Snook, Jr., *Hospitals: What They Are and How They Work*, Aspen Systems Corporation, 1981.

feet with a minimum width of at least 12 feet, 6 inches. As to the two-bed accommodation, a minimum of 160 square feet is usually provided with the beds separated by cubicle curtains. For a four-bed room, the minimum is generally considered to be 320 square feet. The hospital bed is generally 86 inches long, 36 inches wide, about 27 inches from the floor, and can be varied electrically or mechanically into different positions.

Other Components of the Nursing Unit

Among the elements found on nursing units is the nurses' station, which tends to be the focal point of administrative activity. The nurses' station is generally where the nurses keep their records and is centrally located to all the activities of the entire nursing unit. On a nursing unit there is also a medicine preparation room area. Every nursing unit has a utility room. This is a work space where clean supplies, instruments, and equipment and "used" or "dirty" equipment that has been used by the patients are stored. Usually there is also a small pantry, or sometimes even a large kitchen, on the nursing unit, depending on the method used by the hospital to deliver its dietary services. If the food is prepackaged or preplated before coming to the nursing unit, a smaller pantry will suffice. If the food is delivered to the nursing unit in bulk fashion and distributed, there may be a need for a larger kitchen.

Other rooms that might be found on nursing units are a common toilet/bath area (if they are not available individually in the patient rooms), a consultation room where physicians and the families of the patients may meet, and treatment rooms. Some units may also have a pleasant place for visitors to sit down with the patients outside of their rooms.

NURSING CARE

Nursing Care Delivery Systems*

The continuous search for improvement in the delivery of nursing care has provided administrators with four basic model systems: case,

---

*Source: *The Nursing Administration Handbook*, ed. Howard S. Rowland and Beatrice L. Rowland, Aspen Systems Corporation, 1980.

functional, team and primary care. The construction and mechanics of each system reflect a shifting emphasis in the services provided by health care personnel and in the roles of the patient.

Case

The oldest method of delivering nursing care is the *case system* where one nurse is involved in nursing observation and care of a single patient. Considered a one to one relationship, this method is used today primarily for assignments in intensive care units and for educational demonstrations with student nurses.

Functional

The most frequently adopted method is the *functional system* which focuses on the number of tasks that must be provided to the overall patient population and assigns qualified personnel to the appropriate task. This division of labor into interlinking but separate components is based upon the assembly line production concept found in industry, where the worker's repetition of a single activity leads to increased expertise and efficiency. In the nursing unit the breakdown of activities is translated into patient-care assignments which are specific for each staff member: to provide hygienic care, to distribute medication, to administer treatment or therapy, to instruct the patient, to keep records and so on. The central authority resides in the charge nurse who processes all major communications. Though this system has been favored as an economic measure, as in industry, there has been a revision of attitude toward its overall effectiveness in maximum productivity. Comparisons of cost-effectiveness indicate other combinations of nursing care delivery systems are equal to and sometimes superior to the functional method. More important, nurses frequently chafe under this partial involvement, limited to only one aspect of the patient's total health care. Patient-clients are often confused by the endless flow of different care-givers.

Team

The *team system* modifies the depersonalized, skilled-worker approach in a format which focuses on individualized patient health care.

Adopted in the 1950's, this system employs a cluster of health care personnel whose varied skills are directed by a team leader to provide total services for a specific patient case. The formation of a team is a cooperative and collaborative venture which involves a professional nurse capable of leadership and health personnel who are technically proficient in their respective roles and capable of participation in a group effort. The care of the patient is conceived of as a group task, with observations, interpretations and evaluations mutually investigated and shared. The team leader's responsibility is to co-ordinate, supervise and engage the full participation of her co-workers in the construction and implementation of nursing care plans for the well-being of the patient-client. (Patient assignments for teams are made by the charge nurse who also acts as a resource person.)

Primary Care

The most recently developed care delivery method is the *primary care system* which recalls some of the features of the case system but assumes added dimensions in the nurse's increased responsibility in areas such as coordination and range of patient coverage. The primary nurse has full, 24-hour a day, continuous accountability for planning, evaluating and directing the nursing care of a patient case. The primary nurse establishes a direct relationship with the patient, collecting and assessing data, forming plans, making decisions, and representing the patient's total needs in the coordination of activities with other health personnel and disciplines. When she is off-duty, her relief nurse continues to act in accordance with the care plan she has developed. More than one patient case is usually assigned, though this number varies with the nature and treatment of nursing services required and the number of support personnel and systems available in the hospital. The assignment of patient cases is usually the responsibility of the nurse leader who attempts to match professional expertise or special interests with cases. Occasionally the primary nurse is allowed to pick and choose her own patients.

In practice these basic models of nursing care delivery systems have been adapted and altered in new combinations to suit different department needs.

Nursing Care Plans

The following groundwork elements are considered by AHA to be essential to effective utilization of nursing care plans:*

1. Clearly Defined Nursing Care Objectives

Objectives consistent with the purpose and goals of the hospital need to be defined for the nursing service. These will be common objectives for the nursing care given all patients, reflecting what the department of nursing believes good care to be. These objectives should be redefined, in turn, for the several clinical departments and the various patient care units in the hospital. With such overall objectives as guides, the nurse has a basis for determining specific objectives for the individual patient—objectives unique to him and his individualized nursing care needs.

2. Supportive Policies

Seeing and talking with the patient on admission is the first step in the development of a nursing care plan. Does the nurse who will be responsible for the patient's care have the opportunity and responsibility to see the patient as soon as possible after he arrives on the unit? Is she at liberty to talk with the patient, or is she so preoccupied with record forms to be filled out that her initial contact with him is perfunctory or hurried? Admission policies and procedures need to be established to give her the necessary time and opportunity for this important early contact.

There should also be policies delineating the responsibilities and functions of the various categories of nursing personnel. Since nursing care plans include nursing actions to be taken, the responsible nurse must know who can safely carry out the actions and to whom they can be assigned. It should also be understood that the plans cover the full 24 hours of the day. Because the successful development and carrying out of a nursing care plan for a patient depends upon knowledge of the patient's illness as well as on understanding of his background and personality, the nurse must know the physician's plan for

---

*Source: "Practical Approaches to Nursing Service Administration," *Hospitals, Journal of the American Hospital Association,* vol. 6, no. 1, Winter 1967.

care. Therefore the nurse's relationship with the patient's physician and her ability to communicate with him are very important. What are the policies and procedures to facilitate communication between nurse and physician? Do nurses make rounds with physicians? What are the reporting mechanisms? How does the nurse work with other departments involved in the patient's care, such as physical therapy, radiology, dietary, etc.?

3. Administrative Support

If nursing care plans are to be a successful tool in the management of nursing care, the support of hospital administration and of the medical staff is essential. Obtaining this support for the nursing department is primarily the task of the director of nursing, who, as a member of top management and a representative of nursing on patient care and intradepartmental committees, is in a good position to interpret to the administrator and the physicians the aims of the nursing service and the means selected to achieve them.

The director of nursing is also in a position to be influential in bringing about the development of hospital policy and administrative procedures that will facilitate the carrying out of nursing care plans—for example, the procedure for delivery of drugs to the nursing unit; the method of handling patient appointments with radiology; and the policy on control of the progress and sequence of events pertaining to the physician's plan for care.

4. Departmental Policies and Procedures

To facilitate the implementation of nursing care plans, appropriate procedures and policies need to be established within the department of nursing itself.

These should be concerned with such matters as, for example:

- Who has the responsibility for initiating a nursing care plan? (Usually it is the head nurse or team leader, depending on how the service is organized.)
- How are new staff members to be oriented?
- What forms are to be used, and where shall they be kept?
- What disposition is to be made of the nursing care plan after discharge of the patient? Are such plans used for a type of nursing audit?

- What provision is made for periodic evaluation and review of the methods for preparation and use of nursing care plans? What are the supervisor's responsibilities for reviewing and evaluating the plans and for helping the nurse to improve her skill in planning?

Quality of Care

Overview*

Assessing the quality of nursing care is just one part of a total evaluation process. It cannot and does not replace concurrent evaluations or the surveillance of quality in medical record documentation or the vigil to ensure that nursing care plans are maintained and updated. It does not negate patient and physician evaluation or visual observation by supervisors and others. The need for incident reports and investigations remains, as does surveillance work for infection control. Administrative evaluations based on structural standards, such as nursing care hours and income and expense statements, also remain necessary adjuncts.

To assure quality, nursing care must be assessed in terms of outcome, content, processes, resources, and efficiency—in that order or priority.

1. Assessment of Outcome

Quality of nursing care received should principally be measured by the outcome of that care. The assessment of outcome focuses on the alteration in the health status of the consumer. Positive indices that can be used in assessing the alteration in the consumer's health status include the following:

a. An increase in his health knowledge
b. The degree of application of that knowledge
c. The degree of the consumer's participation in his health decision making
d. The degree of responsibility that the consumer assumes for his health behavior
e. His ability to maintain positive health behavior

---

*Source: Wisconsin Regional Medical Board, "Assessing Quality of Nursing Care," *Nursing Administration Quarterly*, Spring 1977.

f. The degree to which the consumer's right to choices that affect his health are assured
g. His ability to utilize health services, both personal and community, with efficiency and economy
h. His ability to function in work and personal roles
i. Longevity

Assessment of the outcome of nursing care also seeks to account for negative outcomes for the consumer of health services which may be attributed wholly or in part to nursing intervention or the lack thereof. Negative indices include the following:

a. Failure to maintain or improve his health status
b. Lack of continuity of care
c. Failure to identify and respond according to factors actually or potentially detrimental to his health
d. Disability
e. Discomfort
f. Dissatisfaction
g. Complications
h. Prolongation of illness
i. Unwarranted death

2. Assessment of Content

Secondly, the quality of nursing care should be assessed in terms of content. Content is the nursing care that is actually given in a specific instance. Content is assessed by the application of standards of nursing practice developed for specific nurse-consumer situations. For example, assessment of content involving a burn patient in an emergency room would differ from an assessment of content involving a coronary patient in the same setting. Similarly, assessment of content to improve the health status of a two-year-old would differ from that of a fifteen-year-old.

3. Assessment of Process

Assessment of process in nursing care focuses on the nature and sequence of events in the delivery of that care. This assessment takes into consideration such aspects as the nature of the interactions among the consumer, nurse, other health care workers, and significant others; the extent to which nursing care objectives have been reached; the specific techniques or procedures used; the degree to which the consumer and significant others have been involved in the entire process; the degree of skill with which nurses have carried out the nursing care as compared with that established by clinical nurse specialists; the coordination among different components of the system and among members of the team; appropriate utilization of each of the available components of the system and the continuity of care.

4. Assessment of Resources

Assessment of resources in nursing care focuses on the properties of the resources used to provide that care and the manner in which they are organized. Nursing care resources include staff, consultants, collaborating disciplines and services, physical structures, facilities, equipment, supplies, administrative structure, operating procedures and policies, and maintenance. A climate conducive to providing quality nursing care is a prime resource. Resources should be evaluated in terms of their accessibility, availability, appropriateness, and acceptability.

5. Assessment of Efficiency

Efficiency is the attainment of quality nursing care reviewed in relationship to the manpower, supply, equipment, space, and other resources of the provider and the appropriateness, acceptability, and cost to the consumer. Efficiency is frequently referred to as the cost-benefit ratio. It is concerned with determining whether there is a less costly way to achieve the same quality nursing care.

ANA Model for Implementing a Nursing Quality Assurance Program*

Many models describe the flow of activities in a quality assurance review process. The ANA Congress for Nursing Practice Model, is a problem-solving process which utilizes process, structure, and outcome criteria as the tools of inquiry.

---

*Source: American Nurses' Association, *Guidelines for Review of Nursing Care at the Local Level,* Bureau of Quality Assurance, DHEW, 1976, Pub. No. (HRA) 76-3004.

1. Identify Values

The first step in implementing this model for quality assurance is to look at social, institutional, and individual values. Any definition of quality implies a consideration of values: What people think of as "good" and as "bad." The values of the culture, the institution, the profession, and the nursing service department will interact to influence the development of the criteria used in the review process. The involvement of nurses at the local level in the establishment of criteria is, therefore, an important aspect of the evaluation system.

For example, identifying values might require consideration of society's values, professional nursing values, and scientific knowledge. A value of the society may be the level of health care the consumers are willing to accept and for which they are willing to pay. Professional values are established standards of the profession, as reflected by such statements as the American Nurses' Association, *Standards of Practice* or the *Code for Nurses With Interpretive Statements*.

Specific institutional values will be reflected in concrete ways in the development of criteria and standards. If a specific nursing service department values prevention as an aspect of patient care, a list of criteria for nursing performance in the gynecology unit might include teaching breast self-examination to each patient.

2. Identify Structure, Process, Outcome Standards, and Criteria

a. Identify the Focus of the Review

Today health is viewed as the ability of the individual to function actively in work, in recreation, and in society. Standards need to be set that define levels of health and establish guidelines to identify how individual patients are progressing toward predetermined goals. These guidelines are developed in the quality assurance review.

The primary purpose of a review system is to assure the patient, the health financers, as well as the profession itself, that patients are receiving health care that conforms to criteria established by nursing peers—care that is effective and efficient. The evaluation can focus on the patients, the providers, or the institution, or in terms of all three simultaneously. The focus will

in part be dictated by the values of the institution and of the individuals within the institution.

If the review looks at the care of patients, the review may be limited to groups of similar patients; or the review may be limited to a specific number of patients. Such variables as age, nursing problems, degree of illness, ecologic factors, or religious orientation may all be used to identify groups of patients.

If the review looks at the nurse, nursing service departments using team nursing may use groups of nurses or patient care units as the focus. Nursing service departments organized using primary nursing or independent nursing practice may use individual nurses as the focus.

If the review focuses on the institution, it may look at the type of services delivered, the administrative structure, the organization, or the flow of activities. In each case, the focus of the review is different. Review of each group will ask different questions and find different answers.

Review committees should be formed within the committee structure of the institution and should carry administrative sanction. Membership on the committee(s) will depend on the focus and activity of the review program. The purpose of the review will dictate whether the committee will be composed of nurses from one specialty (for example, pediatrics) or of nurses from several specialties. A committee limited to practitioners in one specialty would review health care for patients within that specialty. A committee of several specialties might review total care within an institution. Practitioners in similar agencies can form a quality assurance committee within a geographical district.

When institutional review committees are functioning, the results of several institutional groups can be shared. This would result in interagency relationships and might contribute to the development of criteria within a PSRO area.

Multidisciplinary committees composed of representatives from several health professions may pool the results of individual peer review committees and study patient care indepth in one specific area. When the focus of the review is on the patient and criteria are being prepared for health care evaluation studies, multidisciplinary committees would be particularly appropriate. The committee(s) could share in the development of the outcome criteria or coordinate the inclusion of criteria developed by several disciplines into the review process.

b. Identify the Criteria and Standards

After deciding the focus of the review, the patient, the nurse, or the institution, the next step in this review model is to specify the criteria and standards appropriate to evaluate care.

Criteria are defined by the *PSRO Manual* as predetermined elements against which aspects of the quality of a health service may be compared. Criteria are developed by professionals relying on professional expertise and on the professional literature. In a general sense, criteria may be thought of as specific statements of health care that reflect nursing values.

Criteria are statements of structure, process, or outcome that can be measured. For example: (1) Each nurse will have a minimum of 15 continuing education contact hours per year (Structure); (2) A nursing care plan will be written on each patient within 24 hours of admission (Process); and (3) By discharge, patient names medications (Outcome).

By definition:

1. Structure criteria are statements that describe the purpose of the institution, agency, or program. Included are statements about legal authority, organizational characteristics, fiscal resources and management, the qualifications of health professionals and other workers, physical facilities and equipment, and accreditation and certification status. Structure criteria may be written for the patient, for the nurse, or for the institution, e.g., the patient will be situated in a room not less than 10 by 15 feet; the nurse working in a coronary care unit will have successfully completed an ANA approved coronary care course; the institution's staff will have one registered nurse for every ten patient beds.

Other examples of structure criteria can be found in accreditation manuals, in policy and procedure books, and in statements of philosophy and objectives from institutions and nursing service departments.

2. Process criteria focus on the nature, sequence of events, and the activities of health care. Process criteria describe what happens within the institution, during the care and treatment activities, or to the patient, e.g., the patient newly diagnosed as having diabetes mellitus will receive ten hours of instruction; the nurse will collaborate with the patient about his/her nursing care plan; the institution will record data in a problem-oriented system.

3. Outcome criteria pertain to the end results of the health care process and what is focused on the patient. For the patient, an outcome criterion would be a measurable change in the state of his/her health. Outcomes may be positive or negative and are the ultimate indicators of the quality of patient care, e.g., patient has been afebrile for 48 hours before discharge.

If there are existing sets of structure, process, or outcome criteria, the quality assurance review committee will need to decide whether or not modifications are necessary. Whether the review committee writes its own criteria or uses criteria that have already been developed and published, the criteria need to be validated before use in an audit. A common form of validation is by consensus among peers. The rationale for including this step in the identification of criteria is to assure that the criteria are appropriate, relevant, and useful to the nurses working with the subject under review. The nurse who works daily with the content included in the criteria is in the best position to know if the criteria are appropriate and relevant to the group of patients, to the nurses' activities, or to the structural setting.

When criteria have been defined, the review committee needs to agree on the level of performance that will indicate when each criterion has been satisfactorily met. This will establish the *standard* for the review, which, as defined by the *PSRO Manual,* is a professionally developed expression of the range of acceptable variations from norms or criteria.

If a nursing service department decides that each nurse will have a minimum of 15 continuing education contact hours per year, this becomes a structure criterion which defines a level of expected performance. One must then identify an acceptable standard which is the range of acceptable variation from a criterion for a group of patients, providers, or units. If decided that this variation will be satisfactory if 75 percent of the nurses have 15 continuing education contact hours, this is the acceptable standard for the criterion.

3. Secure Measurements Needed to Determine the Degree of Attainment of Standards and Criteria (Gather Information)

The degree to which actual practice conforms to established criteria provides the information used for making judgments about the strengths and weaknesses of nursing practice. Many methods can be used to measure the level of nursing practice according to the established criteria.

The methods include: utilization review, self-assessment, supervisor evaluation, performance observation, and review of records.

Regardless of method, data should be easily accessible and retrievable. The review may either look at what has happened in the past or what is happening in the present. A chart review that looks at what has happened in the past is a "retrospective" review. A "concurrent" review looks at what is happening in the present, that is, while the patient is receiving care.

Specific questions relevant to the topic of study that the review committee needs to answer are:

- What is the source of the data?
- How can the data be collected?
- Who collects the data?
- When can the data be collected?

The answers to these questions should reflect consideration of accuracy and efficiency in data collection.

Each criterion should be stated so that it is possible to recognize immediately whether or not it has been met. The results should be tabulated and a decision made as to whether the percent of yes or no answers corresponds with the standard set for each criterion. When the level of performance does not measure up to the standard established, the criterion for the group has not been met.

4. Make Interpretations About the Strengths and Weaknesses of the Program

The degree to which the identified standards have been met serves as a base for pinpointing the strengths and weaknesses of current nursing programs or practice. Attention must then be given to assure that this information is properly used to effect appropriate changes in practice.

Part of this step involves identifying the factors related to successful or unsuccessful nursing interventions. For example, if one group of nurses meets the criteria for a given group of patients and another does not, a comparison of procedures or practices might provide insight into methods for improving both.

Sometimes the cause may lie outside the area of nursing control—the information may indicate that the problem lies within the administration of the institution (e.g., insufficient nurses) rather than a deficiency in nursing practice (e.g., lack of appropriate knowledge).

5. Identify Possible Courses of Action

When strengths and weaknesses of the nursing practice have been identified, action can be taken to reinforce strengths and to reduce weaknesses. Information from the review should provide a motivation as well as a plan for change. Those who will be affected by this review will see many possible courses of action and should be involved in this process.

The attainment of the standard and available resources serve as the basis for decisions about changes in nursing practice. Alternative actions are numerous. The actions can include continuing education, in-service education, peer pressure, administrative changes, environmental changes, research, reward systems, or self-initiated change. The course of action chosen will be dictated by identified causes of the problem.

Each alternative action will have advantages and disadvantages. Sometimes the mere development of a criteria set by a peer group is enough to change or reinforce the practice of individuals within the group. Likewise, writing of criteria by a multiprofessional group may change the practices of the involved individuals.

6. Choose a Course of Action

After several alternative actions have been proposed and examined in light of existing resources and organizations, the best action is selected for implementation. Decisions need to be made with a realistic consideration of the institution's resources. There may be several contributing causes in any one specific case. Where possible, each of these causes should be identified and action taken to alter each one. In some situations, it will not be possible to clearly identify a single cause for the problem. In that case, many possible solutions will need to be explored and a decision made based on the best possible information.

The individual(s) making these decisions will depend upon the organizational structure of the health setting. The nursing or multidisciplinary review committee may propose several alternatives to the director of nursing or other administrative personnel for final decisions. The authority for action taken may, however, be delegated to the review committee. In such a situation, the results of review and action taken would be provided to the director of nursing and other administrative personnel as points of information. In PSRO review, the results of the nursing review will be incorporated into facilitywide data.

7. Take Action

Improving the quality of care implies a change in behavior. This in turn implies a choice of actions by the decision maker.

Sometimes activities required for change are not controlled by nurses or the nursing service departments. Problems within the organizational structure, such as ineffective policies, inadequate or inappropriate administrators, or environmental conditions should be referred to the appropriate administrators.

Where information is inadequate or skills are lacking, continuing education, in-service education, or staff development will be the appropriate choices. Nurses on the unit may choose to initiate study of a variety of approaches. In-depth studies of the processes of nursing care and the structure in which this care occurs will be frequently appropriate.

8. Reevaluate

At this point, the cycle begins to be repeated. Each time actions are taken, the progress of nursing practice needs to be reassessed and remeasured. Continual reevaluation of practice in light of established criteria and standards can indicate how well a change is progressing and whether the activities taken to implement change are having an effect.

It is particularly important to monitor and document new programs and nursing practice when several actions have been undertaken simultaneously. Decision makers must use cau-

tion in defining a direct cause and effect relationship between a change of policy and a change in behavior of those affected. Careful analysis of the variables in the actions and the results of reevaluation can assure continued improvement of the quality of nursing care.

Difference Between JCAH Approach & ANA Approach

In the JCAH's manual on nursing audit the purposes are:

- To identify those elements of patient care deemed so important that their absence (or presence) serves as a signal that closer examination of a particular chart is warranted.
- To choose standards for the elements and exceptions to the standards.
- To display actual practice data, report variations and appropriate explanations appearing in patient charts.
- To analyze the actual practice and to analyze variations in order to determine justification or deficiency.

The JCAH method is a retrospective approach looking at closed charts. ANA advocates a concurrent approach in the hope that a patient's care will be improved while he is in the hospital. As charts are monitored concurrently, each patient unit will be responsible for evaluating its own care as it is given. An audit committee could be utilized if the individual hospital desired to look at closed charts in order that strengths and weaknesses of practice be identified. In this way, action could be taken to correct deficiencies through educational programs.

- JCAH audit does not concern itself with the total patient; it is only concerned with outcomes of specific diseases.
- The ANA Standards encourage nurses to look at the total patient and his care, to set goals, develop nursing approaches, and evaluate patient responses during hospitalization, to maximize patient capabilities.
- The ANA Standards include guidelines for all patient problems to be assessed, planned for, the plans implemented, and evaluated on an ongoing basis until the problem is resolved or the patient discharged (with referral if needed).

Sources for Development of Criteria and Standards for Quality Assurance*

Four characteristics are desirable in a source: (1) validity, (2) freedom from bias, (3) reliability, and (4) practicality or convenience. The first three are the most important characteristics. Unfortunately, it has been the fourth characteristic, practicality or convenience, that has been used most frequently as the primary determinant of the data source.

Nursing criteria can be derived from many different sources, including of course, methodologies for evaluating quality of care such as CASH, the Veterans' Administration's Nursing Care Quality Evaluation System, the SCALE quality control plan developed at the University of Michigan, and the Quality of Patient Care Scales developed at Wayne State University.

Some other sources include:

American Nurses' Association Publications

- *Code for Nurses with Interpretive Statements,* 1974
- *Guidelines for the Establishment of Peer Review Committees,* 1973
- *Standards of Nursing Practice,* 1973
- *Standards of Geriatric Nursing Practice,* 1974
- *Standards of Maternal and Child Health Nursing Practice,* 1974
- *Standards of Psychiatric and Mental Health Nursing Practice,* 1974
- *Standards of Community Health Nursing Practice,* 1974
- *Standards of Medical-Surgical Nursing Practice,* 1974
- *Standards of Cardiovascular Nursing Practice,* 1975
- *Standards of Orthopedic Nursing Practice,* 1975
- *Standards of Nursing Practice: Operating Room,* 1975
- *Standards of Emergency Nursing Practice,* 1975

National League for Nursing

- *Criteria for Evaluating a Hospital Department of Nursing Service,* New York: National League for Nursing, 1965.

- *Criteria for Evaluating the Administration of a Public Health Nursing Service,* New York: National League for Nursing, 1968.
- *A Guide for Assessing Nursing Services in Long Term Care Facilities,* New York: National League for Nursing, 1968.
- *Standards for Organized Nursing Services,* New York: American Nurses' Association, 1968.
- *New York City Health Code,* New York: The City Record Office, 1964.
- *Quest for Quality: A Self-Evaluation Guide to Patient Care,* New York: National League for Nursing, 1966.

Also:

- Carnegie, M.E. "The Shift of Research Emphasis and Nursing Activity," *Nursing Research,* May–June, 1974.
- Donabedian, A. "Evaluating the Quality of Medical Care," *Milbank Fund Quarterly,* Part 2, July, 1966.
- ———. *Medical Care Appraisal-Quality and Utilization,* American Public Health Association, 1969.
- Haussman, R.K., Director, et al. *Monitoring Quality of Nursing Care Part II—Assessment and Study of Correlates,* U.S. Department of Health, Education, and Welfare, HRA 76-7.
- Joint Commission on Accreditation of Hospitals, *PEP MANUAL,* 1974, *Accreditation Manual* 1978.
- MARCH, The Multidisciplinary Patient Care Audit Project, St. Louis University Hospital.
- Phaneuf, M. *The Nursing Audit: Profile for Excellence,* New York: Appleton-Century-Crofts, 1972.
- Phaneuf, Marie. "Quality Assurance—A Nursing View," *Quality Assurance of Medical Care,* A monograph of the Regional Medical Program Service, 1973.
- "A Plan for Implementation of Standards of Nursing Practice," a report of the Congress for Nursing Practice, 1975.
- Wandelt, M.A., and Ager, J. *Quality Patient Care Scale,* New York: Appleton-Century-Crofts, 1974.
- Wisconsin Regional Medical Program and University of Wisconsin. *Development of Health Outcome Criteria by a Panel of*

---

*Source: *The Nursing Administration Handbook,* ed. Howard S. Rowland and Beatrice L. Rowland, Aspen Systems Corporation, 1980.

Nurse Experts. (Project No. 7) Madison: The Program, 1974.

- Zimmer, Marie J. *Manual: Nursing Quality Assurance*. Madison: University of Wisconsin Hospitals, 1976.

Patient Discharge Planning*

Since nurses have continuous contact with the patient, his family, the doctor, and other personnel participating in his care, they have an opportunity to learn the various expectations and plans each of these people have for the patient's aftercare. Nurses have the opportunity to pull these expectations and plans together, to point out the discrepancies as well as the areas of agreement, and to determine feasibility in terms of resources available outside the hospital. The question, then, is not, Whose responsibility is discharge planning?—everyone is doing discharge planning—but rather, Whose responsibility is the *coordination* of discharge planning? This question can be answered quickly and without hesitation—this is a nursing responsibility.

The sequence of a formal discharge planning process is illustrated in Figure 5-5.

Goals

For the Patient

Benefits will be realized by all involved in the patient planning process if the following patient-centered goals are achieved:

Coordinate the stages of care between illness and recovery

Establish sound admission procedures and policies

Prepare procedures which allow for easy transfer from:

a. An acute unit to another unit within the facility

b. The hospital to home and from home back into the health system

c. One institution to another in the community which will better meet his service needs

___

*Source: Opal Bristow, Carol Stickey, and Shirley Thompson, *Discharge Planning for Continuity of Care*, National League for Nursing, 1976. Pub. No. 21-1604.

Involve the patient and his family in the planning process

Move patient information smoothly and completely to and from various levels of care

Counsel patient and family about facilities and services available to meet physical, social and psychological needs

Strive to attain the development of a unique plan of continuing care for each new patient

Assist the person in returning to society to assume as normal and productive a role as possible

For the Team

Action goals which center on the various members of the professional discharge planning team are as follows:

Initiate discharge plans and teaching of self-care as soon as possible after admission

Maintain current knowledge of available health providers, programs and resources

Identify the need for establishment of new community services and resources

Promote an effective liaison with patient service personnel by written and verbal communication

Furnish utilization data to facility and health planners

Prevent hospitalization benefits such as financial, medical and therapeutic care from being lost

Select the most economical and qualified plan for discharge

Mobilize community resources for specific patient needs

Planning

Discharge planning is dependent upon the following six variables:

1. Degree of illness, health
2. Expected outcome of care
3. Duration or length of care needed
4. Types of services required
5. Addition of complications
6. Resources available

Continuity of patient care must be planned for. Every patient should have the opportunity to reach his maximum potential for recovery. Planning for continuity of care includes planning for the transfer of patients between units within a hospital or nursing home; planning for dis-

Figure 5-5   Discharge planning process

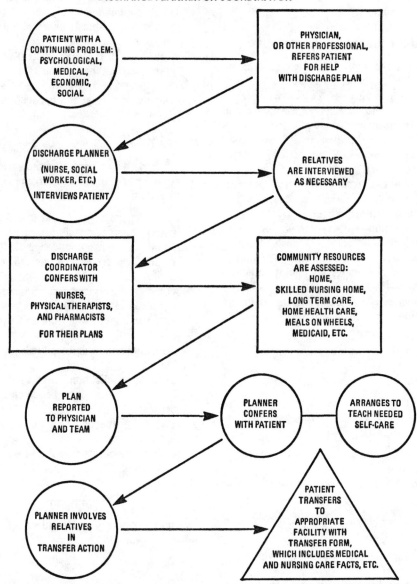

DISCHARGE PLANNING PROCESS
FOR THE
DISCHARGE PLANNER OR COORDINATOR

Source: Opal Bristow, Carol Stickey, and Shirley Thompson, *Discharge Planning for Continuity of Care,* National League for Nursing, 1976, Pub. No., 21-1604.

charge of a patient from the hospital to the home or to another care facility; and planning for use of resources within the community that supplement and reinforce the discharge planning activities of the hospital, nursing home and other post-hospital care facilities.

Nursing Administrator's Role

Without nursing support, the person designated as discharge planner cannot function effectively. The Nursing Service Director should promote an understanding of the needs of such a program:

- Must budget time and money for implementation of a discharge planning program.
- Must provide nursing leadership and involvement in order to insure continuity of patient care. Problems and procedures should be standard items on the staff conference agenda.
- Must require that discharge planning procedures be written and included in a Procedure or Policy Book. They should include these educational concepts:
  - —Provision for someone on the nursing staff to assume responsibility for (1) evaluation of the nursing referral system, (2) development of a program of education and (3) liaison with the administrator of the facility's discharge service
  - —Goals specifically related to: teaching nurses the mechanics of making a referral, clarifying their understanding of home health aides and homemaker services and increasing their awareness of potential candidates
  - —Assistance in eliciting involvement of the physician and paramedical personnel when planning the discharge
  - —Assistance in understanding how nursing's role in discharge planning fits into the institution's total program

A procedure manual should be on every unit. Specifically, information on the mechanics of making a referral, an outline of suggested nursing information to complete a referral and a list of available nursing agencies with their services, addresses and telephone numbers, should be in this manual. A list of potential candidates for referral should also be included. The nursing policies must remain flexible enough to provide for the special needs of a patient. They should also reflect the attitude of the general program objectives.

Functions of the Discharge Planning Staff

1. Screen and study pre-admission records
2. Interview on admission Medicare-Medicaid patients and patients without insurance
3. Assess patient's needs, stimulate and redirect his thinking; encourage self-expression, self-evaluation, and self-determination

4. Assess patient's home situation relative to discharge planning
5. Assist nursing personnel in identifying and assessing patient's needs for discharge planning
6. Identify problems and make appropriate notations on patient Kardex or chart
7. Counsel and involve patient and/or his family in:
   a. discharge planning
   b. acceptance of illness, disability and needed treatment
   c. coping with illness complicated by social and emotional problems
   d. management of finances
   e. self-care and nursing measures in the home situation
   f. reason for transfer to another facility
8. Recommend and assist in placement of patient in nursing home:
   a. arrange transportation if necessary
   b. inform and interpret Medicare, Medicaid, welfare and community resources
   c. use community resources to supplement and reinforce discharge planning activities of the hospital
9. Make referrals to:
   a. community health agencies
   b. public health departments
   c. psychiatric social workers
10. Liaison to maintain continuity of care to:
    a. social service departments
    b. community agencies for post-hospital care
    c. various agencies for welfare assistance and placement
11. Liaison between:
    a. hospital and community
    b. social service department and other community agencies
    c. welfare agencies and voluntary charities
    d. departments in the hospital
    e. doctors, patients and families
    f. hospital and out-patient facilities
12. Resource for:
    a. patient education incorporating available facilities such as the Public Health Nurse
    b. available community facilities
    c. discharge planning for physician and hospital staff

13. Provide in-patient service on a one-to-one basis:
    a. interdepartmental
    b. nursing, ancillary services, chaplaincy and medical services
14. Establish a system of discharge planning
15. Conduct or participate in continuing education sessions relative to discharge planning
    a. hospital personnel
    b. medical social services
16. Work cooperatively with the physician and social service department for comprehensive discharge planning
17. Obtain necessary physician orders for referrals
18. Assist the health team to understand the significance of social, economic and emotional factors in relation to patient illness, treatment and recovery
19. Provide guidance and aid for patient education
20. Evaluate potential obstetrical clinic patients
21. Assist the patient in the emergency room
22. Encourage development of new resources to meet social service needs
23. Review daily census, coordinate needs of patients and advise physician of available services
24. Intake for all referrals from physicians on admissions
25. Participate in studies which will contribute toward improving patient care and health programs in the community
26. Make daily rounds to all nursing units to review discharge plans. Participate in team conferences on units
27. Attend monthly meetings of Audit Utilization Committee
28. Meet regularly with the Utilization Review Committee
29. Formulate and maintain current departmental policies and procedures
30. Meet with public health and social service personnel
31. Attend orientation for new personnel to explain job functions and to offer assistance when needed
32. Decrease average length of stay of patients in hospital and readmission of patients
33. Keep statistical records of activities and referrals
34. Report monthly to director of nursing and administration on hospital stay and discharge plans for those patients for whom she provides help

Evaluating a Discharge Program

Table 5-2 provides a set of indicators and suggests criteria for evaluating a discharge program.

Nursing Practice and Computers

Applications*

In the 1970's more hospitals began to recognize the computer's potential for improving nursing practice and the quality of patient care, especially to facilitate charting, care planning, patient monitoring, interdepartmental scheduling and communication and personnel time assignment.

In many hospitals, information handling by the nurse has become the major problem preventing her from caring for the patient.

Jydstrup and Gross reported in "Cost of Information Handling" that the average time spent in information handling was 7 percent by a nursing aide, 22 percent by a practical nurse, 36 percent by a registered nurse, and 58 percent by a head nurse. Clearly, increased nursing skill is accompanied by increased information handling. Nurses' notes were the single most time consuming written communication.

Nursing Observations

Two general approaches to the automated recording of nursing observations have been developed. The first is a computer-readable form on which frequently-used statements about patient condition or behavior are arranged under general headings. In using this form, the nurse chooses one or more statements that describe the patient that she has been observing under headings such as "sleeping and eating habits," "mood," "appearance."

---

*Source: Adapted from A.J. Hannah, "The Computer and Nursing Practice," *Nursing Outlook*, September 1976. © American Journal of Nursing Company.

Table 5-2 Sample Indicators for Evaluation of Discharge Program

Indicators	Criteria for Determining Degree of Success
Appropriateness of admission (use medical criteria)	___ % decrease in inappropriate admission due to stage of illness in a 6 month period
Appropriateness of length of stay	___ % reduction of overstays in a year or 6 month period
Transfer rates to: home care home nursing home other hospital	Increase from ___ % to ___ % patients going to home care, etc.
Planning needs identified but not met	___ % decrease in unmet needs
Decrease in admission waiting list	___ % decrease in waiting for admission over 6 month period
Follow-up of patients: Utilization of services post-discharge Satisfaction with services Compliance with discharge orders Degree of disability 3 months post-discharge, related to planning goals	___ % increase in use of community services and resources ___ % increase in compliance
Staff acceptance of program	___ % increase in use of planner ___ % inpatients with recorded discharge plans
Feedback from other facilities	___ % decrease in problems of patients accepted due to poor discharge planning information

Source: Opal Bristow, Carol Stickey, and Shirley Thompson, *Discharge Planning For Continuity of Care,* National League for Nursing, 1976, Pub. No. 21-1604.

The second approach has been to develop a branching questionnaire. This approach utilizes a cathode ray terminal (similar to a television screen) on which alphabetical and numerical characters appear. The terminal, activated by a conventional typewriter keyboard, displays a list of choices; for instance, in relation to skin condition, the first choice shown on the terminal might be "skin intact—yes-no." The user selects his answer and indicates it by pressing the corresponding number on the keyboard or touching the terminal with a light-sensitive input device called a light pen.

If the skin is intact, no further choices relating to it appear on the screen, and the nurse can begin recording observations of other aspects concerning the patient. If she records that the skin is not intact, the terminal then displays a further list of choices. Advantages include increased numbers of observations as a result of forced recall; increased accuracy and reliability of observations; legibility, so that the notes take less time to read, are interpreted more accurately, and used more; less time spent writing notes; ready statistical analysis.

Nursing Care Plans

Written patient care assignments are usually accompanied by oral explanations which can be forgotten during a shift.

There are again two general approaches to the automation of nursing care plans. The first approach is to develop computer-readable forms on which the nurse indicates nursing action for a given patient. The forms are then processed by the computer and printouts of the nursing care plan are produced.

The alternative is to design basic care plans for meeting patient-type needs, store them in the computer memory banks, and then adapt them to individual patients. The resulting printout is unique for each patient's assessed needs for daily care.

Automated Monitoring

Automated patient monitoring is so far used mostly in coronary care units and pacemaker clinics to monitor electrocardiograms, analyze the information, and reduce the volume of data to manageable proportions, generally in the form of some type of graph. The computers have also been programmed to recognize deviations from accepted norms and to alert attending personnel to the deviation by an alarm or light.

Scheduling

Various health care institutions have automated the scheduling of personnel work assignments. To accomplish this, patient care needs are first quantified to assess staffing needs, personnel policies are clearly delineated, and a computer program is designed for scheduling of staff within these constraints. When the program is run, the result is a printed staff time schedule.

Administrators have found that automated scheduling makes for easier recruitment and increased job satisfaction, because schedules are known well in advance.

Implementation of a Computer Based Record System*

The implementation of a computer-based record system requires a significant amount of physician and nurse time. It is critical to give a leadership role to one individual who is respected and is experienced in the patient care environment and who has at least minimal skills in information processing. The success or failure of the computer implementation will to a major degree be a function of the ability of this individual to provide leadership in this interface between health care needs and the technical potentials and constraints. It is also necessary to undertake considerable provider education, since no record system, however good the technology, will succeed unless there is understanding and cooperation on the part of the majority of the providers in the use of the technology. Changing long-established habits of medical record keeping requires continuing effort, imagination, and patience. It is essential that there be a competent computer support staff. Because the medical information system is critical to the vitality of the organization, a successful implementation (or transference) requires significant on-site presence of at least a few personnel who have good technical competence and who can work well with medical and management personnel.

The transition from a manually maintained record system to a computer based record system will require considerable planning and a thorough orientation process for nursing personnel. Personnel with specific patterns or characteristics (e.g., female, nurse, little work experience, rural hospital, no prior computer contact, etc.) are more likely to be negatively disposed toward computer applications in health care. The ability to identify these individuals at the outset of planning computer-based systems implementations provides a basis for establishing special training, orientation or counseling activities to insure the success of the project.

Among the specific functions that nurses may be required to fulfill are: admitting the patient into the computer system, daily entering of certain clinical information such as temperature and fluid balance, changing previously entered information, and discharging the patient. In addition nurses would have to learn how to access and manipulate information. For example, in a medications system they might be requesting the printed medication schedule, entering charting information, changing previously entered items, and reviewing the data base.

Checklist for the Nursing Service*

When a computer system is being installed the following questions particularly pertinent to the nursing service should be addressed.

- What information would be retained as nursing input?
- How can nursing input be interfaced with input from others involved in health care?
- What is the value of the information for decision-making?
- What information needs to be available at certain time periods, and what are these time periods?
- What information needs to be temporarily stored?
- What information needs to be permanently stored on-line or by other storage means?
- What information needs to be retained for future reference? Should only transfer or other summary information be retained?
- What information should be available and to whom?

---

*Source: G. Octo Barnett, NCHSR Research Digest Series: Computer Stored Ambulation Record (COSTAR), DHEW, 1976. Pub. No. (HRA) 76-3145.

*Source: Systematic Nursing Assessment. DHEW, 1974. Pub. No. (HRA) 74-17.

- What information needs to be retained for legal purposes?
- What information could be input by the patient and/or family member?
- What type of input, storage, and retrieval devices would best accommodate the information?
- What would be the feasibility and the cost of including the proposed clinical information in a computer-assisted system?
- What orientation programs would be needed to implement such a system?
- Who would input the data?
- If a nonnurse inputs the data, should it be validated by the nurse?
- What effect does the introduction of a data processing system have on the overall hospital structure?
- What action should be taken to:
  —Decrease nurse dissatisfaction or strain due to role conflict?
  —Facilitate nurse acceptance of data processing?
  —Reorient nurse, administrator, doctor, and patient conceptions of the role of a nurse under the conditions of a "new technology?"

NURSE RECRUITMENT*

ABC's of Nurse Recruitment**

A—Acquire an effective nurse recruiter.

B—Budget to allow adequate funds for competitive recruitment programs carefully conceived and based on a realistic projection.

C—Convey a positive image in your ads and literature.

D—Develop strong internal recruitment resources.

E—Encourage promotion from within to fill leadership positions. Appoint the best qualified candidate regardless of source.

F—Foster a climate of openness so that problems surface and are solved before they result in turn-over statistics.

G—Generate effective advertising that reflects not only high professional standards but an administrative philosophy that bespeaks concern for the individual.

H—Heed the advice of advertising experts concerning the selection of media, copy development, timing, and general strategy for placing advertisements.

I—Immediately respond to employment inquiries with a personal letter; a well-prepared, informative, and persuasive brochure; details about specific opportunities available, salaries, benefits, housing, etc.; and a clear statement of qualifications expected. Send follow-up correspondence at regular intervals.

J—Judge the effectiveness of your nurse recruitment efforts in terms of the "average cost per hire." Use this index as a basis of comparison with previous results and with other employers' results.

K—Keep records of each inquiry as received, by origin (journal, newspaper, in-house, etc.) and by summary of their disposition (interviews, hires).

L—Learn which recruitment resources provide the greatest yield in quality as well as numbers of candidates.

M—Maximize the use of these resources.

N—Negotiate with other health care agencies to recommend qualified applicants for whom current vacancies do not exist.

O—Offer assistance to out-of-state applicants in finding convenient, reasonably price housing. This is often essential in metropolitan areas.

P—Promote positive public relations by participating in and sponsoring events which involve potential candidates and present staff members.

Q—Query terminating staff members concerning reasons for resignation. . . . consider their recommendations for improvement.

R—Reward exceptional performance by added responsibility and commensurate authority, compensation, and recognition.

S—Schedule regular performance reviews to assess individual progress, to identify

---

*Source: Except where noted, material in this section on "Nurse Recruitment" is from Tina Filoromo and Dolores Ziff, *Nurse Recruitment: Strategies for Success,* Aspen Systems Corporation, 1980.

**Source: Adapted from Edin Hoffman, "ABC's of Nurse Recruitment," *American Journal of Nursing,* April 1974, pp. 682–83, © 1974 American Journal of Nursing Company.

problems, and to agree on appropriate job objectives.

T—Tell your nurse recruitment representatives and advertising agency about any changes or problems affecting your staffing situation so that suitable adjustments can be made in your recruitment campaign.

U—Understand the hidden costs of inadequate or inappropriate staffing.

V—Vitalize your orientation, inservice, and continuing education programs to provide the latest information.

W—Work with school and college guidance counselors and conduct "career day" programs.

X—X-ray your staffing and scheduling patterns to deploy your present nursing group most effectively.

Y—Yield to constructive criticism in the development of solutions to your recruitment problems and staffing patterns.

Z—Zero in on a unifying theme that distinguishes your hospital as a place to learn and to practice nursing. Promote this theme in all aspects of your recruitment program.

Facts

The National Association of Nurse Recruiters found that 60 percent of hospitals and 53 percent of nursing homes in a survey reported shortages of nurses.

Recruiting a nurse is an expensive proposition. In 1980, according to the nurse recruiters' association, the average cost of recruiting a registered nurse was $731, and the average hospital last year recruited 140, at a cost of more than $100,000.

The American Nurses' Association says the 75 percent employment rate for licensed registered nurses compares with a 56 percent employment rate for all women eligible to work. Of the 25 percent who aren't in the work force, 43 percent are under age 40 and in their childbearing years, while another 25 percent are over age 54 and may not be coming back at all.

Nurse Recruiter

Selection of a nurse recruiter should be based on such qualifications as:

- the ability to sell and persuade,
- the ability to relate well to young applicants,

- an affinity for administrative detail,
- a knowledge of labor laws and general hiring and employment practices,
- a ready knowledge of nursing or the ability to grasp job qualifications and licensure requirements,
- complete honesty in presenting the facts to interested applicants,
- freedom and willingness to travel.

The basic job description offered in Table 5-3 should be helpful to a health care facility in establishing the new position or reevaluating the position as it currently exists at that institution.

Table 5-3   Basic Job Description

Position Title: Nurse Recruiter
Department: Personnel or Nursing
Reports to: Director of Personnel or Director of Nursing

JOB SUMMARY

Meets, screens, interviews, and refers RN applicants. Collects and keeps current listing of RN vacancies. Reviews RN applications and follows up on initial inquiries, interviews, and job offers. Works directly with department heads, supervisors, etc., in establishing rapport and cooperation with, offering jobs to, screening, and employing RN applicants. Periodically assists various members of the department and the director of the department in completing projects and research studies.

DUTIES AND RESPONSIBILITIES

1. keeps in constant contact with department heads to maintain current records of their needs;
2. responds to written inquiries about RN positions available; corresponds with RN applicants regarding interviews, openings, and any other questions applicants may have;
3. greets and initially interviews RN applicants who come to the nurse recruitment office, fully explains hospital benefits, and sees that applicants have a chance to interview with a member of the department of their interest; provides information for callers in regard to RN vacancies; schedules appointments;
4. acts as the coordinator between department heads and RN applicants for job openings and job offers;
5. informs department heads when an RN applicant is acceptable or not acceptable

Table 5-3 continued

by checking references and evaluating results; makes available the references to the department heads;

6. informs the proper departments when an RN applicant does not accept a position;
7. notifies RN applicants if they are unacceptable for employment;
8. keeps a tally of the source of inquiries about RN vacancies and the number of job offers that can be traced back to each source;
9. maintains other files and records as required;
10. works directly with an advertising agency or the hospital's public relations department to coordinate recruitment materials; maintains the materials in up-to-date form;
11. travels to annual RN and student nursing conventions, career days, and other career-related activities to recruit RNs; makes arrangements, assembles materials, attends, and is in charge of recruitment at these conventions;
12. keeps the director of the department informed of any consistent problems and new developments in RN recruitment;
13. performs additional tasks as assigned and requested by the director of the department;
14. adheres to all organizational and personnel policies of the hospital.

Source: Tina Filoromo and Dolores Ziff, *Nurse Recruitment: Strategies For Success,* Aspen Systems Corporation, 1980.

Recruitment Committee

Some institutions have delegated the responsibility to a committee which may include a representative from the personnel department, a member of the nursing administrative staff (at an assistant director level, or a head nurse or supervisor level), and several staff nurses with varying years of service. The committee should have a chairperson to establish regular meeting times, offer an agenda for meetings, and maintain records of decisions for recruitment activities made by the group. It is very important that someone be assigned the task of keeping careful records of recruitment trips and responses to advertising to help the committee evaluate various recruitment efforts.

Many institutions have utilized a committee along with a full-time nurse recruiter. In such an arrangement, the recruiter uses the committee as a sounding board for suggestions and opinions regarding various phases of the recruitment plan.

A Recruitment Program

First, the hospital must decide where the recruiter will travel and where the advertising money will be placed.

One way to begin making these decisions is to research the hospital's past efforts and the results they produced (if there are records). Next, it may be helpful to survey your competitors, if they are willing to share information. Ask where they have placed ads, where they have traveled, and if they have profited from these activities. Finally, survey the nursing staff at your hospital.

The sample survey in Table 5-4 includes questions that will help you compile the information you will need to make decisions about your travel and advertising activities.

Recruitment Budget

Useful guideposts in budget planning are the surveys by the National Association of Nurse Recruiters (NANR). These surveys provide information on budgets allocated for recruitment by hospitals grouped according to size and geographical location.

Basic expense categories to consider when planning your recruitment budget and/or determining your average cost per hire at the end of the recruitment year are the following:

- salaries and fringe benefits for the recruiter and clerical support staff;
- cost of office space and utilities;
- telephone charges (including the flat rate as well as long distance and collect calls);
- postage for first class letters and recruitment packets;
- printing costs for all recruitment materials;
- exhibit costs;
- travel costs to conventions and career programs for the recruiter and assistants;
- booth fees at conventions and job fairs (including rental of furniture for the booth);
- advertising fees (local and national);
- advertising/public relations agency fees for brochures, advertisements, and other materials (if you hire an agency);

Table 5-4 Nursing Staff Survey

Dear Employee:

In an effort to help the office of nurse recruitment identify the most effective sources of possible nursing applicants, I would appreciate your completing the following survey and returning it to my office at your earliest convenience.

Your comments and opinions concerning the development of a nurse recruitment program are greatly appreciated.

Thank you for your time and consideration of this matter.

Sincerely,

1. In what city and state were you born and raised?
2. In what city and state did you attend your nursing program?
3. If you relocated to [name of city or town in which your hospital is located], what influenced you in your choice of this city?
4. How did you learn of nursing job opportunities at this hospital?
5. Why did you choose this hospital?
6. What nursing journal/journals do you receive and read at home? (If you receive more than one, please list the one you read from cover to cover first, followed by the others in order of the next most carefully read, etc.)
7. Do you regularly review the newspaper classified ads?
8. If the answer to number 7 is yes, please list the papers by name and also the day of the week that you read the ads.

Source: Tina Filoromo and Dolores Ziff, *Nurse Recruitment: Strategies for Success*, Aspen Systems Corporation, 1980.

- staff time of the hospital's public relations department;
- staff time for those involved in the interviewing process;
- expenses incurred in interviewing;
- entertainment of prospects, both in-house and on the road;
- cost of preemployment physicals;
- cost of orientation;
- relocation expenses (if your institution offers them).

Recordkeeping

Maintaining detailed records of all aspects of your recruitment program can be very time consuming. But recordkeeping provides you with information that is vital to your future planning. It justifies your budget requests, and it adds validity to your overall recruitment program.

The following information and sample summary sheets will give you some idea of the records you may want to keep.

Monthly Summaries

You should compile a monthly summary of contacts. Table 5-5 should give you some idea of how to put this summary together. This monthly summary will help you estimate your mailing charges, per month, on the packets of information sent through the mail. It will also give you an idea of how many pieces of recruitment information you use each month, so that you can intelligently plan future printing. And it will tell you which recruitment venture is giving you the best return during a particular period of time.

Records of Newspaper Advertising

You should also keep a weekly tally of newspaper ad responses and a cost analysis of newspaper advertising (see Tables 5-6 and 5-7). They will give you information about which newspaper is giving you the best response, which day of the week is best for running your recruitment ads, and a breakdown of the cost per response and eventually the cost per hire from newspaper advertising. Ultimately, these records will enable you to determine if the high cost of classified ads in newspapers is worth your time and money.

Records of National Advertising

You should also keep a cost analysis of recruitment advertising in national media. This record will give you an idea of the effectiveness of a national advertising campaign as it relates to cost per response and cost per hire. Analyzing the cost of advertising in national media is a long-term process, as you may continue to receive inquiries from national ads for several months after the ad appears. The hires may not occur for six months or even a year.

Table 5-5 Monthly Summary of Inquiries
September 1977

Source of Inquiry	RN	Student	LPN	Total for Month
General letters & calls*	22	9	2	33
AJN Ad - September 1977	13	27	0	40
Nursing 77 Ad - September	45	13	1	59
RN Magazine Ad - May 1977	10	15	4	29
Nursing Opportunities 1977	17	32	4	53
AJN Ad - October 1975	3	0	0	3
Totals†	110	96	11	217

*Includes calls and responses to newspaper advertising.
†The summary might also include the number of contacts made on recruiting trips or the total number of packets of information distributed.

Source: Tina Filoromo and Dolores Ziff, *Nurse Recruitment: Strategies for Success*, Aspen Systems Corporation, 1980.

Table 5-6 Weekly Tally of Newspaper Ad Responses

Name of Newspaper Date of Insertion	First Week M T W T F	Second Week M T W T F	Third Week M T W T F

Source: Tina Filoromo and Dolores Ziff, *Nurse Recruitment: Strategies for Success*, Aspen Systems Corporation, 1980.

Records of Programs and Travel

Similar records should be kept for each program you attend. At the very least, keep a record of the number of packets you distribute, so that you can forecast the number you will need for the same or similar programs. Keeping such records, along with the sign-up cards, and, if

Table 5-7   Cost Analysis of Newspaper Advertising

Name of Newspaper Date of Insertion	Cost per Insertion	Total Responses	Cost per Response*	Total Hires	Cost per Hire†

*Cost per Response = Cost per ad ÷ total number of responses
†Cost per Hire = Cost per ad ÷ total number of hires

Source: Tina Filoromo and Dolores Ziff, *Nurse Recruitment: Strategies for Success,* Aspen Systems Corporation, 1980.

possible, coding the applications in packets distributed, will help you determine the effectiveness of recruitment trips in terms of contacts and hires. A cost analysis in relation to number of hires from recruitment trips can also be made, as long as detailed records of travel expenses are maintained.

Geographic Records

Your overall recordkeeping plan should also include a summary of contacts and hires broken down by geographic area. In terms of advertising, you may see a trend in the geographic areas from which contacts or requests for information and hires are coming. Different journals may reach different areas, and this information may be of value when you are deciding where to spend your advertising dollars.

Monthly Reports

This report should provide a summary of applications received, the number of persons interviewed, the number of persons hired, a list of the sources of hires, and a brief summary of the actual recruitment activities that includes a list of where requests for information came from.

The bottom line of all of your recruitment records will help you in planning where to go for nursing applicants, justifying a budget based on the success of various activities, and, finally, determining your cost per hire. Keeping records of

all money spent in the categories designated by your institution, divided by the total number of hires in a given period, will give you your true cost per hire.

Prospect Sources

Staff Members

Staff members are a good source of new employees; they have friends and relatives. Involve your employees in the planning of internal programs, such as designing exhibits and brochures. But, most important of all, take a staff member along on your recruitment trips. For example, if you are traveling to a school career program and a recent graduate of that nursing program is on your staff, take that person with you. Your nurse will be a natural link to the graduating class and will encourage applications to your hospital.

Student Nurses

If your institution has a school of nursing, or trains affiliating nursing students from local colleges and universities, do not neglect these students as a source of recruits. Make sure they know that you are interested in them for future employment. Entertain them at a dinner or a coffee and tea session either at the beginning or end of their affiliation.

In addition, encourage your staff members to put a special effort into making these students feel welcome and a true part of the health care team, whether they are there for only a week or for a full semester.

If your institution does not have affiliating students, but you do have nursing programs in your community, contact the directors of these programs to offer their students experiences at your hospital. Or, if you have any special patient units or programs, offer tours to schools for their students. Set aside some time during the tour for refreshments, and use that period for the recruitment effort. Be sure a representative of your staff is on hand to help. You may even want to consider inviting all of the local schools to send their students to the continuing education programs that you are conducting for nurses at your hospital and in the community.

Alumnae

Another source of prospects is the alumnae association of your hospital's school of nursing if you have one, or had one in the recent past. Some alumnae who were at one time employed at the hospital may be interested in returning, at least on a part-time basis. Let them know such positions are available. Use the alumnae newsletter to reach alumnae with this information.

Yet another source of applicants is the hospital's personnel department, where there are files of past employees. Many nurses leave positions to further their educations or to raise families. It is possible that they are ready to return to work, in either full-time or part-time positions. But they need you to tell them that jobs are available and that your institution wants them back. A personal letter is a worthwhile investment for this group of people.

In this group, however, you may encounter some people who cannot make a regular part-time commitment, but who would like to become part of an on-call or per-diem list. Such lists have worked quite well for some hospitals. People on the on-call list are called to duty whenever someone is needed to fill temporary openings due to vacations, sick days, or unexpected leaves of absence. The individual is under no obligation to accept work, and, at the same time, the hospital does not guarantee any specific amount of work to the individual.

There are some practical reasons for pursuing an on-call list for former employees. These people are already oriented to the hospital and have some understanding of its policies and procedures. They can reduce the use of nurses from temporary agencies, who have little, if any, orientation to the institution. And utilizing these people as part-time or on-call nurses may eventually lead to their full-time employment. (See Table 5-8 for a ranking of job leads that produce results.)

Bonuses

Many health care facilities have tried bonus or bounty systems to encourage their own employees to assist in bringing nurses into the institutions. Some bonuses take the form of an amount of money paid to the employee on the day the new recruit begins work, followed by an additional bonus after the recruit completes a successful probation. In other bonus systems, employees who bring in recruits are rewarded by trips to popular vacation sites, extra time off, or large bonuses after they have recruited three or more nurses.

If you elect to use the bonus or bounty system, plan your program carefully to ensure fair treatment. Keep accurate records to be certain that proper rewards are made to those who earned them. And give serious consideration to broadening the program to include all hospital employees, rather than just the members of the nursing staff.

Table 5-8   Job Leads That Produce Results

Sources Utilized	Total
Faculty	42%
Friends	51
Recruiter	12
Nurses' convention	3
State Nurses' Association Placement Service	2
State employment service	4
Commercial employment agency	3
Placement bureau of school	6
Professional journals	18
Civil Service listings	5
Newspapers	23
Direct application	71

Source: DHEW, 1975.

Individualized Contracts*

In 1980 when Hollywood Medical Center was experiencing severe difficulty in keeping the nurses it had hired, the hospital revamped its nursing administration and, by individual bargaining, established with each RN a special contract fulfilling his or her most important demands. (See Table 5-9 for employment options.)

The approach was uniquely successful. By 1982 this 334-bed hospital was using no outside recruitment agencies yet maintained an inventory of approximately 80 nurses on file for future employment. It no longer had a dwindling nurse pool. It had reduced its operating costs to the point where funds were always on hand for an-

*Source: Neil M. Sorrentino, "An Alternative to Collective Bargaining," *Nursing Administration Quarterly*, Winter 1982.

Table 5-9 Nurse Employment Options at Hollywood Medical Center (1982)

1. **Nursing students** work 4-hour shifts as needed, as their schedules allow, in their role as nursing assistants.
2. **LPNs** in the Seasonal Nurse Assignment Pool (SNAP) program work as needed, at their own schedule, including at least one weekend per month. Rate of pay is $6.25 to $7.75 per hour with no benefits.
3. **Certain RNs** work 4-hour shifts, at their own schedule, and are entitled to half benefits if working at least 24 hours per week.
4. **Other RNs** in the Registered Nurse Remedy (RNR) program work 8-hour shifts, with every other weekend off, with no benefits, at the following rates:
    7–3 shift: $12 per hour
    3–11 shift: $14 per hour
    11–7 shift: $17 per hour
5. **Other RNs** work 12-hour shifts in the ICU/CCU every Saturday and Sunday from either 7 A.M. to 7 P.M. (for which they are paid as if they had worked 36 hours), or 7 P.M. to 7 A.M. (for which they are paid as if they had worked 40 hours); in both instances they receive full benefits. Nurses in ICU/CCU who work 8-hour shifts Monday thru Friday have every weekend off with full benefits.
6. **Most RNs** work 8- or 10-hour shifts, a full 40 hours per week, with full benefits. Salaries are based on experience and responsibilities.

Source: Neil M. Sorrentino, "An Alternative to Collective Bargaining," *Nursing Administration Quarterly*, Winter 1982.

nual increases. It had minimal overtime. It carried no expensive ads. It paid no fees to personnel agencies. Turnover in the intensive care/critical care unit was very low and in other hospital areas was almost nonexistent.

Individual Contracts

The following are some of the terms found in various of these nurse contracts (not all terms are in each contract). The hospital would:

1. provide certain nurses with free temporary housing;
2. give some nurses flexi-time schedules (some working 40 hours in three or four days, some working the least desirable shifts and being paid for 40 hours though working far fewer);
3. allow some nurses to select benefits according to their needs;
4. free some nurses from all weekend shifts;
5. allow discretionary use of compensatory time off;
6. establish four-hour shifts for those who require it;
7. offer variable pay packages to all nurses (such packages to include all, some or no benefits);
8. provide psychological counseling for those requesting this service;
9. offer traditional hours and pay schemes for those nurses who feel completely at home with this sort of remuneration; and
10. open a day-care center within the hospital for the children whose parents are employed by the hospital.

NURSE RETENTION

Increasing Job Satisfaction*

The following suggestions can be passed along to your nursing director for increasing job satisfaction among her nurses and, in turn, helping to increase your hospital's rate of retention.

1. Think of the initial interview as the first step in retention. Be very honest; tell the applicant what you have to offer as well

*Source: Tina Filoromo and Dolores Ziff, *Nurse Recruitment: Strategies for Success*, Aspen Systems Corporation, 1980.

as what you don't have. Avoid creating disappointments and an employee who may resign shortly after orientation.

2. Look at your orientation program as a part of your retention plan. Are you providing the new employee with adequate guidance and direction to function in the manner your institution expects? Provide a comprehensive program for the new graduate that includes intensive management skills instruction and/or review. It will help to make a smoother transition from student to confident practitioner.

3. Reinterview new employees at various times after employment. Such interviews may uncover areas of concern or dissatisfaction that you will be able to deal with at once, and so prevent the individual from leaving your hospital frustrated and needlessly upset.

4. Of course, the exit interview has been traditionally considered the time for learning of employee problems. Be sure that the results of these interviews are directed in a constructive manner to the proper individuals for evaluation and possible action or correction.

5. Good communication can be achieved through regular meetings, newsletters, unit-level meetings (aside from the traditional staff-level meetings) with the director of nursing and the director's staff, and the involvement of all levels of the nursing staff on various patient care committees as well as policy and procedure committees for the nursing department. Make the employees realize that you need their input in matters that involve their work situations.

6. Staff nurses look for ongoing educational opportunities. Be sure that you offer the chance for the nursing staff on all shifts to participate in in-house programs and in programs outside the institution.

7. Be sure your staff members are aware that nursing administration always offers them promotional opportunities before looking outside of the hospital to fill positions. Utilize a well-planned procedure for posting job openings, one that is fair to all employees.

8. Opportunities for horizontal mobility are as important to nurses as traditional vertical mobility. Consider programs that offer the nurse who does not want a leadership position recognition for her clinical excellence.

9. Your mobility plan should also include a well-defined and strictly observed transfer policy that is fair to each employee and allows for mobility within the institution for the purpose of professional growth and development.

10. Last, but certainly not least, be very sure that your salary and benefits plan is competitive for your geographic area of the country.

Inservice Training for Nurses*

To plan for an inservice training program, one hospital in 1979 surveyed its nursing staff to estimate the demand for various programs. The respondents' first choices are reported in Table 5-10. It will be noted that the demand for training differs according to whether the nurse has a diploma, an associate degree or a bachelor's degree.

The survey made it possible to estimate the number of nurses who would take each training opportunity if it were offered.

Some nurses wanted courses for which they could receive college credit. The demand for these courses also varied according to the basic training that the nurse received. These data were also collected so that arrangements could be made with nearby universities.

Career Ladders**

In the early 1970's the National Commission for the Study of Nursing and Nursing Education recognized the benefits of differentiating levels of nurse competency and recommended the following:

- Personnel policies in all health-care facilities should be so designed that they:
  1. Differentiate levels of responsibility in accord with the concepts of staff nurse, clinical nurse, and master clinician with

---

*Source: C. David Hughes, "Can Marketing Help Recruit and Retain Nurses?" *Health Care Management Review*, Summer 1979.

**Source: *The Nursing Administration Handbook*, ed. Howard S. Rowland and Beatrice L. Rowland, Aspen Systems Corporation, 1980.

Table 5-10   Estimated Demand for Various Training Programs

First Choice Training/Experience	Nurse Training Program(%)			
	Diploma	Associate Degree of Nursing	Bachelor's Degree	Total
Practice/Experience				
Anesthesia	0.0	0.0	2.7	1.2
Emergency room	7.7	28.6	2.7	7.2
Inhalation therapy	7.7	0.0	2.7	4.8
ICU/CCU	2.6	0.0	5.4	3.6
Nurse clinics	0.0	14.3	0.0	1.2
Ob/Gyn	0.0	0.0	5.4	2.4
Operating room	5.1	14.3	0.0	3.6
Pediatrics	0.0	0.0	2.7	1.2
Pediatric ICU	0.0	0.0	2.7	1.2
Psychiatry	2.6	14.3	0.0	2.4
Public health	2.6	0.0	2.7	2.4
Other	0.0	0.0	10.8	4.8
Practitioners				
Family nurse practitioner	7.7	0.0	5.4	6.0
Midwife	2.6	0.0	0.0	1.2
Pediatric nurse	0.0	0.0	8.1	3.6
Other	0.0	0.0	5.4	2.4
Further education				
MS	0.0	0.0	8.1	3.6
Other	5.1	14.3	2.7	4.8
Training				
Cardiac	15.4	14.3	10.8	13.3
Leadership	12.8	0.0	2.7	7.2
Management	2.6	0.0	2.7	2.4
Pharmacy	0.0	0.0	2.7	1.2
Physical assessment	5.1	0.0	2.7	3.6
Renal	2.6	0.0	0.0	1.2
Other	15.4	0.0	5.4	9.6
Miscellaneous				
Other	2.6	0.0	5.4	3.6
Sample size	39	7	37	83
Percent in each program	47.0	8.4	44.6	100.0

Source: C. David Hughes, "Can Marketing Help Recruit and Retain Nurses?" *Health Care Management Review,* Summer 1979.

appropriate intermediate grades. These levels should be designed according to the content of the position and the clinical proficiency required for competent performance.

2. Provide for promotion granted on the basis of acquisition of the knowledge and demonstrated competence to perform in a given position.

- Health management administrators and clinical directors of nursing service should build on current improvements in starting salaries to create a strong reward system for remaining in clinical practice by developing schedules of substantially increasing salary levels for experienced nurses functioning in advanced capacities.

- Two essentially related, but differing, career patterns should be developed for nursing practice:

1. One career pattern, episodic, would emphasize the nursing practice that is essentially curative and restorative, generally acute or chronic in nature, and most frequently provided in the setting of the hospital or inpatient facility.

2. The second career pattern, distributive, would emphasize the nursing practice that is essentially designed for health maintenance and disease prevention. This is generally continuous in nature, seldom acute, and increasingly will take place in community or emergent institutional settings.

Model Program

In a plan to reward nursing competence without promoting nurses out of direct patient care and into administration, the University of California Health Care Facilities adopted a four-level clinical nursing ladder. The intention was to provide a system which would:

1. Establish career patterns that provide for quality nursing care
2. Utilize (appropriately) nurses educationally prepared for a variety of levels of practice
3. Provide for recognition and placement of the highly qualified nurse practitioner in direct patient care activities
4. Provide for differentiation of levels of nursing competence
5. Provide explicit expectations for practice that serve as guides for evaluation of performance

In classifying the minimal behaviors for each level, consideration was given to the depth of knowledge upon which nursing decisions are based, the scope of practice, and the degree of responsibility and accountability for patient care. Each level of responsibility is inclusive of preceding levels, and recommended educational and experiential qualifications are indicated. Inherent in each step of the series is the responsibility of the practitioner to evaluate her own performance and identify and take initiative for her continued need for professional growth.

STAFFING

Staffing methods attempt to establish a set of patterns for supplying nurses to patient areas based upon some predicted average workload conditions. Then, when patient demands increase or decrease on a unit during a particular time period, it is necessary to reassign on-duty personnel to balance the staff to patient needs. This dynamic staffing or allocation process is accomplished in one of three ways: the use of float pools, maintaining a call list of part-time nurses or "pulling" staff from one unit to another. Whichever method or combination of methods is utilized, it is important to use some workload measuring system to aid in the reassignment process.

It should be noted that even though staffing processes tend to be effective, the system of providing nursing care also relies heavily upon proper scheduling practices. Scheduling is an important factor in providing sufficient staff to meet patient demands. Therefore, any staffing appraisal should include a reassessment of the institution's nurse scheduling policies and practices as well.

Before any attempt is made at restaffing a nursing service area, it is recommended that a proven workload measuring system be adopted and the data be collected over a sufficient time period in order to understand the patient demand. Also, when collecting workload data, it is recommended that all scheduling policies and practices be reviewed and some effort be made to predict future scheduling criteria. Finally, it is recommended that based upon the workload measurement system and the scheduling policies and procedures, the institutions attempt to devise an allocation process which balances patient need with available personnel while maintaining personal fairness and consideration without affecting patient care.*

Factors Influencing Staffing**

Specifically, here is a list of factors influencing staffing:

- Characteristics of staff. What is the mix of skill levels? Are many on the staff young and inexperienced or is the group more settled, not out to "remake nursing?" What are the levels of educational and experiential preparation? How many are there in total numbers and by position? What are the head nurses' orientations to nursing care? To what extent are registry nurses used for unit staffing (and how are the decisions made as to the number of registry nurses needed)? What is their general social and ethnic background? Are many of them graduates of foreign schools?
- Domain and boundaries of nursing services. What services is the nursing department responsible for? Do these include, for

---

*Source: *A Review and Evaluation of Nursing Productivity*, DHEW, 1977. Pub. No. (HRA) 77-15.

**Source: *Methods for Studying Nurse Staffing In a Patient Unit*, DHEW, May 1978. Pub. No. (HRA) 78-3.

example, the operating room, errand and escort service, out-patient department, emergency services, special research or treatment units? Is the nursing department "extensible" according to the time of day and weekend, e.g., are dietary and pharmacy services on evenings and nights the responsibility of nursing? Are ward clerks or unit managers responsible to nursing administration?

- Place in formal and informal authority structure. Is the informal authority of the nursing department congruent with its place in the formal structure? What actual power does it have?
- Latitude for flexibility. Is the prevailing consensus one of "doing things alike," or is there flexibility for delivery of care by different methods? Can, for example, primary care be used on one unit and team nursing on another?
- Administration. What is the degree of centralization and general organization? Are many persons in middle-management or supervisory positions? What is the prevailing management style; is it, for example, organization or person oriented?
- Teaching programs. Is the hospital associated with a school of nursing? If so, are there joint appointments? How extensive is staff involvement with student teaching?
- Turnover. Are nursing staff attracted to the area for limited times such as for recreational or education purposes? Do new graduates of area schools tend to stay short periods and then move on? What is the turnover rate for differing skill levels?
- Group cohesiveness. How closely knit are the unit staff? Are they "small work groups" or a collective of persons?
- Resources available within the department. Are there persons skilled in staff development, or inservice education? Are there certain individuals with particular clinical skills, research skills, language facility?
- Standards of care. Are the standards clearly spelled out and available to all staff? How many standards are informal, unwritten ones? Do the nursing units set their own objectives and if so, are they reviewed and revised on a routine basis? Are standards of care fairly uniform across the nursing areas?

- Priorities in nonpatient care activities. How much emphasis is placed on formal educational development, participation in research activities, inservice and staff development?
- Professional activity. How much active involvement is there with professional organizations?
- Presence of unionization. Are either nonprofessional or professional staff unionized? If so, what do the contracts cover? What is the resultant climate within the nursing department after election or nonelection of union representation?
- Traditions and history. Although linked with institutional traditions and history, the nursing department may have its own unique blend of traditions and past events that are informally influential in the organization of services and esprit de corps.
- Trends in nursing care delivery. To what extent are emerging and/or unclear roles in existence? Decisions, for example, relative to having clinical specialists in an organizational staff versus line relationship will prompt critical examination of traditional supervisory roles.

All the foregoing factors, as noted, may be seen as having variable influences on the total plan of services to be given in the institution. To get at the overall plan of nursing services and a staffing program that results in individual unit staffing plans and organization of care, however, attention must be focused on what goes on at the unit level in determining the actual care given and the evaluation of nursing care and patient outcomes.

The right side of Figure 5-6 makes more specific the various kinds of daily events and crises that may arise to cause discrepancies between the staffing plan and organization of care and the actual care given to and received by the patient. They include changes in census, patient needs, physicians' schedules, and supporting services available, as well as staff fluctuations due to illness, emergencies, days off, vacations, etc., and the variabilities in the capabilities of total staff on duty because of these unplanned fluctuations. Because very little can be done to alter the occurrence of these types of changes and crises, their influence is depicted as operating in one direction. Personnel needs for satisfaction and

Figure 5-6 Relationship of factors entering into provisions of nursing care at the unit level

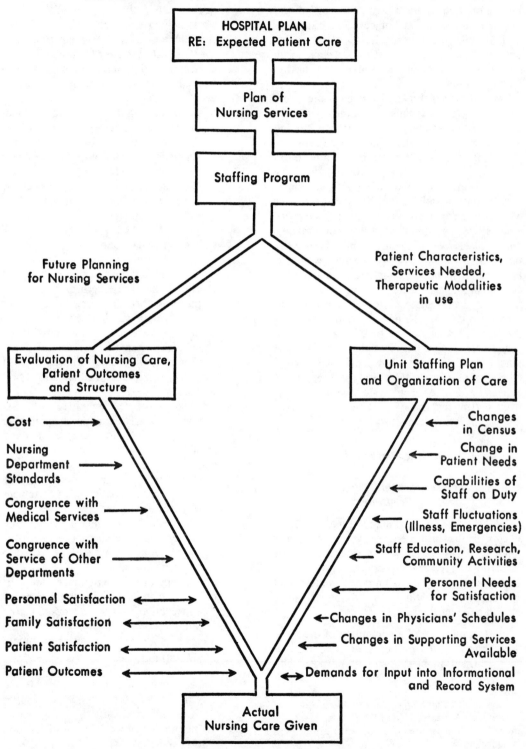

Source: *Methods for Studying Nurse Staffing In a Patient Unit,* DHEW, May 1978. Pub. No. (HRA) 78-3.

demands for organizational maintenance (represented by its subelement: "Demands for Input into Informational and Record System" in the diagram), however, are subject to alteration by "what's going on" and may have a definite influence on the outcome. Thus, they are depicted as having a two-way, or interactive, relationship with the system.

The left side of Figure 5-6 depicts the interdependency of all groups within the hospital in the process of evaluation of the actual nursing care given. As indicated, no one measure of "care" is, or probably could be, employed exclusively, e.g., expected patient outcomes by medical standards may or may not be accompanied by patient satisfaction. Similarly, the level of personnel satisfaction is involved in the process, as are the congruences and coordination with the services of medicine and of other departments. Actual care is always evaluated against certain nursing standards, and, finally, cost of providing the nursing care is a critical factor in the evaluative process. As with the other components, the open system features of the framework allow for the evaluation of the nursing care to feed back into planning for future nursing services, the staffing program, the overall plan of nursing services, and the "negotiated agreement." The open system features also make it clear that the system of events recycles and is repeated continuously.

Staffing Systems

Guidelines for Establishing a Staffing Program*

In order to initiate a staffing program, which includes as its purpose the projection of the amount of staff needed, and in order to begin the educational program associated with building understanding of the comprehensiveness and complexity of staffing, the following steps should be taken:

1. Organization of a committee of the nursing staff for purposes of becoming informed about staffing—its purpose, phi-

losophy underlying the concepts, objectives, methodology—and to gather information about the populations of patients being served.
2. Appointment of an individual to assume responsibility for the program.
3. Collection of data about personnel needed to predict the requirements:
   a. personnel policies;
   b. personnel statistics: average number of workdays; average number of holidays, vacation, illness, leave of absence for various purposes; turnover rates; supply; etc.;
   c. the current number of personnel, by categories, in the department and by individual nursing units;
   d. the cost.
4. Collection of data about patients:
   a. by individual nursing units—admission and discharge rates or visits to clinics; average length of stay; occupancy or turnover rate; and any other type of data which will be useful;
   b. consideration of use of a classification scheme and methodology.
5. Review of staffing patterns currently used by nursing unit, and documentation of rationale employed.
6. Involvement of the committee in the selection of a staffing methodology and the staffing policies and patterns desired and feasible; recognition of constraints that exist in the adoption of the ideal.
7. Introduction of the methodology to collect data regarding patients and statement of why it was selected (the rationale).
8. Writing up of the staffing policies which will be generally applied:
   a. the placement of holidays (attached to weekends or not);
   b. the type of work assignment adopted;
   c. the maximum and minimum number of consecutive days to be worked before a day off;
   d. the number of weekends off per month (or unit of time);
   e. the number of shifts to be worked by each classification (whether all are straight shifts, or two-shift rotation, or three-shift rotation);
   f. the number of weeks per shift, if rotation shifts are used;

---

*Source: *Nursing Staff Requirements for Inpatient Health Care Services*, ANA, 1977, Pub. #NS-18. Reprinted with the permission of the American Nurses' Association.

g. placement of vacation (distributed over the year or not).

9. Calculation of the number of personnel required, by shift, by type of nursing personnel, through use of the methodology adopted. Particular attention should be given to these questions:
   a. For how many patients can one professional nurse plan, supervise and evaluate the care given?
   b. How many associate nurses can one professional nurse direct, supervise, and evaluate?
   c. How many patients will require the direct care of a professional nurse, and how much nursing time will be involved in this care?
   d. How can the autonomy of nursing practice and the acceptance of accountability for results be fostered?
10. Adjustment of the number to provide leadership and coverage to plan for implementation of staffing policies.
11. Planning for how the evaluation of the staffing and scheduling will be made.
12. Implementation of the staffing program.
13. Evaluation of the program.

Using a Staffing Study Committee*

Once it has been determined that a study will be done, a study committee consisting primarily of members of the nursing service administrative group and the hospital administrative staff should be designated. In addition to specifying the number and types of units, the desired schedule, and the nature and scope of the final report, the study committee is responsible for appointing a study coordinator and assigning the necessary supporting people as observers, data clerks, and assistants.

Study Coordinator

The coordinator is the key person in the conduct of the study and should be selected from the nursing service staff.

Since the position of coordinator may require full-time activity, the coordinator's release from regular duties is essential during the time the

---

*Source: *Methods for Studying Nurse Staffing in a Patient Unit,* DHEW, May 1978. Pub. No. (HRA) 78-3.

study is being made and the report written. Some hospitals may want to have the study coordinator continue in a position that will provide continuity for the initiation and supervision of any reorganization decided upon. It is the responsibility of the coordinator to supervise the training of the observers and other members of the study team.

The coordinator carries out the following activities:

1. instructs and supervises the study team,
2. assigns and trains observers,
3. orients other hospital personnel and patients,
4. prepares study materials and data collection forms,
5. selects the patient samples,
6. monitors and edits observers' record taking,
7. assists with the analysis, interpretation and evaluation of the data,
8. prepares the study report.

Other Members of Study Team

The other members of the study team, including data clerk and typist, are selected by the study committee. The data clerk will be needed to assist in preparing statistical tables and is usually chosen from the business office because of experience with business machines and data computation.

Head Nurses/Charge Nurses

The head nurses or charge nurses of the unit or units selected for study are vital members of the study team. They are directly responsible for categorizing patients according to nursing care requirements. They use their nursing judgment to assess the adequacy or inadequacy of the staffing on their unit, and they also assist the study coordinator. Their importance in providing complete support to the study project cannot be underestimated. These nurse leaders set the tone of the units on which the studies are carried out.

Their activities, in brief, are:

1. classify patients according to indicators and guidelines for nursing care requirements,

2. record their perceptions of the adequacy or inadequacy of staffing on their units for the periods studied,

3. assist the study coordinator in checking observer reports,

4. orient patients to the study.

Observers

If the observers are to be selected from the nursing service staff, the study committee appoints the observers. Nurses selected to be observers should carry out their observations on units other than their own.

Responsibilities of Committee

The function of the staffing study committee is to produce a set of staffing policies and procedures that satisfy the unique needs of the nursing service.

Among the policies and procedures that they would be responsible for creating are:*

1. A written statement of the purpose, philosophy, and objectives of the nursing program of care.

2. A written statement of the purpose, philosophy, and objectives of staffing.

3. An identification of the data base, i.e., the information regarding patients, staff, and costs.

4. A written statement of the rationale for the selection of the staffing methodology employed.

5. A coherent set of personnel policies and procedures related to scheduling and plans for implementation.

6. A statement of basic staffing patterns for each nursing unit.

7. A set of performance standards for the nursing staff.

8., A plan for supplementing staff at times of staff illness, emergency leave, and of prolonged heavy work loads, and for reducing the staff when prolonged low work loads occur.

9. A quality assurance program to measure quality of care.

10. A written plan for evaluating the staffing program which includes identification of a system for monitoring the success of the program, for examining the staffing patterns at regular intervals in light of changing conditions, and for initiating appropriate changes.

Selecting a Staffing System*

While it may be tempting to select a staffing system successfully used in another hospital, you should be forewarned that what is appropriate for one hospital is rarely appropriate—without modification—for another hospital.

The difficulty lies in the range of variable factors: organizational systems, patient-unit arrangements, nurse-support systems, levels of technology, employment policies, hospital architecture, etc.

Essentially the parameters of what is being measured in one hospital are different from those being measured in another. These parameters affect the end figures on which staffing calculations are based—that is, the time standards for nursing activities, the total available nursing hours, the actual work-load, the proportionate distribution of nursing hours and work among staff skill levels, the decision rules for patient classification and so on.

The process of gathering information to arrive at these figures is called data collection. It is a process which each nursing service unit should employ, using techniques of measurement which are generally applicable and valid in order to produce the unique figures for particular departments and units. Once these base figures have been established they can then be adjusted to accommodate new conditions or new standards and thus satisfy the changing as well as the continuing needs of the nursing service.

Criteria**

Following are a set of criteria that could be used in selecting the best staffing system for a nursing unit or department [see *The Nursing Administration Handbook,* Rowland & Rowland, Aspen

---

*Source: *Nursing Staff Requirements for Inpatient Health Care Services,* ANA, 1977, Pub. #NS-18. Reprinted with the permission of the American Nurses' Association.

*Source: *The Nursing Administration Handbook,* ed. Howard S. Rowland and Beatrice L. Rowland, Aspen Systems Corporation, 1980.

**Source: *Nurse Staffing Methodology,* DHEW, 1973. Pub. No. (NIH) 73-433.

Systems, pp. 407–76 for model staffing systems]:

- It encompasses enough pertinent variables in its application to produce valid results;
- It utilizes measurement devices that produce reliable and valid data about these variables;
- It is simple, in that it is not time consuming and can be applied by the personnel within the institution with a minimum of consultant specialized personnel in its application;
- It provides baseline data that can be used in comparative studies within the institution or within a set of similar institutions in the delivery system;
- The cost-benefit can be predicted and is worthwhile. A more costly methodology may in the long run be less expensive in terms of benefit; and
- It is responsive to changes in the delivery system, such as the introduction of new positions or elimination of old and the creation of new supporting systems to the nursing care delivery system.

Patient Classification

Overview*

To accommodate fluctuations in census and in the mix of patients needing various amounts and kinds of nursing care, a system of classifying patients can be helpful. Essentially, the system is a method of grading patients according to the amount of nursing time and skill they require.

This assessment can serve in determining the amount of nursing care required during some stated period of time, generally the next 24 hours, as well as the category of personnel (RN, practical nurse, nurse aide) who should provide the required care.

The number of categories in a patient classification range from three or four, the most popular, to nine. These classes relate to the acuity of illness and care requirements, such as minimal, partial, moderate, or intensive. The variables entering into the patient classification systems generally relate to capability of a patient to meet his physical needs to ambulate, bathe, and feed himself. More recent work in classification systems has shown the need to assess instructional needs and emotional support as well.

Patient classification systems have been developed primarily for medical, surgical, pediat-

ric, and obstetrical patients in acute care facilities.

There have been numerous indications of the impact that patient classification and workload methodologies can have in the organization and administration of patient care units. Cost savings through balanced staffing is but one of these benefits. Data on long-range staffing needs for the purpose of budgeting may also be obtained from patient classification and workload information. Patient classification systems may also be shown to have impact in admission scheduling of patients and elective surgery. The assignment of nurses to patients is another area that is directly influenced by classification systems.

Constructing a Patient Classification System*

Classification Categories

The number of classification categories that are used in different systems is not as arbitrary as some might think. For example, the definitions of the classification categories could result from the hospital's policy regarding patient assignment to special care units or a persistent shortage of special unit beds or the absence of a special care unit. Each of these factors would have an effect on the highest level of patient demand on the general nursing care unit.

Unit Differences

Similarly different hospital units have different types of patients with different care requirements. The range of classifications in a minimal care category on a medical-surgical unit is far different than that in a critical care unit or a pediatric unit.

The development of an extended set of specific examples of patients and their care needs in each unit has proved helpful in defining each patient classification category. In this way patient classification will be less a matter of personal opinion than might otherwise result with general definitions. Others have chosen to append appropriate *decision-rule* guidelines for different units. An example of the kind of decision-rules that accompany a classification for a

---

*Source: *A Review and Evaluation of Nursing Productivity,* DHEW, 1977. Pub. No. (HRA) 77-15.

medical-surgical unit can be seen in the following sections.

Using Patient Classification: Decision-Rules for Nurses*

To illustrate the procedure for classifying patients, following are some decision rules used in completing the patient classification sheets in a medical-surgical unit.

Category I: Self-Care

1. *Self-Bathe, Feed, Ambulatory.* Check if patient is "up ad lib," and requires no assistance in bathing or feeding.
2. *To Be Discharged.* If the order has been written, check. Other indicators should be checked also. Includes transfers off the unit.
3. *Surgery—Not Returned.* Check ($\sqrt{}$) if the patient is now in the OR. If the patient is scheduled for today but hasn't gone yet, check the indicators applicable now. (Include heart caths and surgical x-ray procedures.)
4. *Admitted—Except Emergency.* Any non-emergency patient admitted or transferred to this unit during the last 8 hours should have this indicator checked. Also check indicators applicable to the patient now.

Category II: Partial Care

1. *Assist To Bathe or Feed and Assist To Ambulate.* Check for patients who need assistance with bathing, feeding or ambulation.
2. *Oral or Pharyngeal Suctioning.* Also includes patient with N-G tubes connected to suction apparatus. Excludes patients with Penrose drains.
3. *Parenteral Fluids—Up To 3/Shift.* Check for patients with 1, 2, or 3 bottles of IV fluid or blood ordered over eight hours (one shift).
4. *Semi-Conscious.* Self-explanatory.
5. *Slight Emotional Needs Versus More Stable Condition.* Check for patients who are *slightly* confused, anxious, depressed, etc.

---

*Source: J. Segall and J. Wilczynski, "Intensive Care Facility Study," Report 10 16-72, Community Systems Foundation, Ltd.

6. *Vital Signs Ordered—Up To 3/Shift.* Check for any patient with vital signs (blood pressure, pulse and respiratory) ordered 1, 2, or 3 times per shift.
7. *Intermittent Oxygen Therapy.* Includes ultrasonic nebulizer and IPPB treatments. Do not check for O_2 prn orders.
8. *Assist—Hearing/Speech/Vision.* Self-explanatory.
9. *Surgery—Returned.* Check for patients who had surgery today and have returned to floor during the last 8 hours. Check other indicators pertaining to patient now.
10. *Admitted Emergency.* Check for an emergency patient admitted or transferred to unit the last 8 hours. Also check other indicators pertaining to the patient now.

Category III: Complete Care

1. *Complete Bed Bath or Complete Feed for Bedfast Patient.* Check to indicate that patient is a complete bath and complete feed patient.
2. *Frequent Deep Suctioning.* Check for patients who need endotracheal suctioning at least every 30 minutes.
3. *Parenteral Fluids—Over 3/Shift.* Check if patient has 4 or more bottles of IV fluid or blood ordered over one shift (8 hours).
4. *Unconscious.* Check for comatose or unconscious patients. Would also include nonreactive patient following surgery.
5. *Marked Emotional Needs.* Check if patient is *seriously* confused, anxious, depressed, etc.
6. *Vital Signs Ordered—Over 3/Shift.* Check this column if vital signs are ordered more than 3 times on one shift (i.e., q 2 hrs. or more frequently) (blood pressure, pulse, and respiratory).
7. *Continuous Oxygen Therapy.* Check if patient is receiving continuous O_2 via cannula, mask, tent, etc.
8. *Isolation—Complete.* Check only for *complete* isolation, not for patients on stool and needle. Include reverse precaution.
9. *Chest or Abdominal Tubes.* This criteria refers to T, J or chest tubes.
10. *Close Observation for Impending Hemorrhage, Hypo, Hypertension, Cardiac Arrhythmia.* Also check for patients who

need close observation because of convulsive disorders. (Observation required at least every 30 minutes.)

A Model Classification System*

Another example of a classification system appears in Table 5-11. This is *only* an example. Each institution should develop its own criteria and definitions that suit its particular purposes. It is a four class system patterned after JCAH guidelines. To acquire a nursing hours baseline use was made of historical data. The number of hours per patient day was derived by taking the previous year's number of patient days divided

---

*Source: E.A. Schmied, "Nurse Staffing After Hospitals Merge," *Nursing Administration Quarterly,* Fall 1977.

by the number of paid nursing hours; the quotient was 4.2. Since nursing and fiscal affairs both wanted to increase patient care hours, the figure was adjusted to a baseline of 4.3 hours.

Application to Staffing

- Assign proportions of nursing-hour baseline according to skill level and shift-time.
  - —Professional staff are all RNs, including head nurses. Non-professional staff include LPNs, aides, technicians and unit secretaries.
  - —Pro-rate 51% for the day shift; 34% for the evening shift; 15% for the night shift.
  - —Standard = 4.3 manhours per patient day

Professional	= 1.9	44%
Non-Professional	= 2.4	56%
	4.3	100%

Table 5-11 Criteria for Classification According to Nursing Care Requirements

I. (65%) A PATIENT WHO REQUIRES ONLY MINIMAL AMOUNT OF NURSING CARE (An average of 2.8 nursing hours per 24 hours)

Examples

- A patient who is mildly ill (generally termed convalescent).
- A patient who requires little treatment and/or observation and/or instruction.
- A patient who is up and about as desired; takes his own bath or shower.
- A patient who does not exhibit any unusual behavior patterns.
- A patient without intravenous therapy or many medications.

II. (100%) A PATIENT WHO REQUIRES AN AVERAGE AMOUNT OF NURSING CARE (An average of 4.3 nursing hours per 24 hours)

Examples

- A patient whose extreme symptoms have subsided or not yet appeared.
- A patient who requires periodic treatments and/or observations and/or instructions.
- A patient who is up and about with help for limited periods; partial bed rest required.
- A patient who exhibits some psychological or social problems.
- A patient with intravenous therapy with medications such as IV piggybacks every six hours.
- A newly admitted patient, either surgical or medical, who is a routine admission and not necessarily acutely ill.

III. (135%) A PATIENT WHO REQUIRES ABOVE AVERAGE NURSING CARE (An average of 5.8 nursing hours per 24 hours)

Examples

- A moderately ill patient.
- A patient who requires treatments or observations as frequently as every two to four hours.
- A patient with significant changes in treatment or medication orders more than four times a day.
- An uncomplicated patient with IV medications every four hours and/or hyperalimentation.
- A patient on complete bed rest.

IV. (200%) A PATIENT WHO REQUIRES MAXIMUM NURSING CARE (An average of 8.6 nursing hours per 24 hours)

This classification is most often used in intensive care areas.

Examples

- A patient who exhibits extreme symptoms (usually termed acutely ill).
- A patient whose activity must be rigidly controlled.
- A patient who requires continuous treatment and/or observations and/or instructions.
- A patient with significant changes in doctor's orders, more than six times a day.
- A patient with many medications, IV piggybacks, and vital signs every hour and/or hourly output.

The total amount of time required to care for each patient determines his classification.

Source: E.A. Schmied, "Nurse Staffing After Hospitals Merge," *Nursing Administration Quarterly, Fall* 1977.

- Establish "permanent" nursing staff by unit at a number sufficient to service an occupancy level of approximately 70 percent. "Rotating" or "relief" staff is calculated, making up the difference to standard hours calculated above.
- Establish a format whereby the prediction of the number of patients by category and required nursing hours for the *oncoming* shift should be done by the head nurse of the present shift, so that in effect, the head nurses are never involved in planning staff for their own shifts, but instead, do it for each other.

The most valuable feature of this categorization procedure is that it provides for more help when there is a genuine increase in highly demanding patients. Similarly it indicates where and how much staff can be reduced when less acute conditions occur.

How to Estimate Nurse Staffing Needs

How to Calculate Required Nursing Hours*

The workload sheet (see Table 5-12) is used to calculate the mean number of nursing hours required on the unit.

How to Calculate Available Staff Hours By Skill Level*

This worksheet (see Table 5-13) is the companion of the work-load worksheet. It is used to calculate the mean number of hours available from each nursing category. It should be completed each month for each unit being monitored.

CASH Guidelines for Nursing Tasks

In 1967, CASH (Commission for Administrative Services in Hospitals) did a study on the nursing time requirements of patients in various age groups which was designed to give results which would establish time standards of personnel proficiency and quality. The system was also designed so that an audit could be performed on a continuous basis to measure the comparison to the standard. These time standards represent a useful guide to nurse activity (see Table 5-14).

---

*Source: Haussman, Hegyvary, and Newman, *Monitoring Quality of Nursing Care—Part II*, DHEW, July 1976. Pub. No. (HRA) 76-7, Appendix 4.

Table 5-12　Workload Sheet

1. Unit: _____

2. Find the daily average number of patient types 1–4 on the unit. (To do so, add the number of Type 1 patients each day in the month and divide by the number of days in the month. Do the same calculation for Types 2, 3, and 4.) Enter the number of each type in Column A.

		A	B[‡]	C
Average number	Type 1 =		01	
	Type 2 =		03	
	Type 3 =		07	
	Type 4 =		14	

3. Multiply each number in Column *A* by the number in Column *B*. Write the product in Column *C*. (Column *B* is the mean hours required for each patient type, based on previous study; *C* is the number of nursing hours required per type in 24 hours.)
4. Add the four numbers in Column *C*. Enter the number on the blank at the right. _____
5. Divide the total of Column *C* by the sum of the daily average number of patients on the unit (from Step 2 above). This figure tells you the number of hours per patient day required. Enter the answer on the blank at right. _____

Example: Patient unit 3 West
(Steps 2–4) Average patient mix:

	A	B	C
T1 –	08	01	08
T2 –	10	03	30
T3 –	15	07	105
T4 –	02	14	28
	35		171 hours

(Step 5) $\dfrac{171}{35}$ = 4.9 hours per patient day required

---

[‡]Column B lists the mean hours required for each patient type. In this example the ratios are 1:3:7:14. In Schum it was 2.8:4.3:5.8:8.6. Warstler had still another ratio. Each hospital unit must establish its own ratio according to need and available resources.

Source: Haussman, Hegyvary, and Newman, *Monitoring Quality of Nursing Care—Part II*, DHEW, July 1976. Pub. No. (HRA) 76-7, Appendix 4.

How To Develop Staffing Tables*

Staffing tables can be developed so that when the number of patients per classification are known, the number of staff needed can be obtained directly from the table.

---

*Source: *Methods for Studying Nurse Staffing in a Patient Unit*, DHEW, 1978, Pub. No. (HRA) 78-3.

Table 5-13 Available Staff Hours by Skill Level—Work Sheet

1. Unit: _____
2. Obtain a list of *all nursing staff* on the unit. Include all full and part-time employees. Include the head nurse, RNs, LPNs, aides, and any other category you may include in giving nursing care, such as medication technicians. Do not include clerks or unit managers, and do not include nursing supervisory staff who cover more than one unit. Make separate worksheets for each category: (1) RN, (2) LPN, (3) aide and orderly, and (4) other.
3. Starting with the RN category, calculate the *total number of hours* worked by each nurse on the unit this month. Use time cards or staffing roster to ascertain information.
4. Add the hours worked by each person in the category to find the *total number of hours worked by that category* on the unit that month. Enter that number at the right. _____
5. Divide the total number found in Step 4 by the number of days in the month. (Do not divide by the number of days worked. If for December, divide by 31.) Enter the answer at the right. _____
6. Divide the answer from Step 5 by the number of beds on the unit. Enter the number at the right. This number is the mean number of nursing hours of this category available per patient day on that unit. _____
7. Repeat Steps 3–6 for LPN staff. Enter the result from Step 6 at the right. _____
8. Repeat Steps 3–6 for aide staff. Enter the result from Step 6 at the right. _____
9. Repeat Steps 3–6 for "other" category if applicable. Enter the result from Step 6 at the right. _____
   Example:

	RN Staff	Hours Worked This Month		Aides and Orderlies	Hours Worked This Month
(Steps 2&3)	1. (RN name)	168	(Steps 2&3)	1. Name	166
	2. (RN name)	164		2. Name	156
	3. (RN name)	156		etc.	etc.
	etc.	etc.	(Step 4)	Total = 675	
(Step 4)	Total = 1720 hours (for 10 RNs)			(for 4 aides)	

$$(\text{Step 5}) \quad \frac{1720 \text{ hours}}{31 \text{ days}} = 55.5 \text{ RN hours per day}$$

$$(\text{Step 6}) \quad \frac{55.5 \text{ hours}}{35 \text{ patients}} = 1.59 \text{ RN hours per patient day}$$

$$(\text{Step 5}) \quad \frac{675}{31} = 21.8 \text{ aide hours per day}$$

$$(\text{Step 6}) \quad \frac{21.8}{35} = 0.62 \text{ aide hours per patient day}$$

Total nursing hours available per patient day:

RN = 1.59
LPN = 1.85
Aide = 0.62
Total = 4.06

	LPN Staff	Hours Worked This Month
(Steps 2&3)	1. Name	168
	2. Name	170
	etc.	etc.
(Step 4)	Total = 2016 hours (for 12 LPNs)	

$$(\text{Step 5}) \quad \frac{2016}{31} = 65.0 \text{ LPN hours per day}$$

$$(\text{Step 6}) \quad \frac{65.6}{35} = 1.85 \text{ LPN hours per patient day}$$

Source: Haussman, Hegyvary, and Newman, *Monitoring Quality of Nursing Care—Part II*, DHEW, July 1976. Pub. No. (HRA) 76-7, Appendix 4.

Table 5-14 Standard Times for Direct Care Tasks

The following list of standard times for direct care tasks was taken from CASH (C) and Nurse Utilization and Staffing Analysis, Nyack Hospital, Nyack, New York (N). (Source: Hospital Management Engineering Program, Albany, New York). The categories match those in the work sampling form in Figure 28-10.

		Minutes			Minutes
1	**COMMUNICATION: PATIENT/FAMILY**		**33**	Bath: Tub or Shower, Attended	12.00 (C)
1	Admit: Including Patient Orientation	19.98 (C)	**34**	Bed Change: Occupied	10.02 (N)
2	Emotional Support: Reassurance T.L.C.	10.02 (N)	**35**	Bed Change: Unoccupied	4.02 (N)
3	Explanation of Procedure Time Required:		**36**	Dress or Undress: Assist	19.98 (C)
4	Teaching: Patient &/or Family Subject: Time Required:		**37**	H.S. Care (Not including backrub)	2.28 (C)
			38	Incontinent Care: Wash Area	12.00 (C)
2	**MEDICATIONS, I.V., (ADMINISTRATION)**		**39**	Isolation: Gowning, Washing Hands	3.00 (C)
5	I.V.: Start	12.00 (C)	**40**	Oral Hygiene	4.02 (N)
6	I.V.: Check, Adjust, Infiltration	1.98 (N)	**41**	Pre-Meal Care	1.86 (C)
7	I.V.: Add Medication	3.00 (N)	**5**	**PATIENT MOVEMENT**	
8	I.V.: Discontinue	1.98 (N)	**42**	Discharge: Bedside Tasks	4.98 (N)
9	I.V.: Transfusion, Add On	7.50 (C)	**43**	Transfer: Same Unit	12.00 (N)
10	Meds: Injection, Give	2.58 (C)	**44**	Transfer: Other Unit	25.02 (N)
11	Meds: Oral, Give	.90 (C)	**45**	Transport to Other Dept. or Area Where: Time Required:	
12	Meds: Rectal, Vaginal	3.00 (N)			
13	Meds: Topical	4.02 (N)			
3	**NUTRITION AND ELIMINATION**		**6**	**POSITIONING AND EXERCISING**	
14	Bedpan: Give	1.98 (N)	**46**	Assist: Dangle, Ambulate, Exercise (R.O.M.)	7.02 (N)
15	Bedpan: Take, Empty	4.02 (N)	**47**	Assist: To or From Stretcher, Bed, Wheelchair, Chair	7.50 (C)
16	Emesis: Assist Patient, Empty Basin	5.04 (C)			
17	Feed: Complete Assist	19.98 (C/N)	**48**	Position Bed	.42 (C)
18	Feed: Partial Assist	10.02 (N)	**49**	Position Patient: Partial	1.98 (N)
19	Feed: Snack	7.98 (C)	**50**	Position Patient: Turn	3.00 (N)
20	Food: Delayed Trays, Deliver	3.00 (N)	**51**	Turn, Cough, Deep Breathe	5.10
21	Food: Pass or Pick up Tray	2.46 (C)	**52**	Traction: Adjust	3.00 (N)
22	Intake/Output: Record	1.50 (C/N)	**7**	**ROUNDS/ASSIST**	
23	Gastric Tube: Levine Tube: Feed	10.02 (N)	**53**	Assist M.D. With Treatment	25.02 (C)
24	Nourishment: Pass or Give	1.50 (N/C)	**54**	Assist Other Department Persons	4.56
25	Urinal: Give	1.02 (N)	**55**	Rounds with M.D.	3.48 (C)
26	Urinal: Remove or Empty	1.98 (N)	**8**	**PATIENT CHECKS**	
27	Urinary Drainage: Change or Empty	7.62	**56**	Patient Rounds, Nurse	.48 (C)
28	Water: Refill	1.98 (N)	**57**	Symptom Observation	2.52 (N)
4	**PATIENT HYGIENE**		**9**	**SPECIMEN GATHERING, TESTING**	
29	Backrub	3.00 (C/N)	**58**	Specimen Collection: Culture	3.00 (N)
30	Bath: Complete	30.00 (N)	**59**	Specimen Collection: Gastric	15.00 (C)
31	Bath: Partial	19.98 (N)			
32	Bath: Self Care, Assist	4.98 (N)			

Table 5-14 continued

		Minutes
60	Specimen Collection: Sputum	4.02 (C)
61	Specimen Collection: Stool	6.00 (C)
62	Specimen Collection: Urine, Routine	4.98 (C)
63	Specimen Collection: Urine 24 Hour	1.98
64	Stool: Guiac Test	2.16
65	Urine Test: Sugar or Acetone	4.02 (C)
66	Urine Test: Specific Gravity	1.80 (C)
10	**TREATMENTS AND PROCEDURES**	
67	Anti-embolism Stocking	5.00 (N)
68	Catheterization	19.02 (C)
69	Catheter: Irrigate	10.02 (N)
70	Dressing: Sterile	11.04 (C)
71	Dressing: Unsterile	9.00 (C)
72	Enema: Disposable	6.00 (C)
73	Enema: Non-Disposable	12.00 (C)
74	Levine Tube: Insert or Remove	10.02 (N)
75	Levine Tube: Irrigate or Suction	12.00 (N)
76	Oxygen: Start	11.04 (C)
77	Oxygen: Maintain	3.00 (N)
78	Oxygen: Discontinue	9.00 (C)
79	Pre-Op: Bedside Check	5.00 (N)
80	Pre-Op: Shave	15.00 (N)
81	Restraints: Apply or Remove	10.98 (C)
82	Suction: Oral or Nasal	10.02 (N)
83	Tracheostomy: Suction and/or Clean	7.02 (N)
84	Tracheostomy: Change Tube	10.02 (N)
85	Traction: Set Up	15.00 (C)
86	Traction: Remove	4.20
11	**VITAL SIGNS**	
87	Blood Pressure	3.00 (N)
88	Pulse and/or Respiration	1.50 (C)
89	Temperature Only: Oral	3.00 (N)
90	Temperature Only: Rectal	3.00 (N)
91	T.P.R.: Routine	3.00 (N)
92	Weigh: Bed Scale	3.00 (C)
93	Weigh: Floor Scale	4.98 (N)
99	**OTHER: LIST**	

Source: Laurel N. Murphy, Project Director, *Development of Methods for Determining Use and Effectiveness of Nursing Service Personnel*, San Joaquin Hospital, 1976. PHS No. 1-NU 34048.

Suppose that each staff member provides 3 hours of direct patient care while Category I, II, III, and IV patients require 20, 45, 60 and 180 minutes of direct care respectively. A staffing table such as Table 5-15 will enable a user to estimate staff needs as follows:

If there are 15 Category I patients, 10 Category II patients, 5 Category III patients, and 1 Category IV patient, then under I for 15 patients, 1.7 staff are needed. Under II for 10 patients, 2.5 staff are needed. Under III for 5 patients, 1.7 staff are needed, and under IV for 1

Table 5-15 Table for Calculating Number of Staff Personnel Needed (Based upon Patient Class and Staffing During Study Period, Excluding Ward Clerk)

Direct Patient Care Sampling

Hospital ———————— Unit ——— Date of Study ———

Shift ————— Type of Unit ———————

Number of Patients	Number of Staff Members Needed for Category			
	I	II	III	IV
1	.1	.3	.3	1.0
2	.2	.5	.7	2.0
3	.3	.8	1.0	3.0
4	.4	1.0	1.3	4.0
5	.6	1.3	1.7	5.0
6	.7	.5	2.0	6.0
7	.8	1.8	2.3	7.0
8	.9	2.0	2.7	8.0
9	1.0	2.3	3.0	9.0
10	1.1	2.5	3.3	10.0
11	1.2	2.8	3.7	11.0
12	1.3	3.0	4.0	12.0
13	1.4	3.3	4.3	13.0
14	1.6	3.5	4.7	14.0
15	1.7	3.8	5.0	15.0
16	1.8	4.0	5.3	
17	1.9	4.3	5.7	
18	2.0	4.5	6.0	
19	2.1	4.8	6.3	
20	2.2	5.0	6.7	
21	2.3	5.3	7.0	
22	2.4	5.5	7.3	
23	2.6	5.8	7.7	
24	2.7	6.0	8.0	

Source: *Methods for Studying Nurse Staffing in a Patient Unit*, DHEW, 1978, Pub. No. (HRA) 78-3.

patient, 1.0 staff member is needed. Then: 1.7 + 2.5 + 1.7 + 1.0 = 6.9 or 7 staff needed.

The entries in Table 5-15 were prepared as follows:

Multiply a selected number of patients (1 through 24, in this case) by the number of minutes of care determined for a given patient category; convert this to hours by dividing by 60. Divide the result by the number of hours of direct care a staff member provides (three in this case). The resulting quotient is the entry in the table for the given number of patients.

For example, 10 patients in Category II require: $(10 \times 45) \div 60 = 7.5$ hours of care. Then $7.5 \div 3 = 2.5$ FTE staff members.

It is important to note that corresponding tables should be prepared for each unit for each shift, since the entries depend upon the hours of direct patient care given by each staff member in that unit, as well as the minutes of care required by the different classes of patients in that unit.

Staffing tables developed as a result of studies conducted on specific units will reflect the staffing conditions in existence at the time of the study. If the unit was operating in an understaffed condition during the study, the staffing tables will underestimate staff needs. Conversely, if the staff was observed to have excessive personal time during the study, the staffing tables will overestimate staff needs. The head/charge nurse's perception of adequacy is the key to the development of proper staffing patterns. If the unit were overstaffed during the study, staffing estimates from the table could be "rounded down" or decreased. Additional perception of adequacy data could then be taken and comparisons of direct care given per staff member could be made with similar units. Ideally, 6 months after new staffing patterns had been established, repeat studies could be done to determine the impact of these changes.

Using Federal Guidelines for Estimating Nurse Staffing Needs*

In order to establish uniform guidelines for hospitals to project nurse staffing needs, a federally

---

*Source: *Analysis and Planning for Improved Distribution of Nursing Personnel and Services,* Western Interstate Commission for Higher Education, DHEW Pub. No. (HRA) 79-16.

appointed panel of expert consultants made recommendations about: (1) the overall staffing levels required; (2) the desired mix among RNs, LPNs, and aides; and (3) the desired mix of RNs at the associate degree/diploma (AD/DIP), baccalaureate, and advanced degree levels of preparation.

The panel projected a different mix of nursing personnel, within the overall staffing levels required, than that currently existing in most agencies. In making its projections the panel took into account three factors: the number of tasks that can be assigned to other workers, the number of LPNs and aides that an RN can supervise, and the number of patients for whom an RN can care. The panel utilized accepted standards in current practice where these existed and proposed criteria for staffing and educational preparation on the basis of its collective expertise when previous guidelines were unavailable. (See Tables 5-16 and 5-17 for results of this study.)

Basis for Projections

The panel made its projections on the basis of the following assumed conditions: (1) that nurse staffing for a group of patients requires nurses on three shifts for each day; (2) that one FTE nurse will work 1,800 hours per year on the average; (3) that 4.9 FTE nurses are required to provide one nurse for each of the 21 shifts per week, based on the 1,800 hours of work (which allows for the standard work week and holidays, vacation, and actual sick leave taken); and (4) that 20.3 FTE RNs per 100 patients will give one nurse hour for each patient day.

The figure of 1,800 hours was a weighted average of the estimated number of hours worked per year, which the panel adopted, based on surveys by the Bureau of Labor Statistics in selected standard metropolitan statistical areas. The figure corresponds to 45 working weeks, or 225 working days per year.

The derivation of FTE RNs necessary to provide one RN on each shift is as follows:

21 shifts/week $\times$ 52 weeks/year

= 1,092 shifts/year

1,800 hours/FTE RNs/year $\div$ 8 hours/shift

= 225 shifts/FTE RNs/year

1,092 shifts/year $\div$ 225 shifts/FTE RNs/year

= 4.9 FTE RNs

Table 5-16 Criteria for Nurse Staffing and RN Educational Preparation

Field of Employment	Lower Bound RNs	Lower Bound LPNs (Per 100 Patients)	Lower Bound Aides	Upper Bound RNs	Upper Bound LPNs (Per 100 Patients)	Upper Bound Aides	Doct. (%)	Master's (%)	Bacc. (%)	AD/DIP (%)
INPATIENT SERVICES										
General units*	49.0	12.0	12.0	56.5	12.0	12.0			50	50
Rehabilitation units	49.0	12.0	12.0	56.5	12.0	12.0			50	50
Newborn units	49.0	12.0	12.0	56.5	12.0	12.0			20	80
Critical care units	200.0	0.0	0.0	250.0	0.0	0.0			50	50
Extended care units	20.0	20.0	20.0	30.0	20.0	20.0			50	50
All units in hospitals under 100 beds										
Long-term hospitals (psychiatric)	13.0	10.0	30.0	22.0	10.0	30.0			50	50
Psychiatric units in all short-term hospitals	49.0	0.0	24.0	56.5	0.0	24.0			50	50
OTHER HOSPITAL SERVICES										
Operating room	1.5 RNs per 1000 operations (10 RNs/0 LPNs/3 Aides)			1.8 RNs per 1000 operations (10 RNs/0 LPNs/2 Aides)						100
Emergency room	0.22 RNs per 1000 visits (10 RNs/10 LPNs/10 Aides)			0.44 RNs per 1000 visits (10 RNs/10 LPNs/5 Aides)					50	50
Outpatient clinics	0.11 RNs per 1000 visits (10 RNs/10 LPNs/10 Aides)			0.23 RNs per 1000 visits (10 RNs/10 LPNs/5 Aides)				10	80	10

Field of Employment	Lower Bound RNs Per 100 Patients	Upper Bound RNs Per 100 Patients	Doct. (%)	Master's (%)	Bacc. (%)	AD/DIP (%)
CLINICAL SPECIALISTS						
Large teaching (more than 400 beds)	3.0	5.0	Educational preparation for all clinical specialists is at graduate level			
Small (less than 100 beds), and all long-term hospitals	2.0	4.0				
All other short-term hospitals	2.0	4.0	Projections made for 100% master's preparation			
Nursing care homes	0.5	1.0				
Personal care homes with nursing	0.2	0.3				
Hospital ambulatory care	1 per 20 DCC RNs	1 per 20 DCC RNs				
Community health nursing	1 per 20 DCC RNs	1 per 20 DCC RNs				
ADMINISTRATIVE POSITIONS						
Executive/Principal Nurse Administrator						
All hospitals	1 Director of nursing per institution		5	95		
Large teaching (more than 400 beds)	2–3 Assistants and/or associate directors per institution		5	95		
All other short-term hospitals	1–2 Assistants and/or associate directors per institution		5	95		
Mid-level Nurse Administrators/Managers						
All hospitals	1 Head nurse per 30 patients			25	75	
All hospitals	1 Supervisor per 100 patients			25	75	
INSERVICE INSTRUCTORS						
Short-term, large, teaching hospitals	3 RNs per institution			100		
Nursing homes & all other hospitals	0.5 RNs per institution			100		
Community health nursing	0.5 RNs per agency			100		

*General units includes adult medical-surgical, pediatrics, and maternity.
Source: *Analysis and Planning for Improved Distribution of Nursing Personnel and Services*, Western Interstate Commission for Higher Education, DHEW Pub. No. (HRA) 79-16.

Table 5-17   Conversion Chart for Staffing Ratios and Hours of Nursing Care per Day*

	FTE Staff per 100 Patients				RN/LPN/Aide Ratio	Hours per Patient per Day		RN Hours Care (%)
	RNs	LPNs	Aides	Total		RNs	Total Hrs	
GENERAL UNITS								
REHABILITATION								
NEWBORN UNITS								
ALL UNITS IN HOSPITALS								
LESS THAN 100 BEDS								
Lower bound	49	12	12	73	10/2.4/2.4	2.4	3.6	67
Upper bound	56.5	12	12	80.5	10/2.1/2.1	2.8	4.0	70
CRITICAL CARE								
Lower bound	200	0	0	200	10/0/0	9.9	9.9	100
Upper bound	250	0	0	250	10/0/0	12.3	12.3	100
EXTENDED CARE								
Lower bound	20	20	20	60	10/10/10	1.0	3.0	33
Upper bound	30	20	20	70	10/6.7/6.7	1.5	3.5	43
LONG-TERM PSYCH. HOSPITALS								
Lower bound	13	10	30	53	10/7.7/23.1	0.6	2.6	23
Upper bound	22	10	30	62	10/4.5/13.6	1.1	3.1	35
PSYCHIATRIC UNITS IN ALL								
SHORT-TERM HOSPITALS								
Lower bound	49	0	24	73	10/0/4.8	2.4	3.6	67
Upper bound	56.5	0	24	80.5	10/0/4.2	2.8	4.0	70
NURSING HOMES								
Lower bound	9	23	23	54	10/25/25	0.4	2.7	15
Upper bound	20	40	40	100	10/20/20	1.0	4.9	20
PERSONAL CARE HOMES								
WITH NURSING								
Lower and upper bounds	5	10	20	35	10/20/40	0.2	1.7	12

*Figures based on 1,800 working hours per year per one full-time employee.

Source: *Analysis and Planning for Improved Distribution of Nursing Personnel and Services*, Western Interstate Commission for Higher Education, DHEW Pub. No. (HRA) 79-16.

The panel indicated that in hospitals of less than 100 beds, the patient conditions vary considerably. A staffing pattern sufficient to meet any problem is required. Thus, the panel recommended the same criteria for all units in a hospital of less than 100 beds as those recommended for general units in larger hospitals.

Critical care units require intense, complex, and sophisticated nursing care. At times, some patients require continued surveillance and direct nursing care on a one-to-one basis.

Projections for nursing personnel in hospital emergency rooms and outpatient clinics are based on the projected number of visits anticipated. Using the figure of 1,800 hours of work per year, the panel projected a lower range of requirements based on 20 visits per eight-hour day per FTE RN (or 4,500 visits per year), and an upper range of requirements based on 10 visits per eight-hour day per FTE RN (or 2,250 visits per year). The panel projected that the number of outpatient clinic visits an RN can manage range from 20 to 40 visits per day (or a range of 4,500 to 9,000 visits per year).

*Problems of Statistical Staffing Comparisons**

However, there are problems comparing the statistical approach to staffing in one hospital or unit with another hospital or unit—or, of course, with a general standard.

Some of these problems are:

- How well are the patients? New surgical patients require more care than do third or fourth day surgical cases, and chronic cases may have great dependency without being too ill. The degree of illness on each unit is a major determinant in basic staffing needs. Unless this is known, we cannot statistically compare the staffing needs of one unit or hospital to another.
- What types of patients are being cared for? The difference in the type and amount of care exists between medical, surgical, obstetric, ICU, pediatric, etc., patients.

*Source: Thomas R. O'Donovan, "A Penetration Coefficient Approach to Nurse Staffing," *Nursing Administration Quarterly*, Fall 1977.

- How consistent is the census? In some of the services mentioned above, particularly pediatrics and obstetrics, we see great fluctuations in the census. Staffing these units is particularly difficult when trying to use statistical methods.
- What is the layout of each unit? Are there special arrangements on specific units? How far do personnel have to walk to get supplies and equipment and to observe patients?
- How much automation is there on each unit? Does each unit have, for example, bedpan washers, ice-makers, nurse call intercommunication to patients?
- Are medications centralized or decentralized from the pharmacy? Do we have a traditional medication system or a unit-dose system?
- What types of rooms are there on each unit—ward, semi, or private? What is the mix of these types of rooms on each unit? Although patients are often deprived of privacy in ward units, many nurses would comment that the nursing care time in terms of personal services to patients is increased in a ward simply by the proximity of each patient to the nurse. Under certain circumstances, the greater the total square footage of a nursing unit, the greater the staffing needs, if the number of patients is held constant.
- What type of bathroom facilities are there for patients? Are there separate bathrooms or toilets for each room? Are there handwashing facilities in each room? If not, a great deal of wasted time is incurred while nursing staff wash between treating each patient, or when they are required to accompany patients to bathrooms outside their individual rooms.
- Are disposables used and to what extent?
- Is there clerical staffing, and is the desk clerk trained and available for one shift, two shifts or three shifts? To what extent is this clerk trained, and does it relieve the floor nurses of a great deal of time spent in nonnursing tasks?
- Are unit managers being used? What are the total responsibilities of the head nurses? Do they do the unit staffing themselves or does the nursing office perform this function? (All three of these factors affect comparative differentiations.)
- Which shift is being considered? Day and afternoon staffing should definitely be greater than night staffing, and what ratio is considered appropriate among each of the three shifts?
- What are the job descriptions for the nursing personnel? Do LPNs give medications? What is the meeting and conference schedule of the personnel on this unit? Are float nurses available for absenteeism? Does the hospital occasionally use an outside medical pool when short-run needs dictate?
- Is team nursing utilized? This particular method normally requires more staffing.
- Regarding administrative philosophy, does the administration of the hospital desire or require a nearly all RN staff?
- Are patients truly separated? Does the admitting office keep medical patients out of surgical areas (and vice versa)?
- Is there an overall reluctance by the nursing service personnel to float from unit to unit? Or from shift to shift? The index number approach takes large areas into consideration, but it doesn't assist if a particular area is short.
- The managerial ability of each head nurse affects the staffing and the efficiency on each unit.
- The ratio of staffing on days, afternoons and midnights is interrelated. Higher staffing on afternoons may be justified if nights are extremely short staffed. The patients can be settled better by leaving high staffing on afternoons. A ratio of 100 percent staffing on days, 70 percent staffing on afternoons and 30 percent staffing on nights could go to 100, 95, 20, simply because of the night short staffing.
- The difference between units can be exemplified by the ICU theory that the staffing ratio over days, afternoons and midnights would be 100, 100, 100. But because more doctors are around on *days* and they need attention, and the nurses must be available to attend to the orders of the physicians, assist with tests, treatments, dressings and physical examinations, the theory of 100, 100, 100 could possibly be modified to 100, 80, 80. (This point needs further study as to its applicability to the medical/surgical units, etc.)
- Are many versus few private duty nurses utilized? Are student nurses used exten-

sively throughout the hospital? Does the hospital have a good volunteer force which assists the nursing service department? These kinds of points affect differential staffing patterns.

- Policies on linen exchange, leaving the nursing station, patient transportation, and simply whether or not messenger services are available, play a large part in staffing analysis.
- The extent of a high degree of specialization results occasionally in certain nurses being idle in their specialty unit, while nurses in other units are temporarily highly involved or short of help. The problem is how to maximize the advantages of nurse specialization and still have the effective use of them in slack periods. Where feasible, nurses could be trained in two or three specialized areas so that flexibility can be achieved. (PAR, ICU, OB, ER, etc.)
- Differential ability and levels of training among nursing personnel must be considered. The individual nurse competency is a highly relevant issue. (This makes it very difficult to apply arbitrary statistical measures to staffing determinations.)
- The size of the medical staff is certainly an issue at hand. Those hospitals with large medical staffs may find they need more nurses to handle the physicians' orders. Those hospitals with small medical staffs may find that nurses have assumed more and more of the physicians' duties.
- The fringe benefit package at the hospital must be considered. Do employees after five years receive four weeks vacation, three weeks, one week? Do "all" employees after five years receive four weeks vacation? Since fringe benefit policies, particularly vacation, holiday and sick day policies, relate to the hours of each employee throughout a year, the numbers of personnel assigned to each unit are directly affected by these policies. How many coffee breaks are allowed, and how long, and does abuse exist?

ADJUSTMENT TECHNIQUES FOR UNDERSTAFFING AND OVERSTAFFING

Staffing adjustments should not be confused with regular scheduling. Scheduling is concerned with planning for personnel usage throughout the year—taking into account the changing needs due to shifts, seasons, holidays, vacations and the full range of predictable factors.

Staff adjustments, on the other hand, are concerned with unexpected conditions, the day to day variations in need or situation that result in overstaffing or understaffing.

The need for nursing care varies from day to day and shift to shift not only because of the change in the number of patients, but also because of their type and condition. Unfortunately, such variations cannot be accurately forecast. Not only must adjustments be made if supply is to be matched with demand but also if the amount of absenteeism on any given day is to be reckoned with.

The adjustment process can be called the reallocation decision, and it is made centrally (or if decentrally, among divisions of the hospital) each shift, allocating the float pool of nurses and/or "pulling" nurses from the unit to which they were originally scheduled.[1]

The process is in two phases. First the demand for nursing care services must be measured on each unit, taking into account the current number, type, and condition of patients.

The second stage is to adjust such demand to the supply which includes the "core" staff (permanent staff scheduled to a particular unit), the float and/or "pull" staff, and outside resources.

There are a wide range of techniques available for making adjustments for both overstaffing and understaffing.

Handling Understaffing

If a specific station is understaffed while another is overstaffed, a nurse may be floated, i.e. reassigned to another station. Pool personnel can also be used to cover shortages on specific stations. If it becomes apparent that the nursing stations in total will be understaffed for a given shift, several steps can be taken. Part time employees assigned to nursing units and assigned to the nursing pool can be contacted and requested to work an extra shift. In addition, an "on-call" pool has been developed to cover in such situations; these people can also be con-

---

[1] D. Michael Warner, "Nurse Staffing, Scheduling and Reallocation in the Hospital," *Hospital & Health Services Administration,* Summer 1976.

tacted. Another mechanism to add needed personnel is to utilize temporary Professional Nurse Agencies. Basically, the system has been constructed so as to be able to expand on short-term notice; however, anticipation of and planning for these situations are of key importance.*

Floating Nurse

Few nursing administrators like the idea of using floating nurses, yet running a nursing department would often prove unmanageable without them. A national survey by Nursing '75 discovered that 54 percent of all nurses have to float; 42 percent said they are often pulled from one unit to another. Many of them are unhappy doing it; most of those who were against floating felt that nurses couldn't provide quality of care in a variety of hospital units. Others clearly indicated that they liked familiar surroundings and wanted to feel that they were part of a group. Obviously, the use of floating nurses should be minimized.

Nursing Pools—Permanent*

A nursing pool can be of key importance to the staffing system as it provides needed flexibility. The size of the pool can be varied by the staffing coordinator to meet projected patient care needs. For example, in the Methodist Hospital in St. Louis Park, Minnesota, there are three separate area pools—a Medical-Surgical pool, a Pediatrics-OB-GYN pool, and an Intensive Care Pool. Nurses who are recruited for each of the pools receive orientation to all stations within their respective areas and to each nursing station in the hospital. While they may float to any station in the hospital, the nurses in the pools normally float only within their area of training. Each nurse reports to the assistant staffing coordinator before each scheduled shift to receive her station assignment.

They are scheduled on a monthly basis as are all employees in the hospital. As permanent vacancies occur on nurses' stations, pool employees transfer to a nurse's station, thus providing the hospital with a reservoir of trained employees who can fill permanent station assignments.

Flying Squad

An added "wrinkle" to the system normally not seen in many hospitals, is the use of a "flying squad." The flying squad, normally consisting of two nurses, is not assigned to any specific station, but moves from station to station throughout the shift based on varying needs of the stations during the shift. The flying squad members carry pocket pagers so that head nurses in need of additional help can easily reach them. The flying squad will actually work on several different stations during each shift, thus often overcoming the necessity of providing extra staff on several stations just for the purpose of meeting peak activity times. Again, flexibility is added to the system.

Controlled Admissions

The first day of patient stay, particularly for nonelective admissions, imposes more than twice the demand on nurse staff than do subsequent days. Given some choice in placing a new admission plus knowledge of the number of intensive and first day patients on each unit, there is a potential for stabilizing workloads by selective admission to units.

Part-Time Nurses*

A frequent criticism of part-time nurses is their lack of commitment or competence, resulting in many cases from their random assignment to a variety of units or nursing teams. Queensway General Hospital, a 327-bed facility in Toronto, circumvents these problems by using a system which employs a large pool of permanent part-times, each of whom is posted to a specific unit. A second level of fill-ins is labelled casuals.

The system has been used with positive results for over twenty years.

The major factor in determining the competence of a part-time nurse, either permanent or casual, is the number of tours worked. The permanent part-time nurses work an average of 132 tours a year, or about two and a half days a week.

The head nurse annually conducts interviews which enable the department to help those that

---

*Source: Merrill Lehman and Q.J. Friesen, A Centralized Position and Staffing Control Administered by Non-Nursing Personnel, Methodist Hospital, St. Louis Park, Minnesota, 1975.

*Source: Elizabeth Katz, "Flexible Scheduling Using Part-time Nurses," Dimensions in Health Service, Journal of the Canadian Hospital Association, March 1978.

need help and to eliminate those who are not making themselves available often enough to maintain their competence.

Permanent part-time nurses must be available for posting 11 months of the year. They are required to work either on Christmas or New Year's holidays, one weekend out of three, and two of the holiday weekends in the summer. Part-time staff do not qualify for fringe benefits but they do receive vacations according to a percentage of hours worked and shift premiums.

The casual part-time nurses average 60 tours a year.

The competence of the casual nurse is watched over by the nursing supervisors. All casual part-time nurses are divided alphabetically and assigned to a supervisor. The casuals are not identified with one specific unit, but they establish one-to-one contact with the supervisor who, during the course of her tours, is able to observe the casual part-time person at work. The supervisor reports on the competence of the casual to the director of nursing and also sits down with the casual part-time person to determine if she can be available for work more often to maintain her competence, or to recommend in-service programs.

If the casual part-time person does not make herself available for a six-month period, her employment at the Queensway General Hospital is terminated.

Scheduling part-time people is a full-time job. The nursing supervisor is not burdened with the extra work however, since it is handled by a scheduling clerk, who keeps track of the hours worked and seniority, as well as performing other clerical functions.

The head nurse schedules the permanent nurses on her unit and leaves vacant spots to be filled by part-time nurses.

The scheduling clerk in the nursing office fills in the part-time spots with those who have indicated their willingness to work at that particular time. A system of cards is used to keep track of the part-time nurses' availability. The permanent part-time people are posted and then the casual people fill in the remaining time slots.

Because a part-time nurse is permanently assigned to a specific unit, she can become a temporary full-time person when the need arises.

Shared Service Pool*

The Midtown Hospital Association, Denver, a shared services organization composed of seven member hospitals, implemented a program to provide nursing personnel on an on-call or as needed basis to its member hospitals. Under this program, Midtown employs nursing personnel who are sent into the member hospitals upon request to compensate for census peaks, vacations, and employee absenteeism.

In the first year and a half of operation, Midtown filled over 5,000 shifts with registered nurses (RNs), licensed practical nurses (LPNs), nursing aides, speech pathologists, and occupational and physical therapists.

An RN with extensive administrative experience was trained on a consulting basis to assist in getting the program off the ground. A second individual was assigned to develop scheduling and billing procedures and to research the actual needs of interested hospitals.

Three individuals manage the Midtown nursing personnel department: a director, a scheduling coordinator, and an RN consultant.

With few exceptions, utilization on a day-to-day basis does not vary significantly. Requests for personnel usually decrease beginning Friday before any three-day weekend or holiday and are usually higher on days hospital employees are paid. Requests by shifts also remain fairly constant in distribution. Fifty-nine percent of the total requests are for the 7 to 3 shift, 29 percent for the 3 to 11 shift, and 12 percent for the 11 to 7 shift.

Requests for nurses are received by telephone and logged on scheduling sheets by the department coordinator. Requests are received from as little as one hour to up to several weeks before the shift to be filled begins. Although nursing personnel call in for scheduled work at weekly intervals, they are called by the coordinator for last minute requests.

Nursing personnel are oriented in each hospital in which they decide to work. The length and type of orientation depend upon the institution's needs.

---

*Source: Douglas K. Woollard, "Shared Services Organizes Its Own Nursing Pool." Adapted, with permission, from an article originally published in *Hospitals, Journal of the American Hospital Association*, vol. 50, no. 10, May 16, 1976, copyright 1976, American Hospital Association.

All of the participating hospitals have been willing to donate staff time to orient Midtown personnel.

A cost formula has been developed to compute the actual cost of personnel on the basis of current and projected salary levels, shift differentials, and taxes.

Hospitals are charged a flat hourly rate for each classification of personnel regardless of the individual's salary level or the shift worked. However, a shift differential is paid. The rates are calculated to cover personnel costs and program overhead and include a 4-percent contingency factor.

A break-even point was reached after the program had been operative for about 12 months and a sufficient volume had been attained. The current rates for Midtown personnel are about 12 percent lower than those of area commercial pools.

Temporary Help Agencies*

No matter how methodically planned, there will be peaks and valleys and unanticipated discontinuities in either patient census or staffing needs or both. It is just this circumstance, the need to have vacancies filled economically on a per diem basis, that makes privately run temporary help agencies so useful.

These agencies are the legal employers of nurses (and other health service workers) whom they recruit, interview, and place in institutions with which they have agreements. In addition to placement they offer the worker such services as withholding tax accounting, bonding, and malpractice insurance. The hospital pays a fixed amount per shift at a reputed saving of four or five percent relative to what it would cost to use regular staff. Aside from saving on record-keeping and payroll expenses, the hospital is relieved of contributing to social security, unemployment insurance, workmen's compensation, and providing holiday, sick leave, vacation, bonus, health plan, and inservice training for agency people.

Some of the larger temporary help companies are already proposing extensions of their present services. They offer staffing consulta-

*Source: Madalon O'Raew Amenta, "Staffing Through Temporary Help Agencies," *Supervisor Nurse,* December 1977. Reprinted with permission.

tion to client institutions, pointing out the economy and the efficiency of staffing with regular help for only 65 per cent census, then relying on the agency for needs exceeding that. Others suggest putting all new nursing personnel on the agency payroll for a limited probation period. If the hospital then decides to keep them, it has saved hiring and firing expenses.

Advantages

The first and most obvious advantage is cost. Besides a 4–5 percent saving per shift in payroll, clerical work, and fringe benefits, there is a reduction in hidden administrative expenses. Only a minimal full-time staff need be supported and the need for maintenance of a part-time pool is eliminated. The overall efficiency (*ergo,* economy) of matching available part-time personnel in a community with the flexible needs of its institutions' fluctuations in demand or need for staff is a very attractive concept.

Another advantage to hospital management is the fact that agency-employed part-timers can be used as a lever, or disciplinary force. They are a constant reminder to possible balky permanent staff that they can be replaced easily and cheaply. They might help in cutting down absenteeism, turn-over, and over-time pay. The temporaries can't union-organize as a block against the institution. Their persistent presence may act as a deterrent on the regular staff.

There is considerable saving of middle management effort. Supervisors sometimes spend from 60–75 percent of their time securing shift coverage. It takes only a few minutes to call the agency and say, "We need ten nurses for the 11-7 shift Wednesday night." Agencies provide an immediate back-up in emergencies, such as "flu" decimating a staff, holiday absenteeism, local disasters straining the health care system.

Some advantages from the point of view of the regularly employed nurses are unarguable. When the work load is heavy, the staff depleted, just the sight of HELP can be a great boost to morale. Often, the introduction of new ideas and methods or practice by people from diverse backgrounds stimulates more creativity in regulars.

There is always a cadre of nurses in any community who are not able to work at all unless they can have highly flexible self-determined schedules. These are the mothers of young families, students, people between regular jobs, early retirees. Their available time and energy are too unpredictable and sporadic to be built into the regular part-time demands of most hospitals.

Disadvantages

There are, however, many disadvantages in this whole arrangement. Sometimes a nurse's credentials have not been thoroughly checked before she's sent to a job. Even when a nurse has been responsibly certified before she is sent to a facility, there is no guarantee she will be properly oriented once she arrives. Hospitals think agencies should handle it and *vice versa*. While some agencies do keep the orientation literature and the procedure manuals of their client institutions on file, their use is optional.

Other abuses affect patient safety and quality of care. Some hospitals will not hire Associate Degree graduates as regular staff until they have had experience, yet they take whomever the agency sends. Frequently, these temporaries are the same Associate Degree people they wouldn't hire if they came through their own personnel system. They are placed in all units, including ICUs and CCUs, and unless they object, demur, or commit outrageous errors, no one is the wiser concerning their lack of experience or special training.

In general, any temporary people present problems for the head nurse, since they are not familiar with the hospital, the unit, its procedures and policies or routines of care. Some head nurses have a formula: "Two temporaries equal one regular."

A head nurse can spend a minimum of one hour, possibly up to two hours, with each new temporary orientee before the HELPER can even start her work and come up with the inevitable questions that all beginners ask; all orientations need reinforcement throughout the day. At best, the charting of new people has to be checked; at worst, actually done. Extra time slips must be filled out. There may be any number of other added paper work chores, depending on the particular circumstances.

The effect on staff nurses of working with agency help as a rule rather than in emergencies is one of gradual loss of morale. The regulars always end up with the heaviest loads, the sickest patients. The temporaries can and often do

refuse assignments. Not only is the person who is inexperienced in the setting (operating room, emergency room, ICU, working with retardates) apt to experience fear or anxiety, she will surely transmit it to her co-workers.

When management doesn't get the number of temporary workers it needs for nights and evenings (it can only tap what's available through the agencies) it makes the regulars cover. Temporaries always get preferred schedules—days, no holidays, no week-ends—forcing an even heavier dose of less attractive working times on the regulars.

When an institution comes to rely on temporary agency help for a fixed proportion of its staff, not just in the extraordinary situation, there is a documented downward spiral in quality of care and staff morale. In the beginning, regulars welcome temporaries as help in a crisis and relief from imposed overtime. Then, as the temporary-regular mix becomes a stable condition, and the hospital stops hiring new regulars to fill vacancies, more regulars leave and the hospital hires even more temporaries. For the regulars who remain, there are incrementally heavier patient loads and unattractive schedules. Soon they start leaving. To fill the gap, still more temporaries are hired. As soon as a certain ratio (around 33⅓% temporaries) becomes fixed, the difficulties faced by the regulars become so great and the knowledge of it so widespread in the community, that fewer and fewer good nurses are willing to sign on as regular staff. The best people in town stay away; the least able take the jobs. Ineluctably, overall quality of care deteriorates.

This brings us to the most fundamental disadvantage of over-reliance on temporary help, the deleterious effects on patient care. The modern health care system is fragmented enough without patients having to see a different nurse, not just every shift, but for every procedure. Vital energies that otherwise might go into recuperation are used up in the repeated adjustments to relays of people. When a professional nurse doesn't see a patient many times a day or even daily, she can't pick up the significant changes in status that mark improvement or decline. She has no baseline on which to make judgments about the effects of care and treatment. Temporaries barely manage the procedural work; they can't begin to approach teaching and counseling.

*Guidelines for Using Temporary
Help Agencies*

Temporary help agencies do have a place, but that place must be well defined. Criteria should be devised and responsible surveillance imposed.

The ideal arrangement fits the right person to the right temporary job in a bonafide emergency. The agency itself should keep records indicating the specialties, the hospitals and the units nurses not only prefer but for which they seem most suited according to documented feed-back from the facilities they have already worked.

The hospital should be especially aware of the hiring practices of the agencies it uses. Crucial is the knowledge of the quality of a nurse's work experience and her dependability. These should be rigorously investigated and monitored. As a rudimentary precaution, identification should be checked when the nurse first comes to work and a record of her past experience and performance in the hospital should be maintained. If she refuses to work with certain kinds of patients (those with infections, those on respirators, etc.) both the agency and the hospital should know.

When determining which units to staff with temporaries, administration must deliberate long and carefully. Generally it should use regular staff in high pressure units where the pace is swift and new situations arise quickly because these are the areas where orientation is difficult and mistakes with grave consequences are most likely to occur. It is here that the temporary nurse can be most easily traumatized.

As a general rule, it is more sound to restrict the use of temporaries to less pressured areas where vacancies can be anticipated well in advance and a thorough orientation given. Vacations and holidays can be planned far ahead of time in an orderly, reasonable way.

Another safety and quality measure for hospital administration would be for it arbitrarily to limit the total percentage of overall use of temporaries on any given unit. All staffing patterns should be re-evaluated at six-month to one-year intervals and reformulated on the basis of current staffing standards, statistical records, changing needs, values, and practices.

Finally, since nursing administration is liable for the temporary nurse who is not performing adequately, it should provide charge nurses easy access so that problem temps will be identified and will not be reassigned until their defects are dealt with. An agency should know it will be dropped if it persists in not meeting the standards of the hospital or honoring its requests.

Handling Overstaffing

*Requested Absences**

In the Methodist Hospital (St. Louis Park, Minn.) they have been able to contract their staffing to meet short-term decreased patient care requirements. This is done by means of a Requested Absence (RA). If it is found that the nursing stations in general will be overstaffed on a given shift or during a given period, the assistant staffing coordinator will contact scheduled nursing employees, and ask if they would prefer not to work. Often nursing employees are willing to comply with the request. Since this method is mutually agreeable to both Nursing Service and the employee, an efficient means of dealing with temporary overstaffing is created. During the employment interview and the staffing orientation session, employees are notified of this option. The option has proved to be quite popular.

Policies for Implementation

- The staffing office may request that an employee take an RA day or the staff member may initiate the request for an RA day by notifying the staffing office. The RA must be mutually agreeable to both the employee and the staffing office.
- Employees contacted to take an RA day are responsible for notifying the staffing persons if they are to work charge, etc., on the proposed RA day.
- The total RAs taken by one employee may not exceed 20 days (160 hours) for one year.
- There will be no loss of time in calculating benefits during a requested absence.
- RA days may not be used in lieu of leave of absence days.

*Source: Merrill Lehman and Q.J. Friesen, *A Centralized Position and Staffing Control Administered by Non-Nursing Personnel*, Methodist Hospital, St. Louis Park, Minnesota, 1975.

Limiting or Reducing Staff*

A staff reduction is never popular no matter where it takes place, be it in industry or the health care field. However, there are times when the circumstances surrounding this action make it necessary or even mandatory.

There are some general points which should be kept in mind by administrators when considering action leading to staff cuts.

- Staff adjustments should take into account activities and the corresponding skill level required. Wholesale and indiscriminate reductions could purge the nursing service of valuable people having important talents. This should be avoided.
- The total staffing in an area should initially be adequate. A five or ten percent across the board cut in all nursing unit rosters, while of minor consequence to overstaffed areas, can seriously hinder operations where units are already undermanned.
- The means of effecting the staffing reduction should be carefully weighted. Some causes of action have greater impact than others. If the same ends can be achieved through expected normal attrition or encouragement of early retirement, this is certainly a better approach than causing wholesale layoffs on an indiscriminate basis. While the latter is certainly quick and sure, the former, taking some amount of planning and work, would produce the more positive results from a personnel relations standpoint.

Long-Term Techniques*

In the following discussion of how to reduce staff, an attempt has been made to present the less extreme methods first and the more drastic measures last. The exact rank is open to individual preference.

Attrition

If time permits, staffing can be adjusted on a long-term basis through attrition. Such action

can be difficult if

- the rate of attrition, department-wide, is low
- the rate of attrition in a given unit (because of size or type of work) is low
- the time to achieve reduction is short

While attrition is not necessarily the way to end up with optimum staffing in a department (it's possible that the most productive person will leave) it is one of the most "painless" means of reducing staff.

Overtime

Work should be planned in order to be accomplished in a normal work week. In cases where the workload varies because of sudden heavy inputs that cannot be normally handled or deferred, overtime can be authorized. The same argument holds for emergency work.

A review of overtime hours might point out the need for a revamping of personnel scheduling. Too often inflexibility in scheduling can induce overtime where it could otherwise be avoided.

Transfers & Promotions

Where there are apparent cases of under, as well as over staffing, efforts should be made to transfer employees within the hospital and between nursing service units, keeping requirements in mind.

This can be encouraged by posting job openings for which any qualified employee can apply. Worker morale and loyalty can be significantly improved with this type of well administered program. In other circumstances the personnel department may have to act as the agency to match personnel from over—to under—staffed departments.

Promotion from within follows similar arguments and further encourages employee performance on the hope that when appropriate openings occur, they will be filled from within.

Leave of Absence: LOA

The department should encourage the taking of extended leaves of absence such as educational LOA's. The impact on the budget would not be major inasmuch as usually only the barest of benefits are carried in cases of authorized LOA.

---

*Source: "Selected Procedures and Methods of Staff Reduction," Haricomp Guide Series Publication, 1975. Pub. No. 79a.

Re-employment could be contingent on there being positions open at the time a person on leave would seek to return. The exception to such a policy would be with respect to military leaves for which the returning employee is guaranteed a position.

Retirement Phase-outs

Hospitals have long kept employees on the payroll even though they have passed the widely recognized retirement age of 65. Following such a practice unfortunately penalizes the hospital in many ways. The elderly employee may present a picture of marginal productivity [in labor-intensive, nonprofessional positions] and increased injury/illness days; yet often, because of seniority, they enjoy the largest salaries and the most vacation days in their job classification.

Replacement might be possible or a shift to a lower paid position as part of any evaluation of duties and/or departmental organization.

Minimize Part-Time Staffing

An attempt should be made to minimize the use of part-time staff.

This might be done through rescheduling existing full-time personnel or combining the workload of many part-timers to create a lesser number of positions.

Elimination or restriction on hiring of temporary or supplemental staff should be considered. Where the reason for using such personnel is uneven scheduling of workload, attempts should be made to balance the "peaks and valleys" with the resulting loss of need for temporary help. Another common situation which causes a "need" for staff is the failure to preplan vacation schedules. A disciplined policy for taking earned vacation time should cause few if any staff shortages during these times.

Inter-Hospital Transfers

Where severe overstaffing exists, the personnel department might attempt to arrange employee transfers to other hospitals in the area where appropriate positions are open. These workers would be considered as "new employees" in their new employment, but would also enjoy relative job continuity.

Management Engineering

Management Engineering can be of use to the department in indicating performance levels and improvement areas.

A review can be made to determine if, in fact, a valid need exists for the hiring of new or replacing vacant positions in the department.

A check could also be made to determine if positions could be reclassified to a lower level based on existing department requirements.

Usually savings can be effected with the creation of a vacancy since the new employee could be paid at the reclassified, lower rate.

Disciplinary Enforcement

In tight labor markets or when there is a high demand for personnel, enforcement of disciplinary policies tends to become relaxed. A problem worker will be tolerated because replacing him could be difficult. The reverse corollary is also true.

Incompetency and Probation Dismissals

In somewhat of a similar vein, supervisors and head nurses may have identified some of their staff as being incompetent in work required of them. When faced with a staff cut, various means should be taken to encourage these employees to resign.

Also as a prelude to a general layoff, consideration should be given to the dismissal of employees currently on a probationary status.

Layoff

A layoff of staff should be a last resort after all other attempts at trimming personnel have been exhausted.

People affected by the layoff should be given a thorough explanation of the circumstances and be informed of what efforts were made to find positions for them by the personnel department.

They should further be advised that as circumstances change, they would again be considered for employment, but this period of layoff could last for an extended number of months.

Finally, they should be fully informed of their unemployment status and told of their unemployment entitlements.

SCHEDULING

Overview*

The basic problem of scheduling is to provide patient care every day around the clock using nurses who generally work five days a week, one shift per day, and prefer to have weekends off. Scheduling is usually done by nursing supervisors for the units or floors for which they are responsible. They estimate patient care requirements and allocate the available nursing staff to the days of the week so that these requirements are approximately satisfied and hospital personnel regulations observed. They try to schedule the nursing staff so that each nurse gets her share of weekends off and none of the nurses is rotated to evenings or night shifts for an unduly long time, and they also try to accommodate individual nurses' requests for specific days off. Often a schedule is prepared every other week, specifying work days and days off for each member of the nursing staff over the ensuing two weeks.

Preparation of the schedule is a time-consuming task and there is usually dissatisfaction with the results:

1. Coverage tends to fluctuate widely, particularly in the case of RN's; the number of RN's assigned to a given unit on a given shift may vary from day to day by a factor of two or more.
2. In their position of total authority over schedules, supervising nurses are apt to be suspected of favoritism, particularly when they try—as is often necessary and desirable—to take into account the desires and constraints of individual nurses.
3. The attempt to resolve scheduling and allocation problems can result in excessive use of overtime.
4. Schedules frequently have to be changed on short notice because of changes in patient care requirements, illness of a nurse, etc.

The vast majority of hospitals schedule and allocate nurses on an informal basis. The rejection of more systematic methods appears to re-

---

*Source: Christopher Maier-Rothe and Harry B. Wolfe, "Cyclical Scheduling and Allocation of Nursing Staff," *Socio-Economic Planning Sciences,* vol. 7. Reprinted with permission of Pergamon Press, Ltd., copyright © 1973.

flect in part a set of beliefs that nursing, as a profession, is not amenable to formal scheduling and allocation procedures, that too many variables must be taken into account, that most nurses are non-quantitatively oriented and would therefore resist any system involving computers, and possibly in part the failure of previous efforts to take into account some variables that were important to nurses.

Objectives

The objectives of a scheduling and allocation procedure are to assign working days and days off to individual members of the nursing staff so that:

1. Adequate patient care is assured while overstaffing is avoided.
2. A desirable distribution of days off is achieved.
3. Individual members of the nursing staff are treated fairly.
4. Individuals know well in advance what their schedules are.

Factors in Scheduling Decisions

Among the factors that should play a part in scheduling decisions are the following:

1. The different levels of nursing staff—registered nurses, licensed practical nurses, and nurses' aides—have different capabilities; LPN's and aides are legally allowed to perform only certain functions. Even within these categories, individuals can be classified by degree of experience and by the amount of responsibility they are able to assume.
2. Nursing coverage must, of course, be provided 24 hours a day, 7 days a week. Nursing requirements are typically lower during the evening and night shifts than during the day shift. Saturday and Sunday requirements tend to be 20–30 percent lower than weekday requirements, depending on the medical service, due to a lower patient census, fewer new physicians' orders, or both.
3. Vacations and time off for holidays must be staggered to ensure continued patient coverage and equitable treatment for nurses.
4. Weekend days off are highly prized by the nursing staff, preferably both days in a row. Next in preference is two or more days off in a row in the middle of the week.

5. Long stretches of consecutive working days (usually defined as more than five in a row) are undesirable.
6. Despite a salary differential, the evening and night shifts are more difficult to staff than the day shift. As a result, schedules must provide for "rotation"; daytime staff must work on the other two shifts from time to time. Also, staff on evening and night shifts may sometimes have to work on the day shift in order to attend special programs, training courses, etc.
7. Most nurses prefer to remain on one nursing unit, rather than being "floated" or shifted from one unit to another, partly because of the competence and expertise they are able to develop in a particular unit, and partly because of the camaraderie of continued association with the same group. However, there are some nurses who do not mind, and in fact prefer, floating because of the variety of experience it gives them.

Criteria for Evaluation*

A scheduling system can be assessed by observing how well it functions in terms of:

Coverage: The number of nurses (by skill class) assigned to be on duty is in relation to some minimum number of nurses required.

Quality: A measure of a schedule's desirability as judged by the nurse who will have to work it. This measure includes weekends off, work stretches, single days on, split days off, and certain rotation patterns in addition to how a schedule conforms to her requests for days off for a particular scheduling period.

Stability: A measure of the extent to which nurses know their future days off and on duty and the extent to which they feel that their schedules are generated consistent with a set of stable policies (e.g., weekend policy, rotation policy).

Flexibility: The ability of a scheduling system to handle changes, such as from full-time to part-time, from rotation to working only one shift, and special requirements—class

schedules of nurses, requests for days off, vacations, leaves of absence, etc.

Fairness: A measure of the extent to which each nurse perceives that she exerts the same amount of influence upon the scheduling system as other nurses.

Cost: The resources consumed in making the scheduling decision.

Centralized, Decentralized, and Self-Scheduling

Centralized Scheduling

Under centralized scheduling one person in the nursing administration office plans coverage for all nursing units. A master staffing pattern is developed for these units and staffing is based on a pre-established standard. This staffing coordinator has access to clerical help to type, process and distribute the master plan to the units. The coordinator knows the number and availability of staff on any given day and therefore is able to make the necessary day-to-day changes when sickness or other emergencies occur. The coordinator is able to do this by rotating nurses from one floor to another to achieve the best coverage throughout the hospital. Such a person is important in keeping nurses involved in nursing rather than nonnursing functions.

The pitfalls of centralized scheduling are many. The staffing coordinator, unaware of the implications of clinical problems, may not understand that nurses need certain clinical expertise if they are rotated to more specialized units. Nurses are often placed into regimented schedules, offered no choices and few options for change. They are not included as part of the decision-making process, which leads them to frustration and feelings of helplessness and insignificance.

Line vs. Staff Responsibilities under Centralized Scheduling*

Confusion in responsibility and authority may result in staff personnel making decisions in areas where line managers are accountable.

Line positions in the nursing department are supervisory (management positions at the level of head nurse and above); these nurses are ac-

---

*Source: Michael D. Warner, "Computer-Aided System for Nurse Scheduling," *Cost Control in Hospitals,* John R. Griffith, Walton M. Hancock, and Fred C. Munson, eds., Health Administration Press, 1976.

*Source: Gloria Swanberg and Eunice L. Smith, "Centralized Scheduling: Is It Worth the Effort?" *Nursing Administration Quarterly,* Summer 1977.

countable for nursing care of patients on specified units or services. When scheduling is centralized, the employees in the scheduling office are in a staff relationship with management personnel in the nursing department.

• The *line* functions for which the nurses in management positions should be responsible are the following:

1. Establish and control the personnel budget.
2. Develop a master staffing pattern based on patient needs and the method of assignment.
3. Develop procedures for adjustment of staff on a daily basis.
4. Establish requirements for each position on the staff (such as assignment to an intensive care unit or charge responsibility).
5. Develop employees to meet requirements of their position and evaluate their performance.
6. Hire, promote, discipline, and discharge employees.

• The *staff* functions for which the central scheduling office is responsible are the following:

1. Gather facts and prepare reports for line personnel to facilitate budgeting.
2. Schedule employees according to policies in staffing patterns established by line personnel.
3. Implement procedures for reallocation of staff to meet daily needs; consult immediate superior when demand exceeds supply.
4. Implement procedures for position control.
5. Maintain records needed by line managers for evaluation (regarding absenteeism for example).
6. Maintain effective communications with appropriate departments, such as payroll and personnel.

Guidelines*

Effective centralized scheduling is feasible and will work if these guidelines are followed:

• A realistic personnel budget based on master staffing patterns and procedures to ac-

commodate variations in workload is developed with active participation of head nurses;
• Scheduling policies are established, publicized, and enforced;
• Scheduling personnel are carefully selected and oriented to meet the specified needs of the scheduling program;
• Head nurses have opportunities for frequent, meaningful communication with the scheduling staff;
• Line and staff relationships are clearly delineated and understood.

Decentralized Scheduling

Decentralized scheduling has helped to solve some frustrations. Nurses have more input into staffing patterns because the responsibility for staffing is entrusted to the unit supervisor, who is aware of the clinical needs and personal needs of the staff nurses. However, because the supervisor is not an expert in staffing methods and does not have access to clerical help, long tedious hours are spent in nonnursing functions. The schedule remains confusing and inconsistent in spite of sincere efforts.

Self-Scheduling*

Self-scheduling allows the nurses on the unit to assign themselves on the work schedule while assuming total responsibility for daily coverage of the unit and maintenance of the appropriate level of competency. Self staffing involves group cooperation, sensitivity to peer needs, individual accountability and an awareness of the coverage needed in a 24-hour period. Self staffing takes advantage of the best of centralized staffing and decentralized staffing. With this combined system, clerical work and day-to-day problems can be handled by an administrative assistant for staffing with direct input from the unit.

Guidelines

The following guidelines were set up to make self staffing work effectively. In a group meeting, the nurses on a unit decide how many

---

*Source: Gloria Swanberg and Eunice L. Smith, "Centralized Scheduling: Is It Worth the Effort?" *Nursing Administration Quarterly,* Summer 1977.

*Source: Barbara Van Offeren and Carol Glynn, "Staffing Patterns," *Nursing Administration Quarterly,* Fall 1977, pp. 19–20.

nurses are needed to give safe care to their patients. The nurses then identify: full time and part time nurses; nurses working permanent P.M.'s and nights; nurses who will work days with rotations to P.M.'s and/or nights; and nurses working eight-hour or ten-hour shifts.

Given the number of rotations that must be made to P.M. and night shifts, the nurses fill in these rotations prior to filling in day hours. This is important since P.M. and night coverage is the hardest to fill. Rotations are done in blocks of three days to develop some consistency and flow from days to P.M.'s or nights.

Permanent full time and part time nurses fill in their hours making sure their staffing pattern includes every other weekend. Part time nurses working less than 20 hours a week must work one weekend a month. They should try working the weekend where coverage is most needed.

The schedule is usually made out five to six weeks in advance at a group meeting to allow for adequate planning time for staff.

Advantages and Disadvantages

Advantages of self staffing cited by the staff are that it enables them to arrange their personal lives more conveniently; allows flexibility for "moms" who needs days off when children are out of school for teachers conferences; allows for dental and doctor appointments on a more predictable basis and allows for a choice to work with other nurses they are more compatible with.

Disadvantages cited were that nurses filling in the schedule last are not always given first chance on succeeding schedules; there is inadequate coverage or too much coverage on the same days with staff unwillingness to "give and take"; there is not always available staffing to meet the needs of the unit; and the last person to fill in the schedule sometimes has less flexibility unless this can be discussed with other staff members.

Failure in self staffing can be imminent if staff members are immature, do not have a sense of caring for their fellow workers, the ability to compromise, a commitment to their patients and their nursing responsibilities, or if they do not attend the unit meetings.

The clinical director of one of the units utilizing self staffing sees herself as a consultant in identifying the limitations or problems the group does not identify. She facilitates decision making by clarifying the problem and defining alternative solutions.

The clinical director also calls emergency meetings of the unit as a group to solve crises.

Approaches to Scheduling*

The Traditional Approach. Starting "from scratch" each month, the head nurse (or supervisor) makes the decision "by hand," taking into consideration quality and coverage. The major advantage of the traditional approach is its flexibility: since the process is begun from scratch, any changes in the environment can be worked into the new schedule. Its disadvantages include coverage and quality that is uneven, nonstability (unless policies leave little flexibility) and high cost.

Cyclical Scheduling. First a 4-week, 6-week, etc. schedule which provides even coverage and high quality is determined for each unit, then this schedule is repeated period after period. Advantages include high quality (if the quality of the initial schedule is high), even coverage, high stability, and low cost. The overwhelming disadvantage is inflexibility to survive the changes in environment which characterize the majority of nursing units.

The environments where cyclical scheduling seems to have the best prognosis are those that are the most stable, where nurses do not rotate between shifts, and where new nurses can be hired into an open cyclical "slot." [For a full discussion of cyclical scheduling see below.]

Computer Aided Traditional Scheduling. A third approach uses a computer to aid in both keeping track of policies and past working patterns of nurses, and to aid in the fast and more complete search through possible schedules for "good" ones. This approach offers the flexibility of the traditional approach, but reduces operating costs considerably and can produce high quality schedules consistently. It also facilitates incorporation of policies which add stability. The approach's advantages are most dramatic in the situation where nurses rotate among shifts, and where the nursing unit environment is subject to chronic change.

------

*Source: D. Michael Warner, "Nurse Staffing, Scheduling and Reallocation in the Hospital," *Hospital & Health Services Administration*, Summer, 1976.

It has been estimated that approximately 97% of all hospitals use the traditional approach, 2–3% use some version of cyclical scheduling, with only a few using a computer aided approach.

Cyclical Schedules

The cyclical approach is a schedule that covers a designated number of weeks (cycle length) and then repeats itself. The cyclical schedule assigns the required registered nurses, licensed nurses, and total staff to each unit in a manner consistent with average patient care requirements, hospital personnel policies, and the nursing staff's preferences for the distribution of days off.

*Advantages**

- Fairness to All—No Favoritism
- Once Done Doesn't Need To Be Redone Every Week or Two—Saves Time
- Enables Employees To Plan Ahead for Personal Needs, Therefore
- Reduces The Number of Special Requests For Days Off
- Allows Part-Timers to be Scheduled Around Full-Timers
- Vacation, Holiday, and Sick Coverage is Less of a Problem
- Improves Productivity

*Cyclical Schedule Structure***

Table 5-18 shows a simple cyclical schedule. There are five nurses and the cycle length of the schedule is five weeks. Days off are denoted by D. The first line indicates working days and days off for the first nurse, the second line for the second nurse and so forth. The first nurse has the first Sunday off, then a Thursday, then she has Tuesday and Wednesday off, and so on until the five weeks are up at which point the entire pattern of working days and days off begins again. The overall pattern of working days and days off is exactly the same for all of the nurses; the only difference is that it begins in a different week for each nurse. Thus, the schedule followed by the first nurse in the first week is followed by the second nurse the following week, the third the week after, and so on. The weeks start with Sunday and end with Saturday. Each nurse works five days a week, works at most four days in a row, and has two out of five weekends off. Four of the five nurses are always present except on Tuesdays and on weekends, when only three are present.

*Problems***

A schedule must meet staffing requirements and must be consistent with the hospital's personnel policies. Patient care requirements fluctuate from day to day and even from hour to hour; minimum staffing requirements consist of the minimum number and the mix of nursing staff required to accommodate average patient care requirements.

It is not always easy to obtain agreement on minimum staffing requirements. Estimates from nursing supervisors tend to be somewhat biased in favor of more people, while estimates from hospital administration may be biased in the opposite direction. It is thus advisable to consult both sources. If patient care requirements fluctuate widely from day to day, it may also be worthwhile to analyze actual staff coverage over an extended period of time and to conduct interviews to find out what happened on days with a particularly large or small number of nurses on duty.

Hospital personnel policies usually reflect agreements reached between the administration and the nursing staff regarding the distribution of days off for nurses. These agreements specify, among other things, the precise beginning of the work week, the number of days per week that must be given off, the maximum number of working days in a row, how many holidays are to be given off, the duration of vacations, and how many weekends are to be given off. They limit the types of cyclical patterns that are feasible. For instance, if four days off every two weeks are specified instead of two days off each week, the possible range of cyclical patterns is considerably increased.

---

*Source: Thomas C. Kliber, *Modes of Scheduling,* Blue Cross of Western Pennsylvania, Pittsburgh, 1978.

**Source: Christopher Maier-Rothe and Harry B. Wolfe, "Cyclical Scheduling and Allocation of Nursing Staff," *Socio-Economic Planning Sciences,* vol. 7. Reprinted with permission of Pergamon Press, Ltd., copyright © 1973.

Table 5-18 A 5-Week Cyclical Schedule

Nurse	S	M	T	W	T	F	S	S	M	T	W	T	F	S	S	M	T	W	T	F	S
#1	D			D					D	D						D					D
#2		D					D	D				D					D	D			
#3	D					D			D					D	D				D		
#4		D					D	D					D			D					D
#5			D	D				D						D	D					D	

Nurse	S	M	T	W	T	F	S	S	M	T	W	T	F	S	S	M	T	W	T	F	S
#1	D			D					D				D	D				D			
#2		D					D	D						D			D				D
#3		D	D				D					D	D							D	
#4	D			D					D	D				D							D
#5		D				D	D					D				D	D				

Source: Thomas C. Kliber, *Modes of Scheduling*, Blue Cross of Western Pennsylvania, Pittsburgh, 1978.

Cyclical Pattern Alternatives*

Before a cyclical schedule can actually be assembled, patterns of working days and days off must be found which are consistent with requirements outlined.

*Source: Christopher Maier-Rothe and Harry B. Wolfe, "Cyclical Scheduling and Allocation of Nursing Staff," *Socio-Economic Planning Sciences*, vol. 7. Reprinted with permission of Pergamon Press, Ltd., copyright © 1973.

Feasible patterns of working days and days off could be found through some algorithmic approach such as integer programming or a heuristic approach.

In one examination of scheduling for unit coverage by 12 staff members (5 RN, 2 LPN and 5 aides), governed by various weekend, vacation and other policy constraints, there were constructed fourteen feasible alternatives, as shown in Table 5-19. The first four describe a 10-week cycle with a total of four weekends off, the next

Table 5-19 Fourteen Alternative Cyclical Patterns

Length of cycle (weeks)	10				12				12					
No. of alternative patterns	1	2	3	4	5	6	7	8	9	10	11	12	13	14
No. of 4-day weekends off	1	0	0	0	1	0	0	0	1	0	0	0	0	0
Relative frequency (%)	10	0	0	0	8	0	0	0	8	0	0	0	0	0
No. of 3-day weekends off	0	2	1	0	0	2	1	0	1	2	2	1	1	0
Relative frequency (%)	0	20	10	0	0	17	8	0	8	17	17	8	8	0
Total No. of weekends off	4	4	4	4	5	5	5	5	4	4	4	4	4	4
Relative frequency (%)	40	40	40	40	42	42	42	42	33	33	33	33	33	33
No. of 2-day periods off	2	2	2	2	2	2	2	2	3	4	3	4	3	4
Relative frequency (%)	20	20	20	20	17	17	17	17	25	33	25	33	25	33
No. of single days off	6	6	7	8	8	8	9	10	7	6	8	7	9	8
Relative frequency (%)	60	60	10	80	67	67	75	83	58	50	67	58	75	67
No. of 6-workday stretches	2	2	1	0	2	2	1	0	4	2	0	1	0	0
Relative frequency (%)	20	20	10	0	17	17	8	0	33	17	0	8	0	0
No. of 5-workday stretches	2	2	1	0	2	2	1	0	3	4	3	2	2	2
Relative frequency (%)	20	20	10	0	17	17	8	0	25	33	25	17	17	17

Source: Thomas C. Kliber, *Modes of Scheduling*, Blue Cross of Western Pennsylvania, Pittsburgh, 1978.

four a 12-week cycle with a total of five weekends off, and the last a 12-week cycle with four
weekends off. For easier comparison of the individual alternatives, the relative frequencies of
occurrence of four-day weekends off, three-day
weekends off, and so forth, as seen in Table
5-20, show the pattern of days off for four of the
alternatives.

The nurses preferred the cycles with more
weekends off and therefore rejected the 12-week
schedule with four weekends off. They were initially quite excited about the possibility of long
weekends, a feature offered only rarely under
the old scheduling procedures, but their enthusiasm was quickly dampened when they realized,
however, that these could usually only be
achieved by allowing longer stretches of working days in a row.

The advantage of presenting to the nurses alternative cyclical patterns is that the trade-offs
between desirable distributions of days off on
the one hand and undesirable stretches of working days on the other are made quite explicit,
and the choice is made by the nurses rather than
imposed upon them.

Preferences/Constraints*

(The more constraints involved the more
difficult any type of scheduling becomes.)

1. Number of weekends off—1 in four, 1 in
   three, every other weekend.
2. Maximum length of consecutive days
   worked—i.e., no more than six, etc.
3. Whether the days off should be together or
   split.
4. Payroll and overtime considerations (i.e.,
   five work days per week—ten days per pay
   period).

Cautions*

- Giving more or less of one variable affects
  the ability to give more or less of the others.
- There is no one schedule that will work for
  all hospitals and all departments.
- Select several different schedules that complement each other and develop best cyclical schedule for your department.
- Experiment with combination of different
  schedules.

Guidelines*

- Allow for flexibility so that qualified work-
  ers can substitute for each other or trade
  days off
- Establish vacation and holiday policies that
  are fair to the hospital as well as the em-
  ployees
- Allow for in-service programs
- Use part-timers with discretion
  A. Good if they work to the convenience of
     the hospital
  B. Should be scheduled around full-timers
     and not vice versa
- Allow for fluctuations in patient population

Shift Patterns: The 10- and 12-Hour Shifts

Overview**

Within the past few years there has been much
discussion of the benefits of altering the traditional patterns in scheduling, the standard 8-
hour shifts, to new and different configurations.
The most popular of these is the 10-hour day, 4-
day workweek (known as the 4/40 workweek).

For U.S. hospitals in particular, the ten-hour
day, four-day week with predetermined calendar patterns accounts for 83 percent of alternative scheduling. The twelve-hour day, combined
with either the four-day week or the seven day
on-seven day off pattern, accounts for another
11 percent; combinations of the 8-hour, ten-hour
and twelve-hour shifts account for the remainder of the programs.

The ten-hour shift is adopted more frequently
by the larger hospital (measured in beds) and by
the larger experimental programs (measured in
numbers of personnel involved); the more-than-
ten-hour schedule is adopted frequently by the
smaller hospital, and by the smaller program.
Church-related hospitals have a relatively low
number of programs with the more-than-ten-
hour schedule.

*Source: Thomas Kliber, *Modes of Scheduling*,
Blue Cross of Western Pennsylvania, Pittsburgh, 1978.
**Source: William Clint Johnson, "Review and
Analysis of Changed Work Schedules in Hospitals,"
Manpower Administration, Department of Labor,
May 1975. (Unpublished Contract Grant DL 91-48-72-
37.)

Table 5-20 Days Off in Patterns 1, 4, 6, and 11

	Week in cycle											
	1	**2**	**3**	**4**	**5**	**6**	**7**	**8**	**9**	**10**	**11**	**12**
Sunday	1 4		1 4		1	4		1 4				
	6 11		6	11	11	6	11	6		11	6	
Monday		4	1	1		4						
				11		6	6					11
Tuesday				4		1	1 4			1 4		
			11	6	6				11	6	11	
Wednesday	4			4	1	1			1 4			
			6 11		6			11	6		11	
Thursday						4		1	1 4			
			11	6				6 11	6	11		
Friday	1	1	4						4			
	6 11						11	11			6	6
Saturday		1 4		1		4	1 4			1 4		
		6	11		6 11	11	6			11	6	6 11

Source: Thomas C. Kliber, *Modes of Scheduling,* Blue Cross of Western Pennsylvania, Pittsburgh, 1978.

The ten-hour shift appears more concerned with improvement of the level of service and improvement of employee morale (by means of the new work schedule) than does the more-than-ten-hour group. The more-than-ten-hour group, on the other hand, appears more concerned with better recruitment and retention of personnel via the schedule. The ten-hour shifts frequently report inclusion of more man-hours devoted to the case load at the inception of the program, while more-than-ten-hour shifts frequently report programmed decreases in man-hour input. The more-than-ten-hour administrators frequently report an increase in wages associated with the inception of the schedule.

Floor R.N. personnel and charge nurses are usually more favorable in their evaluations of longer shifts while non-nursing professionals are generally the least favorable.

Industrial companies have chiefly cited morale improvements, productivity improvements, and lower unit costs as favorable outcomes of the change. Among the reasons cited for these improvements are fewer start-ups and shutdowns as well as lower absenteeism and turnover, all of which affect unit costs.

Benefits for the worker in addition to the greater bunching of leisure time may exist in changed work schedules. Travel time and transportation costs could be reduced by commuting to and from work four days a week rather than

five. The worker thus would gain a true increase in total leisure time.

Some say that the improvement in morale and reduction in absenteeism and turnover, if any, do not constitute great advantages. They argue that "the advantage of the bunching of leisure time is, in most cases, offset by the disadvantages of the bunching of work. The changed workweek runs counter to a powerful historical trend of shorter working days."

Labor Laws and Unusual Shifts

The Fair Labor Standards Act supplies the basic provisions governing hour and wage regulations, and determines the conditions under which overtime pay is allocated. Two conditions are set for employees working in the hospital services industry:

1. In a one-week period—overtime is paid for time in excess of 40 hours in the weekly period.
2. In a 14-day period—overtime is paid for time in excess of 8 hours in any day or 80 hours for the 14-day period.

These conditions permit a freedom in scheduling arrangements without incurring high additional costs for overtime wages. Depending on which base is chosen and the designated start of the workweek, little or no extra expense is incurred with a ten-hour shift for four days a week; a twelve-hour shift for three days one week and four days the next; or a nine-hour shift for seven consecutive days on and seven off. Two daily meal periods, 30 minutes each, are disallowed from the hour-count on the longer shifts.

Various configurations can be worked out to meet special demands of the nursing units and hospital departments. However, employees must agree in advance to the work-hour arrangements. Statements of the work arrangements should be added as an item of the hospital's pre-employment policy.

The 10-Hour Shift*

Hospitals that have experimented with the 10-hour shift have often found that it has resulted in a reduction in absenteeism and sicktime. Many hospitals have modified the 10-hour day schedules to suit their needs.

The most popular configuration for the 10-hour shift is the 10-hour day, 4 days a week or the 4/40 workweek. Various other configurations include: 2 days of 12-hour shifts followed by 2 days of 8-hour shifts, or 7 days of 12-hour shifts followed by 7 days off. Other institutions have utilized 10-hour days on either one or two shifts. Some have used a 10-hour shift, 5-hour shift, 10-hour shift for days, evenings, and nights respectively, in order to recruit more part-time nurses for the evening shift.

4-40 Combination**

Following are the principal benefits of the 4-40 shift:

- Improve Patient Care
  —Overlapping of Shifts Improves Communication
  —Reduces Tendency To Place Blame on Other Shifts
- Increase Employee Job Satisfaction
- Reduction in Sick Time
- Reduction in Overtime
- Makes Scheduling of Every Other Weekend Off Easier

See Table 5-21 for an illustration of the staffing schedule in use.

To implement the 4-40 shift the following changes would be necessary:

- Establish a New System of Priorities, i.e. Baths No Longer Given in the Morning
- Holidays and Vacations—Scheduled in Terms of Hours Rather Than Days, i.e.

5 Day Week: 10 Holidays × 8 Hours = 80 Hours
4 Day Week: 8 Holidays × 10 Hours = 80 Hours

Weekly Calculation (Each Employee)

5 Day Week: 5 Days × 8 Hours = 40 Hours/Week
4 Day Week: 4 Days × 10 Hours = 40 Hours/Week

Daily Calculation (Total Department)

5 Day Week: 10 Employees × 8 Hours = 80 Hours/Day
4 Day Week: 8 Employees × 10 Hours = 80 Hours/Day

7 on—7 off**

When the longer shift of 10 hours is combined with a pattern of seven days of work followed by seven consecutive days off, you have a 7/70 schedule, a radical departure from traditional schedules.

At Mercy Medical Center in Dubuque, Ia., the same number and mixture of personnel is on duty 7 days a week, with each employee given every other week off. The staff is split into two groups, each nurse working 70 hours in a two-week period (there are two 10-hour shifts and one 5-hour shift each day). Other changes include standard extra pay for working holidays and the scheduling of inservice and educational programs during the employees' time off. Among the administrative benefits of the new schedule have been a reduction (by 26 percent) in employee turnover, nursing care hours and overtime hours. Results of a survey conducted by an independent research group showed that RN satisfaction was 6 percent above industry norms and 8 percent above the hospital employee norm, but less for part-time employees.

Following are the principal benefits of the 7 on 7 off shift:

---

*Source: *A Review and Evaluation of Nursing Productivity*, DHEW, 1977. Pub. No. (HRA) 77-15.
**Source: Thomas Kliber, *Modes of Scheduling*, Blue Cross of Western Pennsylvania, Pittsburgh, 1978.

- Increases Utilization of Space and Equipment
- Improved Service to Patients
- Increased Morale and Efficiency
- Practically Eliminated Absenteeism
- Reduced Personnel Costs

See Table 5-22 for a cost comparison of the 7 on 7 off schedule versus a conventional schedule.

The 12-Hour Shift

One of the most innovative scheduling systems is the 12-hour shift. Full daily coverage is split into two shifts of 12 hours each (from 7 a.m. to 7 p.m., and from 7 p.m. to 7 a.m.) with each staff member working seven days in straight succession followed by seven days off. Instead of head nurse and assistant head nurse being assigned to evening shifts and no night shifts, it is possible to have the busy part of evening shift covered by supervisory personnel and the slow part relegated to limited coverage—a savings for the hospital of at least half of supervisory salaries used formerly for the evening shift.

At the Wyler Children's Hospital* in Chicago:

- Participating RN's receive overtime compensation at one-and-a-half times their basic hourly rate after 40 hours in a calendar week, but are not paid overtime for hours in excess of 8 per day (76 hours regular pay and 8 hours overtime in each biweekly pay period).

----

*Source: Alice B. Underwood, "What a 12-Hour Shift Offers," *American Journal of Nursing*, July 1975. © American Journal of Nursing Company.

- Each participating nurse is granted a 30-minute lunch period and two 15-minute rest periods during each 12-hour shift.
- No shift premium is paid for the 7:00 a.m. to 7:30 p.m. shift. A premium of $9.00 per shift is paid for the 7:00 p.m. to 7:30 a.m. shift.
- Sick leave and vacation time are accumulated with accruals based on each month of completed service.
- Participating nurses receive six paid holidays per year (New Years, Memorial Day, Fourth of July, Labor Day, Thanksgiving and Christmas) and are paid 12 hours of straight time for each holiday.

There are notable benefits and disadvantages to this system. In a survey of "the good and bad aspects" of the 12-hour shift, *RN* (September 1975) reported that:*

Advantages

In terms of efficiency, the total number of sick days taken over the surveyed two month period amounted to the number previously taken in an average week. Communication and interaction improved notably at team turnover time. More time was available for preparing patient records; nurses spent more time with patients, parents and doctors.

----

*Source: "The Good and the Bad of 12-hour Shifts," reprinted from *RN* Magazine, September 1975. Copyright © 1975 by Litton Industries, Inc. Published by Medical Economics Co., a Litton division, at Oradell, N.J. 07649. All rights reserved.

Table 5-21 Personnel Staffing Schedule

No.	NAME	1ST WEEK S M T W T F S	2ND WEEK S M T W T F S	3RD WEEK S M T W T F S	4TH WEEK S M T W T F S
	A-1				
	B-1				
		1 2 1 1 1 1 1	1 2 1 1 1 1 1	1 2 1 1 1 1 1	1 2 1 1 1 1 1
	A-2				
	B-2				
		1 1 2 1 1 1 1	1 1 2 1 1 1 1	1 1 2 1 1 1 1	1 1 2 1 1 1 1

LONG WEEKENDS (rows A-2, B-2)

2 3 3 2 2 2 2   2 3 3 2 2 2 2   2 3 3 2 2 2 2   2 3 3 2 2 2 2

Source: Thomas Kliber, *Modes of Scheduling*, Blue Cross of Western Pennsylvania, Pittsburgh, 1978.

Table 5-22   Cost Comparison of 7 on, 7 off Schedule Versus Conventional Schedule

CONVENTIONAL SCHEDULE

75	Hours (10 × 7.5) 8 a.m.–4 p.m. Monday through Friday
× 26	Pay Periods
1,950	Annual Hours
× $3	a Hour
$5,850	Per Year

NEW SCHEDULE   7 Days On–7 Days Off

Work Week 9 Hours (7 Days) Monday through Sunday 7:30 a.m.–5:00 p.m. (½ Hour Lunch) 63 Hours a Week W - O - W - O - W - O, etc. 26 Weeks Vacation

	7.5	— Regular Hours
	1.5	Time and One-Half
A. Regular Hours	52.5	Hours (7 Days × 7.5 Hours)
	$3	a Hour
	$157.5	× 26 Pay Periods = $4,095
B. Overtime Hours	10.5	Overtime Hours (7 Days × 1.5 Hours)
	× 4.50	a Hour (1½ Times)
	$ 47.25	× 26 Pay Periods = $1,228
C. Vacation Days	10	Vacation Days (in Lieu of Time Off)
	7.5	Hours × 10 Days × $3/Hour = $225
D. Holidays	8	Holidays — (in Lieu of Time Off)
	7.5	Hours × 8 Days $3 = $180
Annual Cost	A + B + C + D = $5,728 Per Year	
	($122 Less Than Conventional Schedule Cost)	

COMPARISON

7 and 7 System = 1,638 Hours (12 hours less work in a pay period)
Conventional = 1,815 Hours (1,950 − 135 Hours) = Vacation Plus Holiday Days

$2.35 Less a Week Than Conventional Set-Up

Source: Thomas C. Kliber, *Modes of Scheduling,* Blue Cross of Western Pennsylvania, Pittsburgh, 1978.

Nurses felt an intense involvement in patient care. They had the opportunity to prepare children for surgery and still be there when they returned post-op. Another benefit was an emotional continuum with patients and parents. Parents, for example, showed less anxiety when the same nurse was present to receive their child after surgery.

Disadvantages

In spite of these benefits, however, the majority of the nurses found that the 12-hour shifts were too exhausting to continue. "By the end of the last day of a four- or five-day stretch, fatigue was close to unbearable," one nurse reported. Cumulative fatigue was the worst aspect of the experiment. During a comparable period the previous year, three minor accidents occurred on the floor, and no medication problems were reported. During the experiment, 10 minor accidents and five medication mix-ups were recorded. The nurses felt the increased incidence was due to extreme fatigue.

The majority felt a 12-hour shift simply doesn't fit the life-style of the average person.

Chapter 6—Materiel Management

OVERVIEW

The desire for improved efficiency has led many hospitals toward a materiel management form of organizing the delivery of materiel services (see Figure 6-1). Materiel management has appeared attractive in part because it offers hospitals an opportunity to consolidate the acquisition, processing, storage, distribution and disposal of supplies and equipment.[1]

The significance of materiel management in overall hospital expenses is larger than might be expected. One study estimated that materiel management accounted for 46 percent of the total hospital budget (Figure 6-2). For a brief view of the procurement process, see the procurement flow chart in Figure 6-3 and a more detailed view of that process with a prime vendor in Figure 6-4.

Functions*

The functions of materiel management include:

- writing and adhering to product specifications;
- procuring all supplies and services through centralized purchasing;
- receiving and accounting for all supplies;
- stocking supplies for "adequate" periods of time only;
- studying and reviewing utilization of the materiel;

- developing and adhering to policies and procedures for product utilization;
- standardizing and evaluating all products and services;
- processing and reprocessing reusable supplies and materiel;
- distributing all goods and services;
- controlling "unofficial" inventories;
- assuming accountability for capital equipment;
- reviewing and servicing patient care equipment;
- controlling printing and all printed matter, including xerography;
- reviewing and evaluating patient charges; and
- disposing efficiently of the waste products of the goods and services purchased.

Advantages of a Materiel Management System*

One of the first and foremost byproducts of initiating the total materiel management concept is centralization of the authority and responsibility for all supply, process, and distribution functions. This is generally accompanied by at least the realization that the major divisions of materiel management should all be located in one area of the building. It is hoped that hospital managers, architects, and designers are learning not to decentralize the materiel functions by lo-

---

[1]Charles J. Barnett, "The Management of Change," *Hospital Materiel Management Quarterly*, August 1979.

---

*Source: Charles E. Housley, *Hospital Materiel Management*, Aspen Systems Corporation, 1978.

Figure 6-1 Organization of a department of materiel management

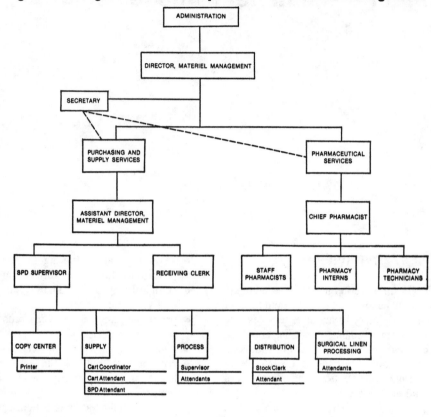

Source: Charles E. Housley, *Hospital Materiel Management,* Aspen Systems Corporation, 1978.

cating, for example, the pharmacy on the first floor, the C.S.R. on the second floor, and the central stores in the basement. All areas dealing directly with supply, process, and distribution of goods and services should, instead, be designed to function together for the sake of efficiency.

Another result of materiel management implementation is a reduction in the number of employees involved in similar functions. Effective materiel management unifies the efforts of all those involved, eliminating expensive duplication of tasks, time, and effort.

Development of the total materiel management concept has other advantageous spinoffs. It puts the responsibility of this function solely in the hands of the trained materiel manager and relieves the nursing staff of supply, process and distribution functions. Paperwork for the materiel management department is greatly reduced

and becomes more meaningful as the departments are freed from the tedious tasks of ordering, stocking, and controlling supplies. Finally, the process of implementing materiel management concepts and principles seems to become contagious as the institution begins to benefit from centralized purchasing and standardization.

Implementing a Materiel Management Program*

There are really two approaches to the organization of a materiel management program. The most prevalent approach is where the decision is made to proceed toward materiel management

_____

*Source: Charles E. Housley, *Hospital Materiel Management,* Aspen Systems Corporation, 1978.

Figure 6-2 Distribution of hospital expenses

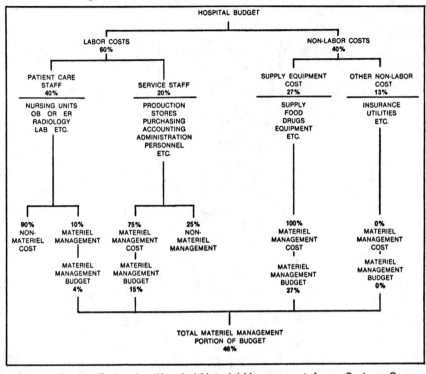

Source: Charles E. Housley, *Hospital Materiel Management,* Aspen Systems Corporation, 1978.

using the current purchasing organization with expanded responsibilities as the basic springboard. This implies that the hospital has the necessary personnel, expertise, and administrative backing to accomplish this managerial feat.

The second approach involves recruiting from outside the hospital. In this situation, top management gives more time to defining objectives, delineating organizational structure, and carefully establishing an effective job description for the new director.

In choosing the director of materiel management, where does one start? In many cases, the person for the job is within the hospital organization, especially in the positions of director of purchasing, director of pharmacy, central supply supervisor, manager of central stores, and supply, process, and distribution supervisor. Their foremost qualification is their experience with supplies and the institution. Nonetheless, they may have no conceptual scheme of materiel management. Other potential sources for consideration are hospital supply buyers, sales representatives and warehouse managers, as well as industrial purchasing agents, marketing managers, and personnel and public relations directors.

The plan should be discussed at a key personnel conference scheduled by top management and including anyone who is either a consumer or a provider of supplies. This will provide credibility and support to the materiel management thrust. It will also be an effective means of communication in that all appropriate parties get the same information at the same time. After introduction of the philosophy by top management, the materiel manager should outline the entire plan, emphasizing all the advantages. Ideas should be solicited from the group, and the notion that materiel management is a group endeavor should be reiterated. Organizational relationships and new policies and procedures should be communicated.

When the program is first instituted, several orientation sessions must be held to familiarize all personnel to the total materiel management

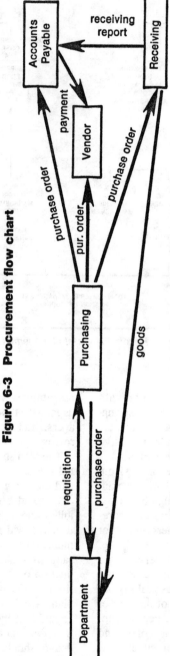

Figure 6-3   Procurement flow chart

Source: Donald F. Beck, *Basic Hospital Financial Management*, Aspen Systems Corporation, 1980, p. 154.

Figure 6-4 Purchase-receipt-payment process (with a prime vendor)

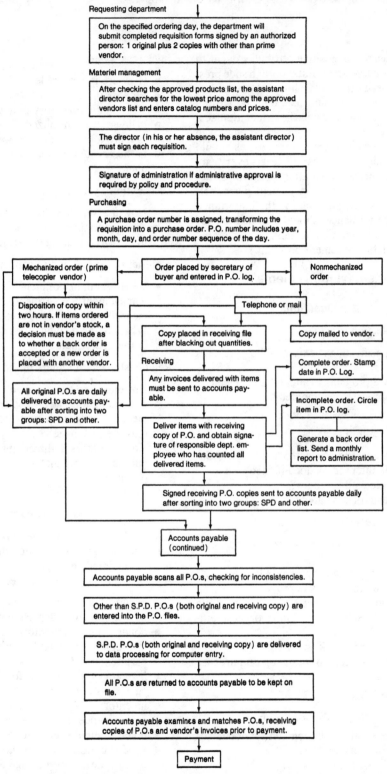

Requesting department

> On the specified ordering day, the department will submit completed requisition forms signed by an authorized person: 1 original plus 2 copies with other than prime vendor.

Materiel management

> After checking the approved products list, the assistant director searches for the lowest price among the approved vendors list and enters catalog numbers and prices.

> The director (in his or her absence, the assistant director) must sign each requisition.

> Signature of administration if administrative approval is required by policy and procedure.

Purchasing

> A purchase order number is assigned, transforming the requisition into a purchase order. P.O. number includes year, month, day, and order number sequence of the day.

Mechanized order (prime telecopier vendor)	Order placed by secretary of buyer and entered in P.O. log.	Nonmechanized order

Telephone or mail

> Disposition of copy within two hours. If items ordered are not in vendor's stock, a decision must be made as to whether a back order is accepted or a new order is placed with another vendor.

> Copy placed in receiving file after blacking out quantities.

> Copy mailed to vendor.

Receiving

> Complete order. Stamp date in P.O. Log.

> Any invoices delivered with items must be sent to accounts payable.

> Incomplete order. Circle item in P.O. log.

> All original P.O.s are daily delivered to accounts payable after sorting into two groups: SPD and other.

> Deliver items with receiving copy of P.O. and obtain signature of responsible dept. employee who has counted all delivered items.

> Generate a back order list. Send a monthly report to administration.

> Signed receiving P.O. copies sent to accounts payable daily after sorting into two groups: SPD and other.

Accounts payable (continued)

> Accounts payable scans all P.O.s, checking for inconsistencies.

> Other than S.P.D. P.O.s (both original and receiving copy) are entered into the P.O. files.

> S.P.D. P.O.s (both original and receiving copy) are delivered to data processing for computer entry.

> All P.O.s are returned to accounts payable to be kept on file.

> Accounts payable examines and matches P.O.s, receiving copies of P.O.s and vendor's invoices prior to payment.

Payment

Source: William Pitts, "How to Negotiate a Prime Vendor Contract," *Hospital Materiel Management Quarterly,* May 1981.

concept. Again, the positive attributes ought to be accentuated. A simple but thorough slide presentation based on actual hospital situational settings would be helpful, as would be written handouts which summarize the orientation session. Furthermore, each newly hired employee should be exposed to these sessions, as should groups of all employees at least every six months. A special orientation program structured just for materiel management personnel, stressing the service aspect and the importance of quality performance, should also be created. (See Figure 6-5 for an implementation timetable for a materiel management program.)

Identifying Problems*

Ask Questions

Product Selection Practices

- Do specifications exist? Who prepares them?
- How are products evaluated and selected? Is the process documented?
- Is there a standardization process?

Vendor Selection Practices

- How are vendors selected? Bids? Negotiation? Is the process documented?
- Who selects the vendor?
- Are vendors evaluated?

Purchasing Procedures

- How do departments requisition purchases?
- Is all purchasing centralized? If not, why?
- How are requisitions approved?
- How does purchasing transmit orders? Is the process time consuming or is it efficient?
- What records are kept? Why?
- Is there a system to follow up on purchase orders?

Receiving System

- Are all goods received centrally?
- Is there good accounting control documentation of every receipt?
- What is the paper flow process?

---

*Source: Marc Hoffman, "Gaining Administrative Support and Respect," *Hospital Materiel Management Quarterly*, August 1979.

Inventory System

- How are inventory levels determined?
- What is the turnover rate?
- What is the inventory policy?
- Is inventory centralized? If not, where is it?
- Is there a perpetual inventory system?
- Is the accounting control of inventory adequate?

Distribution System

- How are supplies distributed? Why?
- Who determines when and how much is delivered to the using department?

Materiel Personnel and Organization

- What functions are included in the materiel management department? What materiel management functions are not included?
- What are the qualifications of the personnel in the department?

Relationships with Others in the Hospital

- Are there are any strained relationships?
- Are there any key department heads or medical staff members whose influence must be recognized?
- How do others in the organization view the purchasing and materiel management departments?

Assemble Facts

Listing the items to be measured involves assembling the list of information that is necessary to make an intelligent decision. Examples of the type of information needed are:

- annual dollar value of materiel purchases by use category, department and per bed;
- dollar value of inventories in all locations, including "unofficial" inventory in user departments;
- inventory turnover rate for the various categories of inventory;
- inventory carrying costs, including interest, obsolescence, shrinkage and storage costs;
- dollar volume spent with all vendors;
- vendor performance, including average delivery time and percentage of line items delivered on first order;
- cost of acquisition, including purchase price, purchase order cost, receiving cost and invoice processing cost;

Figure 6-5 Implementation of a materiel management program timetable

IMPLEMENTATION OF OBJECTIVES
TIMETABLE
MODEL GUIDELINES

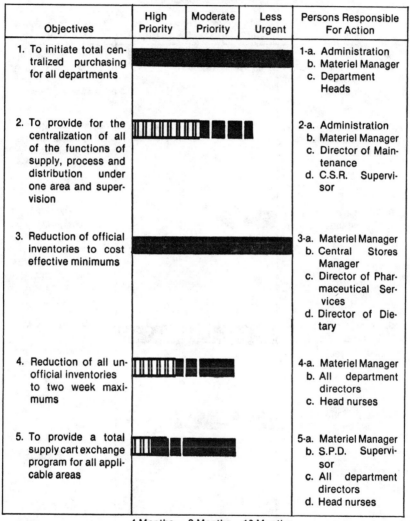

Objectives	High Priority	Moderate Priority	Less Urgent	Persons Responsible For Action
1. To initiate total centralized purchasing for all departments				1-a. Administration b. Materiel Manager c. Department Heads
2. To provide for the centralization of all of the functions of supply, process and distribution under one area and supervision				2-a. Administration b. Materiel Manager c. Director of Maintenance d. C.S.R. Supervisor
3. Reduction of official inventories to cost effective minimums				3-a. Materiel Manager b. Central Stores Manager c. Director of Pharmaceutical Services d. Director of Dietary
4. Reduction of all unofficial inventories to two week maximums				4-a. Materiel Manager b. All department directors c. Head nurses
5. To provide a total supply cart exchange program for all applicable areas				5-a. Materiel Manager b. S.P.D. Supervisor c. All department directors d. Head nurses

4 Months   8 Months   12 Months
12 MONTH PERIOD

Evaluation or Study
Implement
Ongoing

Figure 6-5 continued

IMPLEMENTATION OF OBJECTIVES
TIMETABLE

MODEL GUIDELINES

Objectives	High Priority	Moderate Priority	Less Urgent	Persons Responsible For Action
6. To meet or exceed all of the requirements of the Prudent Buyer concept	■ ■ ■	▬▬▬▬▬		6-a. Administration b. Materiel Manager c. Director of Purchased Services
7. To reduce paperwork in the purchase order process		▥▥▥▥	▬ ▬	7-a. Materiel Manager b. Director of Purchased Services c. Sales Representatives
8. To develop an effective standardization procedure	▬▬▬▬			8-a. Administration b. Materiel Manager c. Director of Purchased Services d. All Standardization Committee Members
9. To explore the feasibility of the prime supplier approach to purchasing	▥▥▥ ▬ ▥▥▥	▬▬▬		9-a. Materiel Manager b. Director of Purchased Services c. Sales Representatives
10. To perform "stockless" purchasing	▬▬▬▬▬▬			10-a Materiel Manager b. Director of Purchased Services

4 Months   8 Months   12 Months
12 MONTH PERIOD

Evaluation or Study
Implement
Ongoing

Figure 6-5 continued

IMPLEMENTATION OF OBJECTIVES
TIMETABLE

MODEL GUIDELINES

Objectives	High Priority	Moderate Priority	Less Urgent	Persons Responsible For Action
11. To reduce and contain all direct and indirect operating costs of the total material management functions	████			11-a. Materiel Manager b. Director of Purchased Services c. S.P.D. Supervisor d. Processing Supervisor e. Director of Pharmaceutical Services f. All applicable departments and units
12. To meet or exceed all accreditation standards that are applicable to the department	▥▥▥ ██ ██	███████		12-a. Materiel Manager b. Director of Purchased Services c. S.P.D. Supervisor d. Processing Supervisor e. Director of Pharmaceutical Services
13. To apply management methods to the supply process and distribution of products and equipment	████████████████			13-a. Materiel Manager b. Director of Purchased Services c. S.P.D. Supervisor d. Director of Pharmaceutical Services

4 Months   8 Months   12 Months
12 MONTH PERIOD

Evaluation or Study
Implement
Ongoing

Figure 6-5 continued

IMPLEMENTATION OF OBJECTIVES
TIMETABLE

MODEL GUIDELINES

Objectives	High Priority	Moderate Priority	Less Urgent	Persons Responsible For Action
14. To establish an evaluation procedure for measuring materiel management effectiveness		▦▦ ▓▓		14-a. Administration b. Materiel Manager c. Fiscal Officer
15. To establish a Property Management System			▦ ▓▓	15-a. Administration b. Materiel Manager c. Fiscal Officer

4 Months   8 Months   12 Months

12 MONTH PERIOD

Evaluation or Study ▥▥▥▥

Implement ▰▰▰▰

Ongoing ▰▰▰

Source: Charles E. Housley, *Hospital Materiel Management,* Aspen Systems Corporation, 1978.

- cost of distribution, including labor and equipment;
- number of personnel involved in the purchase, receipt, processing and distribution of supplies;
- space provided for materiel management functions;
- description of logistics in the institution, including travel distances, elevators and other transportation systems; and
- symptoms of supply problems, for example, the number of walk-on requests in the storeroom, the number of calls for "emergency" needs from using departments and the number of stock-outs.

Find Solutions

1. Collect and categorize the data
2. Compare the data with existing standards
3. Determine the reasons for variance
4. Develop several alternate solutions and list their advantages and disadvantages
5. Select the best alternate solution
6. Prepare a plan of implementation
7. Prepare and present a report to the Administration
8. Implement the plan.

THE MATERIEL MANAGER

Selection*

Before the search for a materiel manager is begun, certain aspects of how materiel management functions should be analyzed. The number of departments in the division, the administrative officer to whom the manager will report and where the materiel manager's position will be relative to the rest of the management hierarchy—all are important factors in the selection process. A thorough analysis of these factors will reveal the degree of expertise, knowledge and education a candidate for materiel manager should possess.

Perhaps individuals in positions within the hospital could fulfill the requirements of the job and become effective materiel managers. The

---

*Source: Larry S. Wrobel and Bruce Rampage, "Administrative Considerations in the Selection of a Materiel Manager," *Hospital Materiel Management Quarterly*, August 1979.

purchasing director, chief pharmacist and supply, processing and distribution manager are all potential candidates. These people bring to the job a unique knowledge and understanding of the hospital's environment and its employees.

Typically the components of the materiel division consist of purchasing, central service, general stores and receiving. The materiel manager at this level of responsibility in an institution over 200 beds should be appropriately considered a part of middle management and should be hired at the department head level. The materiel manager may report to either the assistant administrator for general services or an associate administrator.

If either food service, pharmacy or housekeeping is a part of a materiel division, the manager should be hired at the assistant administrator level and report to the chief operating officer. The materiel manager's effectiveness will be compromised if he or she must supervise several department heads and is not considered a part of top management. Candidates recruited at this level should have the knowledge, background and analytical techniques provided by a graduate program in hospital or business administration.

Qualifications

When applicants for the position of materiel manager are reviewed, the foremost quality to be considered is management ability. Materiel management is in its infancy in many hospitals; consequently, directors for materiel management are confronted with the task of creating and organizing a viable materiel program, rather than the job of maintaining a smoothly running operation. Major project development such as the implementation of exchange-cart programs and inventory-control systems is the rule rather than the exception. A materiel manager must have basic management skills and aptitudes to be effective.

Another essential quality for the successful materiel manager is the ability to relate in both a line and staff capacity to other hospital managers. The individual hired must have effective interpersonal relations skills when acting in a staff capacity. Materiel management will then become a hospital-wide and not a departmental concept.

A viable candidate for the position of materiel manager should have knowledge of the basic concepts of purchasing, inventory control and distribution of materiel within the hospital environment. Specifically, the abilities to relate to vendors and to negotiate contracts successfully are necessary. Familiarity with medical-surgical product lines and fair market prices and capital equipment acquisition [are also desirable.] Also, experience with the requisition method of distributing supplies, par-level-stocking and exchange-cart distribution methods should be required.

The Purchasing Administrator*

As the hospital's purchasing agent, the administrator is responsible for:

* implementing and directing the hospital purchasing program to control the purchase or the lease of all goods and services from outside sources;
* purchasing, negotiating or reviewing and approving all purchase arrangements with outside sources;
* counseling and monitoring purchasing functions in other departments on behalf of administration;
* managing products in general use by establishing criteria for acceptability, cataloging, administering new product review, standardization and working with administration to ensure adequate processing and maintenance of reusable products; and
* managing the capital equipment accountability program.

In addition to the usual departmental management responsibilities, the purchasing administrator has other major functions in the hospital.

Organizational Function

1. Confers on a regular basis with members of administration for the purpose of coordinating the hospital purchasing program with the objectives and plans of top management.

---

*Source: William K. Henning, "Application of the Prudent Buyer Principle to Purchasing Administration," *Hospital Materiel Management Quarterly*, November 1979.

2. Submits monthly reports concerning functional and administrative phases of the program to the assistant administrator.
3. Directs the activities of the standardization committee to assure that it meets at least monthly, is chaired by an appropriate person and that it consistently applies quality criteria and standardization principles to the products it authorizes for general use in the hospital.
4. Maintains a professional rapport with the medical staff, administration, nursing service and all other hospital departments, such that communication is adequate and the agent's expert purchasing skills are applied throughout the hospital.
5. Establishes and maintains proper and appropriate professional and ethical relationships with sales representatives and other outside contacts.

Central Purchasing Management

1. Manages the procurement of supplies, services and equipment for and in the purchasing department.
2. As a staff person and an administration agent, controls all procurement throughout the hospital (with the exception of certain types of purchases reserved by the administrator).
3. Develops, recommends and adheres to policies and procedures relating to the management of purchasing in the hospital.
4. Abides by written hospital procedures on conflict of interest and acceptance of gifts.
5. Orders, bids, negotiates with outside sources and participates in bona fide group purchasing and shared-service efforts with other hospitals.
6. Develops and recommends to administration a purchasing system which identifies department personnel who should be authorized to conduct purchasing.
7. Maintains an up-to-date list of all persons in the hospital authorized to purchase from outside sources and the types of products or services they are permitted to purchase.
8. Coordinates with administration the establishment of procedures necessary for

the administrative approval of purchase orders and contracts, and assures that these procedures are followed in every case within the hospital by direct supervision or by periodic auditing of purchasing activity in other departments.

9. Determines the most cost-effective and prudent method of purchase for every purchase except those reserved to the administrator. Establishes purchasing method guidelines to be followed by department heads in those departments not under the purchasing administrator's supervision.

10. Assures that an appropriately completed purchase order is issued for every purchase or group of purchases in the hospital.

11. Maintains a record of all active contracts for purchases, lease or service and a description of the type of records and location of those records not maintained and filed in the purchasing department.

12. Establishes criteria to determine which purchases should be made for central storage. Defines which purchases should be handled as "specials" and sent directly to departments. Reviews special purchases periodically to identify those which should be shifted from special to central distribution status within the system.

13. Reviews special requests and determines that products are completely and accurately described.

14. Shares with the distribution manager the responsibility of maintaining low inventories in the central area and throughout the hospital by means of a reliable, efficient and low-cost flow of goods from receiving to the various departments. (This is accomplished through purchasing decisions, balancing timely and reliable delivery with the costs of ordering, receiving and storing, cumulatively.)

15. For all important suppliers, establishes a method for periodically monitoring the delivery performance of each; maintains an approved vendor list.

16. Establishes simplified methods of handling repeat orders so that the process is fast, inexpensive and error free.

17. Establishes a method for identifying stockouts and quickly overcoming problems for high-volume consumables.

18. Maintains standard specifications and works with the distribution manager to establish standard purchasing quantities, reorder points (and periodically reviews these standards) for consumables within the central storage and distribution system.

19. Assures that in a department not under the purchasing administrator's control, invoice prices, quantities and terms are matched with similar information on approved purchase orders or contract forms to authorize invoices for payment and that this process is periodically audited by an outside firm.

20. Annually reviews the format and legal conditions on the standard purchase order set and updates this material with appropriate administrative and legal assistance.

21. Supervises the handling of all adjustments and claims with outside sources.

22. Engages in purchasing research and value analysis; studies market trends sufficiently to identify the lowest total-cost purchasing method forecast needs, and shares this information with appropriate hospital personnel.

Regulation and Accreditation

1. Meets or exceeds standards of compliance for all accrediting and regulatory bodies.

2. Monitors all hospital purchasing to assure strict compliance with prudent buyer concepts as defined in the *Provider Reimbursement Manual*.

3. Studies the contractual requirements of hospital third-party intermediaries and determines their methods of applying the prudent buyer concept to hospital audits. Helps the hospital take appropriate action to prepare for the possibility of a prudent buyer audit.

4. Maintains files of analyses and correspondence relating to purchasing decisions such as bids, negotiations and cost benefit analyses.

5. Works with administration to establish procedures to document all prudent-purchasing actions regarding services for departmental management (such as house-

keeping and dietary) and the purchase of financial packages (such as insurance and borrowing).

Product Management

1. Establishes criteria relating to quality, safety, compatibility, labeling and use-life in the case of reusable classes of products (with the assistance of appropriate department heads) for those general-use products which the hospital desires to make readily available and maintain through its materiel system.
2. Writes and assures adherence to product and equipment specifications.
3. Reviews and makes appropriate recommendations on all new supplies and equipment, applying general hospital criteria and the considerations of standardization, cost effectiveness and other general hospital management requirements.
4. Communicates the list of products within the central system to users by means of a printed catalog or a computer system video display.
5. Manages the standardization effort primarily by guiding the standardization committee.
6. As recall coordinator assumes the responsibility of being the focal point for recalls—informing using departments, monitoring the effectiveness of action taken and maintaining all records of recall.
7. Takes appropriate action to assure that adequate maintenance is established for each of the hospital's reusable products.
8. Coordinates the necessary in-service training for new and certain existing products.

Capital Equipment Management

Establishes a system which lists capital equipment by department, value and condition, assuring departmental accountability, and maintains a record for financial and legal purposes.

Disposal of Excess Usable and Salvaged Goods

1. Works with vendors and outside agencies to sell back certain excess supplies and equipment.

2. Works with outside agencies to donate certain usable goods which cannot be returned for credit and destroys the remainder (with the approval of hospital administration).

Evaluating the Materiel Manager*

Guideposts

Guideposts for evaluation of the materiel manager include:

- total control of the acquisition and distribution function;
- centralized authority and responsibility;
- proper receipt and accountability of all supplies;
- reduction and control of inventories;
- elimination of unnecessary stockpiling in work units;
- maintenance of adequate stock levels;
- prevention of lost patient charges;
- quality of centralized purchasing;
- appropriate controls over the disposition of obsolete equipment and excess supplies;
- elimination of excess paper work; and
- overall contribution to hospital cost-containment activity.

Areas of Concern

The manager's performance should be evaluated in the following areas:

1. *System Design.* The materiel manager needs to be held responsible for a well-organized and efficient system. Its design, makeup and organizational development provide the framework on which to build the remaining parts.
2. *Communication of the System to the Staff.* Like other department heads, the materiel manager must be an effective communicator, aware of communication breakdowns and the important role that communication plays in the success of the system.
3. *Ability to Work with Others.* Sounds familiar? Yes, but, clearly, as a staff officer of a hospital, the materiel manager is exposed to the total organization and must possess

---

*Source: Charles B. Stearns, "Getting the Most Out of Your Materiel Manager," *Hospital Materiel Management Quarterly*, August 1979.

tact, diplomacy, empathy and a real ability to work with others.

4. *Problem-Solving Management Style.* An effective materiel manager must have a sound problem-solving management style, detail oriented and sensitive to people's needs.

5. *Willingness to Confront Issues and Follow Through.* Hospital department heads have sometimes been accused of lacking awareness of critical issues on which to follow through. Because of the impact of the materiel management system on the total organization and the reliance that particularly nursing personnel place upon the availability of supplies, a materiel manager's willingness to confront problems, to solve them and to follow up is a must and needs to be judged.

6. *Cost Performance and Budget Development.* The performance of the materiel manager in containing hospital costs, and indeed in reducing them, is the name of the game and the bottom line. If the system and/or the materiel manager fail in this part of the job, one or both should be replaced.

PURCHASING STRUCTURES

Centralized Purchasing*

Centralized purchasing is defined as centralizing the responsibility and authority for the hospital-wide purchasing function under one manager. In many hospitals this is drastically different from the current situation.

In definition, centralized purchasing is quite specific, but in fact there are varying degrees of "centralization" within hospitals. While some hospitals do practice nearly true centralized purchasing, others permit the purchasing of specialized items used by one department (e.g., pharmaceuticals, food) by that department head.

Advantages

Centralized purchasing, when properly established and enforced, allows for both cost savings and improved internal control of the procure-

ment function. Its most common advantages (benefits) include the following.

- Quantity discounts are made possible by consolidating all hospital orders for the same and similar items.
- Product evaluation and standardization efforts are possible.
- Fewer purchase orders are processed thereby reducing purchasing, receiving and inspection time. This also reduces record-keeping and makes that recordkeeping more effective.
- Duplication of effort and poor purchasing practices are minimized through coordination of purchases.
- Purchasing specialists whose primary responsibility is purchasing are developed.
- Department heads are able to devote full efforts to their main responsibilities (i.e., managing their department rather than ordering their department's supplies).
- The number of employees involved in purchasing is reduced.
- The purchasing manager is held accountable by the hospital administrator for the purchasing function.
- The hospital can maximize participation in a group purchasing program due to an increased knowledge of the hospital's needs.
- A unified purchasing policy can be developed.
- Centralized purchasing can attract a high quality purchasing professional because of the opportunities and challenges.

In a typical centralized purchasing environment the purchasing department usually buys for:

- general service departments (those departments that provide service to other departments and do not generate patient revenue);
- nursing care areas (including medical/surgical and special care units); and
- ancillary departments.

Obstacles

The departments that are most difficult to commit to centralized purchasing are those that feel they require too high a level of technical competence for a buyer to procure their equipment and supplies. These departments feel that because of

---

*Source: S. Randolph Hayas, "Total Centralized Purchasing: Can It Ever Be Achieved?" *Hospital Materiel Management Quarterly*, November 1979.

this necessary high level of technical knowledge only they can adequately procure their needs. Departments that are typically most difficult to commit to the concept of centralized purchasing are:

- pharmacy;
- food service;
- maintenance; and
- certain ancillary departments such as radiology or laboratory.

Although department heads may feel their purchases are too technical for a purchasing specialist to perform, through adequately written specifications the purchasing agent can procure at least as effectively as the department head.

How to Establish Centralized Purchasing

The three essential steps to effectively accomplish centralized purchasing are (1) providing full hospital administrative support, (2) "selling" the benefits to department heads to receive their cooperation and (3) establishing the purchasing department's credibility through a slow yet steady implementation process.

Department heads must obtain a complete understanding of centralized purchasing in order for them not to feel threatened by this impending change. It must be understood that centralized purchasing is a method to relieve department heads from purchasing functions in order to spend more time where their specialized talents can be best utilized—managing their department.

The goals established should specifically state dates for implementing the centralized purchasing plan in each department, the date for full centralized purchasing implementation within the hospital, and the savings and other improvements anticipated. It is important to prepare a timetable for implementation of the purchasing program to minimize procrastination on the part of purchasing and other departments.

One department should be chosen as the first area to implement centralized purchasing. It would not be practical to begin on "January 1" a complete (hospital-wide) centralized purchasing program; rather one department should be worked with to define items, specifications, substitutes, vendors, inventory levels, lead times, reorder points, order quantities and appropriate ordering patterns.

When centralized purchasing has been implemented in one department and is fully functional, another department should be chosen for the implementation process.

As centralized purchasing is implemented in each department, ongoing reviews should be conducted of the function of centralized purchasing to identify weaknesses and improvements. This review should be augmented by performance reporting by the purchasing department and by internal and oftentimes objective external audits of the purchasing function. The reviews, performance reporting and audits should be continued periodically after all departments have been fully implemented.

Group Purchasing

The Basic Issues*

The basic premise of group purchasing is that a group of hospitals with a common interest in reducing costs and improving quality can perform the purchasing function better as a group than they can as individual hospitals.

The majority of group purchasing activities have been in competitive bidding and contract negotiations for the purchase of supplies and services. The modus operandi of purchasing groups is usually:

- Standardization is achieved whenever possible between member hospitals.
- Investment in inventory to each hospital is determined by each hospital's current financial position.
- Purchases are ordered as needed by the individual hospitals.
- The supplies are stored in the individual hospitals and distributed to user departments as required.
- Each hospital is responsible for maintaining its own control and reporting systems.
- Individual hospitals do not share supplies, except on an emergency basis.
- Each hospital maintains a staff to meet its day-to-day operational commitments.
- Information is shared between purchasing directors on an informal basis.

---

*Source: Jerry P. Widman, "A Reexamination of Group Purchasing," *Hospital Materiel Management Quarterly,* November 1981.

Advantages

1. Economics on large volume purchases. Buying power is consolidated and better discounts can be obtained. While the hospital will gain a price advantage on many items, not every supply item can be purchased more effectively through group purchasing. In each circumstance, it is important for a hospital to maintain flexibility and benefit from those group prices that are advantageous and ignore the others.

2. Standardization of supply items. Many hospital storerooms stock two similar items when one would serve the need. A group purchasing organization with its overall perspective on the group's requirements is in a unique position to offer guidance and direction in the area of standardization.

3. Exchange of product information and experiences. Through committee meetings and published reports, group members share information with each other to avoid reinventing the wheel in each hospital.

4. Time savings resulting in improved operations. By obtaining items through the group purchasing vehicle, individual hospital purchasing directors have more time to spend in other areas of the purchasing function. This can produce improvements in other purchasing operations such as: response time to users, value analysis of supply items, forecasting supply requirements and standardization efforts.

5. Other benefits. There are other benefits that might be made available through group purchasing.* That method can:

- Make available the services of knowledgeable persons who can provide consultation to members in the current hospital purchasing practices.
- Prepare educational programs to assist members in their continuing educational requirements.
- Assist in disposition of surplus materials.
- Make periodic visits to hospitals to review purchasing programs and assist them in maintaining or improving their programs.
- Monitor and evaluate the effect of group purchasing on each member's purchasing program.
- Assist in preparing specifications for purchasing not covered by group commitments.
- Assist member hospitals in the development of maintenance contracts.

Implementation

Some of the ingredients of successful group purchasing programs are:

- Group purchasing must have the support of hospital administrators, hospital purchasing directors and the health care community in order to be workable.
- While group purchasing is normally a voluntary activity on the part of member hospitals, the concept works best on a committed-volume basis.
- Group purchasing demonstrates success in direct proportion to the enthusiasm of the participants.
- Group purchasing is best geared to the purchase of large-volume items on which agreement can be reached relatively easily among member hospitals.

Myths

1. Group purchasing will bankrupt local suppliers. No hospital will ever purchase all of its supplies through the group purchasing mechanism. There will always be business for local suppliers.

2. Group purchasing deals with "marginal" suppliers. If "marginal" translates into the fact that selected group suppliers may not advertise nationally, then perhaps the myth is true. Some hospital buyers maintain that unless they purchase well-known products, their hospitals are not obtaining good quality. However, as many American consumers have learned, advertising is not always synonymous with quality or value.

3. Hospitals experience late deliveries. Often late deliveries are not the fault of the purchasing organization but are due to hospitals failing to forecast their purchases and, consequently, having an unusually high percentage of rush orders. If "late deliveries" means that deliveries are not accomplished within normal lead time, then group purchasing may indeed be at fault. However, if "late deliveries" means that deliveries

---

*Source: Michael J. Brzezicki and Patricia A. Reed, "What Makes a Successful Group Purchasing Program," *Hospital Materiel Management Quarterly*, February 1982.

cannot be met on a rush order basis, the weakness is not with the group purchasing organization.

4. *Hospitals have no recourse for vendor errors.* Since suppliers are now two steps removed from the hospital, won't they have very little interest in servicing the hospital accounts? If the vendor fails to properly service the individual hospital accounts, the vendor may very well not be asked to submit a quotation for the group's next year's contract.

5. *Hospitals will lose annual contributions and gifts.* Suppliers who are in the habit of giving gifts most often add that cost to the purchase price of their products. The fear of lost contributions and gifts is only justified when prices are not competitive and vendors must rely on the use of gifts in soliciting the bulk of their business.

6. *Purchasing directors will lose their jobs.* The myth here is that under group purchasing, purchasing directors of individual hospitals will become mere order takers and there will be little reason to keep them on. This myth could not be further from the truth. With group purchasing in effect, purchasing directors are free to use their special skills in other areas of purchasing operations: negotiations, new sources of supply, quantitative techniques, standardization, usage rates and other purchasing improvements. Purchasing is still an important management function.

7. *Small hospitals cannot participate.* Many smaller hospitals feel mistakenly that they cannot participate in group purchasing because the minimum quantities are too large. Normally, minimum quantities offered by the group purchasing organizations are in fact not excessive and are attuned to hospitals of all sizes.

Types of Groups*

Groups go by different names, reflecting their organizational differences.

1. Consortiums are formal organizations requiring monetary and personnel commitments. Generally items are delivered to a central location and redistributed to members.

2. Cooperatives are informal organizations requiring little or no monetary or personnel commitments. These are generally the least effective.

3. Corporations are formal organizations that require substantial monetary commitment but little or no commitment of personnel. Generally they offer large savings and arrangements are handled in the same manner as in dealing with an independent surgical supply dealer.

4. Federations are formal organizations requiring considerable administrative, personnel and monetary commitment. Generally substantial savings on selected items are realized because of central delivery and redistribution.

5. Associations are formal organizations requiring little monetary or personnel commitment. This is the organizational structure most often selected. Associations offer many opportunities for savings while requiring few or no purchases.

A purchasing group may be sponsored by nonprofit associations, such as a state or county hospital association, or it may be an independent nonprofit or for-profit organization. A regional purchasing group may be affiliated with other organizations to form a "super group." This larger group may be able to negotiate more favorable agreements than those available to the individual members.

Criteria for Selecting a Purchasing Group*

Your hospital's participation in a group purchasing program increases your buying leverage and offers the expertise of another purchasing professional, the group director, to your staff. Not all groups will suit you and your hospital, and your selection of the right group is one of the important decisions you will make for your institution.

Committed vs. Noncommitted Contracts

Committed contracts ensure for the vendor the purchased volume of the participating hospitals and are apt to receive the most favorable pricing since vendors compete in a win-or-lose contest.

---

*Source: Michael J. Brzezicki and Patricia A. Reed, "What Makes a Successful Group Purchasing Program," *Hospital Materiel Management Quarterly,* February 1982.

*Source: Jack Anderson, "Selecting the Right Group Purchasing Program," *Hospital Materiel Management Quarterly,* February 1981.

In order to participate in a committed volume purchasing program, purchasing or materiel managers must be able to sell their hospitals on the contract brand. Some groups hedge on the committed volume contract by establishing dual vendors for each item.

Noncommitted purchasing contracts require no indication from a hospital of an intent to participate in the agreement. Vendors are simply offering a price in anticipation of increased business, often encouraged by the group purchasing director. The advantage of this style of contracting is that the hospital's purchasing manager does not have to accept specific contract brands. Instead, purchasing agents can ask the group to enter into an agreement with the manufacturer preferred by their hospital. In addition, noncommitted purchasing groups claim that hospitals are able to buy a greater percentage of their needs from group contracts and no hospital is excluded from using agreements because it prefers another brand.

The disadvantage of noncommitted groups is the prices they pay. Why should a supplier offer a discount on existing business when additional sales volume is not assured?

Participation in Contracting

Some group purchasing organizations involve their members in deciding what to contract and where to solicit bids; the ultimate contract acceptance or rejection is voted on by the members. Other purchasing groups occasionally survey their members as to their desires but write agreements without the direct involvement of the hospital representatives.

When a group is writing committed volume contracts, the participation of the members is essential. Vendor approvals and volume commitments are required from each member.

Range of Activities and Prices

An evaluation of purchasing groups does not end with a price comparison of the most common medical–surgical supplies. Many purchasing groups have programs for pharmacy, laboratory, dietary, housekeeping, maintenance and office supplies as well as fuel and medical gases. Some groups have established shared computer programs for inventory and purchasing and have negotiated biomedical repair contracts as well as service agreements for office equipment.

However, comparing the prices of the groups being considered is essential to the selection process. The price survey should include data on the length of contracts with price protection clauses, any delivery, handling and minimum order charges, and any other information you would request from any other supplier.

You should be aware that the representative prices you receive from a purchasing group will be tailored to show its performance in the most favorable light. The shopping list for your hospital will vary, so create your own list of high-volume items for price comparison.

Fee Structure

The manner in which group purchasing organizations derive revenue to sustain their operations will vary among groups. Some popular fee structures are:

1. fixed fee for total program;
2. fixed fee per selected programs;
3. fixed fee per bed;
4. fixed fee per patient day;
5. percentage of hospital purchases (paid by the hospital); and
6. percentage of sales to group (paid by the vendor).

One way to evaluate fees is to calculate the percentage of total contract dollars they represent. A group with $2 million in contracts and a total fee revenue of $50,000 is operating at 2.5 percent of contract dollars. A rule of thumb for a reasonable group purchasing fee is 1 percent of the contract purchases. Groups just beginning or those with ancillary services, such as time-shared computers, would be somewhat higher.

Information Sharing

Do the purchasing groups you are evaluating share price and contract information with other groups? If they do, they are learning valuable information about successes and failures in other parts of the country.

Hospital Personality

The climate within your particular hospital may be a factor in selecting a group purchasing organization. If your hospital staff is receptive to change and to cost-containment efforts, you are likely to achieve good results in a committed volume purchasing group. Also the purchasing group you select should have other members of approximately the same size. Vendors bidding for a contract must factor the cost of servicing each account into their prices, and a large hospital may not improve its pricing by joining a purchasing group made up of very small units.

Specialized hospitals, such as pediatric facilities or burn centers, should look for purchasing groups that represent other hospitals with a similar specialty, since these purchasing groups are more likely to develop contracts for the specialized products used by these institutions.

Making Your Selection

A hospital can belong to several purchasing groups—one for pharmaceuticals, medical–surgical and laboratory supplies, another for a food service program, a third for furniture and office equipment and still another for medical capital equipment.

It would be inadvisable to commit to two or more purchasing groups for the same supply items.

Checklist for Evaluating a Group Purchasing Program*

The Policy Manual

1. Is there a written policy and procedure manual? _____ Yes _____ No _____ Points
2. Does the manual clearly define the purchasing process step by step?
3. Was the policy manual approved by management? committee members? legal advisor? financial auditor?
4. Is the policy manual reviewed and revised at least every three years?

Performance of the Purchasing Group Staff

1. Do the members feel the staff are competent, friendly and interested in their problems? (Contact a sample of member hospital personnel by phone.) _____ Yes _____ No _____ Points
2. Are the communication documents clearly written? (Letters, invitations to bid, contracts, surveys, minutes, etc.)

*Source: Donald J. Siegle, "Evaluation of Group Purchasing Programs; A Proposed Methodology," *Hospital Materiel Management Quarterly,* November 1981.

3. Are contract notices sent to hospitals, and are they clear and informative? (Do they contain price and other order placement information?)
4. Are reports and records accurate and complete? (Survey analyses, annual report, bid analyses)
5. Does the organization enjoy financial stability?
6. Do the staff work well with vendors? (Contact a sample of vendors by phone.)
7. Do the staff attend continuing education programs and stay active with local purchasing associations?
8. Do the staff show initiative on the job? (New projects each year.)
9. Have the staff used research to assist in decision making? (Laboratory tests, written reports, product evaluations, value analysis, etc.)
10. Do reports to management include results of contract negotiations, status of objectives and major conditions affecting the program?
11. Is the program managed at a cost comparable to those of other programs of similar size and age? Note: The average purchasing program has 74 member hospitals with a total of 12,000 beds, is 12 years old, has annual participation of $26 million, average participation of $172 per bed per month and operates at a cost of 0.6 percent of total dollar hospital participation.
12. Do the staff publish a newsletter or participate regularly in a corporate newsletter?
13. Do the staff visit hospitals or have a traveling representative?
14. Are committee members given orientation programs and objectives each year?

Effect on Prices

Does the purchasing program utilize the following methods to effect lower prices?

1. Quantity consolidation resulting in lower vendor cost per unit? _____ Yes _____ No _____ Points
2. Quality standardization resulting in inventory reduction?
3. Negotiation techniques using teams of volunteer hospital personnel?
4. Price stability and longer firm price periods?

5. Reduced freight costs due to quantity consolidation?
6. Better cash terms due to guarantees of groups?
7. Competition from increased number of interested vendors?
8. Contract commitment enabling vendors to plan better?
9. Escalation control, using wholesale market reports?
10. Warehousing, dealing directly with producers and manufacturers and providing distribution?

In addition, other useful questions might be:

11. Does the program document net price trends over multiyear periods?
12. Does the program calculate the dollar savings on each contract total and by hospital?
13. Does the program group products into logical packages that may be competitively bid by many vendors yet be more enticing than individual products? (Example: "total electrical maintenance products" rather than merely "electric bulbs.")

Vendor Potential and Performance

1. Does the group maintain a bidder's list for each contract? _____ Yes _____ No _____ Points
2. Is there a policy for adding and deleting vendors on the bidder's list?
3. Is there a system for recording and assessing the performance of vendors?
4. Is that system of judging performance used as a reference when the next contract with a vendor is negotiated?

The Survey of Market Conditions

The evaluation of a purchasing program is meaningless without a market survey—an array of data and information that portrays the conditions existing before the program was implemented. Such a survey generally requests information on what each hospital is presently purchasing and what the hospital expects the group purchasing program to provide.

1. Was the initial market survey returned by at least 40 percent of the potential participants? _____ Yes _____ No _____ Points

2. Did the survey include a random sample of hospitals by size, services, teaching status and geography?
3. Did the survey determine the quantity and quality of materials being purchased prior to the introduction of group purchasing?
4. Was a survey analysis report compiled and sent to hospital members?
5. Is there a market survey for every new contract negotiated?
6. Does the survey include the price of every item purchased within the product grouping?
7. Does the survey include the name of the vendors being utilized?
8. Is the average price per unit calculated in such a way that it may be compared to national data available?

The Decision-Making Process

1. Are the committees and subcommittees given sufficient specific information to properly make their decisions on the award of the contract?
   a. Are bids systematically compared? _____ Yes _____ No _____ Points
   b. Are results compared to the survey information prior to decision making?
   c. Are prices listed in comparison format?
   d. Do the bids include all sizes and types of products?
   e. Does bid analysis make note of which items have heavy usage?
   f. Does the bid analysis include factors other than price, such as freight, firm pricing, minimum orders, cash discounts and sales service?
2. Is there a democratic process of arriving at the final decision/recommendations with a motion made by the subcommittee and discussion by the full committee?
3. Is there a count made of the membership's vote in order to show the committee the group opinion?
4. Is the decision-making process explained in the policy manual?

Other Services

1. Does the program sponsor continuing education and assist, or help develop, the local purchasing association? _____ Yes _____ No _____ Points

2. Do the program staff assist member hospitals in implementing materiel management programs?
3. Does the program provide product and function research, such as Value Analysis?
4. Does the program provide price review audits or other internal audits to its members?
5. Are there any other byproduct programs?

Shared Materiel Management*

The closest hospitals have come to date in sharing materiel management has been in group purchasing programs, linen and laundry services, and printing services. Group purchasing, although substantially reducing individual hospitals' supply acquisition costs, has not adequately reduced the materiel expense of member hospitals. The real materiel cost reductions and containment are to be realized in the individual hospital's internal materiel management systems for purchasing, inventory control, supply distribution, facility utilization, and the monitoring of patient charges, which goes far beyond the negotiation of purchase price alone.

Services

The shared materiel management services provide participating hospitals with the following:

- purchasing service;
- warehousing and inventory management;
- supply distribution systems;
- patient charge control;
- computerized management information systems;
- biomedical engineering and industrial engineering services;
- printing services;
- capital equipment control; and
- materiel management consulting support to individual hospitals.

The above services are designed to meet individual hospital needs and be provided from a centrally located supply distribution center, staffed by experienced materiel management personnel drawn from member hospitals and materiel management consultants as required.

_____
*Source: Martin H. Purcell, "Will Shared Materiel Management Services Work?" *Hospital Materiel Management Quarterly*, August 1980.

Experienced materiel management support personnel can help each hospital improve its cash flow through inventory control, consolidation, and improved patient supply charge systems. By consolidating storage in a central supply distribution center, it is possible for each hospital to reduce its storage space requirements.

Potential Areas of Benefit

Among the areas that would benefit from shared services are:

Materiel Management
Access to experienced hospital materiel management personnel
Establishment of policies and procedures
Improved management information and performance
Improved service levels from materiel management
Improved control of all resources—money, personnel, and materiel

Purchasing
Savings from group purchasing contracts
Savings from improved purchasing systems
Savings from printing service

Inventory Control
Reduced on-hand inventory
Improved security

Patient Supply Charges
Improved patient supply charge formulation and charge mechanism
Increased patient supply revenues

Supply Distribution
Improved supply distribution systems
Reduced supply distribution expense

Education
Educational training programs for all materiel management personnel
Continuing education programs for hospital staff

Equipment Control
Biomedical engineering services
Capital equipment control program

Facility Utilization
Reduced storage space required at each hospital that can be converted to revenue-producing areas

FUNCTIONS

1. The Receiving Process*

The receiving department should be the point of entry for *all* materiel used in a hospital. The accurate control of materiel must begin at the receiving dock.

The most important function of receiving personnel is the detection of errors. Examples of common receiving errors are receipt of:

1. supplies which were not ordered;
2. items substituted without prior approval by the purchasing department;
3. outdated (shelf life) materiel;
4. damaged or defective materiel; and
5. quantity shortages.

The receipt of materiel is the final point at which the mistakes of the vendor, the shipper and the purchasing department can be detected and readily remedied. The cost of correcting them when the materiel has proceeded beyond this point will be much higher than if they are detected earlier.

Reducing Errors

To prevent errors in the receiving process, the receiving department might be encouraged to follow this procedure:

1. Check the quantity of packages and weights against the shipper's manifest.
2. Inspect and record the condition of containers. Any detected damage should be inspected by the carrier's representative and noted on the receipt which is signed by the receiver. (Failure to follow this process can relieve the carrier of liability.) In the event of damaged materiel which is not found until packages are opened for count verification, the receiver is responsible for notifying the purchasing department of the damage. Although this may be done verbally it should also be noted on the receiving report.
3. Verify receipt of materiel against the supplier's packing slip and the receiving copy of the purchase order to determine that

there are no discrepancies. If the purchase order is unavailable upon receipt of a shipment, it is the responsibility of the receiver to notify the appropriate purchasing authority to process the shipment.

4. Record shortages, overages, incorrect and damaged materiel on the receiving report. *Any deviation between materiel ordered and materiel received must be recorded.* The receiving report should indicate that the order received is complete and should carry the date and the signature of the receiver. The units of measure on the receiving report should be consistent with those on the purchase order; if the purchase order was written as "each" or "case," the receiving report should use these same units of measure.
5. When the equipment is received, the serial number should be recorded on the receiving report. This will assist the accounting department in keeping accurate and complete fixed-asset records.
6. Distribute merchandise to designated departments within an appropriate time period. Upon delivery to designated departments, the recipient should sign the receiving report—thus relieving the receiver of any further responsibility for the materiel.

2. Supply Distribution Systems*

A hospital's distribution system is an intricate network from storage to user points. The goal of any effective distribution system should be to provide the right item to the right place at the right time for the least total cost. Studies have shown that for every dollar spent to purchase an item, another dollar is spent storing and moving it. Administrators should keep in mind when evaluating their distribution system that there is no one best system for all situations (and hospitals).

Requisition System

The requisition system is basically controlled by the user area. Each department functions as a materiel manager and keeps track of its own in-

*Source: Terry D. Rich, "The Receiving Process: A Key to Effective Materiel Management," *Hospital Materiel Management Quarterly,* November 1979.

*Source: Jamie C. Kowalski, "Supply Distribution Options—A New Perspective," *Hospital Materiel Management Quarterly,* November 1980.

ventories. At a given time or when inventory levels get low, a requisition is prepared and presented to the central storage point. The requisition is then filled, supplies are delivered to the user area, and users put the items in their appropriate place.

Par-Level System

A par-level system can be defined as one in which each user department stores supplies in an assigned location in its own area. Physical stock levels in that user area are predetermined, based on a usage rate and the frequency of the replenishment process. At periodic intervals (e.g., every 24 hours, twice a week, or weekly), supply personnel conduct a physical inventory of what is available and order and obtain supplies to return the onhand levels to the predetermined or par level.

Exchange Cart System

The exchange cart system has been the most popular of all systems implemented by hospitals in recent years. The system is basically the same as a par-level system in that there are predetermined levels and predetermined intervals for replenishing inventory to those levels. In the exchange cart system, however, the cart is used for storage and distribution. A duplicate of each cart in the user area is maintained in the storage

area so that at the predetermined time the full cart can be taken to the user area and exchanged for the depleted cart. The cycle repeats itself at the given intervals.

Overviews

A capsulized evaluation of these three options is shown in Table 6-1. It should be obvious that there are advantages in each system and that it is up to a hospital to place a value on the factors involved.

However, the system that requires the fewest steps is the exchange cart system, and it is the least labor intensive.

3. Inventory Control

Functions*

The primary functions of an inventory are twofold: (1) to provide maximum supply service consistent with maximum efficiency and optimum inventory investment; and (2) to provide a cushion between the forecasted and actual demand for a materiel. The goal of any inventory investment should be to support the attainment

---

*Source: Edward D. Sanderson, *Hospital Purchasing and Inventory Management,* Aspen Systems Corporation, 1982.

Table 6-1   Comparisons of Supply Distribution Systems

Distribution System	Total Hospital Inventory Reduction Potential	Labor Utilization	Capital Expense	Space Utilization	Management Control
Par level	High (as high as 50% over requisition system)	Fair	Low	Good	Very good
Exchange cart	High (as high as 50% over requisition system)	Excellent	High	Good	Excellent
Requisition	Low	Poor	Low	Poor	Poor

Source: Jamie C. Kowalski, "Supply Distribution Options—A New Perspective," *Hospital Materiel Management Quarterly,* November 1980.

of the hospital's primary objective (patient care) with the optimum investment in inventory. Optimum inventory investment should not be confused with minimum inventory investment. Optimum investment may or may not be a minimum investment, depending upon various factors. These include the number of patients, patient mix (medical versus surgical), type of services provided, and location in relation to suppliers. Inventory investments are especially important to hospitals since operating funds are usually limited.

The second function, to serve as a cushion between forecasted and actual demand, is largely created by the inability to forecast accurately. This inability to forecast is also created by the same factors mentioned previously (number of patients, patient mix, etc.). All businesses and hospitals have difficulty managing their inventories. Yet no business can operate without one. Inventories protect against unforeseen failures in supply, increased demand, or unanticipated delays in delivery. Thus, inventory is not a luxury, but a necessity to achieve the objective of patient care.

Criteria for Inventory Control*

Many inventory practitioners believe that certain basic criteria must be established in order to determine whether an item will or will not be maintained in the inventory. Table 6-2 illustrates some of the criteria used by inventory managers across the country. These criteria reflect an effort to simplify the decision-making process. There are, however, two other criteria that are more meaningful to this process. They are that (1) there must be available space, and (2) it must be more economical to maintain an item in inventory than to purchase it on demand.

Questions to Be Asked

Inventory practitioners must maintain objectivity in this decision-making process. The following are questions that need to be asked concerning any item:

- What are the anticipated annual usage and associated costs?

Table 6-2 Criteria for Inventory Control

1. Time and extent of probable use
2. Storage costs
3. Obsolescence
4. Shrinkage
5. Transportation costs
6. Investment costs
7. Cost to purchase
8. Quantity price differential
9. Market conditions and price trends
10. Time required for delivery
11. Availability of a substitute
12. Cash flow
13. Alternative investment potential

Source: Edward D. Sanderson, *Hospital Purchasing and Inventory Management,* Aspen Systems Corporation, 1982.

- What is the intended use of the item?
- Is the item applicable for use by more than one department?
- What are the consequences of not having the item available (both real and perceived)?
- What are the economic consequences of allowing the individual department to control the inventory of this item (both real and perceived)?

And more generally:*

- How much space is being occupied by inventory?
- Are materials organized?
- Is security of the storage area adequate?
- Is stock being properly rotated?
- How much of the inventory is obsolete?
- What items are overstocked?
- Are identical items stored in more than one location?
- How are items removed for consumption?
- How are items reordered?
- Are item locations labeled?
- What opportunities exist for improved standardization?

---

*Source: Edward D. Sanderson, *Hospital Purchasing and Inventory Management,* Aspen Systems Corporation, 1982.

---

*Source: Jerry W. Rayburn, "The Art and Science of Inventory Reduction," *Hospital Materiel Management Quarterly,* February 1980.

How to Conduct a Physical Inventory*

Why take a physical inventory? The first important reason to take a physical inventory is to measure how much of each item is actually in stock and compare that to how much the accounting department ledger says is on hand. The physical inventory process allows actual cost adjustments to be made on all the supplies purchased throughout the year. It is also a means of evaluating the efficiency of materiel handling and inventory control for the organization. Other factors related to inventory control are appropriate security for materials that are susceptible to shrinkage, stock rotation, lot control, and environmental conditions affecting shelf life.

Guidelines

The inventory control manager should be encouraged to:

1. Review last year's notes and critique on the physical inventory; assign responsibilities.
2. Set a date to plan the inventory and schedule a coordination meeting 60 days in advance with the internal auditors and computer services: (a) Assign duties to specific individuals in the department for all area clean-up one day before inventory; (b) Conduct a walk-through tour of the area to be inventoried with supervisors to ensure readiness. A tour should be accomplished the day before the inventory.
3. Prepare a schedule of deadlines to be met and communicate these deadlines (closing/cutoff date of inventory) to all using departments within the hospital. Explain how emergency supply requests are to be processed during this period. This schedule shall include cutoffs for receiving as well as for inventory posting.
4. Prepare a written booklet of instructions to be followed for taking the physical inventory. An inventory captain is to be assigned to specific areas. Each inventory captain is to receive these instructions 30 days before the inventory.
5. Training sessions for all count team members shall be conducted at least one week before the physical inventory.
6. All stock items are to be identified with a stock number in the automated or manual inventory system.
7. Clearly mark the stock number in a bright color.
8. Have signs posted on those items not for inventory, reading "DO NOT INVENTORY."
9. Neatly arrange items to facilitate accurate and timely counting.
10. Put material in clean containers prior to the start of the inventory.
11. Identify all items to be inventoried two weeks before inventory.
12. Have location signs posted to eliminate confusion to the count teams.
13. Classify the inventory in separate line stock items, stock keeping units (SKU) per shelf space, bin, or row. Segregate areas within the inventory by drawing chalk marks on the floor to identify the boundaries between adjacent areas.
14. Ensure that all items to be inventoried are on the Inventory Master File so a count card can be printed. (Deadline for entering new items onto the Master File is two weeks prior to inventory.) This is the responsibility of the Storeroom, Inventory Control, and Central Supply Supervisor.
15. Use a pre-printed inventory tag (Count Card) with the stock number written on the tag to be used by the count teams. Use a special tag such as a bright color which is readily noticed to identify "unidentified parts."
16. Request count cards—Two weeks before inventory, submit to Computer Services Operations a separate "Preparation Request Form" #1 for the following items to be prepared at least eight days before inventory:
    a. Central stores cards;
    b. Blank cards—1000; or have signs printed that read "Blank card no. ____ ; ____ items removed after inventory count."
    c. Alpha listing—central stores—eight copies; and

*Source: W. Daniel Cobbs, "How to Conduct a Physical Inventory," *Hospital Materiel Management Quarterly,* May 1981.

d. Numerical listing—central stores—copies.

Causes of Inventory Imbalance*

Factors that can cause inventory imbalance include:

1. failure to review and revise, as necessary, inventory policies on a regular basis;
2. failure to participate in a program of long-range planning and policy determination;
3. failure of the system to react to rapid changes in usage or to accurately forecast future needs and requirements;
4. failure to develop adequate sources of supply, breakdowns in transportation, etc.;
5. failure to gain the cooperation and assistance of using departments and to properly determine their needs and direction of operation;
6. lack of standardization;
7. failure to base buying on actual needs or scientific facts;
8. failure to obtain and train appropriate personnel; and
9. inability to comprehend and to utilize the mathematical and scientific tools of inventory control such as reorder points, economic order quantity (EOQ), etc.

Reducing Inventory*

There is a constant challenge to reduce inventories to a minimum level—not only to maintain the operating efficiency of the institution but also to anticipate delivery problems, maintain maximum discounts for merchandise, anticipate seasonal problems, account for vendor delays, etc. The importance of the total size of the inventories cannot be overstated in terms of its influence on the institution's cash flow, operating expenses and overall fiscal stability. Many industrial companies have failed because of excess inventories. It is important to remember that these inventories represent not only dollar restrictions in cash flow; they also require additional capital for storage, utilities, insurance and the myriad of associated overhead expenses.

Improving the Turnover Rate*

Inventory turnover is the quantitative measurement of the number of times that total inventory dollars are issued and replaced. The turnover rate is calculated by dividing the total annual dollars for supplies issued by the dollar value of the ending inventory. For example, if the dollar value of annual issues is $760,000 and the ending inventory dollar value is $88,500, then the turnover rate is equal to:

$$\frac{\$760,000}{\$\ 88,500} = 8.58$$

The question most often asked by practitioners is: What constitutes a good inventory turnover rate? Many experts feel that an acceptable minimum turnover rate for any inventory is 12 times per year. However, many practitioners in the field believe eight to ten turns per year to be realistic. Conversely, a turnover rate of six or less is inadequate and requires some type of additional analysis and corrective action. Practitioners should also recognize that the hospital's proximity to suppliers and the bed density of the area will influence the turnover rate.

To get a faster turnover rate the inventory manager should be encouraged first, to clean out surplus and reduce slow-moving items, second, to concentrate on increasing the turnover on A items, and third, to reduce the amount of safety stock and the lead time required to order and receive replacement stocks. Practitioners should be aware that reduction in safety stock will increase the probability of a stock-out. If this method is chosen, it should be used selectively.

Management Audit of Equipment and Supply Inventories**

Hospitals have sizable investments in supply inventories and equipment. To be certain they invest no more resources than necessary and yet avoid operating problems requires records that are accurate and planned carefully. The systems and procedures used must be reviewed to ensure

---

*Source: Bruce G. Haywood, "Understanding Economic Order Quantity," *Hospital Materiel Management Quarterly,* May 1980.

---

*Source: Edward D. Sanderson, *Hospital Purchasing and Inventory Management,* Aspen Systems Corporation, 1982.

**Source: Seth Allcorn, *Internal Auditing for Hospitals,* Aspen Systems Corporation, 1979.

maximum control at minimum expense. Thorough internal audits of hospital inventories and inventory procedures can yield substantial savings and reduced risks. Inventory procedures and internal audit checkpoints are available from many sources, and several should be consulted before completing an audit program.

1. Does the hospital have a central receiving area that checks in all supplies and equipment? Is central receiving independent of purchasing, accounting, and ordering departments? Are copies of receiving slips placed in the hands of the person approving disbursements? What control exists over free samples of drugs and supplies? How are narcotics controlled and does the control meet federal standards?

2. Are perpetual inventory records maintained on all major classes of supplies by personnel other than the storeroom's? Are electronic data processing applications appropriate?

3. Have inventory reorder points been established for all supplies? Are the reorder amounts reasonable? Do they take advantage of quantity discounts? How often do stock outages occur?

4. What controls exist over the total number and types of supplies stocked? Is there an unwarranted proliferation of items? Is there stock on hand that no longer is used?

5. What are the procedures for distributing supplies? What documents are used? Do the procedures require proper authorizations? Is adequate information provided to permit the storeroom to bill the right patient or department? What is the procedure for pricing?

6. With what frequency are physical inventories taken? What are the procedures for taking the inventory? Who supervises the inventory counting process? Are spot checks made of the accuracy of counts by disinterested employees or internal auditors? Who may authorize a change in perpetual inventory records? How are shortages and overages reported and to whom?

7. How are supplies stored? Is there enough space that is properly climate controlled and free from spoilage by water or pests? Is the area clean? Are supplies stored in an orderly manner? What condition are the supplies in? Are supplies with limited shelf lives rotated carefully to ensure that none expire before use? How are supplies secured from theft and fire?

8. Is there adequate documentation on purchases of equipment? Are warranties, maintenance agreements, and leases controlled adequately?

9. How is the equipment controlled? Are inventory numbers assigned individual pieces of equipment and affixed securely? How often is equipment inventoried? What procedures are followed and who supervises the process?

10. What are the hospital's policies on equipment depreciation? Is depreciation properly claimed on equipment?

Effective internal control of supply and equipment inventories can yield many benefits for hospitals. Internal auditors must be certain the institutions control and manage their inventories properly.

4. Controlling Theft*

Centralization

Many institutions have unsuccessfully attempted to centralize most purchasing functions. They thought that merely requiring the countersignature of the purchasing agent on purchase orders would prevent or minimize the number of overpriced purchases, inflated invoices or fraudulent payments. In reality, mere centralization usually creates horrendous communications bottlenecks without necessarily improving the quality or integrity of the purchasing process.

Even for those materials that are theoretically purchased centrally by the purchasing department, the purchasing agent usually exercises little authority. Departments such as central sterile supply and x-ray, the numerous laboratories and research facilities may stipulate a specific manufacturer or supplier, along with the price, of a product when submitting their requisitions, leaving the purchasing agent little room for obtaining competitive bids. The backlog of orders

---

*Source: Walter Nagel, "Health Care's Vulnerability to Theft," *Topics in Health Care Financing,* Winter 1978.

to be processed usually means the agent will gratefully accept all the preparatory work done by the requisitioning departments. Thus, even though the purchase order is eventually signed by the purchasing agent, the requisitioning departments are virtually autonomous, no less so than officially autonomous departments such as dietary, maintenance or pharmacy.

Under such purchasing arrangements, the person negotiating with a vendor or placing an order for the payment of a commission or kickback in one form or another has few obstacles. It is immaterial whether payment is made in cash, in the form of a percentage of the purchase price or in kind by the delivery of favors or certain commodities. Invariably such a payment is financed by inflating the invoice—by increasing the price of the invoice, by overbilling on the quantity or, in the case of food products, for example, by skimping on the quality.

Purchasing general storage items, which are purchased on a minimum/maximum inventory control basis, usually involves the purchasing department. These items are often contracted on a yearly basis, and both the purchasing agent and the specific using department jointly negotiate the order. The order may be subject to the countersignature of an administration official who actively compares prices, preventing the purchasing agent or the department staff from arranging a kickback from the supplier and having it financed by inflating the invoice.

Purchases Most Vulnerable to Theft

The purchases most vulnerable to theft are those ordered autonomously by a staff member of a department. These orders may be placed formally in writing or informally over the telephone. Shipments received by the department that placed the order are also very vulnerable to theft. Again these situations prevail in the dietary, maintenance and pharmacy departments.

Under such an arrangement no fictitious price inflation is necessary. The department that places the order receives the shipment and confirms the accuracy of the quantities received. Overstating the quantity is all that is needed. In some instances the same person who places the order receives the shipment, making out whatever receiving document is acceptable to propel the vendor's invoice into the payment process. It is immaterial whether this receiving document

is a copy of a purchase order, an individual receiving slip, a form developed by the hospital itself or simply the packing list issued by the vendor and accompanying the shipment, signed or initialed and dated by the person who placed the order.

Informal purchasing and receiving methods involving only one person are not infrequent. Under these circumstances, it is hard to resist making an arrangement for a vendor kickback or commission payment at the expense of the institution. But even if some lower ranking employee, such as a dietary stockroom attendant, a tool crib attendant or a clerk in the pharmacy, is responsible for receiving orders, it is often easy for higher ranking employees to convince the receivers to make only a casual check of incoming shipments and to see that discrepancies are ignored so that the inflated invoice can be easily processed for payment.

Prevention

This type of manipulative theft involving no physical movement of stolen merchandise is less easy to perpetrate when storeroom items are automatically replenished. Where there is an established minimum/maximum or reorder point method, unexplainable shortages or startling out-of-stock conditions sooner or later will bring such manipulations to someone's attention. Such evidence is never conclusive. The shortages can be the result of miscounts, unrecorded requisitions, undocumented withdrawals, pilferage from the shelves, misplaced stock or faulty min/max calculations. Nevertheless there is at least an indicator that something is wrong if specific items repeatedly show up short on the shelves. Also for specific individual purchases originating in individual departments through itemized requisitions, the opportunities for collusive arrangements between requisitioner and vendor or between purchasing agent and vendor are less tempting and certainly less lucrative.

For these purchases, inflating the price is usually the only feasible method of financing a kickback. Manipulating the quantities by overstating the packing slip and the invoice for isolated shipments going into a specific department is more difficult to achieve. Therefore, by and large, the danger of dishonest manipulations in connection with individual purchases made by or for the various laboratories, x-ray department, operating room, intensive care units or central surgical supply is less significant than for repetitive quantity purchases.

Theft in Receiving and Invoice Payment

Although the receiving process deserves the most attention, it is too often given the lowest priority when protecting the hospital's assets. Many institutions invest enormous amounts of dollars, energy and payroll hours in protecting their employees and clients. But the receiving operation is being given the scantiest attention.

Document control and document matchup are tedious and uninspiring tasks. People responsible for these tasks may have a tendency of skimming through them, with the result that the documentation is not checked thoroughly, and the opportunity for dishonesty is increased. Furthermore, overworked, incompetent or disgruntled receivers may easily be the victims of dishonest drivers. Some drivers simply do not deliver to the hospital all the goods that were ordered. If the receivers fail to notice the shortage, the drivers keep the rest of the shipment, selling it to another buyer for their own profit. If the receivers detect the shortage, the drivers may offer them a bribe or an actual share in the proceeds from the resale. Since drivers often dispose of part of their shipments before they even arrive at the hospital, they are rarely caught in possession of stolen goods, making this form of theft infinitely less risky than the actual removal of stolen materials from the institution.

Collusive theft arranged between receiver and driver is particularly tempting with repetitive deliveries of easily marketable items. In health care institutions these items include food products (particularly meats and expensive canned goods), linen, bulk paper products and widely used chemicals.

Cause

Dishonesty in the receiving process is caused by a combination of factors: weak accountability, low reliability, inadequate personnel and facilities and lack of documentation.

● Weak Accountability

In many institutions the receiving process is so decentralized—more so than the purchasing process—that supervision and accountability of the individual receiving areas are impossible. Receivers report to the storekeeper or in fact are members of the general stores staff. Sometimes they report directly or indirectly to the purchasing agent. This may be a grievous mistake; many receivers are unskilled and are among the lowest paid employees in the hospital. They may be more likely to yield to the temptation of stealing to supplement their incomes. Yet often the receiver's signature is actually the equivalent of a signature on a bank check; sometimes reduced to a mere scribbled initial, it authorizes payment of an invoice that may total as much as $3,000.

Receivers are easily tempted to sign the receipt of a shipment without accurate accountability. This problem is serious enough in the case of a neutral independent receiving department; it is infinitely worse when the same department that autonomously places a purchase order receives the shipment.

● Low Reliability

The level of reliability is also usually low in most institutions. This low reliability level is exemplified by the structural problems encountered in the receiving process. Only in recent years during major expansion projects have major hospitals provided adequate receiving dock facilities with supporting office space and staging areas. In the majority of institutions, space for receiving is inadequate, with single docks often serving institutions with several hundred beds. In many cases a simple alley with no proper unloading facilities serves for receiving of most materials. Inadequate facilities interfere with reliable operation and increase the chance for theft.

A Solution

The principle of dual receiving accountability as a prerequisite for invoice payment is the most powerful device for protecting against buyer/vendor collusion and driver/receiver collusion.

● Method

The accounts payable department should be required to receive two separate pieces of documentary evidence proving that the shipment has arrived as stipulated by the purchase order, the packing slip and the invoice. The first evidence of receipt should be generated by the receiver on the dock who actually assists in or witnesses the unloading of the shipment. The second evidence should be provided by the final recipient. This can be in general stores, central supply, the dietary stockroom, the pharmacy or any one of the laboratories and various other supporting departments receiving individual shipments.

The tools for implementing dual accountability can vary in many ways. There can be two different receiving copies of the purchase orders. Requisitions can have specific copies to serve as receiving documents. Separate receiving documents can be developed, for example, with the original being filled in and signed by the dock receiver while the duplicate accompanies the shipment to its destination. The duplicate is filled in and dispatched to accounts payable, where a matching process takes place.

● Implementation

Many complexities can make the implementation of dual accountability quite difficult. Within a large institution the identical system and paperwork flow will not be practical for all divisions. Variations will have to be devised and exceptions will have to be authorized. The problems may be similar, but the solutions are never the same.

However, by establishing a solidly enforced dual receiving operation, successfully implemented by an alert accounts payable matching process, the institution will curtail two of the major avenues of fraud and theft draining the funds of the institution.

Theft in General Stores

The most serious flaw in a majority of general stores operations is the fact that their staff doubles as receivers on the dock. In fact, in many hospitals the general stockroom is located adjacent to or immediately beneath the receiving dock so that receivers, upon unloading a shipment, can transfer the cartons easily into the general storeroom. Because storeroom personnel alternate working as receivers, frequently the same person who functions as the dock receiver also eventually places the shipment on the storage shelves. This situation offers the most powerful incentive for a receiver to go into collusion with a driver to steal goods.

Hospitals should separate receiving from both general storage and purchasing.

Requisitioning Systems

Most departments order their supplies from general stores through the use of "laundry lists" by product classification. In smaller hospitals, the same person who receives, signs and stocks the merchandise also serves as the dispensing agent distributing the same items to departments and nursing stations. Realizing that most areas, especially nursing stations, never count the items in the supply cart, dispensers can cover by devious short order filling methods any shortage resulting from collusion with drivers in the receiving process.

Supervisors of general stores departments are usually so busy handling special telephone requests or emergency run-outs that they are unable to perform even a ten-percent random spot check of departmental delivery carts. To compound the problem, in certain hospitals computer chargeouts to departments are grouped as a total dollar figure at the end of the accounting month. No department manager can associate a dollar figure with the material received in the department. Also, if a delivery copy is not left with the recipient department, even though charges may be broken down by category, it becomes an exercise in frustration to try to associate every item delivered a month previous to the computer printout.

Par Stock and Cart Replacement Systems

Many hospitals have been experimenting with two methods of general stores distribution—par stock and cart replacement. However, these systems may be causing the proliferation of dishonest actions by general stores personnel. Par stock and cart replacement are both under the control of the person delivering the merchandise, who refills to the par level and itemizes the amount of merchandise stocked. For cart replacement, the filled cart is left and the partially used cart taken away. Thus deliverers have the perfect opportunity to manipulate stock replenishment figures to their own benefit.

Another problem at nursing stations is that nurses sometimes fear running out of critical items. When ordering or having merchandise delivered, they may take supplies and hoard them in a supply area.

Although the dollar value of these items may be insignificant, disposable needles and syringes offer the greatest marketability, and any large quantities of these items should be kept in central locked areas. If central storage space is not available for other items, heavy wire mesh cages might suffice until permanent storage space is allocated.

Before installing a par stock or cart replacement system, administration should clearly define the logistics of such a move. Items selected for either of these systems should fall into the category of disposable stock items or certain sterile kits, or nonchargeables to patients. Take-home types of supplies should be limited. Where possible, random checking of replacements or stock remaining in returned carts should be initiated by nursing administration or storeroom supervision. Also, to prevent hoarding of supplies, nursing and storeroom supervisors should make inspection tours at least once a month and assure that overages are returned to stock.

5. Reports to Management*

Because materiels management interfaces with every department within the hospital, an effective reporting relationship between the materiel manager and the administrator is essential for the institution's effective and efficient operation. As a result, a number of management reports typically emanate from the materiel manager to the administrator.

Financial/Budgetary Reports

The timing of the materiel management reports discussed next is summarized in Table 6-3.

Statement of Revenues and Expenses (Monthly)

The statement of revenues and expenses is typically a written recap of all of the expenses incurred by materiel management and associated revenues that have been generated. It is frequently desirable to have separate reports generated for each component of the department; that is, one for processing, one for distribution, and so forth.

---

*Source: R. Edward Howell, "Administrative Reporting—The Necessary Elements," *Hospital Materiel Management Quarterly,* August 1979.

Table 6-3   Timing of Materiel Management Reports

Monthly Reports
Statement of Revenue and Expenses
Manpower Activity
Lost Charges
Supply Cost Escalation
Supply Usage
Product Standardization
Processing Activity

Quarterly Reports
Linen Inventory and Usage
Pharmaceutical Services
Copy Center Report
Invoice Reconciling
Production Evaluation
Stock-Outs

Semiannual Reports
Contracts Due
Physical Inventory
User Satisfaction

Annual Report
Stock Turns

Source: Compiled from R. Edward Howell, "Administrative Reporting—The Necessary Elements," *Hospital Materiel Management Quarterly,* August 1979.

The statement of revenues and expenses is used by the administrator to obtain a perspective of the financial viability of the department and the hospital. Frequently, this report also includes a year-to-date trends report, which is compared to an annualized budget allocation. This portion of the report is used by administration to determine how well the materiel manager is managing his or her resources and staying within the budgets.

Manpower Activity Report (Monthly)

The manpower activity report is a written recap of the hours worked by employees within the department.

Frequently, the total dollar amount paid for wages and salaries within each employee class is also given. This is used to assess the materiel manager's ability to effectively and efficiently staff the department and to control personnel costs.

Lost Charges Report (Monthly)

The lost charges report is used by those hospitals not using an all-inclusive rate structure. It is usually a written monthly synopsis of the total number of charges lost within each dispensing area, primarily nursing stations and outpatient dispensing. The total number of lost charges is then compared to the total number of items dispensed in an area to determine the magnitude of the inefficiency. The administrator typically uses this report to determine the extent of lost revenues and to pinpoint troublesome areas.

Supply Cost Escalation Report (Monthly)

The supply cost escalation report typically compares the cost of certain high-use items with the cost of those same items in the previous month or reporting period. For those hospitals that have fixed contract prices, this comparison is from contract period to contract period. The cost increase is then expanded by the usage of that item for the reporting period to determine the total increased cost to the hospital for the item. In a time of increasing cost-containment pressure, it is critical that the administrator be able to document the reasons behind the increased costs of health care.

Physical Inventory Report (Semiannually)

The physical inventory report should reflect both the official and unofficial inventories within the hospital. These inventories should be shared with the finance office. It is also desirable to compare this report to previous reports to assess any progress toward predetermined objectives and to monitor any trends occurring within the inventory.

Activity Assessment (Productivity) Reports

Supply Usage Report (Monthly)

The supply usage report provides a written delineation of the supplies used by each department and by the nursing stations. The format of this report is typically arranged so that the user department is identified (usually by name and account number) and the corresponding monthly usage is indicated, both in terms of stock-keeping units (SKUs) and dollar volume. In addition, the supply usage report usually provides the administrator with a total of the supplies within the hospital. The report allows the administrator to identify high-volume users and reduces the potential for indiscriminate cross-charging. The report is also frequently shared with the other department heads within the hospital.

Product Standardization Report (Monthly)

Frequently linked to the product evaluation report, the product standardization report provides the administrator with an assessment of the materiel manager's efforts to condense any duplicative generic items found in stock. This report is usually provided in a narrative form, describing those generic items being consolidated and the projected dollar savings from the consolidation.

Processing Activity Report (Monthly)

The processing activity report provides the administrator with an analysis of the activity occurring within the processing area and is generally viewed as a productivity report. To develop this analysis, the following factors are considered: the category of items being processed, the number of units processed within each category, the predetermined time required to process each piece, the total hours required to process the volume encountered, the hours actually worked and the percentage of staff utilized. This provides the administrator with considerable insight into the appropriateness of staffing within the area and the productivity of its employees.

Linen Inventory and Usage Report (Quarterly)

The linen inventory and usage report indicates the number of pounds of linen used by each area in the hospital, both in terms of pounds and dollar volume, and the total amount of new linen in the inventory that can be placed in circulation when needed. The report provides the administrator with an analysis of linen usage, so he or she may pursue the appropriateness of that usage and a method of monitoring linen inventory levels.

Pharmaceutical Services Report (Quarterly)

This report contains such information as inpatient prescriptions processed, outpatient prescriptions processed, I.V. admixtures filled, the number of hyperalimentations prepared, formulary additions and deletions, the number of pharmacist/physician consults, revenues generated and any other information the pharmacist deems appropriate.

Copy Center Report (Quarterly)

The copy center report provides the administrator with an analysis of the printing and photocopy activity within the hospital. A listing of the copying activity is developed, delineating the user area and volume for each service rendered (photocopy, duplication and so forth). It also usually provides the trends in terms of the total copy center activity. The report provides information about an activity that is easily controlled but frequently abused.

Invoice Reconciling Report (Quarterly)

The simple invoice reconciling report has resulted in the savings of thousands of dollars. It is simply a listing of errors found when invoices were reconciled against vendor billings. The generation of this report forces the reconciling activity to occur and provides an assessment of the billing credibility of your vendors.

Product Evaluation Report (Quarterly)

The product evaluation report provides the administrator with a written description of all supplies and equipment being evaluated in the hospital for possible use. The report should contain the trade name of the items being tested and the name of the supplying vendor, as well as a brief descriptive evaluation of each item and the determination as to whether or not it will be used in the hospital.

Stock-Outs Report (Quarterly)

The stock-outs report is designed to provide the administrator with an assessment of the efficiency of the supply service. The number of stock-outs encountered for each user is indicated, as well as the percentage of stock-outs. The percentage is the relationship of stock-outs to total items issued (stock-out/total items issued) and is perhaps the most insightful indicator of the responsiveness of the supply service. This report is frequently shared with the user department heads.

Contracts Due Report (Semiannually)

The contracts due report is simply a listing of the contracts due to be renegotiated within the next six months and a list of those negotiated within the last six months. This listing should include the generic category of items, the current contract number, the present vendor and the present price paid. The report makes the administrator aware of any potentially sensitive contracts that may be upcoming and provides additional information about the prices paid for these items.

User Satisfaction Report (Semiannually)

The user satisfaction report is simply a narrative report of those activities within the materiel management function and is aimed at determining how satisfied the users are with the services provided and the efforts initiated to correct those concerns that have surfaced. The method of determining user satisfaction will depend upon the needs of the institution and may take the form of surveys, questionnaires, meetings, etc. The user satisfaction report will provide the administrator with some insights into the quality of service being provided.

Stock-Turns Report (Annually)

The annual stock-turns report provides a description of the number of times each stock-keeping unit within the storehouse is issued during the calendar year. The stock-keeping units are grouped into generic categories to facilitate analysis. The stock-turns report provides the materiel manager with the information needed to make decisions as to which items should be deleted from the storehouse inventory. It also provides the administrator with some insight into the activity occurring within the storehouse.

VENDORS

What Hospitals Should Receive from Suppliers*

Beyond competitive pricing, hospitals should demand of their suppliers reliability, service to keep hospital costs low, and assistance in accomplishing the following goals:

1. competitive prices;
2. low ordering, storing, receiving and distributing costs;

*Source: William H. Henning, "Utilizing Suppliers to the Hospital's Best Interests," *Hospital Materiel Management Quarterly*, February 1980.

3. vendor deliveries as promised over 90 percent of the time;
4. ample vendor inventory not far away;
5. reliable inbound transportation;
6. vendor accuracy in products, deliveries and paperwork;
7. vendor systems that simplify the order entry and the paperwork system and offer periodic reports for hospital purchasing and inventory management;
8. personal assistance from vendors to set up and operate the system;
9. broad product lines from vendors permitting multilines purchase orders, receivings and invoices;
10. standardization on quality, cost-effective products;
11. complete, up-to-date product information;
12. minimum amount of handling problems, returns and credits;
13. adherence to codes and regulations;
14. up-to-date information on materiel management systems and procedures.

Evaluating Vendors*

1. Select One Supplier Category to Investigate

The most systems action is in the medical/surgical and laboratory areas, but you may want to start with your office suppliers or forms manufacturers.

2. Know Your Major Vendors

a. What is their track record? Manually or by computer periodically analyze major vendors' delivery performance to separate fact from claims and loose talk.

b. Without computer, your office must perform manual vendor performance ratings by tabulating for each vendor:

- the total number of purchase orders in one month;
- number complete in one shipment/percent complete;
- number completed by date needed;

- average number of items per purchase order;
- number of purchase orders completed within lead time plus safety factor (usually 7–14 days);
- a rating for the period and comparison of vendors in the same product lines;
- evaluation as to whether the vendor sales representative is valuable, efficient, organized, businesslike; whether he or she knows the products, the vendor's own system and materiel management in general; whether he or she is helpful in solving problems and returning goods; whether he or she works with hospitals to reduce handling costs and standardized products.

c. Visit each major vendor.

- Check its location in regard to the hospital.
- Meet the boss and customer service representative.
- How many lines or products are offered and held in stock?
- What is the total dollar value of this inventory?
- Can it reserve stock for your hospital under a systems contract?
- Is the warehouse orderly and clean?
- What is its trucking program?
- Does it have computer capabilities and up-to-date systems?
- Does it offer private-label products as well as national line products?
- Is is aware of the latest products, codes and regulations?

3. Investigate Each Vendor's System Capabilities

a. **Ordering.** For simple product lines, a simple telephone ordering service with standard product ordering numbers and standard forms is effective for small orders and few products. More and more vendors are now recommending that the hospital lease electronic transmission systems, some with card readers, to automatically and accurately transmit orders to vendors. A leading drug distributor is promoting a bar code system that permits the ordering of drugs by simply wanding the bar codes in hospital inventory.

b. **Computer System.** The ordering systems above are being eclipsed rapidly by computer input-output units in the hospital purchasing of-

*Source: William H. Henning, "Utilizing Suppliers to the Hospital's Best Interests," *Hospital Materiel Management Quarterly,* February 1980.

fice that access vendors' computers directly. This is a major breakthrough and the beginning of significant developments in the tying together of hospital and vendor systems. Now, hospitals can place orders directly with vendor computers and receive a printed reply in the form of their own purchase order that indicates which products in the original order were backordered. This not only simplifies ordering and handles the typing of the purchase order, but also indicates, particularly for outlying hospitals, which products will not be received immediately.

c. Reports. Vendors with computers usually provide purchasing and inventory management reports periodically that should be valuable, particularly to hospitals without their own computer capabilities. These reports show monthly usage, update reorder points (ROPs) and economic order points (EOQs) and enable the hospital purchasing agent to perform an ABC analysis of central inventory.

d. Transportation. The hospital should examine the vendor's routine schedules for delivery and the possibility of varying the schedule according to the hospital's needs.

e. Personal Assistance. Investigate the vendor's ability to provide personnel to help the hospital implement its new ordering system and possibly to reorganize its central storage area.

4. Define the System and Estimate Its Cost Impact on the Hospital

For the one or two vendors that look the best, describe the system on paper and try to estimate the differences in cost and performance between your present operation and using the new system. In this way specifications are developed for the negotiating sessions with the vendor. This is the process of prudent buying that evaluates the total cost effect of several alternatives.

This process will lead to the selection of the best one or two systems and the development of specific performance goals for vendor and hospital.

5. Purchasing Methods

The purchasing agent may decide after investigation that it is not necessary for him or her to enter into a large systems contract. Possibly a blanket order will do just as well. He or she may decide to bid some items and contract for others according to which items are most price sensitive and which items benefit most from being handled in a low-cost hospital/vendor system.

It is at this time the purchasing agent should request formal proposals from vendors. Each proposal should be studied carefully and its effect on hospital operational costs examined. If these proposals are vague on service levels and other measures of performance, it is probably because the purchasing agent did not require a specific response. It is important that vendors spell out specifically what they plan to do in the area of service.

6. Monitor Vendor Performance

It is hoped the purchasing agent will have initiated a format for vendor analysis in the initial phases of the search for a vendor system partner. It is then a matter of continuing to measure vendor performance to ensure that the service conditions that everyone agreed to are continued. The beginning of a vendor/hospital system relationship is probably like a new marriage. There will be bad times and happy times, but the important thing is to stick together and work out problems together.

7. Every Year or Two, Repeat the Process

Changes in cost, vendor performance and computer systems occur continually. Prudent buying requires that the purchasing agent look over the field from time to time, and in a cost-conscious way, take a fresh look at each hospital/vendor relationship.

Guidelines for Purchasing Equipment*

The following principles are suggested for planning the purchase of equipment. While they particularly apply to technical equipment, they relate in part to all equipment.

1. Equipment follows function, but the function today may not be the function tomorrow. Needs may drastically change, may increase or may disappear. Consider whether the equipment can then be added to, modified, or easily replaced.

---

*Source: D.G. Sloth, "Selecting Equipment Flexible Enough to Adapt to Changed Needs, Growth," *Hospital Topics*, February 1973.

2. Differentiate between the gadget and the uniquely functional new product. Both are expensive.

3. Most important, look for equipment that is "failsafe"—built so that it will cease to function before it malfunctions dangerously.

4. Try to determine life-cycle cost. This is difficult to ascertain precisely, but the following factors should be considered:

   - Original cost.
   - Operational cost.
   - Maintenance cost and "down-time" potential.
   - Modernization potential. Can the equipment be modified with accessories or new components to increase or improve its function, or has obsolescence been designed into construction?
   - Durability. Can it stand up to the operation (and misoperation) by both skilled and sometimes unskilled personnel? Will temperature, impact, abrasion shorten its natural life?

5. Consider efficiency-effectiveness, the ability of a product to satisfy the need for which it was created. It must be able to accomplish its function easily and quickly. Longevity is not necessarily all-important if the equipment is designed to last the life of its efficiency-effectiveness. If it does not last that long, it was a poor purchase.

6. Find out about availability of parts and service. Equipment that is mechanical or automatic in its operation will eventually require more parts and maintenance. Whether the equipment is an electric bed or an ultrasonic cleaner, the unavailability of parts and service can have serious consequences. Equipment that can be maintained by in-plant personnel is probably not too complicated and well designed. It is ironic that the most simple machine, in terms of performance and operation, is often the most difficult to design and manufacture.

7. If unit or volume investment is large enough, the product should be evaluated before purchase. At the very least, visit another installation. Talk not only to the prime user but also to those responsible for housekeeping and maintenance.

8. Major movable equipment is generally preferred over fixed, long-term equipment. At one time, long life and quality were synonymous, but today the ability to function well may outweigh long life. The owner who can replace worn or damaged components may be better off. More manufacturers can be expected to make this type of equipment. It will be less expensive for the purchaser and will mean more sales over the long run. When equipment becomes obsolete, it can be embarrassing to both purchaser and manufacturer.

9. For certain functions, consider the "systems approach." While a system must be justified economically, in the long run it may be the best way to handle such problems as materials movement, waste retrieval, and convenience foods. The evaluation is much more difficult and often requires collective decisions. The manufacturer has a greater responsibility in planning, simulation, design and postsale contributions. Many state they are qualified; too few are.

10. Can the equipment be cleaned easily? For example, if patients' bedroom furniture is designed to suggest a "home-away-from-home" appearance, such things as sculptured legs and brass pulls may discourage good housekeeping.

11. Does the equipment violate plumbing or electrical codes? If it does, it can create dangerous problems for personnel and patients. Reputable manufacturers build to national and local codes. Others who do not can sometimes offer their equipment at a lesser cost.

12. Does the manufacturer include in the price of the equipment the cost of installation and training the personnel when indicated?

13. Disposables are popular these days. Equipment can be eliminated with their use; however, as process costs decrease, distribution costs increase. For example, the use of disposable linens and packs in the operating room may eliminate one or more sterilizers, but it will require more carts and storage space, and will add to waste-retrieval costs.

14. Medical technology creates more technology, but the development or the availability of the equipment always lags behind technology. It follows that the space to house the equipment, the personnel and the patient that can use the new technology also lags behind. As equipment is developed it is almost always more expensive than what it has replaced.

15. Technical equipment often suffers rapid obsolescence. A piece of equipment may be usable for 20 years, but it also may become obsolete in as little as five years. In some instances, equipment has been obsolete when the hospital opened its doors.

16. Under the worst conditions, equipment should be capable of being replaced with a minimum of disruption; at best, equipment should be designed so that it can be modernized.

NOTE: See Table 6-4 for a form to be completed by vendors before contracting for the purchase of capital equipment.

A Prime Vendor (Supplier) Contract*

A prime vendor relationship comes into being when a hospital enters into an agreement (contract) to purchase the majority of a given class of supplies from one vendor. This contract usually covers a definite period of time and specifies what items are to be purchased. Very few vendors can supply all the items a hospital needs and the prime vendor contract does not affect purchases from other suppliers. For the hospital, the use of a prime vendor can reduce costs, improve service, and allow better use of expensive and limited resources.

One major area in which the hospital can save thousands of dollars is inventory control. The prime vendor can warehouse the supplies and release them as needed for the hospital's use. This keeps in-house inventory low and provides hospital units with supplies as they need them. Buying from one source also takes less total time for materiel management. There are fewer sales representatives to be seen. Performance

*Source: William Pitts, "How to Negotiate a Prime Vendor Contract," *Hospital Materiel Management Quarterly*, May 1981.

specifications in the contract can save money and time by reducing the number of back orders. In addition, with a reduced number of vendors, the receiving process is more efficient. Fewer but larger deliveries come in, and a schedule controls the number of deliveries per day and allocates the work load evenly.

Selection Process

The hospital requests vendors' bids for an estimated committed volume of supplies for a specific time frame (usually one or two years). Lower prices are offered because of the definite commitment of large dollar volumes. The lowest and best bidder who can meet all other prerequisites (inventory, delivery, and service) is awarded the business.

Bids are invited from vendors who can provide a full line of needed products. To facilitate comparison, the hospital may prepare a spread sheet that lists equivalent products from different bidders, annual quantity needed, item prices, and estimated total dollar volume that would be spent on the product.

Before an agreement is made, it is important that hospital representatives visit the physical plant of potential prime vendors. Things to look for are warehouse capacity, cleanliness, organization, and environmental factors (temperature, humidity, insect and rodent control programs). Also, are the personnel hospital-oriented? How many are there? Are products on a computer inventory system? What order-taking processes are used? Is there a good customer service program? What transportation system is used? Do they own their own fleet of trucks or do they use a commercial carrier? How often will they ship merchandise and what emergency contingencies will they respond to? The names of other hospitals serviced by each firm should be acquired and they should be contacted for reference.

After all the bids are in, a final comparison is made to assure that the products listed on the spread sheet are really comparable. Then the lowest bidder who can provide all required services is selected.

Preparing for Prime Vendor Proposals

The prime supplier contract should be built around a three-part proposal sent to suppliers. This consists of a statement of the hospital's terms, a list of major categories for prime sup-

Table 6-4 Capital Equipment: Vendor's Checklist

Note: This form will be referenced in any purchase order issued under this request for proposal. Answer all applicable questions to the best of your ability.

I. *PRICE: MARKET CONDITIONS*

    A. Your price will remain firm for: ——————— days.

    B. What is List Price? ———————

    C. When do you expect your next price increase to occur? ———————.

    D. What do you expect the increase to be? ——————— (Amount or Percent)

II. *WARRANTY-SERVICE*

    A. What is the warranty period on this equipment? ——————— months

    B. When does warranty period begin? ———————

    C. Who will service this equipment during the warranty period? ———————

    D. Do you have service contracts on this equipment? ( ) Yes   ( ) No

        1. Current annual cost? ———————

        2. What is the point of origin of service? ———————

        3. What is the anticipated response time to our facility? ———————

    E. Do you offer a training program for our repair technicians? ( ) Yes   ( ) No

    F. Does this equipment meet the current and applicable requirement or codes of the following:

        1. Occupational Safety & Health Act   ( ) Yes   ( ) No

        2. Underwriters' Laboratory   ( ) Yes   ( ) No

        3. National Fire Protection Association   ( ) Yes   ( ) No

    G. List special tool or equipment requirement to perform preventive and/or repair maintenance to this equipment: ———————

III. *INSTALLATION*

    A. Will installation be the responsibility of: ( ) Vendor   ( ) Medical Center? Is there an additional cost involved? ( ) Yes   ( ) No
If yes, state cost $———————.

    B. Upon receipt of equipment, will your personnel set up the equipment according to the manufacturer's specifications? ( ) Yes   ( ) No
If No, Explain: ———————.

    C. Are there utility requirements?

        1. Electrical Voltage: ——————— Amperage: ———————

        2. Drains: ( ) Yes ———————

            Water: ( ) Yes ———————

            Other: ( ) Yes ———————

            Specifics: ———————.

Table 6-4 continued

    D. Will this equipment have all necessary mechanical, electrical trim or other appurtenances for use upon its arrival? ( ) Yes   ( ) No
       If No, what needs to be done? _____

    E. Will any site preparation be necessary? ( ) Yes   ( ) No
       If Yes, explain: _____ .

    F. Are there supplies necessary for utilization of this equipment?
       ( ) Yes   ( ) No
       If Yes, explain what, from whom, and suggest start-up supply.

       _____
       _____

    G. Is a start-up supply included in the price of the equipment? ( ) Yes   ( ) No
       If so, what: _____ .

    H. Who uncrates the equipment and what must occur upon delivery? _____
       _____ .

    I. Will this equipment require any unloading equipment to make safe receipt at time of delivery? ( ) Yes   ( ) No
       If Yes, specify: _____ .

    J. If installation is involved, will you coordinate delivery and installation to take place on the same date as a term of the Purchase Order? ( ) Yes   ( ) No
       Explain: _____ .

IV. *INSERVICE AND USE*

    A. Do you provide a unit for in-house demonstration or Trial and Evaluation?
       ( ) Yes   ( ) No
       If Yes, specify and state any terms: _____ .

    B. If this equipment is used to perform a patient chargeable service, what is the average charge for this service by other Hospitals? $_____ /treatment.

    C. Will an upgrade be required/available in the forseeable future? ( ) Yes
       ( ) No
       If Yes, explain: _____ .

    D. Will an Inservice on the use of this equipment be required? ( ) Yes   ( ) No
       If Yes, state full specifics: _____
       _____ .

    E. How long has this equipment been on the market? _____ Months _____
       Years.
       List three (3) institutions, preferably in this area, who use this equipment:

          INSTITUTION   *NAME & TITLE OF USER*
       1.
       2.
       3.

Table 6-4 continued

V. *VENDOR*

Use this section below to list any additional information which you feel would be of interest to us in making an award decision.

_____

_____

_____

_____

_____

Completed By: _____ Date: _____

Name & Title

Source: Steven R. Campbell, "Procurement of Major Equipment," *Hospital Materiel Management Quarterly*, February 1981, Appendix.

plier consideration and a supply priority profile (see Tables 6-5 and 6-6 and Figure 6-6).

(a) Supply Categories*

The prime supplier concept is based upon purchasing entire supply categories from one vendor (see Table 6-5). By negotiating total supply categories on an annual volume basis, the materiel manager may actually reduce total supply purchase price by 10 to 18 percent.

(b) Priority Listing*

Priority listing (see Table 6-6) should be those high-dollar-volume items that represent only a small amount of supplies and numbers, but will provide the supplier with a large annual dollar volume. The hospital should be responsible for providing such a list. This priority listing should delineate—

1. name of the item;
2. description of the item;
3. quantity to be purchased at any one time;
4. safety stock requested.

This list of high volume products should become an integral part of the agreement. It specifies the projected quantities to be ordered on a weekly basis and the quantity to be provided for

*Source: Items (a) and (b) are from Charles E. Housley, "The Prime Supplier Contract," *Hospital Materiel Management Quarterly*, February 1980.

safety stock. The vendor should indicate the item price and for how long the price is protected. Procedures and a time frame for making changes in the supply priority profile also should be included in the contract.

(c) Service Provisions

Frequency of deliveries, handling of emergency needs, availability of sales representatives, and other vendor services will be spelled out in the contract. A penalty clause may be included in case the vendor fails to provide an item in a timely manner. The vendor may be required to forfeit a percentage of the price or pay the difference in cost of acquiring the item from another supplier. Or the vendor may be required to obtain the item from another source.

In addition, the vendor may agree to provide periodic usage reports for all items purchased. The reports may include both quantities purchased and dollar volume expended over a specified amount of time.

Last Steps Before Signing Contract

Before signing the contract, care should be taken to prevent initial misunderstandings that might lead to costly errors and confusion. A series of steps is outlined below.

1. Initial meeting: Representatives of the selected prime vendor and the hospital management team review the hospital's entire prime vendor philosophy and the materiel management concept at the hospital. The hospital furnishes the vendor a rough draft of the proposed agreement so the vendor can make its reactions

Table 6-5 Sample Prime Supplier Proposal for Medical-Surgical Supplies

Statement of Terms

The objective of the hospital is to perform purchasing that will provide the Hospital with supplies that are of optimum quality accompanied by excellent service and good prices. To this end, the Hospital is proposing to purchase all or a major portion of all of the Medical-Surgical Category of supplies from a single supplier for a certain period of time, preferably two years. The Hospital is willing to participate in this method of purchasing under the following conditions.

A. *Pricing*

1. In order to be fair and considerate to all parties concerned, the Hospital has developed a brand-name list of supplies called a "Supply Priority Profile" and this Profile becomes an integral part of the proposal. The Profile of the items also delineates the quantities to be ordered and the quantities to be provided for safety stock. The Hospital will be responsible for thoroughly completing the above two columns and the Vendor will be responsible for indicating the price and price protection categories. *The Vendor is urged to complete the proposal as requested and not fragment it with other proposals.*

2. All prices quoted in the Supply Priority Profile will be at Best Quality Prices (BQP) as listed in the most current edition of the Sales Representative's Price Schedule. A copy of this Schedule will be made available to the authorized Hospital personnel.

3. In addition, all prices quoted will be at BQP less a percentage discount of _____% (unless the item is stated in the "Exceptions" category below).

4. All discounts and rebates (including the Motivation Discount) will be reflected in the unit price as stated on the invoice.

5. Furthermore, the Vendor agrees to include a Motivation Discount of _____% if this Hospital's volume annual purchases for the Medical-Surgical Category reach a minimum of $1,000,000.00. This percentage is to be reflected in the prices quoted in the Supply Priority Profile; however, if the Hospital's annual purchases do not meet or exceed the above-stated level, then at the agreed accounting period of one year, the Hospital will refund to the Vendor the stated percentage of the entire dollar volume purchased.

6. The Hospital agrees to pay all monthly invoices to the Vendor within a net 30-day period from the end of that respective month in which the invoices are incurred. (If the Vendor should give a

Table 6-5 continued

2%—10 days, then this should be reflected in the prices quoted under the Supply Priority Profile.)

7. If there are items or categories of items that are exceptions outside of the percentage off the BQP listed in item 3 above, please list these exceptions on a separate page under the column entitled "Exceptions to the Percentage Discount."

8. Since the Hospital agrees to purchase the majority of the Medical-Surgical Category from the Vendor, all such items are presently listed under the Supply Priority Profile. However, as items are added to this category, the Hospital will want to purchase these items from the Vendor in accordance with the above Pricing Schedule. The Hospital agrees to give the Vendor at least 30 days' notice of such items after which the Vendor agrees to supply and keep the necessary delineated safety stock of such item or items. Such requests will be made in writing to the Vendor in the appropriate Supply Priority Profile format.

B. *Service*

1. The Vendor agrees to ship properly ordered supplies to the Hospital at least once per week through its own trucking service, FOB Hospital. The Hospital agrees to limit the number of deliveries; however, if an emergency item is needed, the Vendor agrees to expedite and deliver, FOB Hospital. The emergency situation will be kept to an absolute minimum.

2. The Vendor's sales representative will be utilized for smooth coordination of this Agreement.

3. The Vendor will provide consultation and inservice of any product or piece of equipment without charge under this Agreement as requested by the Hospital.

C. *Price Protection*

The Vendor agrees to provide price protection to the Hospital in accordance with the following schedule:

Category I. These items are price protected for at least a three-month period from the time of Agreement initiation. Any price changes must be executed at the end of a quarterly period and before the next quarter begins. In other words, there will be no price changes until the beginning of a new quarter.

Category II. These items are price protected for at least a period of six months.

Category III. These items are price protected for at least a period of twelve months.

Category IV. These items are price protected for at least a period of eighteen months.

Note: The appropriate category number should accompany each item in the Supply Priority Profile.

Table 6-5 continued

D. *Terms of This Agreement*

1. The terms and conditions of this Agreement shall be in effect for a period of two years.

2. The Hospital may terminate this Agreement with or without cause by giving Vendor 60 days' notice.

3. The Vendor may terminate this Agreement with or without cause by giving the Hospital 60 days' notice.

4. Prices and terms that have been negotiated previously between the Hospital and manufacturers will be honored by the Vendor.

5. If an item appearing on the Supply Priority Profile is at a much higher price than is presently being paid by the Hospital, the Hospital may delete the item from the Supply Priority Profile.

6. All deliveries from the Vendor and/or manufacturer will be FOB Hospital.

E. *Penalty Clause*

If the Hospital should order an item on the Supply Priority Profile in accordance with the quantity listed under the ''Quantity of Order'' and ''Safety Stock,'' and the Vendor does not have that quantity of that item, the Vendor agrees to pay as direct credit to the Hospital the greater amount of (i) the sum of _____% of the total amount of the cost of the item not shipped directly to the Hospital, or, if the item is an emergency, (ii) the difference in cost of having to get the item from another vendor.

Since the Hospital intends to participate totally in the Prime Supplier Agreement, should the Vendor ever be out of an item and that item is needed immediately by the Hospital, then the Vendor or sales representative shall obtain that item from some other source for the Hospital.

F. *Reports*

The Vendor agrees to provide monthly reports of usage, backorders, etc., for all items purchased under this proposal and make them available on a timely basis to the Hospital.

G. *Deadline*

VENDORS' QUOTATIONS MUST BE RECEIVED NO LATER THAN 12 NOON THE _____ DAY OF _____, 19___. THE QUOTATIONS THAT ARE LATE WILL NOT BE CONSIDERED. FURTHERMORE, VENDORS WHO ALTER THIS PROPOSAL WILL STAND THE RISK OF HAVING THEIR PROPOSAL NOT BEING CONSIDERED.

Source: Charles E. Housley, ''The Prime Supplier Contract,'' *Hospital Materiel Management Quarterly,* February 1980.

Table 6-6 Major Categories for Prime Supplier Consideration

A. Medical-Surgical
 1. Medical-surgical supplies in general
 2. Intravenous solutions and sets
 3. Dressings
 4. Cardiac and vascular implants
 5. Orthopedic implants
 6. Surgical instruments
 7. Bulk oxygen
 8. Cylinder and tank gases
 9. Monitoring equipment
B. Pharmaceuticals
 10. Direct drugs
 11. Indirect or wholesale drugs
C. Office Supplies
 12. Office supplies in general
 13. Office equipment
 14. Typewriters
 15. Copiers
 16. Paper supplies
D. Printed Matter
 17. Single page forms
 18. Business forms
 19. Envelopes and stationery
E. Dietary supplies
 20. Staples
 21. Fruits and vegetables
 22. Meats and poultry
 23. Frozen commodities
 24. Bread and bread products
 25. Beverages
 26. Paper products
 27. Dietary disposable items
 28. Silverware and utensils
 29. Dietary equipment
 30. Vending contracts
 31. Milk and milk products
F. Maintenance
 32. General supplies
 33. Plumbing supplies
 34. Electrical supplies
 35. Heating, air conditioning, ventilation supplies and equipment
 36. Biomedical engineering items
G. Linen
 37. Patient care items
 38. Surgical linen
 39. Uniforms
 40. Draperies and curtains
 41. Contract laundry
H. Housekeeping
 42. General housekeeping items
 43. Detergents and cleaning compounds
I. Radiology
 44. Film and chemicals
 45. General supplies
 46. Diagnostic and therapeutic equipment

Table 6-6 continued

J. Laboratory
   47. Miscellaneous/general supplies
   48. Chemicals
   49. Sera
   50. Blood and blood products

Source: Charles E. Housley, "The Prime Supplier Contract," *Hospital Materiel Management Quarterly*, February 1980.

known. Copies of the hospital's brochures on sales representatives and statement of services are given to the vendor representatives for their information and review. The hospital's written policies and procedures that govern the relationship between the hospital and its vendors should be made an integral part of the contract.

2. Second meeting: Any changes in the proposed contract are made final. The vendor group is given an overview of the materiel management departments and systems.

3. Third meeting: The contract is reviewed and signed by the vendor representatives and the hospital director of materiel management.

4. Classroom orientation to materiel management: A two-day orientation on the hospital's materiel management systems is given to designated vendor representatives.

5. "Hands on" practical materiel management orientation: A one-week vendor orientation is attended by designated vendor representatives. It covers all materiel management areas, policies and procedures, theory and practice. It involves demonstrations of how the systems are used so the vendor gains a better idea of how items are ordered, received, stored, and placed on carts; how the products are distributed; and what problems occur in a hospital environment.

COST CONTAINMENT

Materiel management represents approximately 46 percent of the hospital's annual operating costs, with about 19 percent of these costs allocated to materiel labor and 27 percent allocated to supply expense. Therefore, there is a lot of room to bring about savings and cost containment efforts. These cost containment efforts can be in many forms and different variations such as reduction of inventories; better utilization of personnel; better buying habits; utilization of less space for materiel efforts; amalgamation of

the supply, process and distribution functions; better negotiations; shared services; simpler methods of purchasing; group purchasing; stockless purchasing; and innovative methods of purchasing such as prime supplier and corporate prime supplies. The list seems to be endless.*

Guidelines**

The following suggestions are offered as areas for consideration in containing and controlling the costs of hospital supplies and equipment.

1. Where possible, deal directly with manufacturers.
2. Refuse to pay vendor price increases without prior notification.
3. Purchase supply items on a competitive basis.
4. Negotiate with vendors for better prices and terms.
5. Reduce inventory levels.
6. Establish a standardization or product evaluation committee for supply items.
7. Incorporate cost containment as part of an employee's performance evaluation and encourage suggestions for improved supply utilization.
8. Reduce linen usage by rotating top sheet to bottom, thereby using one clean sheet rather than two every day.
9. Eliminate the fourth daily meal ("nourishment").
10. Standardize items and avoid brand name preference (e.g., duplication of items under different trade names).
11. Conduct educational sessions on purchasing and inventory control policies and procedures for user departments.
12. Sell excess and unneeded equipment.
13. Rotate stock of perishable items.
14. Establish a pharmaceutical services center to purchase and warehouse drugs on a nonprofit basis for participating hospitals.
15. Participate in group purchasing efforts.
16. Reduce the number of "stock" items in

---

*Source: Charles E. Housley, "From the Editor," *Hospital Material Management Quarterly*, February 1980.
**Source: Jerry P. Widman, "101 Ways to Contain Hospital Supply Costs," *Hospital Materiel Management Quarterly*, May 1980.

Figure 6-6 Supply priority profile

	Item	Description	Order Unit	Order Quantity	Safety Stock	Unit Price	Previous Dollar Volume	Price Protection Category				
								1	2	3	4	5
1	Electrodes	Long-term, adult	each	500	1,000		$120,000					
2	Admission Kits	Made to order	each	600	1,000		99,000					
3	Sutures	Ethicon 811H	dozen	15	10		87,000					

(List 350–500 medical-surgical supplies based on volume priority. For example, No. 1 is the largest dollar volume item purchased, No. 2 is the second largest dollar volume item purchased.)

To be completed by the Vendor

Source: Charles E. Housley, "The Prime Supplier Contract," *Hospital Materiel Management Quarterly*, February 1980.

the storeroom or catalog by eliminating similar items and purging slow-moving items.

17. Increase inventory turnover rates for major supply commodities.
18. Negotiate blanket orders by commodity for a specified period and firm price.
19. Change linen every other day.
20. Reduce wasted food from inpatient meals by examining returned patient trays for reusable items.
21. Pursue the sale of scrap materiel.
22. Establish a drug utilization review program.
23. Tighten requisitioning practices and security procedures to reduce pilferage.
24. Establish a forms control program.
25. Instigate an exchange cart or par level system for supply items to reduce storage and handling costs.
26. Concentrate purchasing efforts on major dollar items rather than wasting time on minor items.
27. Print forms in-house.
28. Centralize and control photocopy requirements.
29. As linen items wear out, replace them with those of more durable quality.
30. Make arrangements for equipment and supplies to be utilized on a "trial basis" before making a commitment.
31. Establish a materiel management center to serve several hospitals for functions

such as purchase of supplies, warehousing, distribution.

32. Freeze capital expenditures.
33. Carefully control the inventory investment on single-use items.
34. Obtain supplies from vendors on a delayed-invoice payment basis.
35. Promptly return rejected materiel to vendor for credit.
36. Establish blanket orders for high usage items.
37. Where possible, discontinue supplying slow-moving items to user departments.
38. Conduct a monthly review of purchasing statistics to determine poor vendor deliveries or quality.
39. Conduct a weekly executive review of all purchases valued above a set amount (suggested maximum: $500).
40. Buy on a supplier "make and hold" basis.
41. Review all A items daily, B items weekly and C items monthly for excess coverage.
42. Compile a list of slow-moving materiel for return to vendors.
43. Use the quick-delivery flow principle: tell suppliers to the day and time when to deliver materiel.
44. Annually review order points and order quantities for appropriateness.
45. Categorize and control parts by an ABC inventory classification method.

46. Reduce ordering costs by combining requirements on one form when possible.
47. Buy on a consignment basis.
48. Request vendors to stock goods for quick delivery to a local warehouse.
49. Encourage the proper use of supplies and discourage their waste by improving employee awareness of costs.
50. Reject all overshipments in excess of 10 percent.
51. Set up inventory level charts and monitor them by major commodity grouping.
52. Consolidate the number of hospital storage locations.
53. Reschedule purchase orders for later deliveries when demand decreases.
54. Reduce the safety stock level of storeroom items.
55. Obtain cost-saving suggestions from the medical staff for frequently used items.
56. Discourage hoarding of supply items.
57. Calculate and control, by item number, how many months the materiel will last.
58. Avoid overstocking supplies in user departments.
59. Purchase all major or routine supply items through competitive bidding.
60. Evaluate the cost-benefit relationship of prime vendor contracts to major supply categories.
61. Periodically audit the quantity of supplies requisitioned by user departments.
62. Discourage the ordering of "special" supplies for user departments and hospital employees.
63. Conduct cost-benefit analysis studies prior to making major supply and capital equipment commitments.
64. Require properly authorized requisitions prior to issuing materiel from the storeroom.
65. Schedule regular deliveries of supply items to key user departments.
66. Maintain an up-to-date perpetual inventory system.
67. Train and instruct all purchasing department personnel in the performance of their duties.
68. Encourage materiel management personnel to attend educational programs, seminars and workshops to acquire information on current developments in the field.
69. Insist that supplies be used for the purpose for which they were purchased.
70. Contract for an independent objective review of the purchasing system at least every five years.
71. Reduce the number of different using departments involved in the selection of vendors and the buying process.
72. Number, control and account for all purchase orders.
73. Provide to the administration a monthly statistical report on purchasing activities.
74. Conduct formal vendor performance analyses regarding price adherence, quality and delivery; report results to individual vendors.
75. Supply to vendor representatives a policy statement (e.g., a welcoming booklet) with guidelines covering vendor relations, ethics and visits to hospital employees.
76. Compare all information on invoices to purchase order and receiving report.
77. Assure that vendors are not charging sales taxes.
78. Control all distribution of supplies under a single materiel management department.
79. Have buyers change commodities at least every three years in order to obtain a fresh look.
80. Establish a follow-up system of vendor delivery pledges.
81. Review weekly open purchase orders and back orders for past-due items.
82. Establish one central location for vendor catalogs and insist that vendor representatives be responsible for their update.
83. Disallow salesmen from contacting user departments without prior authorization.
84. Do not issue a purchase order without an authorized requisition.
85. Refuse unauthorized split shipments from a vendor.
86. Use preprinted weekly requisitions for user departments.
87. Limit storeroom access to authorized employees.
88. Periodically compare the perpetual inventory with the physical inventory by cycle counting inventory items (particularly high-value items).

89. Require that all incoming merchandise, materiel and supplies pass through a central receiving point.
90. Insist that every item in inventory be there for a specific purpose.
91. Maintain an up-to-date storeroom inventory catalog.
92. Reduce the number of vendors.
93. Reduce the number of deliveries per year.
94. Simplify the storeroom identification system and properly identify and label storeroom items.
95. Record all competitive bids obtained from vendors and maintain a price inventory record.
96. Establish rules for items which are candidates for blanket purchase orders (e.g., three times a year or more).
97. Meet with other hospital purchasing personnel to discuss common problems and exchange information.
98. Review the legal aspects of purchase order terms and conditions.
99. Analyze each purchase order with respect to quality, delivery and pricing.
100. Prenumber and control patient charge tickets to ensure that they are not lost and that all appropriate costs are charged to the patient.
101. Learn to say "no."

The Prudent Buyer*

In April 1979 the GAO distributed 20,000 copies of a two-volume publication to every hospital in the United States and every member of the American Society for Hospital Purchasing and Materials Management of the American Hospital Association. Volume one deals with the results of a joint study of the GAO and the AHA on the state of the art of hospital purchasing and materiel management practices. It contains recommendations for such hospital purchasing practices as competitive bidding, standardization, and group purchasing.

Volume two is a self-administered checklist and audit guide (that includes simplified audit

_____
*Source: Jerry P. Widman, "Effects of the 1980 GAO Study on Hospital Purchasing," *Hospital Materiel Management Quarterly*, February 1981.

programs) for evaluating and improving purchasing practices and other materiel management functions.

The GAO analysis indicated that:

1. Some hospitals paid twice the price paid by other hospitals.
2. Some vendors sold the same item to hospitals in the same geographic area at different prices.

As a result of the report it is likely that hospital purchasing practices will be subjected to closer review by fiscal intermediaries and that intermediaries will intensify their audit of hospital purchasing practices. Hospitals will need to review their purchasing functions and determine whether they are obtaining the most appropriate prices, consistent with good service and high quality, especially for routine supply items. If a hospital has sound purchasing practices and procedures it should have no problem justifying the prices paid. However, if such practices are not in place, hospitals should reexamine their existing purchasing policies and practices and change them accordingly. At a minimum every hospital should have a stated policy that addresses prudent buying.

The Checklist

The GAO checklist (Table 6-7) offers a tool for directors of materiel management, internal auditors, and outside auditors in evaluating purchasing and materiel management practices. A self-assessment program, using the checklist, will highlight those specific areas that deserve management attention and corrective action. The GAO checklist consists of over 250 questions. Each question compares existing practices to preferred ones. It is organized according to the following major subject areas:

- Authority and responsibility;
- Purchasing;
- Inventory management;
- Supply distribution—medical/surgical supplies;
- Supply distribution—linen;
- Pharmaceutical purchasing;
- Pharmaceutical inventory management;
- Food service; and
- Audit and evaluation.

Table 6-7 Prudent Buyer Checklist

- Hospital policy specifying administrative approvals by dollar level..
- One uniform purchase set and one uniform policy/procedure for all hospital purchases.
- Purchase order bearing a certificate of pricing requirement: Seller warrants and certifies that prices under this order for like-quantities and like-goods shall be as low as, or lower than, those charged seller's most favored customer, in addition to any discount for payment.
- One control point for all purchasing, assuring—even for purchase orders not originated in the purchasing department—that purchasing policies and procedures have been followed.
- A purchase order covering every purchase of goods and services.
- Purchase orders numbered and issued sequentially.
- Purchase orders showing terms, prices or reference to pricing agreement.
- Comparison of quantities, prices and terms on invoices with purchase order.
- Standard specifications written for frequently purchased products. (Specifications updated periodically.)
- Establishment of Economic Order Quantities and Reorder Points for stocked products.
- Contracts specify scope of activity, terms, termination and specific price. Legal review advisable. Long-term contracts reviewed periodically.
- Nonstock purchases made upon receipt of signed requisition.
- Signature cards in purchasing for every department head authorized to requisition.
- Purchasing done in hospital departments outside of purchasing:
  - Signature card for each person authorized to purchase, indicating products or services to be purchased.
  - Blocks of purchase orders provided. Record of numbers in purchasing.
  - Design of departmental purchasing procedures by purchasing agent.
  - Adherence to system, documentation of decisions and prudence monitored by purchasing agent.
- Prudent procedures for purchasing services:
  - A written plan for the review and purchase of services.
  - Alternatives comparing quantitative and qualitative factors carefully analyzed.
  - Service provider's proposals must be related to hospital objectives and costs must be delineated in writing.
  - Proposals shall be reviewed by administration and/or trustees.
  - Reasons for purchasing decision shall be documented.
  - Contract.
- Purchasing policies to include:
  - Definition of prudent buying.
  - Conflict of interest.
  - Acceptance of gifts statements.
- Regular procedure for reviewing departmental supply expenses and inventories.
- Criteria established for vendor performance. Vendor performance monitored and an approved vendor card file maintained (updated periodically).
- Internal audits to ensure procedures are followed.
- Accounts payable rules; method of approving invoices for payment. Method for changing invoices to agree with POs.

Source: William K. Henning, "Application of the Prudent Buyer Principle to Purchasing Administration," *Hospital Materiel Management Quarterly*, November 1979.

Other Anticipated Effects

So far the major emphasis of third party intermediaries has been on price and price comparisons. While perhaps not as obvious as the aforementioned effects, the GAO report suggests some other effects (side effects of the GAO study) on hospital purchasing practices. These side effects are:

- Regular or periodic reviews of purchasing operations to determine compliance with the prudent buyer concept;
- Higher expectation of the materiel management function by hospital administration;
- Increased competition within the hospital supply and manufacturing industry;
- Improved documentation pertaining to rea-

sons and justification for purchases of capital equipment and routine supply items;

- Use of more sophisticated inventory control techniques, such as economic order quantity (EOQ) methods, A-B-C analysis, and other quantitative techniques;
- Renewed emphasis on value analysis and standardization;
- Tighter accounting and internal controls aimed at reducing waste, pilferage, and obsolescence;
- More frequent audits of effectiveness and efficiency of purchasing, supply distribution, and inventory management; and
- Increase in the number and quality of educational programs and publications on purchasing and materiel management techniques.

Evaluating the Prudent Buyer*

To evaluate the strengths and weaknesses of the purchasing department with respect to the prudent buyer principle, an administrator can use the following approaches:

- interviewing purchasing employees and key members of user departments;
- examining the contents and design of key documents and records;
- evaluating the functional goals, policies and procedures of materiel management; and
- conducting random samples of selected records and documents.

Specific review steps for purchase transactions might include:

1. Determining the filing practices for all basic purchasing documents (e.g., requisitions, quotations, purchase orders, purchase order revisions, purchase history records).
2. Conducting a purchase order review by obtaining a representative sample of purchase orders over the past 12-month period. The representative sample should be a cross-section by buyer, by commodity category, by dollar value, by user department, etc.
3. Pulling all documents related to each purchase and preparing a worksheet to evalu-

ate each of the purchase orders under consideration.

The objective of reviewing purchase transactions is to determine whether sound purchasing practices are being followed: Are the actions those of a prudent and cost-conscious buyer?

THE PRODUCT STANDARDIZATION COMMITTEE*

One of the things a hospital can do to support cost-containment efforts is establish a product standards and evaluation committee. With the proliferation of products and continual innovation affecting the technology of health care, it is essential that there be a formalized function to carry out an evaluation process. If it is left to the physicians or others involved directly in patient care, the evaluation may be relegated to a hit-or-miss approach because of other pressing demands on the time of these individuals. Often, decisions are made that are based on emotion, on past experiences or on pressure from sales representatives.

The chairperson should be a dynamic individual capable of generating enough interest in the evaluation process to maintain viability. Committee members should include the purchasing agent and ad hoc members as may be necessary, and a representative from administration, nursing and the physicians. Meetings should be frequent enough to review any new products and should also be held whenever major equipment contracts expire. This will facilitate the efforts of the purchasing department in the evaluation of bid specifications. Sample products should be available for evaluation during and after the meetings for inservice or trial use by the medical staff.

Examples of items to be evaluated include electronic thermometers, infusion pumps, catheters, etc. Ideally, the representative from nursing would spearhead an evaluation on the nursing units on a formalized basis. This would involve physicians' input as well. The results and the analysis would be documented and reported back to the product standards and evaluation committee during a subsequent meeting.

---

*Source: Jerry P. Widman, "Development of a Product Purchasing Program," *Hospital Materiel Management Quarterly*, November 1979.

*Source: Dale R. Gunnell, "The Mechanics of Cost Containment," *Hospital Materiel Management Quarterly*, May 1980.

As various products are evaluated, all salient points would be recorded in order to eventually obtain an acceptable product for the least cost.

Because meetings would generally take place during the regular workday, participants must be given time away from their regular duties to allow them to participate in product analysis.

Objectives

Generally the objectives of the committee are:

- To provide the mechanism to ensure an improved level of patient care through product evaluation with emphasis on the quality of care and the containment of costs;
- To evaluate the voluminous and continuous flow of new and improved products;
- To reduce the expense of educating and training personnel to many and varied products and techniques through standardization;
- To keep administration and department heads informed and abreast of changes in equipment and products;
- To assist department heads in understanding mutual problems in reference to supplies and equipment; and
- To minimize the quantities of inventory by reducing the variety of products.*

More specifically the objectives have been stated as:

1. Primary and Secondary Objectives:
   a. The primary objective is to identify the *products* best suited for department use after consideration of factors involving cost, standardization, availability, source, etc.
   b. Secondary objectives are to reduce the number of different items used to accomplish a given task, eliminate wasteful duplication of products and achieve economy through standardization.
2. Other Objectives:
   a. Review all proposed product changes including additions and deletions of inventory and other standardized items, including yearly contract items.
   b. Evaluate products as deemed necessary

to determine their acceptability as a result of bidding or prior to bidding.
   c. Determine which departments or nursing units should be involved in given evaluations.
   d. Identify when need exists and select ad hoc members.
   e. Approve length of product trial periods.
   f. Establish criteria for product evaluations.
   g. Make recommendations to purchasing, including all supporting justification data.
   h. Review information on new products which warrant committee consideration.

Representation and Responsibility

The committee is to be composed of the following representatives:

a. assistant administrator, materiel services;
b. nursing representative;
c. physician;
d. purchasing agent; and
e. ad hoc members.

The chairperson will schedule and conduct all meetings and also keep committee members advised of all requests by any department that requires product evaluation.

a. *The assistant administrator, materiel services,* is to provide administrative support and keep other administrative staff informed on proceedings. In the absence of the chairperson, the assistant administrator may act as the chairperson.
b. The *nursing representative* is to coordinate all necessary nursing involvement and provide technical input as products relate to nursing in the evaluation process.
c. The *physician representative* is to provide technical clinical input and coordinate or suggest which clinical areas and which physicians should be involved with the evaluations.
d. The *purchasing agent* is to provide technical information as well as cost, source and availability data on all products evaluated. He or she shall also arrange for product detailing and/or samples as requested by the committee. The purchasing agent will also keep the chairperson advised of all

---

*Source: Charles E. Housley, *Hospital Materiel Management,* Aspen Systems Corporation, 1978.

new products and all requisitions or other requests routed to the purchasing department that would result in a change in inventory items, yearly contract items, or other standardized products in use in the hospital.

e. The *ad hoc members* will be assigned as necessary to assist with specific evaluations. The committee may request information or assistance from any department in the hospital that is a primary user of the products involved in any given evaluation. Appropriate personnel from these departments will be assigned as ad hoc members for evaluation of products concerning their departments.

Product Standardization Guidelines*

Subject

Administrative policy for products and equipment evaluation and standardization.

Objective

To monitor and control the use of supplies and equipment within the hospital with emphasis on the quality of care and the containment of costs.

Policy Statement

It shall be the policy of this hospital that any product or piece of equipment which is proposed for use within the hospital must first undergo evaluation and approval by the Evaluation and Standardization of Products Committee.

Procedural documentation

- All potential products (either for use or evaluation) must be submitted to the Department of Materiel Management by physicians, hospital personnel, sales representatives, patients, etc.
- The department will initially screen all items before submitting them to the Standardization Committee.
- The materiel manager will contact the concerned departments for their recommendations and comments before the item is brought to the committee for review.
- A product standardization profile (Figure 6-7) is prepared for each item to be reviewed. The profile of each item is distributed to each committee member at the meeting.
- An agenda is prepared and distributed at least one week prior to the next committee meeting.

- The committee shall meet at least monthly and also on an "as needed" basis.
- If the requesting department is not represented on the committee, then it may send a representative to present the item. This representative may vote in this one case.
- Possible committee actions are:
  a. Acceptance of the product
  b. Nonacceptance of the product
  c. A 30-day evaluation
  d. A 60-day evaluation
  e. A 90-day evaluation.
- The products to be evaluated are to be paid for by the supplier if at all possible.
- Once an item has been reviewed and rejected, the product will not be reconsidered by the committee for at least a year unless there is a favorable price or product change.
- If an item is approved, the respective department is responsible for submitting a product orientation and utilization procedure to the Standardization Committee for review before the newly accepted product is actually purchased.
- The Committee also shall submit a list of all newly proposed items to the Patient Charge Committee for their review and determination of patient charge (if applicable) before the item is reviewed by the Standardization Committee.
- The minutes of all committee meetings must be sent to the administrator or his delegate before any action is taken. If the administration does not approve of the stated action or actions, this is communicated back to the committee and the item or items are not purchased.

Exceptions

All items must undergo the above procedure with one exception. If the product is requested on an emergency basis by a physician, it can be purchased. However, this item and action will be reviewed at the next committee meeting.

Review and Comment

At least annually.

Authorized Signature

Administrator.

*Source: Charles E. Housley, *Hospital Materiel Management*, Aspen Systems Corporation, 1978, pp. 121–122.

Figure 6-7 Product standardization profile

DATE:_____   HOSPITAL PRODUCT NUMBER_____

REQUESTED PRODUCT:_____

MANUFACTURER:_____

SUPPLIED BY:_____

REQUESTED BY:_____

REQUESTED ITEM WILL:

       ☐   BE AN ADDITIONAL ITEM

       ☐   REPLACES:_____

       ☐   REDUCES USE OF ANOTHER ITEM:_____

       ☐   OTHER:_____

PRODUCT COMPARISONS:

CHARACTERISTICS	PRESENT ITEM	REQUESTED ITEM
MANUFACTURER		
SUPPLIER		
ANNUAL USE		
USE AND/OR EVALUATION RESULTS		
AVAILABILITY		
PATIENT CHARGE		
PACKAGING DATA		
HOSPITAL STOCK ITEM		
MINIMUM ORDER QUANTITY		
ADVANTAGES		
DISADVANTAGES		
QUANTITY ON HAND		
COST PER UNIT		
NET SAVINGS (OR LOSS)		
OTHER		

PRODUCT RECALL PROCEDURE*

Recall Notification

There are various means through which the hospital may be notified of product recalls, alerts,

and hazard notifications; these could be notification by the company letter or mailgram directed to the administrator or member of the medical staff, by verbal or written notice to a particular department, or by phone.

Another immediate means of notification is through subscription to the National Recall Alert Center, a service that provides immediate notice by way of mailgram (directed to the attention of the purchasing department) of all recall

---

*Source: Ronne Patt Teselsky, "Centralizing Product Recall Notification and Documentation," *Hospital Materiel Management Quarterly*, May 1981.

Figure 6-7 continued

STANDARDIZATION COMMITTEE ACTION:

☐ ACCEPTED

☐ NOT APPROVED

☐ APPROVED FOR 30 DAYS EVALUATION

☐ APPROVED FOR 60 DAYS EVALUATION

☐ APPROVED FOR 90 DAYS EVALUATION

☐ TABLED PENDING FURTHER INFORMATION

☐ OTHER:_____

ADDITIONAL COMMENTS:_____

_____

_____

_____

DATE:_____

SIGNATURE OF CHAIRMAN:_____

Source: Charles E. Housley, *Hospital Materiel Management,* Aspen Systems Corporation, 1978.

actions taken by the Food and Drug Administration.

Another subscription-type service available to the health care industry is ECRI bulletins which deal with medical products and devices where problems have occurred. (The ECRI bulletins are put out by the Emergency Care Research Institute, a special testing laboratory operated by and with Health Devices. Health Devices is a subscription service which provides hospitals with test-result data as well as information regarding products that have been recalled.) These bulletins for the most part are geared toward the medical staff since they pertain mainly to particular test findings and recommendations.

In-Hospital Procedure

There should be a single department in the hospital responsible for handling all recall notifications, whether it be the purchasing department, risk-management division or administrative area.

By policy and formalized procedure, any department or individual receiving a recall notification must forward a copy of the notice to the purchasing office where immediate investigative action begins.

Using the product recall/alert notification form (Figure 6-8), the buyer for the product in question (completing the top portion of the form) indicates the date and using departments. The buyer also notes what type of notification it is (recall, alert, or hazard notice), giving product description and all other applicable information such as catalogue or model number, lot number, and manufacturer.

A brief statement as to the reason of the notification is provided along with a copy of the notification. The form and notice are sent to the probable users as well as the SPD stores and central supply areas where it is determined whether or not there is a supply of the product in the hospital. Where the recall notice may involve equipment, a copy of the form and notification would be sent to the instrumentation (or biomedical en-

Figure 6-8   Product recall/alert form

Date: _____

To: _____   FROM: PURCHASING DEPARTMENT

_____

_____

_____

We have received a Recall _____ Alert _____ Hazard _____ notification for the following:

Product Description: _____ Catalogue/Model No. _____

Lot No. _____ Manufacturer _____

Reason for Recall/Alert: _____

_____

PLEASE INVESTIGATE TO SEE IF YOU HAVE THIS PRODUCT ON HAND , COMPLETE THE LOWER PORTION OF THIS FORM AND RETURN IT TO PURCHASING IMMEDIATELY.

Date: _____   TO: PURCHASING DEPARTMENT

From: _____
               (DEPARTMENT)

By: _____

We do _____ do not _____ have this product in our department.

Quantity on Hand: _____   Lot No. _____

NOTE: IF YOU DO HAVE THE PRODUCT IN YOUR DEPARTMENT, PULL ALL QUANTITIES OUT OF USE AND AWAIT INSTRUCTIONS FROM PURCHASING FOR RETURN OR CORRECTIVE ACTIONS TO BE TAKEN.

FOR PURCHASING DEPARTMENT USE ONLY

Vendor Notified _____ Via _____ Attention: _____
                   (DATE)   (NAME)

Return/Corrective Action Instruction: _____

_____

_____

Recall/Alert procedures completed: _____ By: _____
                                       (DATE)   (NAME)

Form #PUR—094 7/78

Source: Saint Mary of Nazareth Hospital Center, Chicago. Reprinted with permission.

gineers) and/or maintenance department for follow-up with the using department for proper verification.

When a department receives a recall notification form, they have the responsibility to examine their supply (or equipment) and report back to purchasing, using the center portion of the form, as to whether or not they have the product on hand. If they do, they must record the quantity on hand and list the lot (or model and serial) numbers. At that point the product is removed from use pending return or corrective action instruction from purchasing.

Upon receipt of the completed recall forms from the departments, purchasing notifies the vendor of quality status, completing the last portion of the recall form. Here the date the vendor was notified, how the vendor was notified and to whom the information was given are recorded. All return or corrective action instructions are obtained from the vendor and recorded where indicated.

Where hospital staff receive recall or hazard notifications for products that have not been used by the hospital, they maintain a separate file for 18 months. They do this as a reference source since there has been occasion when the Food and Drug Administration has asked if hospital staff were notified of a recall of a particular product that they should have received whether they used the product or not. Staff members have not found the need to maintain recall notification records beyond the point at which the hospital is affected.

In addition to the documentation retained in the purchasing office, hospital staff provide to the risk-management department a monthly report and accumulative quarterly update of all recalls affecting the hospital.

EVALUATING MATERIEL MANAGEMENT OPERATION*

There are basically four methods to measure the effectiveness of the materiel management efforts in today's hospitals.

1. The Supply Performance Review

This method answers the question how well materiel management is meeting the needs of the individual institution and how well it is meeting the needs of each department and function of the institution.

It is recommended that a supply performance review be completed at least once a year, and preferably every six months.

The unit or department requiring the supply or materiel services must delineate, along with the materiel manager, the specific needs of that department or unit. Then supply standards and criteria can be developed so that a performance review can be completed.

---

*Source: Charles E. Housley, "Evaluating the Effectiveness of the Materiel Management Effort," *Hospital Materiel Management Quarterly*, August 1979.

Specific performance standards must be established for each area in need of materiel services in conjunction with designated responsible members of materiel management.

A clear understanding must be brought about between the department's needs and its wants. After the department's supply needs have been established materiel management should forecast for these needs and have the right supply at the right place, at the right time and in the right quantities.

Supply standards for most departments are very dynamic and should be updated frequently.

2. The Supply-Price Comparison

With every purchasing agent, buyer and materiel manager, there is an innate reservation to openly share supply prices with fellow purchasing colleagues. Today everyone is looking for the best price for hospital commodities, and almost everyone thinks he or she has obtained it. On the other hand, how can you tell if your hospital is getting the best price or even a good price? Prices for the same product vary from hospital to hospital, from region to region and from dealer to dealer. Why do prices for identical supplies differ? There is much speculation about this question; however, the major reasons are:

1. In some cases, volume is a factor of price. The greater the volume, the lower the price should be.
2. Location can make a difference. The greater distance the supply must be transported, the higher the price.
3. The negotiation skill of the purchasing agent is a definite factor.
4. The type of supply sometimes makes a difference.
5. The prestige of the institution can have a distinct effect on prices. Large teaching hospitals often get their products at cost because there is the likelihood that these products will become standards of practice for future physicians.
6. The supplier's need to make a quota or promotional sale is a factor.

The primary objectives of the supply-price comparison are to gather uniform price information from as many hospitals as possible in reference to the large-dollar-volume supplies, coordinate or computerize the data, then distribute this information back to the hospitals with a high price, average price and low price paid for each identical supply at a local, state, regional and national level. In the future, one may want to use some type of correlation coefficient to compare the prices to such hospital materiel programs as centralized purchasing, group purchasing, prime suppliers, and so forth to determine just how these programs and other factors such as size and location affect the prices paid for hospital supplies. The supply-price comparison can be an extremely valuable negotiation and containment tool for hospitals.

3. Management Audit

The management audit is a very helpful tool for the materiel manager. It can be the impetus and catalyst for the implementation of plans. For the department it can also mean the beginning of credibility and responsibility for the manager of materiels. (See the Management Audit Checklists at the end of this chapter.)

4. The Materiel-Cost-Per-Patient-Day Formula

The fourth and final method of evaluating the effectiveness of the materiel efforts is the use of the materiel-cost-per-patient-day (MCPPD) formula. It tells you how you and your materiel efforts uniformly compare with those of other hospitals irrespective of size, location, age, and the like.

Purchasing, receiving, distribution, central supply, pharmacy, print shop, linen processing and property management all fall within the purview of materiel management. Therefore, any attempt to measure the quality and quantity of materiel management must take into consideration all of these functions.

This is what the MCPPD does! Totaling all materiel costs, one can use this figure as the numerator and divide it by the total hospital patient costs per diem as a denominator and project a ratio of materiel costs to hospital costs. This ratio will be relevant to all sizes of hospitals.

Summary

The supply performance review is a subjective method of evaluation but a useful one. The sup-

ply-price comparison is very objective but is severely limited because it deals with only one small segment of materiel management—the purchased price. The management audit is for the most part a very objective endeavor. Its importance to the materiel manager and the administrator will definitely increase in the future. The MCPPD formula is probably the most inclusive and objective method of evaluating materiel management's effectiveness. It deals with quantifiable entities to which there can be little exception or argument.

Management Audit Checklists

Materiel Administration

1. Is the department under the direction of a trained materiel manager?
2. Is the materiel manager directly responsible to the administration or a member of the administrative team?
3. Are there carefully delineated policies and procedures for the materiel administrative functions?
4. Are they written?
5. Are they kept revised and distributed to the appropriate departments and units?
6. Is there a policy and procedure manual?
7. Have all of the key materiel functions been amalgamated and centralized into one single department?
8. Is there a materiel master plan?
9. Does it include materiel planning for at least five years?
10. Is there a products evaluation committee?
11. Are physicians represented on the committee?
12. Is the materiel manager a member of the administrative team?
13. Does the materiel manager have a copy of the Joint Commission on Accreditation of Hospitals standards?
14. Does the department meet or exceed all of these standards?
15. Is the materiel manager responsible for a departmental operating expense budget?
16. Does the materiel manager have both line and staff responsibilities in reference to the hospital budget?
17. Does the materiel manager stay abreast of all of the trends in health care materiel management?

18. Is the materiel manager represented on the area shared services committee or the group purchasing committee?
19. Does the materiel manager have interdepartmental responsibilities for the management of materiels?
20. Are personnel performance appraisals done on a regular basis?
21. Is there an effective means of communicating materiel news to all appropriate departments, units and members of the medical staff?
22. Is there a materiel literature library which is available to all personnel of the department?
23. Is there an area or regional supply disaster plan?
24. Is there an effective materiel orientation program for the hospital and departmental personnel?
25. Is there an administrative reporting mechanism?

Purchasing

1. Does the hospital truly practice centralized purchasing?
2. Is there an administrative policy in reference to centralized purchasing?
3. Has this policy been distributed to all appropriate parties?
4. Are any departments allowed to bypass the centralized purchase process?
5. Are major equipment purchases made through the purchasing departments?
6. Does the department purchase all supplies according to hospital product specifications?
7. Does the department always use purchase orders even for service contracts?
8. Are certain persons in each department designated to initiate departmental requisitions?
9. Is there an approved supply list for each department?
10. Do special requisitions take a separate approval?
11. Is there an administrative or board policy and procedure for capital equipment requests?
12. Are major equipment items purchased through a competitive bid process?
13. Are standing purchase orders discouraged or forbidden?

14. Are prime vendor contracts negotiated for all major supply classifications on a periodic basis?
15. Does the hospital participate in group purchasing efforts?
16. Has the blank check form of purchasing been eliminated?
17. Are the personnel exercising purchasing responsibility trained in all phases of purchasing, especially the legal aspects, so as to avoid controversy or litigation?
18. Are all contracts, agreements, leases and rental agreements involving multiple payments easily available for review and audit as to payments being in accord with the purchase document?
19. Are electronic ordering devices utilized effectively in the purchasing process?
20. Is stockless purchasing practiced for the pertinent departmental purchases?
21. Are standardized requests for quotations and bids utilized for substantiating buying decisions and for developing and maintaining a vendor file?
22. Are warranties and guarantees utilized until fully expired?
23. Are there policies and procedures in reference to departmental visitation by sales representatives?
24. Is there a published list of approved vendors that the hospital does business with?
25. Is there a skilled and competent negotiator involved with the purchasing process?
26. Are there policies and procedures for conformance with the prudent buyer concept?

Receiving

1. Is there a set of policies and procedures for the receiving process?
2. Is there a specified person in charge of all receiving?
3. Is the receiving process centralized?
4. Are deliveries of major purchases scheduled in advance with the receiving area?
5. Are supplies that were ordered without a purchase order ever received?
6. Do all of the departments know about the receiving policies and procedures?
7. Are they adhered to?
8. Are all quantities of supplies ordered blanked out on the receiving copy of the purchase order?

9. Is there proper filing of all receiving documents along with back-order documentation?
10. Are all back orders routinely reviewed to ensure their proper delivery?
11. Does the receiving program provide for accurate and prompt receiving so that accounting can take advantage of earned discounts?
12. Is there a receiving procedure for equipment brought into the hospital on evaluation?
13. Is shipping a part of the receiving program?
14. Are there policies and procedures for returned goods?
15. Are there effective internal controls in reference to the receiving process?
16. Is the receiving process checked periodically for the proper accounting of received goods?
17. Are supplies ever left on the receiving dock overnight or over weekends?
18. Are there policies and procedures for receiving radioactive materiel?
19. Are there policies and procedures for handling damaged goods?
20. Is there sufficient space for properly receiving supplies and equipment?
21. Is there a mechanism for receiving goods and services after regular hours and on weekends?
22. Are only authorized personnel allowed into the receiving area?
23. Are proper security measures taken in the receiving area?
24. Does the hospital receive goods and equipment for areas other than the hospital such as physicians' offices, the gift shop, etc.?
25. Is there a training and orientation program for the receiving personnel?

Supply, Process, and Distribution

1. Are there effective current maximums and minimums for all approved supplies?
2. Are physical inventories taken at least every six months?
3. Is supply cost coded and dated before being put in the central stores?
4. Has a total inventory maximum for the central stores area been established by administration?

5. Has official and unofficial inventory been defined in your hospital?
6. Are unofficial inventories physically taken at least annually?
7. Is an in-use linen inventory taken at least annually?
8. Are all supplies broken down into issue units before being placed in central stores?
9. Is there a thorough and frequent cleaning schedule for the central stores area?
10. Have all supply, process and distribution functions been amalgamated into one area?
11. Does a supply item have to be reviewed and approved by the products standardization committee before it is placed in central stores?
12. Is central processing under the supervision of a trained and capable supervisor?
13. Does central processing meet and exceed all of the pertinent JCAH standards?
14. Are there written procedures for the processing of all trays and instruments?
15. Are separate soiled and clean divisions of the central processing area maintained?
16. Are autoclaves and sterilizers maintained on a frequent preventive maintenance schedule?
17. Have policies and procedures for the entire SPD department been delineated and distributed to the appropriate personnel?
18. Is a total supply-cart exchange program utilized for supply distribution?
19. Are cart-supply quotas reviewed and revised on a frequent basis (at least quarterly) by the appropriate materiel and nursing personnel?
20. Do nurses and unit personnel ever come to SPD to pick up supplies?
21. Is the SPD area open and staffed seven days a week, 24 hours per day?
22. Is an effective supply charge system maintained for all supplies issued from SPD?
23. Does a lost-charge report go to nursing and administration at least monthly?
24. Do the supply carts contain all supplies for an entire nursing unit?
25. Has all other supply inventory, except what is on the supply carts, been removed from the nursing units?

Chapter 7—The Pharmacy

OVERVIEW

The hospital pharmacy has the role of manufacturing, compounding, and dispensing drugs and other diagnostic and therapeutic chemical substances that may be used in the hospital. Smaller hospitals may not have a regular pharmacy department; they may purchase items from a local pharmacist and maintain only a limited supply under lock and key. In larger hospitals, a full-time pharmacist is available, sometimes with one or two assistants. The pharmacist who heads the pharmacy department must be licensed and be able to provide a full range of pharmacy activities. Whether the pharmacy department manufactures certain solutions or drugs is a matter of hospital policy.

Though the pharmacy and therapeutics committee (see box on page 256) recommends the standard drugs to be dispensed in the hospital, it is the pharmacist's responsibility in the vast majority of hospitals to select the brand or supplier of drug dispensed for all medication orders and prescriptions unless a specific notation to the contrary is made by the prescriber.*

Pharmacy Director: Job Duties**

● Supervises and coordinates activities of personnel in hospital pharmacy, and compounds

---

*Source: Edward D. Sanderson, *Hospital Purchasing and Inventory Management,* Aspen Systems Corporation, 1982.

**Source: *Job Descriptions and Organizational Analysis for Hospitals and Related Health Services,* U.S. Training and Employment Service, Department of Labor, 1971.

and dispenses medications by means of standard physical and chemical procedures to fill written medication and prescription requests issued by physicians, dentists, and other qualified prescribers.

● Plans, organizes, and supervises activities in hospital pharmacy according to hospital policies, standard practices of the profession, and State and Federal laws. Interviews, employs, and orients trained Pharmacists. Establishes work schedules and assigns Pharmacists to specified areas of responsibility in the administration, dispensing, or preparation functions of the department. Supervises work performance of the Pharmacists and related personnel to insure adherence to established standards.

● Supervises and, as necessary, assists Pharmacists in compounding and dispensing medications to fill written prescriptions and medication requests. Reviews written prescriptions to determine that overdoses or toxic compounds will not result from prescribed ingredients. Weighs, measures, and mixes ingredients or prepares medications through such procedures as blending, filtering, distilling, emulsifying, and titrating. Selects prepackaged pharmaceuticals from pharmacy stock when available. Places compounded medications in bottles, capsules, or other package form and types and affixes labels to container showing identifying data and instructions for use. Completes written records of each prescription filled for pharmacy files; for control file on narcotics, poisons, and habit-forming drugs; or for billing purposes of the Financial Management Department.

● Supervises inventory of pharmacy stock periodically, to determine stock needed and assure use of stock before expiration date recommended by manufacturer. Places orders for supplies with salesmen or drug wholesalers, verifies receipt of merchandise, and approves bills for payment by Financial Management or Purchasing and Receiving.

• Maintains formularies, sources of information on preparations, standard compendia on pharmaceuticals, reference texts, and journals in department for use of qualified personnel. Consults with and advises medical staff concerning information obtained on medications, such as warnings issued on drugs currently on the market, incompatibility of certain drugs, or contraindications of drugs or other pharmaceuticals.

• Initiates, develops, and carries out rules and regulations pertaining to administrative and professional policies of department with the approval and cooperation of hospital administration and Pharmacy and Therapeutics (P & T) Committee, respectively. Establishes and maintains system of records and bookkeeping in accordance with hospital policy for recording patients' charges for prescriptions and pharmaceutical supplies and for maintaining adequate controls over requisitioning and dispensing of all pharmaceuticals, including control file of narcotics, poisons, and habit-forming drugs received and issued. May serve as member of hospital Pharmacy and Therapeutics Committee in formulating department policies.

• Prepares departmental budget.

• May serve on civic committees to inform public on uses and abuses of drugs.

Pharmacy Technician: Job Duties*

Under the supervision of the pharmacist, assists in the technical aspects of preparing and dispensing medications. Duties include the following: Maintaining patient medication profile records; setting-up, packaging, labeling, and distributing medication doses; filling and dispensing routine orders for stock supplies of patient care units; maintaining inventories of drugs and supplies; mixing drugs with parietal fluids and related aseptic manipulations; and packaging and manufacturing drugs.

*Source: *Industry Wage Survey: Hospitals and Nursing Homes, September 1978,* Bureau of Labor Statistics, Bulletin 2069, November 1980.

HOSPITAL FORMULARY SYSTEM*

Since the typical patient receives approximately ten prescription orders during each confinement, the potential role of a formulary in supporting both rational drug therapy and cost-containment merits critical review.

A formulary represents the official compilation of drug products that have been sanctioned for use within a given environment. A list of preparations found on the pharmacy shelf, or a printout of drug orders dispensed during a recent time period, cannot be construed as a formulary.

When a drug list is expanded beyond "what is available" to include one or more specifications indicating "how a product should be used," the realm of the "formulary" has been entered. Several formularies merely designate the recommended daily dosage while others, routinely or selectively, add information on cautions, warnings, restrictions, pharmacology and similar aids to facilitate appropriate use.

The Formulary Manual

More than 80 percent of the large hospitals place limited or extended compilation of authorized products within a manual that includes one or more supplemental sections. These sections describe how the drug list/formulary was prepared: procedures for amendment; prescribing regulations established by the institution; technical aids, rules and advice to facilitate cost-containment efforts; services offered by the pharmacy department; special instructions covering therapeutic categories or particular pharmaceutical products; data on selected medical conditions; and/or hospital regulations.

Regardless of the manual's scope, the approved pharmaceutical preparations constitute the central component which is commonly referred to as the "drug monograph section."

The Formulary System

The administrative process by which the drug list/formulary and manual is implemented is

*Source: T. Donald Rucker, "Effective Formulary Development: Which Direction?" *Topics in Hospital Pharmacy Management,* May 1981.

called a formulary system. Although procedures vary by institution, the system, at a minimum, involves (a) an organized method by which a committee composed primarily of practitioners evaluates the therapeutic credentials of competing drug products; (b) periodic publication of the authorized preparations; (c) methods for revising the list; (d) interim communication techniques—usually the drug bulletin—to inform members of the medical, pharmacy, nursing and administrative staff regarding modifications in approved drugs and drug use policies; and (e) guidelines controlling the use of drugs outside the formulary such as nonformulary items and investigational products.

Organization

Drug approval may be based upon one or more of the following criteria: relative safety and efficacy, economic advantages, administrative ends and a residual category labeled "all other reasons." Since an optimum formulary implies that no other combination of therapeutic agents will yield a higher level of patient health, it is evident that the question of drug acceptance must be addressed first before additional factors are employed.

Flexibility

A hospital formulary must be able to carry unique products sufficient to accommodate the medical needs of its service population. Flexibility also implies that certain therapeutic categories may require auxiliary items to provide treatment options for controlling patient conditions that are not responsive to the drugs of first or second choice.

Flexibility also recognizes that some pharmaceutical preparations—perhaps no more than a dozen—may be admitted to the formulary to satisfy "political considerations" within the institution. It should be equally apparent that any such additions, along with all nonformulary drugs, become prime candidates for follow-up studies under a drug utilization review program.

Updating

The formulary should be updated and revised frequently to reflect scientific advances in both product discovery and clinical usage.

Reliance on a periodic drug bulletin is a very ineffective means of updating the formulary after 18 to 24 months have elapsed. A complete revision of these formularies should be undertaken at least every two years.

Limitations

The formulary should not be expected to serve as a surrogate for institutional drug policy. Formularies cannot be held accountable for the prescribing of agents for unlabeled or unapproved conditions, excessive use of drugs admitted for reserve purposes, selection of the most appropriate dosage form, ensuring the appropriate duration of therapy and so forth. Thus it is imperative that the P&T committee, or companion authority, conduct related programs designed to attain rational drug therapy.

Secondly, the administrator and hospital staff should not be led to embrace a formulary on the premise that all cost-containment problems pertaining to pharmaceuticals have been brought under control. Although restricting prescribing orders to the drugs-of-choice model will generate savings in the areas of pharmacy expense and total patient cost, a formulary is not a substitute for prudent purchasing policy, the prospective impact that clinical pharmacists located on the floor can have on rational prescribing, the gains inherent in a continuing program of drug utilization review, the benefits of a unit dose distribution system, or the services of a drug information center. In fact, a formulary may be a prerequisite for realizing several of these objectives.

Factors Influencing Drug Selection

Direct factors influencing which drugs will be carried on the formulary include: type of medical problems seen at the institution; general administrative policies established by the P&T committee; screening criteria that have been adopted to determine product acceptance; scope and quality of documentation efforts developed to support formulary changes; and the fidelity with which committee members follow established protocols in making their decisions.

An approach to the development of screening criteria is found in the explicit standards used by a highly ranked hospital formulary:

1. it is the only drug that is effective for the purpose used;
2. it is superior to other drugs in use because:
   - it is effective for all patients, or for selected patients, taking into consideration variations in patient response
   - it causes decreased toxicity, or greater patient tolerance
   - it is less expensive although as effective as other agents
   - it is easy to administer

Cost Efficiency

Can a formulary based upon the drugs-of-choice model simultaneously support cost-containment goals? Fortunately, a formulary maximizing therapeutic criteria also will minimize the number of chemical products maintained on the shelf. Deviations from this model, of course, automatically lead to an increase in inventory expense. This point is illustrated by the findings of a national study where the poorest performing formulary carried nearly four times as many dosage forms as the best one.

Furthermore, a well-controlled formulary will yield an economic bonus due to higher turnover per drug. Thus many products may be purchased in larger rather than standard quantities. Finally, the concept of relative safety and efficacy supports maximum efficiency in helping patients regain their health.

Additional economic implications arise when product interchangeability is considered within the context of therapeutic equivalency. Not only can savings be effected by listing the cheaper equivalent item, as in the case of cephalosporins and total parenteral nutrition, but by enforcing a tight policy in the procurement of nonformulary items as well. In this latter instance, one investigation reported a net saving of nearly $3.00 per prescription and about $6.40 per order when adjusted to reflect authorized refills.

Pharmacy and Therapeutics Committee*

The core of the formulary system is the pharmacy and therapeutics committee or equivalent committee composed of both pharmacists and physicians. The purposes, organization, and functions and scope of this committee are set forth in another professional policy document, the *Statement of the Pharmacy and Therapeutics Committee*, adopted by the American Society of Hospital Pharmacists and the American Hospital Association. It is also dealt with by the Joint Commission on Accreditation of Hospitals and the Social Security Administration. Basically, the duties of this committee are:

A. To serve in an advisory capacity to the medical staff and hospital administration in all matters pertaining to the use of drugs.

B. To serve in an advisory capacity to the medical staff and the pharmacist in the selection or choice of drugs which meet the most effective therapeutic quality standards.

C. To evaluate objectively clinical data regarding new drugs or agents proposed for use in the hospital.

D. To prevent unnecessary duplication of the same basic drug or its combinations.

E. To recommend additions and deletions from the list of drugs accepted for use in the hospital.

F. To develop a basic drug list or formulary of accepted drugs for use in the hospital and to provide for its constant revision.

G. To make recommendations concerning drugs to be stocked in hospital patient units or services.

H. To establish or plan suitable educational programs for the professional staff on pertinent matters related to drugs and their use.

I. To recommend policies regarding the safe use of drugs in hospitals, including a study of such matters as investigational drugs, hazardous drugs, and others.

J. To study problems involved in proper distribution and labeling of medications for inpatients and outpatients.

K. To study problems related to the administration of medications.

L. To review reported adverse reactions to drugs administered.

M. To evaluate periodically medical records in terms of drug therapy.

*Source: Carl T. DeMarco, *Pharmacy and the Law*, Aspen Systems Corporation, 1975, pp. 78–79.

DRUG DISTRIBUTION SYSTEM

Once the hospital receives the drugs, they must be distributed. Distribution is primarily to the nursing units where inpatients receive the majority of the drugs dispensed by the pharmacy.

Generally the drugs fall into one of three categories:*

1. Items sent to the nursing units for floor stock inventory. These are items regularly stored in the unit and not charged to the patients directly. Examples of such non-chargeable items are rubbing compounds and antiseptics for wounds and bandages.
2. Patient-chargeable stock items kept in the nursing unit. These include disposable enemas and other disposable external preparations.
3. Common prescription drugs that are dispensed and charged only upon the receipt of a prescription by a physician. This category of prescription drugs represents the vast majority of drugs used and also represents the greatest cost in the pharmacy.

Unit Dose Drug Distribution System**

The unit dose drug distribution system (UDDDS) represents a considerable refinement over the individual prescription order and ward stock methods of dispensing medications. It has been shown to be the safest, most efficient means of delivering drugs from the pharmacy department to the patient.

Hospitals should consider the implementation of a unit dose program because of its inherent advantages over traditional systems in packaging and systems improvement. The hospital will experience a reduction in medication errors, savings in nursing time associated with medication-related activities, and decreased raw drug costs.

Of course, these benefits should be balanced against capital equipment costs and increased pharmacy personnel requirements necessary to operate a unit dose system.

The starting point of the medication distribution cycle in UDDDS is the writing of the prescription order. The nurse removes the order from the chart and forwards it to the pharmacy; the pharmacy will interpret the order and profile

the medication on a patient profile card. This drug profile is maintained for every patient receiving drugs within the hospital.

A quantity of drug in ready-to-administer form, sufficient to last until the next time the unit dose cassettes containing each patient's medication drawer are exchanged, is sent to the nursing unit. The nurse places the initial quantity of drug in a patient drawer corresponding to his or her room number in the unit dose cart cassette. At a specified time each day the unit dose cassettes are exchanged by pharmacy personnel. Usually this occurs every 24 hours; however, in some hospitals cassettes are exchanged more frequently.

The pharmacy, in either case, will have placed enough doses of medication in the drawer of the cassettes for each patient on the unit to suffice until the next time the cassettes are exchanged. The nurse rolls the unit dose cart to each individual patient room, removes the dose of medication to be given from the patient drawer in the cart, and administers it to the patient.

The administration of the drug is recorded in the medication administration record at that time. A physician order will notify the pharmacy when the patient is to be discharged or the medication is discontinued. This alerts the pharmacy not to dispense any additional dosages to this patient. Under this system, medications are billed at the time of discharge or at the end of a specific time interval as required by the billing cycle.

Advantages

In a traditional distribution system the nurse must prepare the drug for administration. One of the major differences here is the dispensing of the drug by the pharmacy in a unit dose package. A unit dose package is defined as "one which contains the particular dose of the drug ordered for the patient."

Better Controls

Advantages of using unit dose packaging are many. The package identifies the drug name, strength, expiration date, etc. up to the point that it is administered to the patient. Liquids and injectables are more accurately measured because of the rigid controls utilized when repackaging medications in unit dose form. There are no such controls available to the nurse to ensure

---

*Source: Edward D. Sanderson, *Hospital Purchasing and Inventory Management*, Aspen Systems Corporation, 1982.

**Source: Larry S. Wrobel and David Burris, "Implementing Unit Dose Drug Distribution System," *Hospital Materiel Management Quarterly*, November 1980.

that every dose of medication is accurately prepared.

Minimum Waste

Drug waste when utilizing a unit dose package is minimized. Under a traditional system, when the medication is discontinued and the unused portion of a three- to five-day supply of the drug is returned to the pharmacy for safety reasons, it must be discarded. The unit dose package can be placed back into inventory, because the drug has been maintained in sanitary form. Packaging improvements in UDDDS reduce raw drug costs and increase patient safety.

Fewer Steps

There also are fewer steps involved in the unit dose system. The nursing staff no longer has to transcribe orders to a patient treatment and medication profile and medication card. The medication comes from the pharmacy in ready-to-administer form, and therefore nursing time spent in preparing doses is drastically reduced.

Charting is simplified because it is done immediately after the dose is administered to the patient instead of when medication rounds have been completed, as is the case in the traditional system. The need to reorder medications is eliminated since the pharmacy will automatically send to the nursing unit the amount of doses necessary for the next time period. The need to process credits no longer exists because the billing under a unit dose system is most commonly performed at the time of discharge.

Reduced Errors

Implementation of the UDDDS therefore results in a simpler and less complex method of dispensing drugs. This will lead to a system where there are checks to decrease the opportunity for making a mistake, and consequently a reduced potential for medication errors. The increase in patient safety occasioned by a reduction in medication errors is the single most important reason for implementing a unit dose system. A significant study compared errors of commission (drugs incorrectly administered to the patient) between a multidose dispensing and a computer-based unit dose system. Disguised observers in this study examined 428 doses given on the multidose dispensing unit and 1,243 given on the unit dose dispensing unit. The errors observed are indicated in Table 7-1.

The data in Table 7-1 categorically demonstrate that the unit dose system reduces medication errors.

Saved Time

Another major advantage of a unit dose system is the saving in nursing time associated with medication-related activities. Another study, conducted to quantify the time spent by nursing personnel in both the Unit Dose Drug Distribution System and traditional drug distribution system, showed that nursing time spent in medication-related activities was reduced by 50 percent.

Reduced Drug Costs

There are three primary ways in which UDDDS can reduce drug costs. First, drug inventory can be reduced by restricting drug storage to the pharmacy except for current drug doses, emergency drugs, and a few drugs needed on specialty nursing units. The pharmacy dispenses a one-day or less supply of medication as opposed to a three- to five-day supply. Fewer drugs are in the system; therefore, unofficial inventory of medications on the nursing units is decreased

Table 7-1   Percent Reduction in Medication Errors under a Unit Dose System

	Multidose	Unit Dose	Difference
Wrong dose given	5.32	0.56	4.76
Unordered drug given	1.26	0.40	0.86
Extra dose given	0.56	0.24	0.32
Time wrong ± 1 hour	9.80	4.02	5.78

Source: B. Means, H. Derewicz, and P. Lamy, "Medication Errors in a Multidose and Computer-Based Unit Dose Drug Distribution System." *American Journal of Hospital Pharmacy* 32:2 (February 1975) pp. 186–191.

significantly. Drug loss due to the discarding of unused portions of medications returned to the pharmacy after the drug is discontinued can be reduced.

Second, sound pharmacy practice dictates that any medication dispensed to a patient that was exposed to the environment must not be reused. Bulk tablets, liquids, unused portions of multidose injectable preparations, and any refrigerated medications are discarded when returned to the pharmacy. Under the unit dose system these medications are placed back into the pharmacy stock and redispensed. In addition, the increased controls in the system decrease pilferage.

Finally, certain supply items, such as medication cups, prescription labels and vials, and certain forms that are necessary under a traditional drug distribution system, do not have to be purchased.

As a result of the aforementioned factors, savings from $0.23 to $2.00 per patient day have been shown.

Comparative Costs

The advantages of the unit dose system must be compared to the costs involved in the operation of the program. The unit dose system requires a relatively large initial cash outlay for capital equipment. Primary costs involve the purchase of unit dose carts and packaging equipment. These costs are of a one-time nature, and when amortised over the life of the asset become almost negligible.

Personnel costs necessary to implement a unit dose system are of greater concern and are more difficult to justify. The unit dose system necessitates the hiring of additional pharmacy personnel because of the increased workload. However, the increased workload can be performed by pharmacy technicians as opposed to pharmacists. The pharmacist can then serve more effectively in a quality control capacity to monitor patient profiles for allergies, check for potential drug interactions, and review the work of pharmacy technicians. Some directors of pharmacy have justified the hiring of additional personnel by having a portion of the nursing personnel budget transferred to the pharmacy. The rationale for this is the estimated savings in nursing time caused by the implementation of the unit dose system.

Gaining Acceptance

Support from the medical staff, nursing staff, and pharmacy staff is essential before embarking on a unit dose system. A UDDDS can be justified to these groups on the basis that it will enhance patient care through the following:

1. Increased patient safety through decreased potential medication errors and adverse drug reactions.
2. Reduced time spent by the nursing staff in medication-related activities, thereby allowing more time for direct patient care.
3. Compliance with the JCAH standards for pharmacy distribution systems.
4. Participation of the pharmacist in drug monitoring services.
5. Control of pharmacy inventory and reduced drug cost per patient day.

Drug Distribution (JCAH Standard IV)*

Written policies and procedures that pertain to the intrahospital drug distribution system shall be developed by the director of the pharmaceutical department/service in concert with the medical staff and, as appropriate, with representatives of other disciplines.

Interpretation

Drug preparation and dispensing shall be restricted to a licensed pharmacist, or to his designee under the direct supervision of the pharmacist. A pharmacist should review the prescriber's order, or a direct copy thereof, before the initial dose of medication is dispensed (with the exception of emergency orders when time does not permit). In cases when the medication order is written when the pharmacy is "closed" or the pharmacist is otherwise unavailable, the medication order should be reviewed by the pharmacist as soon thereafter as possible, preferably within 24 hours.

The use of floor stock medications should be minimized; the unit dose drug distribution system, which permits identification of the drug up to the point of administration, is recommended for use throughout the hospital.

---

*Source: Joint Commission on Accreditation of Hospitals, *Accreditation Manual for Hospitals*, 1983 ed., Chicago, 1982. Reprinted by permission.

Written policies and procedures that are essential for patient safety and for the control, accountability, and intrahospital distribution of drugs shall be reviewed annually, revised as necessary, and enforced. Such policies and procedures shall include, but not be limited to, the following:

- All drugs shall be labeled adequately, including the addition of appropriate accessory or cautionary statements, as well as the expiration date when applicable.
- Discontinued and outdated drugs, and containers with worn, illegible, or missing labels, shall be returned to the pharmacy for proper disposition.
- Only a pharmacist, or authorized pharmacy personnel under the direction and supervision of a pharmacist, shall dispense medications, make labeling changes, or transfer medications to different containers.
- Only prepackaged drugs shall be removed from the pharmacy when a pharmacist is not available. These drugs shall be removed only by a designated registered nurse or a physician, and only in amounts sufficient for immediate therapeutic needs. Such drugs should be kept in a separate cabinet, closet, or other designated area and shall be properly labeled. A record of such withdrawals shall be made by the authorized individual removing such drugs and shall be verified by a pharmacist.
- There shall be a written drug recall procedure that can be implemented readily and the results documented. This requirement shall apply to both inpatient and ambulatory care patient medications.
- Drug product defects should be reported in accordance with the ASHP-USP-FDA Drug Product Problem Reporting Program.
- Medications to be dispensed to inpatients at the time of discharge from the hospital shall be labeled as for ambulatory care patient prescriptions.
- A system designed to assure accurate identification of ambulatory care patients at the time they receive prescribed medications should be established.
- Unless otherwise provided by law, ambulatory care patient prescription labels should bear the following information:
  - Name, address, and telephone number of the hospital pharmacy;
  - Date and pharmacy's identifying serial number for the prescription;
  - Full name of the patient;
  - Name of the drug, strength, and amount dispensed;
  - Directions to the patient for use;
  - Name of the prescribing practitioner;
  - Name or initials of the dispensing individual; and
  - Any required Drug Enforcement Administration cautionary label on controlled substance drugs, and any other pertinent accessory cautionary labels.
- In the interest of effective control, the distribution of drug samples within the hospital should be eliminated if possible. Sample drugs brought into the hospital shall be controlled through the pharmaceutical department/service.

A QUALITY ASSURANCE PROGRAM*

The complexity of the systems necessary to provide pharmacy services in a hospital would seem to mandate the development of a quality assurance program.

Here is how one hospital went about setting up such a program. First it agreed on four principles:

1. High-quality pharmaceutical services begin with established policies and procedures, which are adhered to during *all phases* of preparation or dispensing of the end product (U/D, I.V.s, purchasing, etc.).
2. A quality assurance program should determine the correlation between what is actually occurring in *all areas within a department* and what is stated in established policies and procedures.
3. Results from the quality assurance program should be used to evaluate the program or system being reviewed for the effectiveness of established policies and procedures and the department's personnel.
4. The audit of the quality assurance program becomes a repetitive cycle that constantly

---

*Source: Matthew J. Land et al., "A Comprehensive Quality Assurance Program for Hospital Pharmacy Departments," *Topics in Hospital Pharmacy Management,* November 1981.

measures compliance, evaluates departmental programs and systems, and guarantees a high-quality end product.

Criteria for the quality assurance program were then developed on the basis of the pharmacy department's existing policy and procedure manual, laws pertaining to pharmacy practice and published standards of practice.

Methodology of Complete Program

The entire pharmacy department is reviewed bimonthly except for processes for which monthly audits are desirable—e.g., small population size or better retrievability over a longer period of time. The review of nonformulary requests represents such a sample.

The Audit Form for Quality Assurance

The audit form (Figure 7-1) is used as a permanent record of each audit performed. On the quality assurance audit form the criteria are listed specifically and numbered for ease of identification. There is space for recording the relative compliance for each sample. Each sample is judged individually for compliance (+), noncompliance (−) or an inability to effectively measure (0). The consistent appearance of 0s indicated that the criterion needed to be reevaluated and restated for ease of measurement.

When the sample population is large, a sample of ten is randomly selected using a random numbers table for each audit period. Where populations are small, every sample must be assessed.

Each audit form has ample space for "comments" concerning judgments that need to be made during the audit or to define the nature of the deficiency. In some cases professional judgments must be made or additional information provided; however, certain criteria have been identified that can be sufficiently assessed by clerically oriented pharmacy technicians. These functions are handled by supportive personnel familiar with basic legal requirements and departmental policy, provided the quality assurance auditor is readily available for any questions. The quality assurance audit form is clearly marked as to which criteria may be assessed by a technician (T) versus a pharmacist (P). This facet of the program provides for a less biased audit and results in financial savings in terms of pharmacist time.

Certain audits of specific structures and processes have been scheduled to minimize disruptions in the daily work-flow pattern. For example, the inpatient department is reviewed before 8 A.M., when the volume of personnel and orders is minimal.

Criteria for Evaluation

All samples are evaluated for each audit on the basis of a predetermined standard. Standards have been set up in terms of percent compliances. For example, for criteria that are particularly critical to the system a standard of 100 percent is assigned. These include such things as correct labeling of drugs and medication bins. In some cases a range of acceptable compliance is permissible and standards are then set below 100 percent. The lowest standard set by the system is 75 percent and includes such criteria as the placement of the allergy and diagnosis on the patient profile. The standard in this particular case is not ranked higher because this information is often missing from the patient record.

Criteria which are judged on the basis of a set completion time were also assigned a standard below 100 percent and an acceptable time range was indicated for overall compliance.

Overall compliance ratings for each of the criteria are recorded on the quality assurance audit summary form (see Figure 7-2). This form provides an organized record of each of the audits completed and their corresponding dates identifying possible trends and patterns of noncompliance for each of the criteria. Follow-up actions to criteria that are not in compliance are also identified chronologically on the form, and each is surveyed for improvement. In this manner results of audits are compared on a regular basis and the effectiveness of follow-up action is evaluated more objectively.

Follow-Up Record

Each month a quality assurance follow-up record is generated. It is based on all audits completed for that month. The form identifies each audit period, dates of audits completed during that period and the name of the auditor. It also lists the criteria of noncompliance by reference number. Wherever overall compliance is identified as being substandard on the summary form, the original audit form is reviewed to complete the quality assurance follow-up record. In this

Figure 7-1 Quality assurance audit form

Process		Process criteria	Sample compliance					Standard %	Overall compliance	Comments
			1 2	3 4	5 6	7 8	9 10			
Patient profile system	T	a. Patient name, room number recorded on profile						100		
	T	b. Medication starting day indicated on top of profile						100		
	T	c. Patient number is readily available						100		
	P	d. Order transcribed into profile according to protocol • transcription date • automatic stop order date • generic name • strength and dose • interval • mode • initials • doses/bin • "PRN" separated • anticoagulants "on call" • schedules less than every other day noted								
	T	e. Additional profiles initiated as required by protocol						100		
	P	f. PRN orders • entered at bottom • dosing interval • minimal doses available						100		
	P	g. Discontinued drugs yellowed out						100		
	P	h. Change orders entered as new order						100		
	T	i. Unexpired automatic stop order dating						100		
	T	j. Stat single doses and topical preparations in miscellaneous section with details						100		
	T	k. Old profile cards labeled DEAD						100		

Structure: _____ 1.   6.
Date: _____ 2.   7.
Auditor: _____ 3.   8.
Sample identification: _____ 4.   9.
    5.   10.

Source: Matthew J. Land et al., "A Comprehensive Quality Assurance Program for Hospital Pharmacy Departments," *Topics in Health Pharmacy Management,* November 1981.

Figure 7-2 Audit summary form

Structure: patient profile system

Process criteria	Date	Overall compliance								
		7/14	8/5	8/15	8/26					
a. Patient name and room number		100	100	100	100					
b. Medication starting date		100	80	100	100					
c. Patient number		70	90	90	100					
d. Order transcribed		90	95	100	100					
e. Additional profiles		100	100	100	100					
f. PRN orders		100	100	100	100					
g. Discontinued drugs yellowed out		100	100	100	100					
h. Change orders		100	100	100	100					
i. Unexpired automatic stop order		90	90	90	100					
j. Miscellaneous section		100	100	100	100					
k. Old profiles labeled		100	100	100	100					

Source: Matthew J. Land et al., "A Comprehensive Quality Assurance Program for Hospital Pharmacy Departments," *Topics in Health Pharmacy Management*, November 1981.

manner time is conserved by focusing only on necessary audit form entries. Criteria that are not in compliance are reported in terms of positive recommendations directed toward correcting deficiencies to the administrator or supervisor. The original copy of this form is then submitted to the appropriate departmental administrator for follow-up action and dating. A copy of all materials is retained by the quality assurance auditor.

When Noncompliance Calls for Fast Action

In instances where noncompliance is serious enough to warrant immediate action, the area administrator is notified in an urgent action communication form. Examples of applicable situations include the lack of removal of outdated or damaged medications, incorrect labeling, and quick resolution and prevention of potential problems in patient care.

Data generated from each audit are then given to each of the primary pharmacists working on a regular basis in the area audited. The primary pharmacist presents the results of the audit at the monthly staff meeting for open discussion. The area administrator then documents all actions completed to correct noncompliance or deficiencies in the systems. Documentation of all meetings, policy and procedure revisions, corrections, etc., is included on the monthly follow-up record and is used as a permanent record for JCAH and other inspections.

MANAGEMENT CONTROLS

Cost Consciousness*

The pharmacy usually ranks in the top three revenue-producing departments of the hospital. It therefore carries a heavy burden to maximize its revenues while minimizing expenses.

*Source: Frank M. Braden, "Viewpoint: Hospital Pharmacys' Changing Role," *Topics in Hospital Pharmacy Management*, May 1981.

There are many avenues to approach this end: the introduction of therapeutic equivalents and formularies, the use of less skilled technicians, the application of computer profiles, the utilization of computerized billing, and inventory control offer other ways of maximizing revenues and minimizing expenses.

Specifically, the hospital pharmacy must maximize reimbursement. The pharmacist must be aware of maximum allowable charges, what is not currently being reimbursed at this level and what should be reimbursed at this level to cover costs and produce the needed profit for the hospital.

Another area that demands innovative management is cost control. The first step should be to institute a generic therapeutic substitutions formulary. Competitive bidding with a best-buy list (a listing of vendors that will offer the best overall price and service to the hospital) must also be instituted. This should be accomplished with group purchasing which offers real cost savings.

Loss prevention is another area that the pharmacy must embrace. Good accounting-control systems to minimize the loss of revenue must be instituted. The pharmacy has several unique problems in this area. First is the high volume of individual revenue items. Second, the pharmacy's revenue items are not all stored within the physical confines of the pharmacy department. The goal must be to turn these dispersed drug inventories into revenue rather than operating costs through loss.

Purchasing*

In 1977 the U.S. General Accounting Office (GAO), with assistance from the American Hospital Association, surveyed 21 short-term general-purpose hospitals concerning pharmaceutical costs.

The study found that:

- "Pharmaceutical purchasing improvements . . . lagged behind the improvements made in the hospitals' general purchasing activities."

---

*Source: Fred M. Eckel and James C. MacAllister, "Impact and Implications of the GAO Report on Hospital Purchasing Practices," *Topics in Hospital Pharmacy Management*, August 1981.

- "Procedures were generally very informal" because "purchases were often made by simply calling a vendor when stocks were low and ordering what was needed."
- "Decisions on what constituted low stock and how much to order were based on judgment with no formal criteria and few records to guide the decisions."

The study concluded that "regardless of which department purchases pharmaceuticals, sound purchasing principles should be followed. Thus, hospitals should assure that formal purchasing and inventory control procedures consistent with those used for its general purchases are developed for pharmaceuticals. These procedures should include a system of internal controls to safeguard the integrity of all transactions and a mechanism for monitoring the pharmacy's purchasing performance. Maximum advantage should be taken of cost reducing techniques, such as group purchasing and competitive bidding."

The study lends support to administrators and purchasing agents who wish to remove authority and responsibility for purchasing pharmaceuticals from the pharmacy. While the report briefly recognizes the specialized nature of pharmaceutical purchasing, it is clear that the pharmacist is not recognized as possessing adequate purchasing expertise. Competitive bidding, standardization, group purchasing, accountability and control practices were some of the areas identified as major weaknesses in pharmacy purchasing.

Administrators and purchasing agents may eventually insist that greater cost reductions can be achieved if responsibility for pharmaceutical purchasing is assumed by institutional purchasing agents.

This philosophy should not necessarily threaten the pharmacist. If the pharmacist continues to make the basic decisions on acceptable vendors, drug products available and inventory required, and the purchasing agent officially negotiates contracts, then the best possible situation exists. It establishes the pharmacist as the professional and primary decision maker while creating an atmosphere of fairness and non-favoritism.

Another useful publication is a GAO checklist and audit guide titled:

Checklist and Guidelines for Evaluating Purchasing and Materials Management

Functions in Private Hospitals—Opportunities for Improving Hospital Purchasing, Inventory Management, and Supply Distribution, Part II (PSAD-79-58B) (Washington, D.C.: GAO, April 1979).

The checklist format promotes an organized, constructive and systematic procedure for evaluating purchasing functions. The audit section describes how to complete the checklist for each function. The checklist and companion audit guide are management tools that can be used effectively by hospital administrators, managers and auditors in gathering information, surfacing problems, and improving purchasing and other materials management functions. It also could form the basis for a quality-assurance program in pharmacy purchasing and inventory control.

Theft in Pharmacy*

Like a cashier's booth, a pharmacy in these days of lucrative narcotics traffic is vulnerable to theft not only by employees, but by violent intruders. Holdups and burglaries may not be very frequent, but they do occur and their success is essentially dependent upon the precautions in existence.

Pharmacy thefts have spread with the proliferation of satellite pharmacies, a definite trend in hospital construction and renovation. While the unit dose system may have reduced the total volume of critical drugs in accessible patient care areas, concentration of the drugs has spread with the dispersion of satellites. There are more targets for holdups and burglaries.

Safeguards

In large installations there is usually a back door leading to a deserted corridor where the drug shipments arrive. These areas are highly vulnerable to theft. To protect against collusive removal of drugs in quantity, as well as against holdups and burglaries, a wide range of measures are available. These range from panic buttons and bulletproof teller windows to videotape television cameras, conventional burglary alarms and sophisticated intrusion detectors.

In the central pharmacy it is also essential to protect the receiving process from theft. Dual verification prior to payment of the manufacturer's and distributor's invoices is vital. At the same time steps must be taken to prevent messengers or delivery staff from removing quantities of drugs and pharmaceutical products from the pharmacy. Therefore, an alarm and television surveillance installation is sometimes an advisable step.

Purchasing Process

Even with these protective measures, the purchasing process remains vulnerable. Substantial losses may continue for a long time without being discovered if the pharmacy director or whoever is responsible for purchasing is in collusion with vendors or manipulates to supply privately owned drug stores from hospital stock. This is particularly true if the stock is diverted in the receiving process. Such activities are not infrequent.

But even with a strong purchasing department, to exercise meaningful control over the procurement of drugs is a difficult task. The trend of automating staple drug purchases is likely to prove a step in the right direction, not only improving the efficiency and reducing payroll cost, but also narrowing the risks.

Productivity*

Hospital pharmacy computer systems provide a data collection capability significantly beyond the range of the manual systems they replace. Increased data collection capability creates the conditions necessary for implementation of effective management control systems.

The majority of pharmacy productivity reporting systems compare units dispensed to labor hours expended. Hospital pharmacy computer systems generally have the capability to economically collect the workload statistics either per shift, per day, per week or per month. Capabilities for payroll interface and report generation are generally available only through an institution-wide system supported by the hospital's in-house computer.

---

*Source: Walter Nagel, "Health Care Industry's Vulnerability to Theft," *Topics in Health Care Financing,* Winter 1978.

*Source: Christopher Adams, Beverly A. Tuck, and Max L. Hunt, Jr., "Departmental Productivity through Computerized Systems," *Topics in Hospital Pharmacy Management,* February 1982.

In one community hospital, Lutheran General Hospital, a 700-bed teaching hospital located in northwest suburban Chicago, pharmacy services are provided 24 hours per day through a centralized pharmacy. A pharmacy satellite serves the critical care units. The total personnel budget includes approximately 70 full-time equivalents (FTEs).

Lutheran General Hospital initiated an institution-wide productivity reporting system in 1978:

- to support managers' requests for additional resources; and
- to highlight opportunities for improved use and allocation of personnel.

Choosing the minimum number of output measures to represent the maximum amount of pharmacy workload is the key to an efficient control system.

Nine output statistics are recorded at Lutheran: inpatient orders filled in central pharmacy, inpatient orders filled in satellite pharmacy, outpatient orders, I.V. admixtures filled in central pharmacy, I.V. admixtures filled in satellite pharmacy, adult TPNs, perinatal TPNs, hours providing clinical services and hours for special projects and liaison.

Tracking by job position provides a sufficiently large aggregation to minimize distortion created by persons performing functions that are not regularly assigned while, simultaneously, focusing on the productivity levels of specific work groups.

Degree of Precision

Standard times are the core element of a productivity reporting system. They are also the average time in hours required to perform one unit of workload volume. Standard times are multiplied by workload volumes to obtain required hours. Required hours are then compared to available hours to yield a utilization rate. The formula is as follows:

Utilization rate =

$$\frac{(\text{workload volume}) \times (\text{standard time})}{\text{available hours}} \times 100$$

This utilization rate is always expressed as a percentage (e.g., 95 percent).

Productivity reporting system validity is an important factor in system acceptance. Validity is dependent on the accuracy of the standard times forming the system parameters. Work methods, physical location and service mix vary by hospital, and therefore internally developed standards usually reflect more accurately the time required and thus help ensure system acceptance.

The appropriate methodology for standards development is a result of the number of times a function is performed and the number of people performing the function. Various methods of developing standard times are available.

- Time study or work sampling is generally appropriate for functions performed many times by many people—for example, unit dose dispensing. (Personal, fatigue and delay allowances of 15 percent, as well as a break allowance of 6.7 percent, were established at Lutheran General Hospital as part of hospital policy.)
- Self-logging is generally appropriate for functions performed many times by few people—for example, prepackaging. This assumes that a high degree of trust is placed in the employees doing the logging. (A 6.7 percent break allowance would be added.)
- Estimation is generally appropriate for functions performed relatively few times— for example, cleaning the pharmacy. (A 6.7 percent break allowance would be added.)

Segmentation of Information

The first level of reporting segments workload volume, required hours, available hours and utilization rates by program and job position to constitute a detailed report. The second level of reporting displays program and job position subtotals on a summary report for quick review of each pharmacy unit. This summary report is further distilled to track key factors for major units within the pharmacy.

Three levels of reporting allow for different management control at different management levels. The detail report is used most effectively by pharmacy supervisors, the summary report is used most effectively by pharmacy assistant directors and the key factor report is used most effectively by the pharmacy director and hospital administration.

Setting of Limits

Control systems need formal limits to highlight deviations that signal operational problems. The indicator for pharmacy productivity is the utilization rate range. Utilization rate ranges can be set by using 100 percent as the base point, and standards can be modified upward or downward to account for productivity changes. Alternatively, the utilization rate range can be modified downward to account for day-to-day workload peaks or it can be modified upward to account for expectations of improved productivity. For example, the pharmacy's base point is 97.5 percent with the utilization rate range constituting plus or minus 7.5 percent or 90 to 105 percent.

The determination of utilization rate limits ultimately becomes a negotiated process between pharmacy management and hospital administration. All considerations of medical care cost and quality trade-offs are not amenable to quantifiable resolution.

Communication of Information

For limits to be used effectively by the pharmacy manager a consensus must exist between the manager and hospital administrator. Once consensus is achieved, pharmacy utilization rates can be used as managerial shorthand to speed and enhance decision making. Hospital administrators are trained in the use of quantitative analyses. These analyses assist the administrator in sorting out objective facts from subjective impressions.

Cost-Effectiveness

Pharmacy productivity reporting has been used successfully by pharmacy management for both operational and strategic planning. It was used to plan FTE requirements for new unit dose and satellite pharmacy programs, to justify staffing increases because of increased workload and to reallocate staff more equitably within the central pharmacy. The pharmacy productivity reporting system ensures that all areas of the pharmacy are functioning productively and that no area is overutilized to the extent that patient service and patient safety are jeopardized. Pharmacy is also prepared to respond to the increased reporting and justificational requirements that a state rate-review program may require.

Management Audit

For a review of the factors involved in a complete management audit of the pharmacy department, see Table 7-2.

PHARMACY AND THE LAW*

Hospital Liability

In providing drugs to patients, hospitals may incur criminal or civil liability. As an employer of pharmacists, nurses, and physicians, hospitals also may be liable for the acts of these professionals or employees under their control.

The hospital will be liable not only for negligence occurring in the pharmacy, but also for negligence in the handling and administration of drugs anywhere in the hospital.

The pharmacist, as well as the hospital, may incur vicarious liability based upon the acts or omissions of hospital employees under his control and supervision. There could be liability for the improper selection, training or supervision of technicians. Written standards and a policy and procedure manual should be developed for selection, training and supervision of personnel. Formal academic training and state certification are also desirable safeguards against liability.

Use of Support Personnel

In a hospital pharmacy supportive personnel may be used as called for by the standards of the Joint Commission on Accreditation of Hospitals and the federal government's Medicare regulations. However, such personnel may not direct or manage a hospital pharmacy. Nor may they exercise the consultative or decisional powers of the pharmacist concerning compounding, dispensing and drug usage. Their tasks should be restricted to manipulative or mechanical tasks with appropriate checks and quality controls in effect.

Clinical Pharmacy

In addition to the traditional activities of drug ordering, preparation, distribution, pharmacy administration, and recordkeeping, hospital

---

*Source: David G. Warren, *Problems in Hospital Law,* 3rd ed., Aspen Systems Corporation, 1978.

Table 7-2 Management Audit of the Pharmacy Department

Practice	Yes	No	Proposed Plan of Action	Responsible Parties
1. Is the pharmacy under the direction of a trained, competent pharmacist?				
2. Is the pharmacy open and staffed 24 hours per day, seven days per week?				
3. Are code blue carts processed in the SPD area?				
4. Does the pharmacy meet or exceed all of the pertinent JCAH standards?				
5. Are all drugs unit dosed from the pharmacy?				
6. Are drugs supplied to all nursing units via the cart-exchange or transfer program?				
7. Are all pharmaceuticals purchased through the central purchasing program?				
8. Is there an effective pharmacy and therapeutics committee?				
9. Is there an effective drug formulary that is kept up to date?				
10. Are there effective policies and procedures for drug recalls?				
11. Is a physical inventory taken in the pharmacy at least semiannually?				
12. Is there a total pharmacy inventory maximum that has been established and enforced by administration?				
13. Is there an effective charge procedure established for drugs?				
14. Does the total inventory in the pharmacy turn at least 18 times per year?				
15. Do nurses and unit personnel ever come to the pharmacy to pick up drugs?				
16. Is the I.V. admixture program supervised and operated by the pharmacy?				
17. Is there a drug information system?				
18. Has an effective orientation program for hospital and pharmacy personnel been established?				
19. Is there a clinical pharmacy program?				

Table 7-2　continued

Practice	Yes	No	Proposed Plan of Action	Responsible Parties
20. Is there a policy and procedure for outdated drugs?				
21. Are drugs purchased through group purchasing endeavors?				
22. Are generic equivalents approved by the pharmacy and therapeutics committee?				
23. Have therapeutic equivalents been established by the pharmacy and therapeutics committee?				
24. Does the pharmacy operate within or below its established budget?				

Source: Charles E. Housley, "Evaluating the Effectiveness of the Materiel Management Effect," *Hospital Materiel Management Quarterly,* August 1979.

pharmacists are becoming involved in other activities generically referred to as "clinical pharmacy." "Clinical pharmacy" includes activities such as taking medication histories, monitoring drug use, contributing to drug therapy, drug selection, patient counseling, drug administration programs, and surveillance for adverse reactions and drug interactions. In addition to improving patient care or providing it more efficiently, these activities are important from a legal standpoint and may possibly create problems regarding scope of practice under professional practice acts.

Drug Laws

The entire stock of the hospital pharmacy is subject to governmental control at all levels, but perhaps the most rigidly regulated items are the various drugs. It is imperative that the administrator, pharmacist, medical staff and all employees who are authorized to deal with drugs understand the manner in which they are regulated. The hospital attorney should be prepared to aid in the interpretation of laws and regulations dealing with drugs, and he should keep the administrator informed of changes and revisions as they affect the hospital.

New and Investigational Drugs

The general law of negligence governs in cases involving use of new drugs in a way other than provided for in the official labeling. In applying these principles to hospital practice, it appears prudent for a pharmacist to question a physician prescribing a drug in a manner that deviates substantially from the package insert. In really questionable cases, an acknowledgment and assumption of liability form could be obtained from the physician to provide protection to the pharmacist and hospital and possibly serve as an element in the defense of any subsequent liability suit.

Controlled Substances

The Comprehensive Drug Abuse Prevention and Control Act of 1970, commonly known as the Controlled Substances Act, replaced virtually all pre-existing federal laws dealing with narcotics, depressants, stimulants and hallucinogens.

Hospitals are included under regulations that implement the Controlled Substances Act as "institutional practitioners," and as such must register with the government in accordance with the provisions of the Act. Each registrant must take a physical inventory every two years. In maintaining inventory records a perpetual inventory is not required. However, a separate inventory is required for each registered location and for each independent activity which is registered. In addition to inventory records, each registrant must maintain complete accurate records of all controlled substances received and disposed of.

All registrants must provide effective controls and procedures to guard against theft and diversion of controlled substances.

STANDARDS

Safe Administration of Drugs (JCAH Standard V)*

Written policies and procedures governing the safe administration of drugs and biologicals shall be developed by the medical staff in cooperation with the pharmaceutical department/service, the nursing service, and, as necessary, representatives of other disciplines.

Interpretation

Written policies and procedures governing the safe administration of drugs shall be reviewed at least annually, revised as necessary, and enforced. Such policies and procedures shall include, but not necessarily be limited to, the following.

- Drugs shall be administered only upon the order of a member of the medical staff, an authorized member of the house staff, or other individual who has been granted clinical privileges to write such orders. Verbal orders for drugs may be accepted only by personnel so designated in the medical staff rules and regulations and must be authenticated by the prescribing practitioner within the stated period of time.
- All medications shall be administered by, or under the supervision of, appropriately licensed personnel in accordance with laws and governmental rules and regulations governing such acts and in accordance with the approved medical staff rules and regulations.
- There shall be an automatic cancellation of standing drug orders when a patient undergoes surgery. Automatic drug stop orders shall otherwise be determined by the medical staff and stated in medical staff rules

and regulations. There shall be a system to notify the responsible practitioner of the impending expiration of a drug order, so that the practitioner may determine whether the drug administration is to be continued or altered.
- Cautionary measures for the safe admixture of parenteral products shall be developed. Whenever drugs are added to intravenous solutions, a distinctive supplementary label shall be affixed to the container. The label shall indicate the patient's name and location; the name and amount of the drug(s) added; the name of the basic parenteral solution; the date and time of the addition; the date, time, and rate of administration; the name or identifying code of the individual who prepared the admixture; supplemental instructions; and the expiration date of the compounded solution.
- Drugs to be administered shall be verified with the prescribing practitioner's orders and properly prepared for administration. The patient shall be identified prior to drug administration, and each dose of medication administered shall be recorded properly in the patient's medical record.
- Medication errors and adverse drug reactions shall be reported immediately in accordance with written procedures. This requirement shall include notification of the practitioner who ordered the drug. An entry of the medication administered and/or the drug reaction shall be properly recorded in the patient's medical record. Hospitals are encouraged to report any unexpected or significant adverse reactions promptly to the Food and Drug Administration and to the manufacturer.
- Drugs brought into the hospital by patients shall not be administered unless the drugs have been identified by the attending physician, another responsible prescribing practitioner, or a pharmacist (preferably the hospital pharmacist), and unless there is a written order from the responsible practitioner to administer the drugs. If the drugs are not to be used during the patient's hospitalization, they should be packaged and sealed, and either given to the patient's family or stored and returned to the patient at the time of discharge, provided such action is approved by the responsible practitioner.

---

*Source: Joint Commission on Accreditation of Hospitals, *Accreditation Manual for Hospitals,* 1983 ed., Chicago, 1982. Reprinted by permission.

- Self-administration of medications by patient shall be permitted on a specific written order by the authorized prescribing practitioner and in accordance with established hospital policy.
- Investigational drugs shall be properly labeled and stored, and shall be used only under the direct supervision of the authorized principal investigator. Such drugs should be approved by an appropriate medical staff committee. Investigational drugs should be administered in accordance with an approved protocol that includes any requirements for a patient's appropriate informed consent. On approval of the principal investigator, registered nurses may administer these drugs after they have been given, and have demonstrated an understanding of, basic pharmacologic information about the drugs. In the absence of an organized pharmaceutical department/service, a central unit should be established where essential information on such drugs is maintained.
- Orders involving abbreviations and chemical symbols should be carried out only if the abbreviations/symbols appear on an explanatory legend approved by the medical staff. In the interest of minimizing errors, the use of abbreviations is discouraged, and the use of the leading decimal point should be avoided. Each practitioner who prescribes medication must clearly state the administration times or the time interval between doses. The use of "prn" and "on call" with medication orders should be qualified.
- Drugs prescribed for ambulatory care patient use in continuity with hospital care shall be released to patients upon discharge only after they are labeled for such use under the supervision of the pharmacist and only on written order of the authorized prescribing practitioner. Each drug released to a patient on discharge should be recorded in the medical record.
- Individual drugs should be administered as soon as possible after the dose has been prepared, particularly medications prepared for parenteral administration, and, to the maximum extent possible, by the individual who prepared the dose, except where unit dose drug distribution systems are used.

Unless otherwise provided by the medical staff bylaws, rules and regulations or by legal requirements, prescribing practitioners may, within their discretion at the time of prescribing, approve or disapprove the dispensing of a nonproprietary drug or the dispensing of a different proprietary brand to their patients by the pharmacist.

Practice Standards of the American Society of Hospital Pharmacists

In addition to codes of ethics, professional societies also develop standards of practice that amount to pronouncements concerning the manner in which the practice should be conducted. The American Society of Hospital Pharmacists has been very active in this area. Some of the statements the Society has prepared include:

Guidelines for Institutional Use of Controlled Substances

Statement on Unit Dose Drug Distribution Systems

Statement on Supportive Personnel in Hospital Pharmacy

Statement on Clinical Pharmacy and its Relationship to the Hospital

The Hospital Pharmacist and Drug Information Services

Guidelines for Single-Unit Packages of Drugs

Statement on Hospital Drug Control Systems

Statement on Research in Hospital Pharmacy

Statement of Guiding Principles on the Operation of the Hospital Formulary System

Statement on Principles Involved in the Use of Investigational Drugs in Hospitals

Statement on the Competencies Required in Institutional Pharmacy Practice

Minimum Standard for Pharmacies in Hospitals with Guide to Application

Statement on Pharmacy and Therapeutics Committee

Guidelines for Scientific Research in Hospital Pharmacy

DEA Guidelines for Controlled Substances

All hospitals must provide effective controls and procedures to guard against theft and diversion of controlled substances. The DEA (U.S. Drug Enforcement Administration) has outlined fourteen factors which it takes into account in determining whether a control system is suitable.

(1) The type of activity conducted (e.g., processing of bulk chemicals, preparing dosage forms, packaging, labeling, cooperative buying, etc.);

(2) The type and form of controlled substances handled (e.g., bulk liquids or dosage units, usable powders or non-usable powders);

(3) The quantity of controlled substances handled;

(4) The location of the premises and the relationship such location bears on security needs;

(5) The type of building construction comprising the facility and the general characteristics of the building or buildings;

(6) The type of vault, safe, and secure enclosures or other storage system (e.g., automatic storage and retrieval system) used;

(7) The type of closures on vaults, safes and secure enclosures;

(8) The adequacy of key control systems and/or combination lock control systems;

(9) The adequacy of electric detection and alarm systems, if any, including use of supervised transmittal lines and standby power sources;

(10) The extent of unsupervised public access to the facility, including the presence and characteristics of perimeter fencing, if any;

(11) The adequacy of supervision over employees having access to manufacturing and storage areas;

(12) The procedures for handling business guests, visitors, maintenance personnel, and nonemployee service personnel;

(13) The availability of local police protection or of the registrant's or applicant's security personnel, and;

(14) The adequacy of the registrant's or applicant's system for monitoring the receipt, manufacture, distribution, and disposition of controlled substances in its operations.

Central storage for drugs in the hospital should be under the direct control and supervision of pharmacists. Only authorized personnel should have access to this area.

When controlled substances are stored at nursing units, they, likewise, should be kept securely locked, and only authorized personnel should have access to these drugs. A question arises concerning medication carts and unit dose carts. If these carts are used merely for delivery purposes, it would seem they need not be locked; however, if they are used for storage, they may require locking for security reasons.

Generally, if medications are on carts for brief periods, if they are designated for specific patients and if they are not part of a bulk storage unit, the carts probably do not need locks. On the other hand, safety factors may dictate locking all medications.

Medicare Pharmacy Standards

The following regulations set forth the conditions that must be met in order to qualify for Medicare reimbursement for pharmaceutical services provided in hospitals.

Condition of Participation—Pharmacy or Drug Room.—The hospital has a pharmacy directed by a registered pharmacist or a drug room under competent supervision. The pharmacy or drug room is administered in accordance with accepted professional principles.

(a) Pharmacy Supervision.—There is a pharmacy directed by a registered pharmacist or a drug room under competent supervision.

(1) The pharmacist is trained in the specialized functions of hospital pharmacy.

(2) The pharmacist is responsible to the administration of the hospital for developing, supervising, and coordinating all the activities of the pharmacy department.

(3) If there is a drug room with no pharmacist, prescription medications are dispensed by a qualified pharmacist elsewhere, and only storing and distributing are done in the hospital. A consulting pharmacist assists in drawing up the correct procedures, rules, and regulations for the distribution of drugs and visits the hospital on a regularly scheduled basis in the course of his duties. Wherever possible the pharmacist, in dispensing drugs, works from the prescriber's original order or a direct copy.

(b) *Physical Facilities.*—Facilities are provided for the storage, safeguarding, preparation, and dispensing of drugs.

(1) Drugs are issued to floor units in accordance with approved policies and procedures.

(2) Drug cabinets on the nursing units are routinely checked by the pharmacist. All floor stocks are properly controlled.

(3) There is adequate space for all pharmacy operations and the storage of drugs at a satisfactory location provided with proper lighting, ventilation, and temperature controls.

(4) If there is a pharmacy, equipment is provided for the compounding and dispensing of drugs.

(5) Special locked storage space is provided to meet the legal requirements for storage of narcotics, alcohol, and other prescribed drugs.

(c) *Personnel.*—Personnel competent in their respective duties are provided in keeping with the size and activity of the department.

(1) The pharmacist is assisted by an adequate number of additional registered pharmacists and such other personnel as the activities of the pharmacy may require to insure quality pharmaceutical services.

(2) The pharmacy, depending upon the size and scope of its operations, is staffed by the following categories of personnel:

(i) Chief pharmacist.

(ii) One or more assistant chief pharmacists.

(iii) Staff pharmacists.

(iv) Pharmacy residents (where a program has been activated).

(v) Nonprofessionally trained pharmacy helpers.

(vi) Clerical help.

(3) Provision is made for emergency pharmaceutical services.

(4) If the hospital does not have a staff pharmacist, a consulting pharmacist has overall responsibility for control and distribution of drugs and a designated individual(s) has responsibility for day-to-day operation of the pharmacy.

(d) *Records.*—Records are kept of the transactions of the pharmacy (or drug room) and correlated with other hospital records where indicated. Such special records are kept as are required by law.

(1) The pharmacy establishes and maintains, in cooperation with the accounting department, a satisfactory system of records and bookkeeping in accordance with the policies of the hospital for:

(i) Maintaining adequate control over the requisitioning and dispensing of all drugs and pharmaceutical supplies, and

(ii) Charging patients for drugs and pharmaceutical supplies.

(2) A record of the stock on hand and of the dispensing of all narcotic drugs is maintained in such a manner that the disposition of any particular item may be readily traced.

(3) Records for prescription drugs dispensed to each patient (inpatients and outpatients) are maintained in the pharmacy or drug room containing the full name of the patient and the prescribing physician, the prescription number, the name and strength of the drug, the date of issue, the expiration date for all timedated medications, the lot and control number of the drug, the name of the manufacturer (or trademark) and (unless the physician directs otherwise) the name of the medication dispensed.

(4) The label of each outpatient's individual prescription medication container bears the lot and control number of the drug, the name of the manufacturer (or trademark) and (unless the physician directs otherwise) the name of the medication dispensed.

(e) *Control of Toxic or Dangerous Drugs.*—Policies are established to control the administration of toxic or dangerous drugs with specific reference to the duration of the order and the dosage.

(1) The medical staff has established a written policy that all toxic or dangerous medications, not specifically prescribed as to time or number of doses, will be automatically stopped after a reasonable time limit set by the staff.

(2) The classifications ordinarily thought of as toxic or dangerous drugs are narcotics, sedatives, anticoagulants, antibiotics, oxytocics, and cortisone products.

(f) *Committee.*—There is a committee of the medical staff to confer with the pharmacist in the formulation of policies.

(1) A pharmacy and therapeutics committee (or equivalent committee), composed of physicians and pharmacists, is established in the hospital. It represents the organizational line of communication and the liaison between the medical staff and the pharmacist.

(2) The committee assists in the formulation of broad professional policies regarding the evaluation, appraisal, selection, procurement, storage, distribution, use, and safety procedures, and all other matters relating to drugs in hospitals.

(3) The committee performs the following specific functions:

(i) Serves as an advisory group to the hospital medical staff and the pharmacist on matters pertaining to the choice of drugs;

(ii) Develops and reviews periodically a formulary or drug list for use in the hospital;

(iii) Establishes standards concerning the use and control of investigational drugs and research in the use of recognized drugs;

(iv) Evaluates clinical data concerning new drugs or preparations requested for use in the hospital;

(v) Makes recommendations concerning drugs to be stocked on the nursing unit floors and by other services; and

(vi) Prevents unnecessary duplication in stocking drugs and drugs in combination having identical amounts of the same therapeutic ingredients.

(4) The committee meets at least quarterly and reports to the medical staff.

(g) *Drugs To Be Dispensed.*—Therapeutic ingredients of medications dispensed are included (or approved for inclusion) in the United States Pharmacopoeia, National Formulary, United States Homeopathic Pharmacopoeia, New Drugs, or Accepted Dental Remedies (except for any drugs unfavorably evaluated therein), or are approved for use by the pharmacy and drug therapeutics committee (or equivalent committee) of the hospital staff.

(1) The pharmacist, with the advice and guidance of the pharmacy and therapeutics committee, is responsible for specifications as to quality, quantity, and source of supply of all drugs.

(2) There is available a formulary or list of drugs accepted for use in the hospital which is developed and amended at regular intervals by the pharmacy and therapeutics committee (or equivalent committee) with the cooperation of the pharmacist (consulting or otherwise) and the administration.

(3) The pharmacy or drug room is adequately supplied with preparations so approved.

One section relating to nursing from the conditions of participation for hospitals is also relevant for it deals with administration of medications. For example:

20 C.F.R. 405.1024(g)

(5) Only (i) a licensed physician or a registered professional nurse or (ii) a licensed practical nurse, a student nurse in an approved school of nursing, or a psychiatric technician, when these three classes of personnel are under the direct supervision of a registered professional nurse, is permitted to administer medications, and in all instances, in accordance with the Nurse Practice Act of the State.

Chapter 8—Central Supply, Property, Housekeeping, and Laundry Management

CENTRAL MEDICAL AND SURGICAL SUPPLY SERVICE

The Central Medical and Surgical Supply Service (CMSSS) is the department responsible for providing supplies and equipment required by all other departments that render patient care. It is the hospital department that renders service by collecting, receiving, processing, storing, issuing, and distributing supplies and equipment used in the care and treatment of patients. This department serves the entire hospital including related outpatient services.

Functions*

• Process, maintain, and dispense supplies and equipment required by medical, nursing, or paramedical personnel in designated departments for the care, diagnosis, or treatment of patients.
• Provide modern equipment maintained in optimum working condition and utilize best known methods and techniques for the processing of materials.
• Develop processing and supply control methods which will provide supplies and equipment most efficiently and economically.
• Provide effective training programs and competent supervision to assure high standards of performance for CMSSS personnel.

*Source: *A Manual for Hospital Central Services,* DHEW, Pub. No. (HRA) 75-4012, 1975.

• Participate in inservice education programs for all hospital personnel.
• Maintain representation on nursing care procedures, standardization, and infections control committees.
• Participate in supply and equipment research in an effort to provide the most suitable information available to nursing, paramedical, and medical groups.
• Maintain an accurate inventory of supplies and equipment.
• Reduce total cost of the department by cost analysis of personnel, supplies, and equipment.

Organization*

In many hospitals, Central Service is attached to the department of nursing service; in others, the Central Service Supervisor may report to the chief of pharmacy, the head of the operating room, the purchasing department, or to an associate administrator.

There is a growing trend toward consolidating Central Service to include a central cleanup area where all soiled supplies are processed. In the dispensing area, general stores and Central Service are combined and headed by a Central Dispatcher, who may or may not be the Purchasing Agent. Laundry and Pharmacy are adjuncts to this area but have separate department heads.

*Source: *Job Descriptions and Organizational Analysis for Hospitals and Related Health Services,* U.S. Training and Employment Service, Department of Labor, 1971.

Central Service should be located centrally to those nursing units which it serves. The number of workrooms and amount of storage space required will be determined by the size of the hospital and degree of centralization. Dumbwaiters, pneumatic tubes, and other mechanized means of transferring supplies are standard equipment in new hospitals to facilitate service and reduce time in transporting needed supplies. This department may require separate areas for decontamination, packaging, glove preparation, linen preparation, sterilization, sterile and nonsterile storage, and dispensing.

The staff of Central Service may include one or more registered nurses or practical nurses; the remaining staff typically consists of assistants, technicians, aides, orderlies, and messengers trained on-the-job. The size of the staff will depend on the size of the hospital, degree of centralization of supply, extent to which disposable articles are purchased, and extent to which supplies are assembled by the department.

In many hospitals, Central Service is headed by a registered nurse, but opinions differ among hospital experts on whether this is necessary. There is a growing trend toward heading the service with an experienced manager not trained as a nurse, with a professional nurse as a member of the advisory committee.

Central Supply Supervisor: Job Duties*

● Supervises and coordinates the activities of personnel engaged in furnishing sterile and nonsterile supplies, equipment, and services for the care and treatment of patients:
● Establishes methods and work performance standards for preparing and handling sterile items. Demonstrates to personnel procedures such as proper use of sterilizing equipment, setting up treatment trays, and maintenance of equipment of department. Insures that aseptic techniques are employed in preparing and handling sterile supplies, whether reusable or disposable. Prepares instruments for repair and maintains regular schedule for checkup of electrical equipment by the maintenance department.

*Source: *Job Descriptions and Organizational Analysis for Hospitals and Related Health Services,* U.S. Training and Employment Service, Department of Labor, 1971.

● Insures that work and storage areas are clean and orderly. Takes microbiological samples of air, surfaces, and equipment and sends to laboratory for sterility check.
● Supervises personnel engaged in decontaminating, assembling, packaging, and sterilizing linens, dressings, gloves, treatment trays, instruments, and related items; preparation of standard irrigating solutions; rotation of stock; and requisitioning, issuing, and controlling supplies and equipment. Maintains adequate stock on hand by visual inspection and by consulting inventory records. Recommends changes in budget and inventory level to meet current demands. Prepares and submits requisitions for additions and replacements, and stores received stock in appropriate areas of supply room. On presentation of proper authority, dispenses stock for delivery to various hospital departments, and inspects returned equipment to insure that all parts have been returned. Keeps inventory of items issued and maintains a schedule of charges to be billed to the using department or patient.
● Prepares reports on activities of the department and maintains necessary records on assigned personnel. May interview applicants and conduct inservice training for department personnel.

Departments to Be Serviced*

Nursing Units

All nursing units within the hospital that administer general or special nursing care to the patients are serviced by the CMSSS. This service includes the processing of all basic supplies and equipment that may be required during the patient's period of hospitalization. It may also include those supplies required for home care that may be given on discharge in hospitals that make such follow-up provisions.

Surgical Suite

The department may provide the surgical suite with the following basic items:

● Dressings
● Parenteral solutions
● Administration sets

*Source: *A Manual for Hospital Central Services,* DHEW, Pub. No. (HRA)75-4012, 1975.

- Gloves
- External solutions
- Special trays
- Needles
- Syringes
- Miscellaneous supplies and equipment, such as armboards and drains

The department may also provide the following special sterile items and anesthesia supplies if needed.

- Linen
- Linen packs
- Basin sets
- Basic instrument sets
- Air ways
- Suction catheters

Labor-Delivery Unit

The department may process and supply all items that may be required by the patient from the time she is admitted into the labor room until she has delivered.

Basic items:

- Examination equipment and supplies
- Preparation equipment and supplies
- Dressings
- Administration sets
- External solutions
- Needles
- Gloves
- Parenteral solutions
- Syringes
- Special trays

Special sterile items:

- Linen packs
- Basin sets
- Basic delivery instruments
- Special delivery instruments

Nursery

The department may process and supply all items and equipment necessary for the individual care of all infants in the nursery. This includes the equipment used in the care of the premature infant and those who may require special treatment.

Basic items and equipment:

- Bathing sets
- Sterile linen

- Thermometers
- Examination equipment

Special equipment and service:

- Special trays, such as exchange transfusion, resuscitation, and circumcision
- Processing of nursery equipment, such as incubators and resuscitators

Outpatient Department

The outpatient department includes the emergency room and is serviced with all supplies and equipment necessary in the treatment and care of all patients in this area. If hospital policy provides supplies, these may include those necessary for the patient to continue his care at home until the next visit to the department.

Basic items and equipment:

- Examination equipment
- Diagnostic procedure trays
- Rubber goods, such as gloves and catheters
- Treatment trays and sets
- Dressings
- Miscellaneous supplies

Radiology

All supplies and equipment for the diagnostic procedures and the care of the patient while in the radiology department are supplied by the CMSSS. Special procedure trays are considered as basic equipment when supplied to this specialty department.

Basic supplies and equipment:

- Diagnostic procedure trays and sets
- Needles and syringes
- Inhalation equipment
- Rubber goods, such as gloves and rectal tubes
- Miscellaneous supplies

Pharmacy

Solutions and supplies such as needles and syringes required for preparation of drugs are provided to the pharmacy.

Clinical Laboratory

The service to be provided to the clinical laboratory by the CMSSS has been a subject of much discussion. Each hospital will have to decide whether or not to wash and sterilize all equipment, including laboratory glassware. Among other things it depends on funds available for capital equipment since duplication of such equipment would be needed to make provision for the processing of laboratory supplies. However, due to the high degree of contamination, it is advisable to provide a sterilizer for the laboratory.

If disposable supplies are used, each hospital should decide whether or not this department shall be provided with supplies from the CMSSS or receive the supplies directly from general stores.

Basic supplies:

- Needles and syringes
- Dressings
- Rubber goods

Research Department

The extent of service that is provided to this specialty area will depend on the amount and type of research that is carried on in the hospital. The supplies and equipment that would ordinarily be provided would include the following:

- Linen packs for animal surgery
- Instrument sets
- Gloves
- Dressings
- Solutions
- Basin sets
- Needles and syringes
- Miscellaneous

Economic Aspects*

Labor-saving devices are being installed in hospital areas. In the area of distribution pneumatic tubes may be used for small items, dumbwaiters for standard items, and the elevator for portable equipment. A system of vertical conveyors that automatically discharge the requested items at a special place is the latest contribution to hospitals in automatic dispensing.

Cost analysis should be made of the time and effort expended in effectively dispensing supplies manually as compared with the cost of automatic distribution. In many instances the automatic method would prove to be more economical over a given period of time. Further

losses in the CMSSS are frequently the result of poor controls, inefficiency in operation, and overstocked inventory.

Control*

The first factor to consider in establishing centralized control is a good orientation program for new employees. This should be followed by a continuing departmental inservice program for all hospital personnel in the proper use of supplies and equipment. This can be accomplished by having written policies governing dispensing. Control may be facilitated by a record of all items dispensed, and by developing a definite system for the requisitioning and dispensing of supplies and equipment.

Suggestions for improving control systems include:

- Hold individual nursing unit or specialty department accountable for lost equipment.
- Have a perpetual "follow-up system."
- Through cooperative effort inform users of supplies and equipment of the importance of control.
- Do periodic equipment control study to determine frequency of use of "special" equipment.
- Mark all equipment legibly and where it can be seen.
- Number all trays and portable equipment.
- Reduce the amount of outdated supplies by proper rotation.
- Use peg-board method for location of each piece of equipment and special tray dispensed from the department (see Table 8-1).

Inventory

Establishing maximum and minimum levels of inventory has many advantages; among them are: (1) bookkeeping is simplified, (2) overstocking and depletion of stock are negated, (3) more economical means of purchasing is possible, and (4) the availability of supplies when requested is enhanced. Control of inventory and accurate records within the department aid in the maintenance of the perpetual inventory.

---

*Source: *A Manual for Hospital Central Services,* DHEW, Pub. No. (HRA) 75-4012, 1975.

Table 8-1 Sample of Index to Supplies and Equipment— Equipment Storage Room

Items	Section	Shelf	Items	Section	Shelf
Portable Equipment			*Orthopedic Supplies*		
Alternating Pressure Mattress	H	6–7–14–15	Adjustable Crutches	F	
Aquamatic Motor	H	4	Bed Boards	I	
Aquamatic Pads	H	5	Bed Cradle	I	
Aspirator—Gastric	A		Bed Lifter	L	
Aspirator—Oral	A		Belts—Pelvic, Traction	C	3–4
Barron Pump	H	3	Bradford Frames	K	
Cradle Bed	B		Bryant's Traction	K	
Electric Room Deodorizer	I	16	Buck's Extension Apparatus	D	4
Heat Cradle	B		Buck's Extension Bracket	D	4
Heating Pad—Electric	G	14	Buck's Extension Hooks	D	4
Lamp—Perineal	B		Blocks—Shock	E	1–2–3–4–5

Source: *A Manual for Hospital Central Services*, DHEW Pub. No. (HRA) 75-4012, 1975.

Theft of Surgical Supplies*

Surgical instruments and medical supplies do not normally offer a target for massive diversion. Even petty pilferage is rarely significant in this area in terms of total quantities, and most of it is not preventable. Disappearing thermometers can amount to a substantial loss over a long period, but stolen bandages, adhesive tapes, gauze bandages, pins and needles will never amount to more than a negligible fraction of the total expenditure for surgical supplies. The notorious loss of stethoscopes and ophthalmoscopes at the end of the residents' term usually is substantial, but it occurs once a year and again is not completely preventable.

In central surgical supply itself scissors may be the one major target. Most staff who work in these departments have little use for other surgical instruments. There have been occasions where a connection was established between an employee in the central supply room and a privately owned surgical supply house, but those incidents are infrequent.

Central Services Glossary**

Antiseptic: Any chemical agent that is usually applied to living tissue and which inhibits the growth of microorganisms without necessarily destroying them.

---

*Source: Walter Nagel, "Health Care Industry's Vulnerability to Theft," *Topics in Health Care Financing*, Winter 1978.

**Source: *A Manual for Hospital Central Services*, DHEW Pub. No. (HRA)75-4012, 1975.

Aqueous solution: A liquid in which a chemical is dissolved in water.

Aseptic: Sterile, free from any living microorganisms.

Aseptic technique: Performance characterized by precautions for constant exclusion of microorganisms.

Autoclave: A sterilizing apparatus that uses saturated steam under pressure.

Bacteria: One category of microorganisms. This is the type of microorganism which is of greatest concern to hospital personnel because it is difficult to destroy and produces many different diseases.

Bagged: Method of enclosing supplies and equipment. This may be done by plastic or paper to prevent spread of infection or to maintain sterility.

Capital equipment: Expensive items that have an investment value such as sterilizer, water still, and some mechanical cleaning apparatus.

Communicable disease organism: A pathogenic microorganism which is readily transmitted from person to person by direct or indirect contact.

Contamination: Soiling with microorganisms or other harmful agents.

Detergent: A cleaning agent which facilitates removal of grease or soil. A suitable detergent must be selected; it must clean but not injure the surface of the article.

Diagnostic procedure: The method or manner of determining the presence, nature or cause of a disease.

Disinfectant: Any chemical agent, used on inanimate materials, which inhibits or destroys most microorganisms.

Ethylene oxide gas sterilizer: An apparatus using gaseous ethylene oxide, with or without added inert gas, as the sterilizing agent.

Equipment: Items of durable nature such as instruments and suction apparatus.

General stores: The facility of the hospital which stores in bulk form all supplies and equipment required within the hospital.

Germ: A microscopic or submicroscopic organism capable of producing disease.

Heat resistant: Not affected by heat.

Heat sensitive: Will be affected or destroyed by heat.

Hemostat: A clamp forceps to control the flow of blood.

High-vacuum steam sterilizer: A pressure apparatus, employing saturated steam as the sterilizing agent, which operates on the principle by which air is removed from the chamber with the aid of a vacuum pump or other mechanical device.

Infection: Invasion of human body tissues by pathogenic microorganisms.

Microorganisms: Organisms visible only with the aid of a microscope.

Moisture sensitive: Will be affected or destroyed by excessive moisture.

Pathogenic microorganism: A microorganism which produces disease.

Process: A series of procedures designed to prepare supplies and equipment for use in rendering patient care.

Pyrogen: Fever-producing bacteria that may be found in water which is not freshly distilled.

Sanitization: A process whereby microorganisms present on an object are reduced in number to a level considered safe for human use.

Sanitizer: An apparatus employing a sanitizing agent such as hot water, steam, or chemicals.

Solutions:
  External: Sterile liquids that may be used as irrigation or cleansing agent.
  Parenteral: Sterile liquids that are administered internally. Commonly referred to as intravenous solutions.

Spores: Certain microorganisms which usually form a thick cell wall enabling them to survive in adverse environments.

Sterile: Free from all microorganisms.

Sterilizer: Apparatus using saturated steam *under pressure*, ethylene oxide, or dry heat as the sterilizing agent. These include gravity and mechanical types.

Supplies: Items ordinarily consumed by use in rendering patient care. However, such items as needles, glassware and linen are also classified as supplies.

Thumb forceps: Pincer-like instrument with smooth tip to grasp objects.

Tissue forceps: Pincer-like instrument with teeth to grasp tissue.

Ultrasonic washer: An apparatus in which the cleaning of equipment, principally instruments, is accomplished by the compressional force of the ultra-sound waves.

Washer: An apparatus in which glassware, instruments, utensils, and other items are cleaned.

Washer-Sterilizer: An apparatus in which instruments and utensils are washed and then sterilized, employing saturated steam under pressure.

PLANT AND PROPERTY MANAGEMENT

Superintendent of Plant Operations: Job Duties*

[May also be called administrative engineer, chief engineer, director of buildings and grounds, or plant engineer.]

● Administers and directs program to maintain buildings, grounds, and equipment and to procure or generate all utilities and their distribution systems; coordinates these activities with the other departments to insure safe and efficient operation:

● Attends staff meetings to ascertain hospital policies, assists in their development, and interprets these policies to his staff.

● Plans and recommends development of physical facilities. Reviews and recommends ap-

---

*Source: *Job Descriptions and Organizational Analysis for Hospitals and Related Health Services,* U.S. Training and Employment Service, Department of Labor, 1971.

proval of plans for construction. Advises on structural changes and additions or modifications to buildings. Interviews contractors to receive and analyze bids, including blueprint analysis of proposed changes. Submits bids and recommendations to the administration, basing recommendations on economy and feasibility of bids. Provides liaison with contractors, architects, engineers, and material and equipment suppliers.

• Prepares department budgets. Approves orders for equipment and supplies, as authorized.

• Establishes and administers preventive maintenance program. Analyzes costs and work schedules; sets priorities; expedites operations and repairs.

• Periodically inspects buildings and utility systems to determine need of alterations and repairs. Approves contracted work. Accompanies appropriate State and local authorities inspecting buildings and utility systems.

• Is responsible for departmental personnel matters pertaining to the employment, training, termination, and grievances of employees.

• May direct safety, fire control, security, and civil-defense programs and participate in hospital infection-control program.

Requirements

• Graduate degree in engineering, preferably civil, mechanical, or electrical, supplemented with specialized training in business management or related experience.

• And/or 5 to 10 years' progressive experience in supervision and maintenance in installation, construction, and maintenance of equipment, utilities, and buildings.

• Able to assume overall responsibility for engineering and maintenance of hospital utility services, buildings, and grounds.

• Able to make emergency decisions in respect to failure of plant utilities or other delegated responsibilities.

• Able to comprehend wide range of technical subjects and coordination of details.

• Facility to communicate with people under his supervision as well as other department heads and public.

• Ability to work to standards set by applicable national, state, and local building codes.

Plant Maintenance*

Users and management can eliminate a tremendous amount of maintenance cost by:

1. Buying equipment that is not unreliable, expensive to repair or that will create internal building damage.
2. Limiting and controlling use of the building by staff, patients and others to prevent physical damage (will nurses ever learn adhesive tape was not meant for the hanging of pictures?).
3. Setting sensible standards for color, signs, door exits, private, public areas, etc.
4. Using the technical expertise of maintenance people or allowing them to acquire it themselves.
5. Ensuring that purchased materials and equipment are not obsolete.
6. Having clear-cut policies as to responsibilities in who pays for what and why.
7. Hiring qualified, experienced and mature maintenance staff to avoid the lost time and damage cost of nonproductive workers.
8. Having adequate equipment to work with. One may lose here on savings temporarily, but make it up later in reduced labor costs. Do not buy if you can contract more cheaply.
9. Ensuring that adequate and complete records are kept of materials used and time taken by whom and for what, a process that will involve the help and co-operation of accounting, stores, purchasing, etc.
10. Encouraging upgrading, training, education and field visits by the maintenance staff to keep them abreast of modern methods, materials and equipment.

Procedures

• Department heads, unit heads and directors should countersign all maintenance re-

*Source: H.D. Plunkett, "Good Maintenance Management Means Big Savings," *Dimensions in Health Service,* Journal of the Canadian Hospital Association, pp. 32–34, © 1977.

quests going to the maintenance department.

- Have a maintenance request form in duplicate showing location, date, requester, approval of department head and the requested action.
- The maintenance department should have a repair order (in duplicate) to redefine the job in trade jargon, stating worker to do the repair, time, materials used (or material requisition number), special instructions, etc. The original goes to the trade, the other is an office control copy.
- Institute a hospital-wide order that workmen report to maintenance supervisory staff only. How many "ten minute jobs while you are here" have blossomed into economic monstrosities and derailed the regular maintenance schedule?
- Enforce hours of work, break times and regulate holiday times.
- Establish a strong emergency repair system to permit fast efficient emergency repairs. Sometimes in the heat of an emergency an unknowing person can create greater havoc by not acting in a sensible way. This can increase costs, damage, down time, etc.
- Off-hour coverage by maintenance is a questionable matter. Is it more economical to call in trades for evening, night and week-end repairs or is it better to set up a work schedule and rotate staff? Each individual hospital or facility would have to analyse this situation for itself.
- Record areas worked in, the number of jobs done, by whom, and develop a cost per repair ratio.
- Set up a preventive maintenance program (not only for equipment but the building as well).

Equipment Maintenance*

One way of helping keep costs down is to control the maintenance of hospital equipment through a Hospital Equipment Control Procedure. Following is one such procedure which has been used with success. The system provides minute information as to equipment location, date

equipment was last serviced, next service due date, and description of equipment. The annual report derived from the permanent record system provides total labor cost, total cost of replacement parts, and projected cost for the next fiscal year's maintenance.

Objectives

1. to ensure proper maintenance of equipment to avoid down time;
2. to inform health care personnel of the availability of equipment;
3. to designate equipment location;
4. to allow proper library and file control for each type of equipment service and operator manual;
5. to allow control of spare parts needed and prevent purchasing problems by avoiding stocking useless parts, supplies, etc.;
6. to allow proper amortization for tax allowances on five-year and ten-year depreciation periods, etc.;
7. to supply information to obtain total asset value of all hospital-owned equipment.

Procedure Plan

Control and inventory will be conducted by a designated equipment control coordinator (ECC). The ECC will initiate scheduling of calibration and maintenance of all hospital electrical/mechanical and operational equipment. To ensure that equipment is properly maintained and controlled, the following action will be taken:

- All equipment under this system will be assigned a control number by the ECC. This number will be affixed to the equipment and will be used for scheduling calibration and preventive maintenance and for asset inventory control. For accounting purposes, the department holding the equipment will assume accountability for the equipment.
- Lease and rental equipment can be incorporated into the procedure to ensure that preventive maintenance is being performed per the lease/rental agreement.
- No equipment under this system will be removed from the hospital without the approval or concurrence of the ECC. The ECC will be responsible for transferring the

---

*Source: Oscar L. Marryott, "A Procedure for Controlling Hospital Equipment," *Hospital Materiel Management Quarterly,* May 1981.

equipment to other departments, returning equipment to the manufacturer, or obtaining any outside calibration or maintenance required.

- Electrical/mechanical equipment coming into the hospital for the first time must go to a calibration area where it will be logged, functionally tested, and assigned a control number by the ECC. While in this calibration stage, the equipment will be evaluated for safety and availability for usage. It will also be checked for certification, in compliance with hospital-approved electrical safety standards recommended by the National Fire Protection Association.
- The ECC will start a technical history file for electrical/mechanical equipment and will assist in setting up for usage, ensuring that the operator is satisfied that equipment is fully functional.
- The ECC must be notified of any obsolete or unused electrical/mechanical equipment by supervisors having such equipment in their department. This will allow proper disposition of the equipment.

A Specific Control Method

From the inventory data, an electronic data-processing (EDP) printout for distribution will be accomplished showing the following information:

- equipment description
- model number
- manufacturer
- serial number
- control number (asset number)
- area location
- source of procurement (new, used, or leased)
- last calibration date

Future EDP printouts for distribution can show as time allows:

- due date of next calibration
- calibration time required by technician
- repair time incurred
- parts cost for maintenance

The existing department number can be used for the area location number. Inventory data will

be recorded on a 3″ × 5″ card. Cards can be preprinted to aid filling in required information.

Upon recording inventory data, a control (asset) tag will be affixed to the equipment. For ease of location, the tag should be secured next to the manufacturer's name plate or serial number when possible. Tags preprinted with consecutive numbers can be purchased. The number should be large enough for ease of maintenance and inventory reading, but the tag should be small enough to accommodate small pad locations inconspicuously.

Distribution of EDP printouts from data processing will be based on departmental management requirements (safety department, accounting, laboratories, plant maintenance, materiel handling, biomedical engineering, etc.).

The EDP printout will also be the guide for the ECC to compile or establish the location of all service and operator manuals for equipment listed.

The annual ECC report should: evaluate equipment performance; analyze the quality of service received; indicate the amount and type of equipment down time; show what equipment was determined obsolete and how the equipment was disposed of; indicate the required maintenance time in hours; and show proposed changes for the next year.

Using a Clinical Engineer*

As health technology expands, medical instrumentation is rapidly becoming one of the most significant factors in influencing the quality of patient care. The proliferation of medical "hardware" over the past few years has been accompanied by increased procurement expense, greater installation cost and more complexity in operating and maintaining the equipment. As instrumentation is more widely used, a new member of the health team needs to be addressed: The Hospital Clinical Engineer.

It has gradually become more important for administrators of health care facilities and their staff to be assured that a knowledgeable person is responsible for the current condition of the medical instrumentation within the institution,

---

*Source: Earl Simendinger, W.S. Topham, and Dennis Wong, "Keep Up with . . . New Roles in Health Care: Clinical Engineer," *Health Care Management Review,* Fall 1976.

especially since the Board, the physicians, the administration and the nursing staff are all legally responsible. The Joint Commission on Accreditation has made it clear that the hospital and its staff are liable for injuries to the patient found to have resulted, both directly and indirectly, from noncompliance with safety regulations. A contract with an outside equipment management agency does not exempt the hospital from liability.

There are approximately 2,000 hospitals in the country with 200 beds or more. It is primarily these institutions who have a need for an in-house engineer who can contribute to both patient education and patient safety. The range of academic credentials that clinical engineers bring to the hospital runs the gamut from electrical, biomedical, mechanical, chemical and industrial engineering.

The clinical engineer can:

- provide training programs on medical electronic equipment
- provide equipment repair service
- provide a comprehensive preventive maintenance equipment program—short and long range
- inspect newly purchased equipment before official acceptance and payment
- provide consulting information to physicians on patient equipment
- provide input before purchasing all medical equipment
- maintain a filing system for medical equipment
- provide information and assistance on the' real need for equipment replacement or repair
- assist in setting job related priorities relative to patient safety items
- design, develop, and modify equipment for special needs
- check out and authorize implant devices before surgery
- complete appropriate reports and projects as assigned by administrators
- be an active member of the hospital safety committee, including internal inspection for safety hazards
- assist in the planning, design, and supervision of installation of special care units, ICU, CCU, etc.

Calibration Procedures*

Calibration procedures provide for the establishment of a calibration system to control the accuracy of equipment used in the hospital.

In general, all equipment will be calibrated or given a preventive maintenance check at intervals established on the basis of degree of use; accuracy or stability; type of service; and probability of a continued, unimpaired and useful service life, including wear. Calibration should normally be performed during the week prior to the due date or at least by the due date.

(Note: When an instrument malfunctions, has been damaged, or no longer meets the accuracy specified by the manufacturer, it will be repaired and recalibrated.)

Written calibration procedures will be prepared or provided and used for calibrating all equipment calibrated at the hospital. These procedures may be on the hospital's format or may be supplied by the equipment manufacturers.

The procedures will contain the following minimum information:

- the specific equipment or group of equipment to which the procedure is applicable;
- fundamental types of calibration information such as calibration points, environmental requirements, standard calibration conditions, and accuracy requirements;
- a brief description of the scope, principle, and theory of the calibration method;
- a list of all standards and accessory equipment required to perform the specific calibration (if possible, a block diagram layout of the testing setup shall be included);
- a complete and accurate description of the calibration procedure arranged in a step-by-step manner;
- directions for completing necessary documentation.

The recall card file (or EDP printout) will be reviewed at least once each week. Calibration of an instrument will be initiated during the week prior to its expiration date. The recall card, instrument file folder, and the hospital's calibra-

---

*Source: Oscar L. Marryott, "A Procedure for Controlling Hospital Equipment," *Hospital Materiel Management Quarterly,* May 1981.

tion procedure manual or the manufacturer's repair and calibration manual will be removed from the file.

Calibration and Repair Records*

Records should be kept regarding calibration and repair of equipment.

In general, all electrical/mechanical equipment purchased and received by the hospital will be processed through calibration services prior to release for use.

A recall card will be initiated and maintained for each instrument and filed according to the date recalibration is due. (Note: A recall card is used with the calibration/maintenance recall method. When the EDP printout method is used, an EDP system printer form is used in place of the recall card.) The following information will be entered on the card:

- description
- model number
- serial number
- control number
- manufacturer
- accuracy (if applicable)
- calibration
- calibration date
- recalibration date
- remarks

Each week the recall file (or EDP printout) will be reviewed.

An instrument calibration record will be completed for each instrument calibrated and will include:

- description
- manufacturer
- model number
- serial number
- calibration interval
- accuracy
- location
- control number
- lease/rental number
- drawing number and revision
- calibration date
- date due

- equipment used for calibration
- characteristic being checked
- standard value
- measured value
- allowable tolerance
- actual tolerance
- remarks
- calibration technician number and initials
- date
- equipment owner

Mechanical equipment unless otherwise specified requires calibration every six months; therefore, a mechanical calibration record will be initiated once a year. Each additional calibration will be entered on the same type form.

When an instrument requires adjustment or repair, the information will be recorded on an instrument history record.

When an instrument is found to be inoperative (in part or completely) the operator or technician will initiate an equipment repair request tag.

A calibration tag will be affixed to each instrument which has been calibrated or has gone through preventive maintenance.

Theft in Engineering and Maintenance*

Tools and maintenance materials are some of the items most frequently stolen from health care facilities. Many mechanics and maintenance and repair personnel work in the evenings and during weekends when there are fewer health care staff on duty in the institution. It is not difficult for them to steal equipment and materials without being observed. The only way to prevent massive disappearance of tools and equipment is through a rigid system of documentation of materials requisitioned, specifically those charged to an individual work order.

The greatest opportunity for diversion of maintenance material exists in the requisitioning, purchasing and receiving process. Next, the transfer of materials from building to building offers the greatest opportunity. These types of losses are impossible to curtail altogether, but the procedures for storage, inventory control

*Source: Oscar L. Marryott, "A Procedure for Controlling Hospital Equipment," *Hospital Materiel Management Quarterly*, May 1981.

*Source: Walter Nagel, "Health Care Industry's Vulnerability to Theft," *Topics in Health Care Financing*, Winter 1978.

and issuance control can limit the opportunities drastically.

Payroll Fraud

Another area of substantial drain on hospital funds is the maintenance payroll. Since maintenance personnel, skilled and unskilled, often have to work for prolonged periods of time in outlying buildings, away from the foreman, it is difficult for even the most loyal and most efficient foreman to keep strict control over the staff. As a result, there is a constant risk of staff disappearing for periods of time to perform moonlighting jobs elsewhere while on hospital time. The most serious loss in this area stems from staff completing jobs on overtime which were not completed during regular daytime hours because crew members were moonlighting.

Only rigid detailed scrutiny by the chief of maintenance of hours spent on individual work orders can narrow the chances of substantial loss through this type of payroll fraud.

Abuse of Professional Privilege

Finally there is the pattern of abuse of executive and professional privilege. When maintenance staff members, including the leader, are dishonest, they soon give in to requests from administrators, physicians and innumerable department heads. They may first make small repairs in the private homes of executives and professionals. Next they may agree to minor construction for these professionals—all on hospital time and with hospital tools and equipment. In some institutions these abuses have been minor; in others they have assumed startling proportions before being uncovered.

Audit of Facility Property*

There are many reasons why an audit of all facility property is worth its cost. Identification and itemization of each item can aid in future insurance claims, accurate tax accounting, discouragement of employee theft, proper maintenance scheduling of machines and appliances, long-range planning of replacement schedule estimates, etc.

The actual responsibility for the program can rest with the accounting department, with the security department maintaining control. Audit review and update should be conducted on a regular basis throughout each facility department.

Proper organization of the actual audit process will require the cooperation of several people. A detailed procedure should be established, published, and enforced as company policy. Key individuals should be informed in a memo which:

1. outlines the objectives and importance of property control
2. describes the use of the record forms
3. establishes a uniform system of installation of permanent identification tags
   Suggestions:
   a. machinery: prominent, eye-level, on front if possible
   b. desks, tables, etc.: left side of back, immediately below top
   c. files, bookcases: front upper left-hand corner
   d. chairs: rear edge of seat or center of back
   e. warehouse trucks, etc.: prominent position, yet not where subject to being removed or defaced by movement or wear
4. assigns responsibility for installing and maintaining the system

When establishing the audit inventory procedure, consider the future of the program as well as the present requirements. Decide what is required now and what might be required by property records as the facility expands. The following is an outline of various functions to be covered:

I. Physical Control
   A. Identification/ownership
   B. Location
   C. Custody
   D. Maintenance and repair records
II. Tax Accounting
   A. Original cost date—reconcile with actual conditions
   B. Depreciation method
   C. Group accounts or units
      1. Straight line
      2. Sum of life

---

*Source: A. Michael Pascal, *Hospital Security and Safety*, Aspen Systems Corporation, 1977.

3. Declining balance
4. Guideline lives
5. Determined reserve ratios
III. Corporate Accounting
   A. Verification of asset values
   B. Cost accounting
   C. Distribution of overhead burden
IV. Fire Insurance
   A. Replacement cost (new/adjusted)
   B. Evidence of value
   C. Items excluded from coverage
V. Plan for capital expenditures (near and long-term)
   A. Tax considerations
      1. Investment tax credit
      2. Guideline lives
   B. General considerations (moves, etc.)
   C. Equipment leased and/or purchased (list of all pertinent facts for each item)
      1. Inventory number
      2. Description
      3. Location
      4. Date of purchase/lease
      5. Cost (acquisition and installation)
      6. Depreciation (cost, method, and provision)
      7. Unrecovered cost
      8. Estimated remaining life
      9. Investment credit
     10. Asset classification

The actual decision as to what should be included in the property audit varies. Ideally every piece of property should be inventoried by the system. For each item an individual card should be created, classified by asset category, listing:

Equipment number
Description
Location
Date of purchase/lease
Cost of acquisition/installation
Depreciation reserve
Uncovered costs
Estimated remaining life
Investment credit
Depreciation method
Depreciation provision

All records and the item numbering system should be kept short and unencumbered. Numbering should be sequential and, unless absolutely necessary, uncoded. Only simple codes to identify specific locations, billing dates, etc., should be added to the numbering system, and should be simply indicated by use of a letter preceding the number. Such coding could also be indicated by different color identification plates.

ENERGY MANAGEMENT*

The Energy Management Committee

The committee approach is necessitated by the interdepartmental character of energy management. The use of energy in a health care institution cuts across all departmental lines; all departments have some degree of control over the amount of energy consumed. The energy management function will address few if any problems that are completely solvable by a single manager from a single discipline. Rather, the most commonly encountered situations will be those that require decisions by administrators and others and implementing actions by engineering, maintenance, finance, and several medical, service, and support departments.

Activities and Goals

It is up to the energy management committee to communicate the top management's commitment to energy management to all other elements of the organization. The committee's active pursuit of energy conservation should be visible; in this way the committee will be publicizing management's commitment through its actions.

The committee must also promote communication with all of the organization's end users of energy. Conserving energy in small, individual ways—that add up to significant savings when multiplied by all users—comes largely through attitude change. In the past, an institution's employees considered energy seldom or not at all; now, however, an organization needs all its employees to be aware of the importance of energy and the need to conserve it whenever possible. The committee must provide for the energy awareness that leads to attitude change.

**Source: John W. Janco, Robert D. Krouner, and Charles R. McConnell, *The Hospital Energy Management Manual,* Aspen Systems Corporation, 1980.*

Generally, the energy management committee should be expected to set realistic but challenging goals for energy conservation, formulate plans for the achievement of these goals, and then operate, monitor, and evaluate the energy management program.

The Energy Audit

The energy audit—or survey, or study—should seek to identify all factors that affect energy consumption within the institution. The people performing the audit must know what to look for, and the extent of the expertise required will be directly related to the complexity of the systems involved. It will be necessary to identify all the energy-using systems in the facility, understand how they are operated and maintained, and assess their condition in detail.

The auditors must also possess knowledge of the various codes and regulations that essentially dictate energy consumption in certain aspects of health care delivery and thus place limits on some potential energy-saving actions.

As a start, the auditors should have the utility bills for the preceding few years. The auditors will need architectural, mechanical, and electrical drawings and specifications for the entire facility in order to familiarize themselves with the building and the layout and operation of all its energy-consuming systems. If such drawings and specifications do not exist, as may be the case with some older structures, it is recommended that sketches of the building and its systems be developed.

The auditors will also have to have available all operating and maintenance procedures furnished by the manufacturers and installers of the facility's fixed equipment or by the designers of the structure. In some cases, it will be necessary to contact equipment manufacturers and installers and request operating and maintenance information for equipment put in place years earlier. Lacking such procedures or the ability to obtain them, it may be necessary to assemble the best possible procedures in house by calling upon the knowledge of operating and maintenance personnel.

The audit surveyors should also be aware of the scope and timing of any planned programs of modernization, renovation, change of use, or expansion. It will be of limited value to concentrate on the shortcomings of certain existing systems if they are to be altered in the foreseeable future.

Types of Audits

There are two basic types of audits: (1) the preliminary audit, (2) the complete energy audit (see Tables 8-2 and 8-3).

The Audit Report

Administration may allocate certain organizational resources based on the audit report; the institution's trustees may also use the report as a basis for capital funding decisions. Most certainly the energy management committee will base much of its program direction on the contents of the report.

Recommendations should be listed in some logical order of priority. A reasonable approach would be to present first the no-cost and low-cost actions that can be taken with existing resources, then go on to rank those actions that require investment by the length of the payback period (giving highest priority to those with the shortest payback period).

Each project that requires investment should be evaluated on the basis of full financial cost versus full financial return over its useful life. This brings absolute cost and funding factors into consideration along with simple payback. Any assumptions made in the cost-benefit analysis should be clearly stated. For appropriate items of significant cost, life-cycle costing should be considered.

Using an Energy Management Consultant

The primary benefits to be obtained from the use of an outside consultant are objectivity, experience, analytical expertise, innovation, and full-time commitment.

There are several degrees of involvement possible for the qualified energy management consultant. Moving from the level of most to least involvement, the consultant can:

- perform the entire energy audit, prepare a comprehensive report and action plan, and participate in implementation;
- perform the energy audit and prepare a report outlining all recommended actions; or merely
- review an internally prepared audit report and make recommendations.

When the institution makes the decision to employ an energy consultant, management should be prepared to supply guidelines to prospective consultants so that they will respond uniformly to requests for proposals. Five major

Table 8-2 Federal Government Definition of a Preliminary Energy Audit

I. A preliminary energy audit provides a description of the building or complex audited and its energy-using characteristics, including:
- The size of the building in gross square feet.
- The age of the building.
- Hours of operation, including periods of partial use and vacation periods, if applicable, and the average number of occupants during each period.
- Identification of major energy-using systems, including:
  1. Primary heating and air conditioning (gas-fired steam boiler, oil hot-air furnace, etc.).
  2. Terminal heating and air conditioning (radiator, unit ventilator, fan-coil unit, double duct, etc.).
  3. Domestic hot water (electric, natural gas, etc.).
  4. Special systems (food service, laundry, etc.).
  5. Lighting (incandescent, fluorescent, etc.).
- Energy use and cost data by type of fuel for the preceding 12-month period; by month, if practicable, using actual data, or estimates if actual figures are unavailable.
- Total annual energy use expressed in btu's, using established conversion factors from engineering manuals.
- Total annual energy use expressed in btu's per gross square foot (the EUI) and energy cost per gross square foot.

II. A preliminary energy audit provides a brief description of activities that have been undertaken to conserve energy in the facility being audited, including whether:
A. A person has been designated to monitor and evaluate energy use.
B. Work partially or fully satisfying the requirements of an energy audit has been performed.
C. Detailed studies of energy use and conservation have been conducted.
D. Any major conservation measures have been considered or implemented (if so, a list of such measures should be provided).

Source: U.S. *Federal Register.*

Table 8-3 Federal Government Definition of a Complete Energy Audit

I. An energy audit should contain all the information required of a preliminary audit, plus descriptions of the following:
A. Major changes in functional use and mode of operation planned in the coming 15 years (renovation, demolition, etc.).
B. For buildings of more than 200,000 gross square feet, if available:
  1. Peak electric demand, both daily and annual cycles.
  2. Annual energy use by fuel type for each major mechanical or electrical system, if information is available or can be reasonably estimated.
C. A description of general building conditions.

II. An energy audit should provide a determination of appropriate energy-effective maintenance and operating procedures for the facility through:
A. Demonstration based on actual records of energy use that consumption has been reduced not less than 20 percent annually through implementation of changes in operations and maintenance.
B. Recommendations, on the basis of on-site inspection, of energy-saving changes, including a scheduled preventive maintenance plan and a general estimate of energy and cost savings resulting from one of the following:
  1. Effective operation of ventilation systems and control of infiltration conditions, including: (1) repair of caulking or weatherstripping around windows and doors; (2) reducing outside air, shutting down ventilation in unoccupied areas, or both; and (3) assuring central or unit ventilating controls are operating properly.
  2. Changes in the operation of heating and cooling systems through: (1) lowering or raising indoor temperatures, (2) locking thermostats, (3) adjusting supply or heat-transfer medium temperatures, and (4) reducing or eliminating heating and cooling at night or at other times when a structure is unoccupied.
  3. Changes in the operation of lighting systems through: (1) reducing illumination levels, (2) maximizing use of daylight, (3) using higher-efficiency lamps, and (4) reducing or eliminating evening cleaning of buildings.

(Continues on page 290.)

Table 8-3 continued

4. Changes in the operation of water systems through: (1) repairing leaks, (2) reducing the quantity of water used (for example, with flow restrictors), (3) lowering settings for hot water temperatures, and (4) raising temperature settings for chilled water systems.
5. Changes in the operation and maintenance of the utility plant and distribution systems through: (1) cleaning equipment; (2) adjusting air-to-fuel ratios; (3) monitoring combustion; (4) adjusting fans, motors, and belt drives; (5) maintaining steam traps; and (6) repairing distribution pipe insulation.
6. Such other changes as may be determined to be useful or necessary.

III. An energy audit should indicate the need, if any, for the acquisition and installation of energy conservation measures and should include an evaluation of the need and potential for retrofit based on consideration of one or more of the following:
A. An energy-use index or indexes, for example, the EUI.
B. Annual energy cost per gross square foot.
C. Physical characteristics of the building envelope and major energy-using systems.

IV. An energy audit may include:
A. An assessment of the estimated costs of and savings from all suggested energy actions.
B. The projected simple payback periods likely to be involved in the purchase and installation of energy-conserving systems and equipment.

Source: U.S. *Federal Register.*

areas of effort must be considered in a comprehensive energy management program: how many of these are presented as proposal guidelines will depend on management's assessment of the institution's ability to cope with perceived problems without outside assistance. Depending on individual need, the request for proposal should ask prospective consultants to quote on some or all of the following:

1. A complete examination of the physical plant, including mechanical equipment, aimed at the identification of specific ways to increase energy efficiency and reduce energy cost.
2. An economic and functional appraisal of plant and equipment that will provide the institution with data to use in developing intermediate and long-range capital equipment plans and budgets.
3. A comprehensive assessment of all institution policies and procedures affecting energy consumption.
4. The establishment of the means for monitoring energy consumption, energy efficiency, and the continuing effectiveness of the energy conservation program.
5. The establishment of information and education programs to ensure that institution employees will be aware of proper conservation practices and to encourage widespread participation in the total energy conservation effort.

HOUSEKEEPING

Key Responsibility Areas*

Among the key responsibilities of the housekeeping department are to:

1. Clean floors
2. Clean furniture
3. Discharge cleaning
4. Move furniture
5. Remove garbage
6. Replace mattresses
7. Replace disposables in washrooms (paper towels, soap, etc.)
8. Replace supplies in utility rooms
9. Clean housekeeping equipment
10. Clean isolation rooms
11. Inservice training
12. Orientation
13. Clean fixtures
14. Clean walls and ceilings
15. Exterminate bugs and pests
16. Clean curtains
17. Clean windows
18. Wash canopies
19. Clean bathrooms
20. Defrost refrigerator in nursing station
21. Clean elevators
22. Water plants.

(NOTE: See Table 8-4 for the goals of a housekeeping department in a typical hospital.)

*Source: Alberta Education, *Management Planning and Appraisal Systems Manual*, Edmonton, Alta., Canada, Alberta Education, 1976, p. 9.

Housekeeping Services Director: Job Duties*

• Directs and administers the housekeeping program to maintain the hospital environment in a sanitary, attractive, and orderly condition.
• Establishes standards and work procedures for the housekeeping staff in accordance with the established policies of the hospital. Plans work schedules and assigns hours and areas of work to insure adequate service for all areas of the hospital. Interviews, selects, hires, evaluates, and terminates personnel and is responsible for their training and supervision.
• Inspects and evaluates the physical condition of the hospital; recommends painting, repairs, furnishings and refurnishing, relocation of equipment, and reallocation of space to improve sanitation, appearance, and efficiency. Reports any unsafe conditions. Conducts research to improve housekeeping technology. Investigates and evaluates new housekeeping supplies and equipment. Takes, processes, and analyzes microbiological samples of air and surfaces to evaluate housekeeping methods and materials.
• Conducts staff meetings and meets with members of other departments to coordinate housekeeping activities with those of other departments. Serves on the Infection Control Committee and on other committees as requested.
• Prepares budgets, work reports, and other administrative guides. Inventories housekeeping supplies and equipment, and selects and requisitions new or replacement supplies and equipment. Is responsible for maintaining the records of the Housekeeping Department.

Theft in Housekeeping**

In most hospitals, housekeeping supplies and equipment are purchased centrally and stocked in general storage. The numerous cleaning fluids and paper products used by housekeeping crews are rarely a prevalent target for mass diversion. Petty theft is easily accomplished, but there is a

---

*Source: *Job Descriptions and Organizational Analysis for Hospitals and Related Health Services,* U.S. Training and Employment Service, Department of Labor, 1971.

**Source: Walter Nagel, "Health Care Industry's Vulnerability to Theft," *Topics in Health Care Financing,* Winter 1978.

good chance that waste is a greater source of loss in the housekeeping department than pilferage.

The difficulty of supervising a cleaning crew that is widely dispersed throughout the hospital or health care institution aggravates the waste problem. Even fresh linen is not safe, since instead of walking some distance to the housekeeping closet for a supply of rags the housekeeping crew often pick up towels and pillowcases to wipe walls, etc.

Cleaning equipment is occasionally removed, particularly in a campus-type hospital where control of car and truck traffic is difficult to achieve. Usually, however, all the floor polishers and vacuum cleaners stolen do not represent a very substantial loss.

The biggest risk with the housekeeping crew is their exposure to other supplies and equipment. Cleaners, sweepers and polishers often work in deserted departments where office equipment, microscopes and other items are easily accessible. Trash disposal offers the housekeeping staff the biggest opportunity for concealing and eventually removing valuable equipment. Without concealment in the trash, removal of heavy equipment is usually too difficult and too risky. For that reason trash compacting equipment is one of the best investments not only for efficient trash disposal, but also for narrowing the chance of valuable equipment and supplies being concealed in huge trash disposal units.

LAUNDRY MANAGEMENT

As central laundries and linen supply firms have become more common, the laundry manager's role has expanded to include buying linen, warehousing, issuing new linen, delivering, collecting and sometimes repairing linen. In addition to managing people and equipment, the modern laundry manager also has to manage large quantities of supplies. Shortages and linen abuse have thus become major worries.

Linen Use Management*

Linen management can effect improvements in two ways: first through linen control—that is,

---

*Source: Jim Summers, "Beyond Dirty Linen: Linen Management as an Innovative Asset," *Health Care Management Review,* Spring 1979.

Table 8-4 Goals of Housekeeping (Misericordia Hospital)

Goal categories	Goals
Physical structure	• Assess need for change in the physical structure of the hospital.
	• Inform the appropriate hospital management where a modification in the physical structure of the hospital would facilitate maintenance of a clean, safe environment.
Equipment and material	• Continuously investigate the acquisition of new cleaning equipment or cleaning agents which will facilitate the development and maintenance of a clean, safe environment.
	• Maintain adequate supplies of materials in the service rooms.
	• Maintain the equipment in proper working order.
	• Make equipment readily accessible to those who need it.
Work processes and methods	• Standardization processes and methods of cleaning.
	• Provide consistent uniform instruction on how to do jobs and utilize equipment.
	• Evaluate staffing patterns such as whether staff should be rotated through all areas or be assigned permanent areas of responsibility.
	• Continuously evaluate methods in terms of effectiveness and safety.
	• Open communication with other departments about factors interfering with housekeeping functions.

Safety
- Provide adequate safety training.
- Ensure that equipment meets acceptable safety standards.
- Continuously assess and if necessary improve the safety of work processes and methods.

Education
- Institute an orientation
  (a) to hospital
  (b) ways of supporting housekeeping department.

Management and staff relations
- Foster and maintain an attitude of cooperation and respect among staff members.
- Improve communication through
  (a) regularly scheduled meetings
  (b) constructive criticism
  (c) consultation with staff
  (d) prompt action on grievances, complaints, etc.
- Assign work equitably and fairly.
- Assess staffing patterns.

Relations with other departments
- Assess the functions presently performed by housekeeping and reduce those which are inappropriate.
- Endeavor to achieve an optimal amount of cooperation with other departments through mutual understanding of each department's roles.

Source: Merla H. Dyck, Clarence Weppler, and Allen Woodruff, "Goal Setting in Hospital Departments," *Health Care Management Review*, Summer 1981.

by lowering linen use levels and reducing replacement costs; and second, through providing good management information to use areas.

Reducing Replacement Costs

Many institutions spend $.05 or more per year in replacement costs per pound of linen processed. Proper linen use management can reduce these costs to less than $.03. A mere $.0075 per pound reduction will save $30,112.50. Replacement costs are not the only area in which proper linen use management can create savings; controlling levels of linen use is also important.

Reducing Use Levels

Properly controlled institutions are able to contain linen use at approximately ten pounds per patient day without any patients being short of linen. This is accomplished by eliminating linen abuse in various forms.

Providing Management Information

A linen use manager should be able to cut linen replacement costs and to lower linen use per patient day. Given a 500-bed occupancy rate, if per-pound replacement costs could be lowered by $.0075 per year and use per patient day by a mere two pounds, total annual savings should approach $49,457.

Linen use managers can produce variance reports that identify high-use and high-cost areas, along with low-use and low-cost areas. In either, abuse may have occurred, either of the linen or possibly of the user (radically different linen use ratios for units providing similar treatment may be an indication of different care patterns).

Linen Theft*

Not only do all people use sheets and pillowcases in their homes, but linen, if it is in good condition (particularly factory new) is very marketable. Linen has even been accepted as currency in the dope traffic market. One heroin addict was told exactly where to find linen in a certain hospital. He was told, "You come back with one sheet or three pillowcases, and I'll give you a fix."

---

*Source: Walter Nagel, "Health Care Industry's Vulnerability to Theft," *Topics in Health Care Financing,* Winter 1978.

Linen, wherever possible, should be stored so that only personnel who have access to it as part of their actual duties can pilfer it. Linen supplies in stock should be made inaccessible to a large crew of stock people and order fillers by being kept under lock and key. The keys must not be submastered. In fact, where possible, access to unused linen storage would best be protected by a dual keying operation where no one individual in possession of one key can have access to the stock.

The difficulties in protecting linen in transit are numerous. The linen on top of the cart is inviting to potential thieves. Zipped plastic or canvas covers, even padlocked at one end, have been more successful. At least they have brought about an obstacle to the temptation to rifle the carts in elevators, on elevator landings and in corridors.

Positioning the closet or linen cart alcove directly facing the nursing station is the best way to deter pilferage. In this way, even during thinly staffed hours, the linen is within a reasonable line of vision of the nursing staff. This is the most practical and reasonably enforceable method of protecting linen from pilferage by people walking through the hospital corridors (patients, visitors, professional staff, housekeeping staff and intruders).

Keeping the supply of linen very low to correspond with bed occupancy on each floor in theory would limit the quantities of linen accessible to patients and visitors, thereby eliminating the temptation for theft and reducing the losses. In practice, more often than not these tactics have resulted in massive hoarding by the staff, with nurses tucking linen away in a variety of closets and corners, including patient rooms. Thus limiting accessibility quickly results in increased accessibility and consequently increased losses.

The use of commercial or cooperative laundries serving numerous health care institutions changes the pattern of exposure. Trucks hauling soiled linen in one direction and bringing back clean linen offers a new dimension. Soiled linen is not a significant target of theft. But diversion of clean linen involving truck drivers in transit can amount to substantial losses. Control by weighing, the prevalent method of keeping track of linen, is notoriously unreliable due to delays in the turnaround (caused by equipment breakdowns, labor problems, etc.). Locking or sealing trucks at the point of departure is not feasible when trucks make frequent pickups and deliveries.

Locking or sealing of individual hampers or carts wheeled onto the truck, however, is a workable protective measure. It makes it necessary for the driver to be in collusion either with a loader at the laundry or the unloader at the hospital before the linen can be successfully diverted. Seal number accountability or custody of the keys to the hampers is a tedious task, yet often worth the effort to prevent massive losses while trucking clean linen.

Internal Audit Checkpoints*

Hospitals must handle the cleaning of large volumes of soiled and contaminated bed linen, robes, gowns, towels, blankets, and other reusable cloth items. For large hospitals, the volume may reach many thousands of pounds a month. Efficient and economical laundry handling is essential to keeping adequate supplies of clean items on hand at all times at a reasonable cost. Internal auditors must be alert for procedures or problems that add unnecessary costs or produce unsanitary processing and missed opportunities for improvement. In hospitals that contract for laundry services, auditors must evaluate the terms of the contract and the quality of the service to ensure that the institution is receiving good results at a reasonable cost. Below are ten sets of checkpoints on laundry handling.

1. Is the laundry adequately staffed? Does labor turnover appear to disrupt operations?
2. What has been the laundry's safety record? How many injuries have been reported? Are there any obvious safety hazards? Is the laundry clean and adequately lighted and ventilated?

---

*Source: Seth Allcorn, *Internal Auditing for Hospitals*, Aspen Systems Corporation, 1979.

3. Are the employees supervised properly? Does the laundry manager report to management on operations? Does the manager communicate freely with all hospital areas that generate laundry as to needs and problems?
4. How well is the laundry equipped? Is the equipment in good operating condition? Who is responsible for maintaining it?
5. How are inventory records of linen in storerooms and in circulation maintained? How often is it inventoried physically? What is the expected life of linen in service? What costs are associated with repair and replacement? Is there an adequate amount of inventory, too little, too much?
6. How is laundry processed? How is contaminated, stained, and infected linen washed? Are detergents suited to water hardness and do they contribute to pollution? What is the usual processing time required to have linen back in service?
7. How do operating costs compare with commercial laundry services? Is accurate cost information available for comparison? Are utilities used by the laundry metered separately?
8. How is laundry transported? How are soiled items delivered to the laundry? How is contaminated laundry marked and separated from regular laundry? What records are kept of laundry received and delivered?
9. How is damaged linen detected and repaired? Is there a sewing room for repairs? What other services are offered by the sewing room? Is the sewing room equipped properly?
10. What is the overall quality of the laundry's service? Do nursing personnel believe the laundry service is good?

Chapter 9—Dietetic (Food Service) Department

OVERVIEW*

Functions

The Dietetic Department is responsible for planning, organizing, and directing all phases of the dietetic operation which includes menu planning; food preparation and service; budget estimates; cost control and administrative recordkeeping; patient therapy and education; analysis and appraisal of personnel requirements; and safety and sanitation programs. The department is responsible for keeping informed of advancements and changes in equipment and food for possible application.

It is a responsibility of the Dietetic Department to specify quantity and quality of food through use of commodity specifications. Meals must supply basic physiological needs and also have aesthetic appeal to the patient. For efficiency in operations, all diets can be built around general diets by additions and modifications.

Files of recipes for quantity cooking are maintained to facilitate preparation and cost control. The recipes should contain formulas to be followed and indicate yields in terms of number and size of servings, and costs of both total recipe and single servings. A diet manual, prepared or recommended by the department and approved by the medical staff, must be available for use by physicians and nurses.

Food preparation and service constitute a large part of the work of the Dietetic Department. All foods should be prepared under strictly sanitary conditions in accordance with local and State public health regulations. Food should be prepared preserving full color, flavor, and nutritional value; meals should be attractively served. Trays must be inspected so that patients on modified diets will receive proper meals. Dishwashing and housekeeping in main kitchen, floor kitchen, and other dietetic areas usually are also functions of this department.

Another function is that of formal and informal education. Dietetic interns are trained in many hospitals. Nurses, medical and dental students, and interns and residents are instructed in principles of nutrition and diet therapy. The department is also responsible for teaching patients and their families nutrition and modified diet requirements.

Other dietetic services include visiting patients in nursing units to determine their food preferences both as to type of food and manner in which it is prepared; advising patients with special dietetic problems prior to their discharge from the hospital, or as referred from the outpatient clinic; cooperating with medical staff in planning, preparing, and serving metabolic research diets.

Standards

The Joint Commission on Accreditation of Hospitals has developed minimum standards for Di-

---

*Source: *Job Descriptions and Organizational Analysis for Hospitals and Related Health Services,* U.S. Training and Employment Service, Department of Labor, 1971.

etetic Departments in hospitals, which include standards on organization, facilities, personnel, foodhandling practices, records, and policies.

The American Dietetic Association has developed standards for the education of dietetic interns and has established specified educational requirements for qualified dietitians.

In most States, it is required by law that those involved with food service shall be subject to physical examination to determine that they are free of communicable diseases. Local or State Health Departments require that the premises and personnel conform to ordinances and regulations. All employees must wear hair nets and/or caps when handling and preparing food.

Organization

The Dietetic Department (see Figure 9-1) is under the direction of a Food Service Director who usually reports directly to the Administrator or to an Associate Administrator. Administrative policies, budgetary controls, and procedures for carrying out the dietetic program are determined by the Administrator in cooperation with the Food Service Director and heads of other departments involved such as Nursing, Housekeeping, or Laundry. The Food Service Director is then delegated full authority for implementing the dietetic program. The number of staff is determined by such factors as average number of hospital patients, number of modified diets, type of service, number of personnel served, extent of educational programs, and physical capacities of the department.

*Director of Food Service (Dietetics): Job Duties**

● Plans, directs, and coordinates activities of Dietetic Department to provide dietetic service for patients and hospital employees:
● Establishes departmental regulations and procedures, in conformance with administrative policies, and develops standards for organization and supervision of dietetic service. Deter-

---

*Source: *Job Descriptions and Organizational Analysis for Hospitals and Related Health Services*, U.S. Training and Employment Service, Department of Labor, 1971.

mines quality and quantity of food required, plans menus, and controls food costs. Reviews regular diet menus as to cost and suitability to type of hospital, and standardized recipes for menu requirements. Makes frequent inspections of all work, storage, and serving areas to determine that regulations and directions governing dietetic activities are followed. Recommends or institutes changes in techniques or procedures for more efficient operation. Develops and prepares policies and procedures governing handling and storage of supplies and equipment, sanitation, and for records and compiling reports. Prepares job descriptions, organization charts, manuals, and guidebooks covering all phases of departmental operations for use by employees. Makes final determination of kinds and amounts of supplies and equipment needed.
● Interviews and makes final selection of applicants for employment. Reviews work schedules for personnel and job performance ratings.
● Selects, upon recommendation, personnel for transfer, promotion, and special training to insure most effective utilization of individual skills and employee development.
● Reviews records and reports covering number and kinds of regular and therapeutic diets prepared, nutritional and caloric analyses of meals, costs of raw food and labor, computation of daily ration cost, inventory of equipment and supplies. Develops and directs cost control system. Prepares and submits department budget.
● Confers with other department heads regarding technical and administrative aspects of dietetic service. Establishes effective relationships with medical staff, nursing, and other patient care services. Attends hospital staff conferences and transmits information to department staff regarding new developments and trends.
● Delegates authority to supervisory staff for task details to facilitate smooth flow of materials and services.
● Attends professional meetings and conferences to keep informed of current practices and trends in fields of dietetics and nutrition. May prepare articles for publication in professional journals and lecture on various aspects of dietetic operations. May discuss dietetic problems with patients or their families and explain diet therapy for specific case.

In smaller hospitals the duties of Dietitian may be combined with this job.

Figure 9-1   Dietetic department

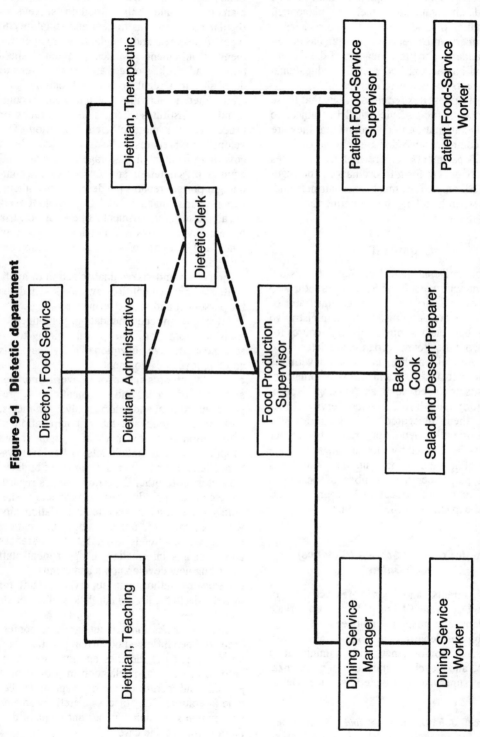

Source: *Job Descriptions and Organizational Analysis for Hospitals and Related Health Services*, U.S. Training and Employment Service, Department of Labor, 1971.

Administrative Dietitian: Job Duties*

[Also known as assistant director of food service or as food production manager]

● Directs and supervises hospital personnel concerned with planning, preparing, and serving food to patients, staff, and visitors:

● Plans basic menus considering such factors as variety, season of the year, availability of foods, known food preferences of the group, nutritional and caloric content, and food costs. Estimates number of people to be served and computes quantity of food to be prepared to insure that individual portions will be in conformance with dietetic standards. Prepares daily menus and portion specification orders for guidance of the staff and inspects prepared food to insure adherence to specifications, observing appearance, quantity, and temperature, and sampling the food to estimate its palatability.

● Develops and implements work standards, sanitation procedures, and personal hygiene requirements consistent with institutional rules; local, State and Federal regulations; and foodhandling principles. Inspects food preparation and serving areas, equipment, and storage facilities, observes the appearance and personal habits of the staff to detect deviations and violations of current health regulations, and orders corrective measures as necessary.

● Prepares daily work schedules and assigns duties and responsibilities, through supervisors, to dietetic staff. Employs dietetic personnel, directs orientation and training, and initiates, recommends, and approves personnel actions, such as transfers, promotions, and separations, according to procedures established by hospital administration.

● Responsible for records and reports concerning technical and administrative operations, such as number of meals served, menus, analyses of diets, food costs, supplies issued, repairs to dietetic equipment, maintenance service and costs, personnel data, and continuous inventory of supplies on hand. Suggests revisions or adaptations of procedures for more efficient performance of department and for training of employees.

---

*Source: *Job Descriptions and Organizational Analysis for Hospitals and Related Health Services,* U.S. Training and Employment Service, Department of Labor, 1971.

● Reviews technical publications, studies journals, and confers with food industry representatives regarding new developments in food packing and processing, new and modified equipment, and new nutritional concepts. Selects those with merit for possible incorporation into the hospital programs.

● Depending on the size and organization of the Dietetic Department, may directly supervise the food preparation personnel, overseeing the cooking, serving, and cleaning tasks. May also supervise all dietetic personnel not specifically assigned to patient food service or modified diet preparation. May direct the employee food-service activity.

MENU PLANNING*

Cycle Menus

Most health care institutions have capitalized on the advantages cycle menus can provide. Cycle menus are defined as carefully planned menus which are rotated according to a definite pattern. Cyclical menus offer numerous advantages, such as:

● Minimizing menu planning time,
● Coordinating preparation,
● Reducing repetition of menu items,
● Promoting standardization of preparation procedures,
● Increasing labor efficiency due to improved coordination and organization planned into the menus,
● Simplifying purchasing,
● Taking advantage of purchasing seasonal variation of foods,
● Improving inventory control and cost control, and
● Maximizing utilization of equipment—potentially resulting in reduction of energy expenditures.

Seasonal menu cycles can vary from two to several weeks. However, experience indicates that the maximum amount of variety with the minimum amount of repetition can be incorporated into a three-week seasonal menu cycle.

---

*Source: Judy Ford Stokes, *Cost Effective Quality Food Service: An Institutional Guide,* Aspen Systems Corporation, 1979.

Some institutions prefer four three-week cycles per year while two three-week cycles (fall/winter, spring/summer) are suitable for others.

Selective v. Nonselective Menus

One menu consideration that surfaces periodically is whether to provide patients with a choice of foods. While this may be an admirable goal, a realistic appraisal must be made that balances the benefits against the changes required.

The following points review the advantages inherent in the selective and nonselective menu.

Selective

- Patient satisfaction could be improved, since there is a positive psychological impact when the patient chooses specific foods.
- Menu variety could be increased, which could minimize special food orders.
- Special diet orders by physicians could be limited because special diets would be ordered only as a therapeutic measure, rather than to cater to a specific patient.
- Knowledge of favorite menu items could be improved and used in future menu planning. Patient contact would be fostered if the dietician or food service director offered written guidance in marking the daily menu selection.
- Food waste could be reduced *if* menus were carefully tallied and *if* leftovers could be used on the cafeteria line.

Nonselective

- Food and labor costs would be minimized at least 15 percent.
- Demand on skill and quantity of labor would be decreased due to the reduction in number and types of foods to be prepared.
- Time required for meal preparation and service would be reduced, which would generally enable the food to reach the patient at a more optimum temperature.
- Storage and preparation areas required would be reduced.
- Quantity and types of equipment required would be minimized.
- Quantity of supervision required would be decreased.

- Food waste would be minimized with the nonselective menu, since closer control on all aspects of food service could be maintained.

Many of the advantages inherent in the selective menu are labor-intensive and increase food service costs. However, special institutional circumstances may dictate and justify the need for such an increased expenditure.

LABOR COSTS

Contributing Factors*

The cost of labor is a major consideration in planning and controlling total food service costs. Labor represents approximately 50 percent of total food service costs.

The following food service areas must be carefully evaluated when labor budgets and staffing needs are determined.

- Amount of labor-saving equipment available
- Physical plan of the kitchen area (Does the placement of the preparation and serving areas require extra walking or movement?)
- The use of china as opposed to disposables
- Menu pattern (selective or nonselective menus as well as menu size and complexity)
- Form in which food is purchased (convenience or "homemade" foods)
- Number of meals served per day, seating capacity
- Working conditions in the kitchen (including temperature, humidity, lighting, and noise)
- Personnel training programs, motivation, and skill of employees
- Amount and adequacy of supervision
- Current wage rate
- Rate of labor turnover
- Personnel productivity
- Performance standards required in production and service (Maintaining high standards will require more supervision.)
- Employee morale (low morale may result in

---

*Source: Judy Ford Stokes, *Cost Effective Quality Food Service: An Institutional Guide*, Aspen Systems Corporation, 1979.

substandard performance, low productivity, and/or absenteeism)

- Number and complexity of therapeutic diets
- Quantity of nourishments and/or between-meal feedings to be prepared and served
- The department that dispenses trays to patients
- The department that is responsible for maintaining sanitation standards in the dining room
- Type of food service (self-service, length of daily operation, number and type of special services provided)

True Hourly Costs*

It is important to remember that the hourly employee wage rate is only the beginning of actual labor costs incurred by the employer. Although this cost may be considerable, especially with the rising minimum wage, it can become the least costly component of labor when the hidden costs are considered.

Table 9-1 graphically presents the expenses incurred by the employer on an hourly basis per employee. Assuming that an employee were paid $3.35 per hour, the following expenses incurred by the employer would yield an actual productive cost of $9.74 per hour, almost triple the base wage.

NOTE: Food service productivity has been estimated at approximately 50 percent—compared to other industry productivity rates of 80 percent.

Development of a Food Service Productivity Index**

Because the food service department operates continuously throughout the year, it is not uncommon to maintain constant dietary department staffing to meet peak utilization requirements. This staffing rigidity limits the ability of the food service managers to respond effectively and efficiently to fluctuations in the daily census and resulting food service demand. As a result,

---

*Source: Judy Ford Stokes, *Cost Effective Quality Food Service: An Institutional Guide,* Aspen Systems Corporation, 1979.

**Source: Karlton Brehm, "Developing a Food Service Productivity Index," *Topics in Health Care Financing,* Winter 1977.

Table 9-1 Actual Hourly Employer Costs Per Employee[1]

Base Rate Paid to Employer per Hour	$3.35
FICA (employer's share)	.20
Workmen's Compensation	.07
Unemployment Compensation	.11
Medical and Hospital Insurance	.13
Uniform Allowance	.05
Meals (two, each costing employer $1.00)	.27
Meal Breaktime (30 minutes)	.24
Coffee Breaks (2 @ 15 minutes each)	.24
Vacation (one week)	.07
Time Off for sickness (7 days)	.07
Holiday Pay (7 days)	.07
Total Cost Per Hour	4.87
Total Productive Cost Per Hour (50% Productivity)	$9.74

[1]The figures do not include additional employer costs incurred for supervision, pilferage, payroll preparation, bookkeeping, overtime, institutional maintenance for employees, life insurance, or other employee benefits.

numerous periods occur throughout the normal operating cycle when the food service department's staff is underutilized.

Following is a system to assist health care managers in monitoring and controlling the productive efficiency of a food service department.

Individual Measurement System

This measurement system should:

- Establish labor efficiency standards.
- Provide an accountability system for both management and staff use.
- Serve as a basis to establish departmental labor goals and objectives.
- Measure those aspects of labor utilization controllable by the dietary department's management.
- Establish the bases for interperiod comparison and evaluation.

Routinely Compiled Information

A partial list of the relevant data routinely compiled by the accounting system include:

- Labor hours—normally accumulated according to job classifications, shifts and functional areas.
- Labor dollars—accumulated by job classifi-

cation (for example, preparation, cafeteria, etc., shifts and functional areas).

- Gross food purchases—recorded and segregated by major classifications (e.g., meat, poultry, dairy products and dry goods).
- Meals served—statistically accumulated for each functional service area (for example, inpatient routine, special dietary and cafeteria).

Labor hours and the number of meals served appear to be the most suited to the development of a productivity measurement system. A correlation between the number of labor hours required to produce a given number of meals and the number of meals produced should be consistent regardless of cost or price increases. As the volume of meals produced varies, so should the manhours required and the efficiency of the manhours employed.

Example

The first step in compiling a productivity measurement system is to list each employee who worked during the period, separating the employee list into functional areas (inpatient routine, special dietary, shared classifications, etc.) and job classifications (dishwasher, cook, supervisor, etc.). Next, identify the department's employees by name, job classification, individual hours worked during the period and the total hours worked by the department.

Third, compile the total meals and equivalent meals served by each functional area for the period.

1. Record each employee and the number of hours worked by functional area and job description.
2. Record the number of meals or equivalent meals served.
3. Subtotal the manhours worked for each job classification and total all manhours worked in each functional area.
4. Calculate the index value by dividing the number of meals served by the number of manhours worked. The resulting index value represents the number of meals produced per manhour by individual employee, job classification and functional area (see Table 9-2).

Chris Jones' index value indicates that 25.5 meals per hour were produced for each manhour

(a total of 12.0 per preparation manhour). The functional area, inpatient routine, produced 6.1 meals per manhour. The entire food service department produced a total of 2,625 meals, using 587 manhours, or approximately 4.5 meals per manhour.

Cumulative Results

After several periods of data have been accumulated, an average or "normal" relationship between manhours and meals served will become apparent. This average can be used as the standard by which each subsequent period can be evaluated. The establishment of a relevant range of acceptable results at varying activity levels will facilitate more efficient staff utilization and manpower planning.

The information developed by the measurement system can be correlated with the census forecast and other future activity information to determine future staff requirements. Vacations or other employee time off can be scheduled in advance so that the manhours to be worked correspond to the estimated production levels.

THEFT*

Petty Pilferage

In terms of petty pilferage, food is the most diversified target in any hospital, with much food being dishonestly consumed on the premises. This type of pilferage may be relatively harmless, resulting in little or no loss to the hospital, particularly when employees eat food left on patients' trays. Attempts to curtail this type of eating on the premises for contamination reasons usually are without success. In spite of attempts at locking up food supplies in the kitchen, employees can pilfer food by invading the kitchen's storerooms and the pantries on the inpatient floors. This usually occurs at night. It is the guards and maintenance and housekeeping personnel who are often the biggest offenders in this area, since they are in charge of submaster keys which allow access to these areas.

---

*Source: Walter Nagel, "Health Care Industry's Vulnerability to Theft," *Topics in Health Care Financing,* Winter 1978.

Table 9-2   Sample Worksheet to Calculate Meals Per Manhour

Job Classification and Functional Area	Hours Worked	Total No. of Meals Served	Index Value
Inpatient routine		1,800	
Preparation:			
Chris Jones	70		25.7
Steve Snyder	80		22.5
Subtotal preparation hours	150		12.0
Cooks:			
John Smith	87		20.7
Subtotal cook hours	87		20.7
Dishwashing:			
Ralph Armstrong	60		30.0
Subtotal dishwashing hours	60		30.0
Total inpatient routine hours	297		6.1
Special Dietary		150	
Cooks:			
Bill Reynolds	65		2.3
Total cook hours	65		2.3
Total special dietary hours	65		2.3
Cafeteria		675	
Cashiers:			
Linda Burr	30		22.5
Total cashiers hours	30		22.5
Busboys:			
Tom Peters	35		19.3
Total busboy hours	35		19.3
Total cafeteria hours	65		10.8
Shared Classifications		2,625	
Purchasing department:			
Bill Allen	80		32.8
Total purchasing hours	80		32.8
Management:			
Alex Lang	80		32.8
Total management hours	80		32.8
Total shared classification hours	160		16.4

Source: Karlton Brehm, "Developing a Food Service Productivity Index," *Topics in Health Care Financing,* Winter 1977.

Organized Pilferage

Some food pilferage involving eating on the premises is more organized. In large cities, hospital employees, particularly the unskilled employees of the dietary department, have on occasion brought in whole families from their neighborhoods to feed them in deserted corridors or hidden stockroom corners of the hospital.

However, even in the inner-city hospitals where such activities can assume sizable proportions, the total volume of pilfered food is rarely enough to raise the food cost per patient per day significantly. Therefore, if the buildings lend themselves to easy concealment and the traffic is essentially uncontrollable, as in most campus-type institutions, it is usually a waste of energy to cope with this type of theft.

Highest priority should be given to diversion of food in quantity. To curtail this type of theft there is only one principal method—lockup—to achieve very limited accessibility. High-priced items such as meats and poultry, canned fish, coffee and any packaged foods that are highly desirable and easily concealable, must be locked in freezers, coolers, stockrooms or cages where only the personnel assigned to these areas have access. Specifically, nighttime lockup must be very strict, with hardware not keyed to submasters available to nondietary personnel. Personnel who allow access to unauthorized persons must be subject to severe disciplinary action.

The biggest losses always result from collusive actions between requisitioner and vendor or between receiver and driver. The most vulnerable items are those which are both purchased and received by the dietary department. In most hospitals this applies to all perishable foods, including the most high-priced products such as meats, poultry and fish. But even shipments of lettuce and other produce have been known to be received short, with drivers pilfering and selling them to the taverns around town and splitting the proceeds with the receiver. For that reason, it is indefensible to have a process where the payment of an invoice for food products requires only the signature of a dietary employee. The principle of dual accountability in receiving, difficult as it is to accomplish in many institutions, is always a step in the right direction.

CHECKLIST FOR CONTROLLING COSTS*

Since food service costs generally represent the second highest expenditure of health care institutions, proper management in this area requires serious consideration. By responding to and analyzing the cost-control checklist which follows,

managers should be able to maximize cost savings *and* reimbursement for food services in health care institutions.

Cost Accounting & Budgeting

1. Are food service cost components budgeted and compared to actual costs on a monthly basis, including raw food, labor, and supplies?
2. Are these costs examined in terms of cost per meal and/or cost per patient day?
3. Has an inventory cost-control system been initiated, monitored, and maintained?
4. Are revenues generated by the food service reflected in the cost per patient meal or per patient day?
5. Are periodic conferences held with administration and other pertinent departments to compare the actual food service expenditures with the food service budget?

Menu Planning

1. Is there a seasonal menu cycle?
2. Is a selective menu essential to maintaining or improving current patient census?
3. Is a selective menu cycle economically feasible?
4. Are therapeutic diets coordinated specifically with the general diet menu to minimize additional preparation?
5. Are menus planned to maximize labor and time efficiency?

Purchasing and Receiving

1. Are firm price quotes obtained on all food purchases?
2. Are these prices obtained through a competitive mechanism (such as a cooperative buying service)?
3. Have monthly purchasing ceilings been established for specific food items such as milk, eggs, bread?
4. Are meat and produce weighed to compare the invoiced quantity with the ordered quantity?
5. Are invoiced prices checked for agreement with quoted prices?

Food Preparation and Service

1. Is portion control consistent and effective?
2. Are specific systems monitoring food quantity established? (For example, how many cans of vegetables are used for each meal?)

*Source: Judy Ford Stokes, *Cost Effective Quality Food Service: An Institutional Guide*, Aspen Systems Corporation, 1979.

3. Are leftovers utilized effectively?
4. Has the actual cost of nutrition-related medical requirements (therapeutic diets, mechanically altered diets, and nutritional supplementation) been determined?
5. Are records kept of the cost of nutrition-related medical requirements?
6. Is the necessity for all therapeutic and mechanically altered diets periodically evaluated?
7. Are ancillary food services (such as supplementary nourishments, special catering functions, and activities) specifically cost detailed?
8. Has policy been set for gross cafeteria receipts to reflect accurately the number of meals served?
9. Do records reflect the actual cost of meals served in patient food service (hospital and/or hospital-based skilled nursing facility) compared to cafeteria food service?

Labor Efficiency
1. Have the number of labor-minutes per meal for the food service been determined?

2. Has the rate of employee turnover been determined?
3. Is the employee turnover rate periodically determined and evaluated?
4. Are job descriptions drafted and reviewed at least annually with respective personnel?
5. Are detailed duty schedules drafted and reviewed at least quarterly with respective personnel?
6. Are records kept of duties performed for at least two weeks each quarter?
7. Is the daily work distribution periodically reviewed to maximize labor efficiency?
8. Are employee and guest meals periodically evaluated for cost effectiveness?

Energy Efficiency
1. Has an energy audit been conducted of the facility?
2. Is energy efficient equipment planned into future equipment replacement budgets?
3. Has each department been trained in methods of energy conservation?
4. Has an effective preventive maintenance program been established?

Chapter 10—Security (Loss Prevention)

OVERVIEW

Controlling the Opportunity*

The three necessary elements to a criminal act are motive, opportunity, and means. Although management can put various restraints on each, only *opportunity* can be controlled. Motives can be curbed by an effective program of positive morale building and company loyalty and built-in reminders of the consequences of illegal acts. The means to steal can be controlled to a certain extent by routine checks at various doors, and by limiting employee access to high-risk areas. But the internal thief, aware of facility policy regarding door checks, will still manage to circumvent the system by getting stolen items out through "secured" doors. Therefore, the only controllable element is opportunity. It will diminish significantly with effective controls.

It is impossible to list all the things that might trigger an employee theft. However, experience shows that the following individuals have the most opportunities:

1. Supervisors and other authority figures
2. Guards
3. Night and weekend employees who are generally unsupervised for long periods
4. People with keys
5. Long-time trusted employees
6. Storekeepers and receivers
7. Clerks handling money and payroll or equipment records
8. Service department personnel
9. Terminating employees

This list is included not to suggest guilt or to exclude other potential thieves, but to generalize the profile; keys, time, lack of supervision or accountability, and authorized access to materials and records represent opportunity. Twenty-five percent of all employees will steal to some degree if they feel they can get away with it, and only a very small percentage are ultimately caught. It is upsetting to note that within that 25 percent, the management-level thief is responsible for over 60 percent of the total loss.

Types of Internal Dishonesty*

NOTE: Also see "Theft" in the separate chapters covering specific hospital departments.

Embezzlement and Fraud

Embezzlers are successful primarily because they are respected employees who handle financial records. Embezzlement is the most costly white collar crime. One expert outlined that embezzlers leave their place of employment each working day with more than $8 million of employers' cash and merchandise, a total of more than $2 billion annually. Regular burglars and robbers do not do half as well.

An effective security system will reveal embezzlement before it becomes disastrous. The use of security audits and document control has proven highly effective.

_____
*Source: A. Michael Pascal, *Hospital Security and Safety,* Aspen Systems Corporation, 1977.

Pilferage

Too many administrators fail to see the folly of stationing a guard at the front door of the facility to monitor members of the public who enter and leave, while leaving the employees' entrance and the shipping and receiving areas open with no security present at all. The amount of money that is lost through your front doors over a ten-year span will in no way match the loss you suffer in one year through your back doors. In general, the following represent materials most often vulnerable to employee pilferage:

1. Linens: sheets, towels, blankets, curtains, draperies
2. Clothing: uniforms, aprons, robes, and gowns
3. Food: patient trays, cafeteria and dietary department supplies
4. Maintenance supplies: paint, hardware, light bulbs, lumber, hand and power tools, plumbing supplies
5. Paper goods: stationery, office supplies, housekeeping supplies
6. Capital equipment: electric fans, projectors, typewriters, furniture, floor polishers
7. Drugs and pharmaceuticals
8. Money: facility and personal
9. Patients' and employees' belongings: jewelry, luggage, clothing, personal appliances
10. Medical supplies and equipment: stethoscopes, surgical instruments, laboratory equipment
11. Gift shop supplies and equipment
12. Housekeeping supplies: soaps, brooms, pails
13. Photographic supplies and equipment: cameras, film, projectors, enlargers
14. Time: intangible, but costly

The term "pilferage" usually means small-scale theft of insignificant items. However, regular or long-term pilferage will rapidly add up to a major loss.

Kickbacks and Collusion

Collusion, the cooperative meeting of two thieves, can be present anywhere in the facility. For example, it could involve a document falsification scheme between members of the shipping and accounting departments; it could involve an authorized keyholder's "loaning" keys to someone else; and it could involve a major kickback operation between the facility purchasing agent and an outside supplier.

The purchasing department requires special attention, as it is an area particularly vulnerable to kickback. In brief, management must monitor long-term relationships between inhouse purchasing agents and outside suppliers. Be wary of the agent who prefers to deal with an established supplier in any new transactions rather than to receive competitive bids; while in reality merely extending the kickback, the agent may argue that the established supplier's quality of service and fair prices are known. The unchallenged, long-term relationship can lead to many abuses. The supplier, now assured of business, becomes lax in the accounts. Orders may be neglected and quality reduced, while top-line materials are channeled to another facility where the purchasing agent is not on the take. It might be more profitable for the supplier to court the other hospital.

Responsibility for Security*

It is usually a mistake to place the primary responsibility for preventing loss of hospital assets on the security director, captain of the guards or a similar individual. A capable security chief or captain of the guard can make essential contributions in the area of perimeter protection, internal lockup effectiveness, traffic control in all its dimensions and investigative activities, including contact with law enforcement agencies. However, the most competent security chiefs, whether they enter the hospital field with a police background or other law enforcement experience, cannot with any degree of effectiveness assume the responsibility for the numerous loss prevention problems involving systems and procedures.

The responsibility for procedural security must be assumed by a person well versed in the problems of materials handling, paperwork documentation and accounting procedures. In a medium-sized or small hospital, the controller would be the logical choice. However, control-

---

*Source: Walter Nagel, "Health Care Industry's Vulnerability to Theft," *Topics in Health Care Financing,* Winter 1978.

lers are "desk-bound" accountants, with little knowledge of materials handling, truck traffic, receiving operations, distribution methods, etc.

The Assistant Administrator

The ultimate choice therefore should be an assistant administrator whose talent, exposure and interest permit the merging of procedural accountability problems with physical security problems in arriving at overall solutions protecting the assets of the hospital.

Rarely does one person possess the talents and the experience that would allow him to accept total responsibility for all phases of loss prevention, procedural as well as physical. Hospitals with at least 750 beds usually have an industrial engineering staff or a systems and procedures department. Often these are the people best suited for assuming a comprehensive responsibility for loss prevention programs. But they will require strong efforts at coordination.

Committees

The establishment of a committee can be an excellent approach to coordinating industrial engineering staff or systems and procedures staff. The committee, for example, could consist of the controller, an industrial engineer and the security director.

Controller's Role

No matter how broad the responsibilities of the security chief, and regardless of who in the administration has the ultimate loss prevention responsibility, the controller has to take an active part in the vast majority of the loss prevention measures. This active part must include influencing the procedures and the policies as they are generated, and using the audit staff as the most effective potential enforcement tool.

In smaller hospitals, where the budget does not permit a sizable audit staff, the same principle should prevail. But in practice, controllers in small hospitals, with the help of external auditors under contract, will have to function as internal auditors would in larger institutions.

SCOPE OF A SECURITY PROGRAM*

There are two basic facets of security, physical and procedural. Physical security involves protecting the facility against intrusion from without and diversion of goods from within. It involves the integration of a large variety of protective measures including control of the facility's perimeter, lockup techniques, electromechanical devices, electronic surveillance and traffic control including employees, visitors, drivers and contractors.

Procedural security involves developing specific accountability controls directed at the flow of hospital supplies and materials, especially all receiving functions and regulating the operation of the dock. The most far-reaching security problems are procedural in nature. The most sophisticated electronic equipment cannot prevent people from diverting supplies and materials over a receiving or loading dock. It is the procedural accountability controls governing the flow of these goods which must provide the strongest basis for security. All other security measures should be built around those controls.

The "inventory-of-exposure" method is one of the best approaches to developing a comprehensive, practical loss-prevention program. This approach involves distinguishing between the two principal categories of hospital supply diversion: petty pilferage perpetrated by employees, visitors, contractors or intruders; and large-scale theft committed through collusive effort—collusion among deliverers, receivers, material handlers, maintenance people or janitors, or collusion among higher-level hospital employees such as purchasing agents, vendors, bookkeepers and data processing personnel. The inventory-of-exposure approach realistically assesses the relative risks and potential losses in both categories of diversion.

Practical targets of vulnerability that should be addressed include:

- the procurement process—curtailing collusion between buyers and vendors;
- receiving-dock operations—attacking the numerous risks of mass diversion;

---

*Source: Walter Nagel, "A Total Approach to Loss Prevention," *Topics in Health Care Financing*, Winter 1978.

- the facility's perimeter—protecting sites and buildings from intrusion, and channeling traffic patterns (includes the use of electronic devices and an effective guard force); and
- internal security—cutting back access to easily marketable supplies and materials.

Optional targets include:

- contractor collusion;
- abuse of equipment and materials;
- payroll fraud;
- computer fraud;
- expense account abuse;
- diversion through scrap disposal; and
- compromised information (research material, financial data, patient records).

For a complete survey of areas of potential security problems, the hospital administrator may find the "Hospital Security Questionnaire" (Figure 10-1, on page 310) useful.

Perimeter Traffic and Employee Theft

The ease with which theft of larger pieces of equipment and sizable quantities of supplies can be curtailed varies. One factor determining this is the level of existent protection of the perimeter of individual buildings or the total complex. Modern hospitals consisting of one major single structure are easier to protect than huge campus-type facilities consisting of innumerable buildings, some completely separate, others connected by tunnels and bridges. Some campus-type installations covering several city blocks lend themselves to effective fencing; others do not.

Controlling Traffic

It should be difficult for people entering or leaving the institution, especially employees, to carry stolen equipment or supplies out of the building. Controlling pedestrian traffic is not impossible but is usually very costly. It is also time consuming and may affect the attitude of hospital personnel. Costly measures may include a centrally monitored burglary-type alarm system, a carefully planned and rigidly enforced lockup schedule, and strategic guard coverage of all unlocked exits.

Channeling of different types of traffic through different entrances and exits is also an excellent method. Ideally, no staff members should enter or leave by the same exit reserved for patients and visitors. Entering or exiting vendors, salespeople, delivery people, contractors and service personnel should not be allowed to mingle with patients and visitors; rather they should be routed through a permanently guarded entrance where they can be identified, scrutinized and properly directed. No pedestrian traffic of any kind should be permitted to cross receiving docks, trash docks, morgue exits or truck gates.

Visitor passes have been abolished in many institutions, even in some inner-city hospitals. Drastic structural variations, which have become the fashion in recent years, have made visitor control close to impossible in some institutions. This is especially true when outpatient services (treatment areas and private physicians' offices) intermingle with inpatient areas. Thus coping with intruders has become the task of a patrolling guard force, aided by ward managers and the nursing staff.

Alarm Systems

No two hospitals are alike, no matter how similar they are in design, and no two hospitals require the same alarm system. In certain hospitals—especially rural hospitals that are protected by total fencing, and those that have a type of vehicular and pedestrian traffic which is easily controlled—any capital budget or maintenance expenditure for an alarm system would be a total waste. Other hospitals may require the most sophisticated and near foolproof burglary alarm systems to protect the entire perimeter, supported by strategically located internal intrusion alarms of the microwave, ultrasonic or photoelectric cell variety.

Guard Coverage

The best trained and best organized guard force will at most provide only a fraction of required security in any hospital. However, the guard force can be a valuable supporting agent in many of the areas comprising the total program, including materials movement, dock security, and traffic control and its many aspects.

Figure 10-1   Hospital security questionnaire

Purchasing	Which departments are almost autonomous in purchasing their supplies?

Dietary ☐   Maintenance ☐   Pharmacy ☐

OR ☐   X-ray ☐   Central supply ☐

Labs ☐   Laundry ☐   Housekeeping ☐

Others:

Receiving	Which departments listed above do their own receiving, directly from vendors?

Payment of Invoices	What type of document supports a vendor's invoice?

	Packing Slip	Receiving Record	PO Copy
Received at Central Dock			
Received by Department			

Construction

Are competitive bids from contractors mandatory?

For all construction ☐   For projects over $_____

What documentation is required for contractors' invoices?

for labor_____

for materials_____

for equipment rental _____

Whose approval will authorize payment?

Chief engineer ☐   Chief of maintenance ☐

Administrator (associate or assistant) ☐

Figure 10-1   continued

Stores

Easy Access versus Reliable Lockup

Storage Areas	Accessible to Roving Guards, Janitors, Aides, Maintenance People, Construction Crews	Reliable Lockup
General Stores		
Central Supply		
Dietary		
Pharmacy		
Linen		
Maintenance		
Laboratories		
X-Ray		

Distribution

Supply Categories	Manual by Carts, Hampers Flat Trucks, Baskets	Mechanical		
		Dumb-waiters	Con-veyors	Auto-mated Lifts
General Supplies				
Surgical Supplies				
Meals				
Drugs				
Prescriptions				
Linen				

Other means _____

Inpatient Floors

Risky Exposure versus Reasonable Protection

Supply Categories	Open Storage		Reliable Lockup
	Dispersed	Part of Nursing Station	
Surgical Supplies			
General Supplies			

Figure 10-1 continued

Inpatient
Floors Cont.

Risky Exposure versus Reasonable Protection Cont.

Open Storage			
Supply Categories	Dispersed	Part of Nursing Station	Reliable Lockup
Linen			
Nonprescription Drugs			
Purses—Nursing Staff			

Hold-up
Risks

Are Cash and Drugs Protected by Holdup Devices?

	Panic Alarms	TV Surveillance
Main Cashier		
Satellite Cashiers		
Main Pharmacy		
Satellite Pharmacies		
Cafeteria Cashiers		
Vending Machines		
Gift Shop		
Garage Cashiers		

Parking

What Protection Is Available against Theft, Vandalism or Personal Attack in Parking Lots and Garages?

	Guard Patrols	Audio Surveillance	TV Surveillance	Panic Alarms
Open Lots				
Covered Garages				

Equipment

Are electric typewriters bolted down?   Yes ☐   No ☐

Are tape recorders, projectors locked up?   Yes ☐   No ☐

Is it easy to conceal such equipment in trash hampers?   Yes ☐   No ☐

Will guards intercept employees or intruders departing with such equipment?   Yes ☐   No ☐

Figure 10-1 continued

Security
Devices

Does the hospital rely heavily on

CCTV ☐   Intrusion alarms ☐   Door contact alarms ☐

Guard coverage-fixed posts ☐   Patrols ☐

Source: Norman Jasper Associates, "Hospital Security Questionnaire," *Topics in Health Care Financing,* Winter 1978.

Internal Security

The system of internal security, as opposed to perimeter security, should be based on selective inaccessibility, i.e., selected lockup or alarming, which in turn must be based on an evaluation of the vulnerability of specific equipment and materials.

An integral part of the security program is a clearly defined set of regulations governing the issuance of individual keys, submaster and master keys, and grand masters. The system must include a method of authorization for key issuance and an easily enforceable procedure for retrieving keys.

Petty Pilferage

Patient care areas are notorious sites for storing a large variety of items, many of them useful to almost everybody—pencils and paper clips, aspirins, bandaids, various surgical supplies. Although petty pilferage is unavoidable, the total loss even over a long period of time represents a small percentage of the entire outlay for supplies in any health facility. There is no profit in locking up pencils and paper clips and issuing them out on request because the nuisance and the payroll costs of such issuance far outweigh any amount of losses that could conceivably occur. These items are usually not removed in quantity.

The best method of protecting the supplies should be the same as applied to linen. Storage facilities, whether they are desk drawers, wall closets or cabinets, should be within the circumference of the nursing station if at all possible.

On floors that are very thinly staffed at nighttime, it would be a good measure to provide for lockup of the storage facilities when the day shift goes off duty.

In any outpatient clinic or emergency room, standard surgical supplies have to be within easy reach, virtually in every treatment area. This in itself will contradict any attempts at making accessibility difficult. Lockup will prove unnecessary. Under the circumstances the wisest approach to these patient areas is to consider all supplies expendable and written off whether used judiciously, wasted, or pilfered.

Equipment Theft

Office equipment is infinitely more vulnerable to theft than medical equipment. Late-model electric typewriters and dictation machines bring a very high price, sometimes as much as 60 percent of the prevailing retail price, when sold to "fences." Microscopes are practically the only lab equipment that has a considerable attraction, but they are rarely stolen for financial profit. More often they are taken by employees or intruders who want them for personal use. There is no significant market offering a worthwhile price for second-hand medical equipment, at least not for the type of equipment that can be carried from the premises.

Under these circumstances a health care facility is well advised to expend the greatest effort in protecting their office equipment. While the bolting or lockup of office equipment is essential, it is not enough to protect the equipment. If it is practical, traffic in and out of the hospital should be controlled through effective guard coverage and package or equipment transports should be monitored. The guard force should also aggressively challenge personnel suspected of stealing. Rigid measures like these are usually called for in urban institutions.

Parking Lot Theft

Incidences of car vandalism and theft increase at night and occur more frequently in covered parking garages that have many levels. Slashed tires, stolen spare tires and stolen CB radios are the most frequent incidents, but the highest priority problems involving covered garages and parking lots not adjacent to the hospital include purse snatching, mugging and rape.

Effective curtailment of these combined risks is possible, although quite costly. The best approach is a combination of steady patrolling, preferably motorized, and massive closed-circuit television surveillance.

Personal Property Theft

All hospitals are easy targets for purse snatchers and wallet thieves. Personnel are usually more frequent victims of this type of theft than are patients. Female nursing staff and secretaries are often careless about leaving pocketbooks in easily accessible places. Female patients sometimes fall asleep with their pocketbooks at the foot of the bed. Male employees, particularly the professional staff, often hang up their jackets with their wallets inside, making them easily available to the potential thief.

Employees' Goods

Personal property theft can be avoided only with the provision of lockup facilities. For example, unless the nursing staff has reasonably adequate storage space in lockers, cabinets or desk drawers that are lockable or located in constantly attended areas, no degree of care and alertness will prevent theft.

Patients' Goods

Safes for patient's valuables substantially reduce the risk of theft of patient's belongings in most institutions. However, patients may at first refuse to turn in their valuables, surrendering them only before going to surgery. When this happens, jewelry and dentures may be temporarily locked up in nurses' desks or even in the narcotics cabinet, and are exposed to theft. A better method, although a considerable burden to the staff, would be to dispatch these personal belongings to the valuables safe as the patient goes into surgery.

Payroll Theft

Time Clock Fraud

Punching the time clock for someone who is absent, who arrives late or departs early is one of the most common forms of payroll fraud. A more serious form is when an employee deliberately avoids work during regular working hours and stays overtime to get the needed work done.

Abuse by Supervisory Staff

The most damaging payroll fraud in industry, in construction and perhaps in hospitals, is usually perpetrated by the supervisory staff themselves. These people may receive pay for "ghosts" on the payroll—nonexistent or retired employees. Employees who have quit may continue to receive their pay and split it with their former supervisors. Any variety of schemes can work.

Cash Theft

The cashiering unit usually adjoins a business office, a financial office or the admissions office. Minimum precautions should be to keep the door between the cashier and these other offices locked at all times. When used, the door should automatically close, with a lockset provided for keyed entry only from the outer office. A small window in the door and a low voltage bell and buzzer can be provided to enable recognition by the cashier before allowing authorized personnel to enter the area.

More sophisticated arrangements may be necessary if the cashier's door is in an area traversed by the public, such as an admissions office or a hospital corridor. The door should then be alarmed or made inaccessible to unauthorized personnel 24 hours a day. Entry or exiting equipment can be controlled through a shunt key or magnetic card key. After it has been opened legally, the door should automatically return to the alarmed or inaccessible mode and returned to a closed position.

At each of the cashiering positions, the minimum protection that should be provided is a "panic button" or holdup alarm that can be foot, knee or hand operated. This alarm should be silent and should annunciate by both a light and a bell or buzzer at a different location in the hospital. The alarm should be relayed (preferably automatically or by telephone) to a local law enforcement agency. In all cases, even if the guard force is armed, the relay should be made to police authorities. The police are usually much better equipped to handle these situations than a guard force empowered only with the rights of "citizens arrest." The cashier should be taught to comply with the burglar's request not to try to be a hero, but at the same time follow the prescribed routine for activating the alarm.

For nighttime protection, a roll-up grill could be designed to enclose the cashiering location, or the cashiering function could be made a separate room removed from a main corridor with a doored entrance. Lockup protection should at least include a padlock for the roll-up grill and a lock for the door of the room.

Naturally small equipment such as digital calculators should be placed in locked drawers or cabinets, while items like electric typewriters in open areas should be bolted to desks.

Security Tactics in Urban Hospitals

1. controlled entrance to the cashiering office, which is protected by alarm 24 hours a day and which has limited access;
2. a bullet-proof glass enclosure with small pass-through windows;
3. a panic button at each cashiering location tied into hospital alarm system, if any, and simultaneous relay to local police authorities;
4. an optional videotape camera triggered by an alarm condition when the cashier uses the panic (or holdup) button;
5. if collections are made from other hospital departments after hours or on weekends when the cashiering office may not be staffed, a commercial night depository safe that has an outside opening constructed through either a reinforced wall or a cut-out slot in the bullet-proof glass.

Main Cashier

Through modern advanced systems technology, cashiers may be equipped with electronic means such as a CRT to view the customer account status. The cashier's function would be to collect the monies owed to the hospital at the time of discharge. Whether the receipt is electronically printed or manually written by the cashier, it should be fully auditable and numerically controlled. This applies to all payments of cash, checks or charge card, whether they are processed through a cash register or collected in a cash box.

Most hospitals are on a nine- to 15-day cycle for final billing (except for terminal billing,

which might be immediate). Whether the system is manual or data processed or a modern CRT approach is used, the cashier should not possess the means manually to remove a patient account from the file by keypunching or by access coding. The cashier should act only as the collection agent and should not be able to feed information into the patients' account system. This input to the system should be accomplished by another person in the control division of the hospital.

Cafeteria

Of course, the most complicated type of cashiering is in the general employee cafeteria, which serves visitors, volunteers and medical staff. Visitors might pay a slight additional surcharge, volunteers may receive discount or no-charge meals and medical staff may receive free late night dinners. Discounts may occur with meal coupons, paper punch cards, passes or sign-out sheets. Whatever the system, the recipient of the discounted or free meal rarely watches what the cashier rings into the register. The cashier could benefit easily by ringing lower rates and having the recipient sign for a larger total or punching a higher total on the meal ticket. On a sign-out sheet, the cashier could insert a false name and employee identification number.

The best defense against this type of theft (besides eliminating all uncontrolled free or discounted meals) is to constantly test cashiers to assure they are ringing and collecting the right amount for each item. This testing can be performed by an outside specialized service which employs professional "shoppers" familiar with cashiering practices, or by hospital security personnel trained in "shopping" techniques. This will ensure against direct theft from the cashiering unit, but it will not prevent cashiers from charging friends less than they should for meals.

Register Thefts

The biggest mistake made by hospitals is to allow the cashier to have both keys needed to operate the register. The first key unlocks the mechanism for register operation and gives total readings for money and number of transactions. (This is usually termed an "A" total, or if two or more different drawers or separate cashier operating keys, there can be "B," "C" and "D" totals.) The second key produces totals, either by cashier or classification, and resets all totals back to zero. This is commonly termed the "Z" total or "Zed" total.

When a simple type of register is used, as in most hospitals, if the cashier has control of both keys, the hospital is probably losing money. For example: a cashier starts at breakfast, rings up about $20 worth of sales, "Zeds" out the register, removes that part of the detail tape, takes out the $20 and starts to ring all over. In a large hospital, this would go unnoticed. Since cafeterias are part of food service, the cost of the cafeteria is partially hidden in the cost of patient meals per day.

In smaller cashiering areas, such as a gift shop, shortages might be revealed by losses discovered by physical inventories. However, if the gift shop is combined with a coffee shop which does not maintain its own inventory and is serviced by the dietary department, there is still room for the cashier to pocket some of the proceeds.

In both of these examples and other similar situations, the financial division rather than departmental personnel should obtain "Zed" totals and reset registers. The financial division should retain the second keys to the register(s) and should be the only ones able to zero out the registers and obtain the final readings. In single drawer registers used by more than one cashier during a day, separate cash tills (banks) can be provided for each cashier. If registers are to be reset only once a day, balancing by cashier can still be achieved.

Safeguards Against Kitchen Pilferage

The administration should investigate the economic extent of personnel pilferage and institute appropriate safeguards to minimize theft that may be small initially but can substantially pervade every department in time. Listed below are several guidelines.

- Institute a perpetual inventory system to protect the institution against a majority of its potential losses.
- Conduct unexpected inventories by employees other than storeroom personnel.
- Secure all storage areas, maintaining a close check on keys.
- Recommend that the food service director periodically check storage areas unannounced.
- Lock the kitchen at night.
- Maintain tighter security near the loading dock.
- Restrict nonfacility personnel from wandering through the premises.
- Prohibit employees from storing personal belongings such as purses in the kitchen.

Source: Judy Ford Stokes, *Cost Effective Quality Food Service: An Institutional Guide*, Aspen Systems Corporation, 1979, p. 56.

Chapter 11—Ancillary Services

OVERVIEW

The hospital's ancillary departments may also be called professional service departments. Literally, ancillary means a department that assists the physician in diagnosis or in the treatment of the patient. Ancillary is defined as a cost (having expenses) and revenue center (able to bill the patient for services) within the hospital which requires, either by regulation or third party urging, either that a physician direct the department or that a physician provide guidance and supervision over the department. In other words, what differentiates an ancillary service department from other hospital departments is that it is able to charge the patient directly, thereby generating revenue for the hospital, and it must be under the direction of a physician.

Ancillary departments are very complex because their charge structure is different and consists of many individual tests. In addition, the departments have highly sophisticated equipment and a variety of well-trained technical staff. Another factor that makes these departments complex for management is physician compensation. There are a variety of ways in which the physicians who direct these departments may be reimbursed.

A typical large community hospital will have the following ancillary departments: clinical laboratory, radiology (x-ray), physical therapy, inhalation therapy, anesthesiology, EKG (electrocardiography, heart station), and EEG (electroencephalography).*

Physician Compensation*

[Also see Chapter 2: Medical Staff] Generally, ancillary physicians are under some form of contractual arrangement with the hospital. There are a wide variety of contractual arrangements available to an administrator and a board of trustees when hiring a physician for the laboratory. These arrangements are also applicable to other ancillary service physicians. Common contractual arrangements include the following: the physicians could receive a percentage of the department's gross charges or a percentage of the department's net income; they might be given a professional fee-for-service; or they could be paid as hospital employees. In some hospitals the physicians lease the ancillary department, managing it somewhat as a franchise.

It should be noted that, unlike many of the other physicians who serve patients, these hospital-based specialists work under special contracts. These specialists—radiologists, anesthesiologists, and pathologists—could be considered to have a monopoly within the hospital, since, once they sign a contract, other competing specialists in their discipline outside of their group are not allowed to practice in the hospital.

Hospital Facilities: Ancillary Services

Hospitals frequently are gauged on the quantity of specialized services they provide. In the

*Source: I. Donald Snook, Jr., *Hospitals: What They Are and How They Work,* Aspen Systems Corporation, 1981.

American Hospital Association's 1980 survey of hospitals, 55 specialized facilities and services were reported as being available (Table 11-1).

Table 11-1   Hospital Facilities: Ancillary Services

Percent of hospitals	Provide facility/service
85.6	respiratory therapy department
85.3	physical therapy department
84.5	postoperative recovery room
80.7	social work department
78.1	pharmacy/registered pharmacist (full time)
72.7	hospital auxiliary
72.6	emergency department
71.5	blood bank
65.8	intensive care unit (mixed)
63.3	electroencephalography
60.8	histopathology laboratory
59.6	volunteer services department
58.9	dental services
58.8	diagnostic radioisotope facility
50.9	organized outpatient department
43.4	speech pathology services
42.5	patient representative services
39.5	occupational therapy department
37.1	podiatric services
35.0	premature nursery
30.9	intensive care unit (cardiac only)
27.9	abortion inpatient service
26.8	rehabilitation outpatient services
23.7	therapeutic radioisotope facility
22.5	radioactive implants
22.1	hemodialysis inpatient
19.8	CT scanners
18.4	x-ray therapy
17.8	pharmacy/part-time pharmacist
15.2	cardiac catheterizations
14.8	abortion outpatient service
14.5	megavoltage therapy
12.5	hemodialysis outpatient
11.7	home care department
11.0	family planning service
11.0	long-term care (skilled nursing)
9.8	open-heart surgery facilities
8.8	alcoholism/chemical dependency outpatient
8.0	alcoholism/chemical dependency inpatient
7.2	genetic counseling service
7.1	orthopedic service
6.6	intensive care (neonatal)
5.9	hospice
5.8	long-term care (other than s.n.)
4.8	rehabilitation inpatient service

Table 11-1   continued

Percent of hospitals	Provide facility/service
3.5	organ bank
3.6	intensive care (pediatric)
2.1	burn unit

Percent of hospitals	In psychiatric/ psychology services
34.8	clinical psychology services
34.0	consultation and education
30.6	emergency services
24.2	outpatient services
19.8	inpatient unit
15.5	partial hospitalization program
3.7	foster and/or home care

Source: American Hospital Association.

Hospitals have tended to increase the scope of their offerings, even to the point of duplicating expensive services.

Internal Audit Checkpoints*

These internal auditing checkpoints are common to most ancillary services.

1. What procedures have been established to ensure tests, procedures, and therapies are performed by licensed and qualified staff?

2. What are the procedures for assuring that the correct service is performed on time and properly? What procedure exists to ensure that patients do not receive a service not ordered by the physician?

3. Are the results of test procedures and therapy reported promptly and in a manner that is controlled so as to make sure the physician receives the information?

4. Are test results and films retained in an orderly fashion? Have record retention schedules been prepared and are they followed?

5. Do the various laboratories maintain logbooks that provide positive control over specimens and patients? Do the labs adequately control all processing and do the controls ensure processing on a timely basis?

---

*Source: Seth Allcorn, *Internal Auditing for Hospitals,* Aspen Systems Corporation, 1979.

6. How are drugs controlled on the wards? Do medical records reveal instances of patients receiving drugs not ordered and of other patients being billed for drugs never administered?
7. Is it clear to all ward and laboratory personnel and physicians how services are to be requested and reported?
8. Are personnel friendly and courteous to patients? Do patients frequently complain about the quality of care?
9. What system is used to transport patients to and from tests? Does it provide for prompt pickup and delivery?
10. Do the laboratories and therapy areas coordinate the times patients will be called for tests? Do the ancillary service areas frequently schedule their work at the same time making it difficult to get patients to all appointments?

Clinical Laboratories Department*

Functions

The primary function of the Clinical Laboratories Department is to perform laboratory tests in the six main fields of bacteriology, biochemistry, histology, serology, hematology, and cytology, in order to assist medical staff in making or confirming diagnoses. In addition to specialized tests, clinical laboratories in all general hospitals are responsible for making routine tests that are agreed upon by medical staff and hospital administration. These usually include urinalyses for all patients on admission, blood cell and hemoglobin count, and gross and microscopic examination of all tissues removed at operations. The laboratories also determine causes of communicable diseases and, upon request, render bacteriological service as a control and continual check on all apparatus used for sterilization. In larger hospitals, the clinical laboratories will be divided into a number of specialized units (see Figure 11-1 for an organizational chart for a clinical laboratories department).

Histopathology: Prepare and examine tissue to provide data on cause and progress of dis-

---

*Source: *Job Descriptions and Organizational Analysis for Hospitals and Related Health Services,* U.S. Training and Employment Service, Department of Labor, 1971.

ease; make microscopic examinations of tissue pathology; engage in research to develop new histopathological methods and new stains to produce greater clarity during examination of special tissue structures or chemical components; perform autopsies and interpret gross and microscopic autopsy findings in conferences with medical staff and technologists for future diagnoses and treatment of patients.

Biochemistry: Perform chemical tests of body fluids and exudates to provide information for diagnosis and treatment of disease; investigate chemical processes involved in functioning and malfunctioning of the human body; and study effects of chemical compounds upon physiological and biochemical functions of the body to provide information on optimum methods of treating pathological conditions.

Hematology: Analyze and test blood specimens and interpret test results to provide a basis for treatment of diseases; and engage in research related to hematological methods and diagnosis. The blood bank, in a hospital having these special units, is usually a part of hematology. The bank provides for storage and preservation of blood plasma. Blood may be procured either directly from donors or from other blood banks. When obtained from donors, this unit extracts blood and makes necessary laboratory tests.

Microbiology: Cultivate, classify, and identify micro-organisms found in body fluids, exudates, skin scrapings, or autopsy and surgical specimens to provide data on cause, cure, and prevention of disease; engage in research to develop new or improved bacteriological methods for discovering and identifying pathogenic organisms; and investigate biology, distribution, and mode of transmission of bacteria and nature and efficiency of chemotherapeutic treatment.

Serology: Prepare serums used to treat and diagnose infectious diseases and immunize against these diseases, and identify diseases based on characteristic reactions of various serums; investigate safety of new commercial antibiotic products and accuracy of therapeutic claims; direct immunology tests and injections; investigate problems of allergy; and conduct tests to determine therapeutic and toxic dosages and most effective methods of administering serums, vaccines, antibiotics, antitoxins, antigens, and related drugs.

Cytology: Examine human cells to detect evidence of cancer in its early stages and other dis-

Figure 11-1 Clinical laboratories department

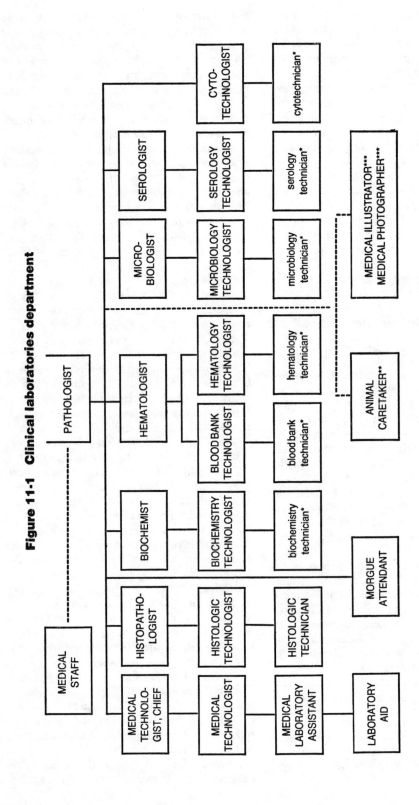

* This job is combined with MEDICAL LABORATORY ASSISTANT.
** This job has been included in this department for convenience.
*** This job is usually found in a research laboratory.
NOTE: This chart is for illustrative purposes only and should not be considered a recommended pattern of organization.
Source: *Job Descriptions and Organizational Analysis for Hospitals and Related Health Services*, U.S. Training and Employment Service, Department of Labor, 1971.

eased conditions; engage in research to develop new cytological methods, and new stains to produce greater clarity during examination of cell structures.

The clinical laboratories may be responsible for a number of other functions, such as basal metabolism tests; activities of clinical photographic laboratory, medical illustration unit, and morgue; and care and treatment of animals used in research. Teaching programs for student nurses, interns, residents, and medical technologists and other laboratory personnel may also be a function of this department.

Organization

The physical facilities of this department will depend on its workload. The very small hospital, which performs only routine examination in its laboratory, requires a minimum of space and equipment. In the large hospital, the laboratory space may be divided into a number of divisions, including an office for the pathologist and a central workroom for facilities that may be utilized in common by all laboratory units. Where a great deal of outpatient work is performed, a small branch laboratory may be set up in the Outpatient Department or Clinic for routine tests.

The director of this department is a doctor of medicine or osteopathy with qualifications in pathology acceptable to the Council on Education and Hospitals of the American Medical Association or the Committee on Hospitals of the Bureau of Professional Education of the American Osteopathic Association. Where it is not possible to secure the full-time services of a pathologist, arrangements should be made for the services of a pathologist for tissue and post mortem examinations and for the interpretation of tests and examinations.

Depending upon the hospital, requirements for a clinical laboratory director can be met by: (1) A full-time clinical pathologist, (2) a part-time clinical pathologist (frequently, arrangements can be made for a pathologist to serve two or more hospitals within a given area), (3) a consulting pathologist to whom materials can be sent for diagnosis and who will come to the laboratory periodically to supervise the services and meet with the medical staff, or (4) a member of the medical staff who has had training in clinical pathology and will direct the laboratory in those

cases where the volume of work is insufficient to warrant the full-time services of a specialist. In the latter instance, tissue examinations requiring extensive equipment and skill can be sent to the nearest clinical laboratory which is headed by a qualified pathologist.

The hospital pathologist reports to the associate administrator on administrative functions and supervises all personnel assigned to the laboratories. For professional standards, the pathologist is responsible to the chief of the medical staff. He may delegate certain administrative duties to the chief medical technologist. All regularly employed laboratory technologists and technicians should be on the registry sponsored by the American Society of Clinical Pathologists.

Relationships with Other Departments

Laboratory services must be coordinated with all other diagnostic functions of the hospital, which requires consultation with members of the medical staff, the associate administrator or the administrator, and other department heads. A system should be established for performing all routine tests within a specified period of time after admission of a patient. Emergency laboratory service must be available on a 24-hour basis.

Laboratory services are important to the work of the Outpatient Department, and close cooperation is necessary between these services. Personnel in the laboratory have occasional contact with patients; medical, admitting, and nursing staff; and with other employees. The pathologist may lecture to students, professional societies, and medical organizations. There is cooperation with other department heads, private physicians, and personnel in other laboratories and related activities in radiology and technical services.

Pathologist: Job Duties

● Supervises and directs activities of the clinical laboratories in accordance with accepted national standards and administrative policies of the hospital.
● Establishes department procedures and methods. Assigns and supervises activities of department personnel. Directs training of resident physicians, interns, technologists, and technicians assigned to the department. Requisitions sup-

plies and equipment. Serves as consultant to other department heads and visiting physicians, to interpret laboratory findings and assist in determining appropriate method and extent of treatment necessary. Participates, along with personnel of other departments, in planning joint administrative and technical programs and recommends methods and procedures for coordination of pathological services with related patient care services. May engage in research projects and prepare scientific papers on the nature, cause, and behavior of diseases. Investigates and studies trends and developments in pathological practices and techniques and evaluates their adaptability to specific needs of the pathological program. Lectures to students, professional societies, and organizations in the medical field. Prepares budget for the fiscal year and submits to administrative officials for approval.

• Provides pathological services to aid in the diagnosis of diseases and the treatment of patients and to assist in post mortem diagnoses.

• Supervises all laboratory work, demonstrating new techniques to staff and performing difficult tasks demanded by complex or unusual situations. Conducts macroscopic and microscopic examinations of specimens of body tissues, fluids, and secretions, and diagnoses nature of pathological condition. Prepares report on each case, incorporating recommendations for treatment, such as surgery, chemotherapy, or roentgen-ray therapy. Prepares vaccines and immune serums. Conducts autopsies, performing macroscopic anatomical examinations and microscopic studies of all tissues or fluids showing evidence of pathological conditions. Prepares complete report on post mortem study, including description of pathology performed; post mortem diagnosis conditions; and statement of cause of death.

Chief Medical Technologist: Job Duties

In large hospitals, and those engaged in research, the chief medical technologist would be responsible for supervision and performance of tests in only one of several fields of clinical pathology. Thus, he would be classified according to field of specialization, such as histologic technologist, biochemistry technologist, microbiology technologist, hematology technologist, serology technologist, cytotechnologist, or blood bank technologist.

In smaller hospitals the medical technologist would be responsible for supervision and the performance of tests in any one or a combination of areas of specialization depending upon the size and scope of the laboratory activity.

• Supervises, coordinates, and participates in activities of workers performing various chemical, microscopic, and bacteriologic tests of body fluids, exudates, skin scrapings, or autopsy and surgical specimens to obtain data for diagnosis and treatment of disease.

• Consults with pathologist to plan priorities of work to be completed each day. Prepares work schedules and assigns duties to workers in the laboratory. Supervises workers in assigned section or area of specialization in clinical laboratory. Checks validity and accuracy of test results obtained by laboratory personnel on a sample basis by performing the same test and comparing results. Keeps records pertaining to tests performed and charts test results to insure that variation in test results and standards are within acceptable quality control ranges. May keep time records and make ratings and recommendations for promotions. Gives instructions to new workers in procedures and techniques of performing tests. May direct training and instruction of students of medical technology. May interview and hire new laboratory workers.

• Performs experimental testing procedures and submits reports to pathologist suggesting changes to increase validity and reliability of tests. Demonstrates to personnel newly approved methods to implement standard procedures. Studies current medical laboratory literature to obtain information on new test methods and procedures.

• May assist pathologist during autopsies. May schedule appointments. Orders replacements to maintain stock of equipment and supplies.

Radiology Department*

The principal functions of the radiology (x-ray) department are to assist the physicians and other health team members in the diagnosis and therapy of a patient's disease through the use of radiography, fluoroscopy, and radioisotopes. High energy machines such as linear accelera-

*Source: I. Donald Snook, Jr., *Hospitals: What They Are and How They Work,* Aspen Systems Corporation, 1981.

tors, employing high particle acceleration, are also used in radiotherapy.

In the average community hospital, 90 percent of the workload in the x-ray department consists of radiography (making a record on x-ray film by means of radioactivity) and fluoroscopy (x-ray examinations of deep structures by means of roentgen rays using a fluorescent screen).

A secondary mission of the radiology department is to engage in essential research for medical advancement and to participate in educational programs for hospital residents and in inservice programs for the medical staff.

Organization

In large hospitals, the radiology department may be organized into three separate sections: diagnostic radiology, therapeutic radiology, and nuclear medicine. In small hospitals, these may be arranged in one organization. The department is under the general direction and supervision of a competent radiologist, a graduate of a medical school who is licensed to practice in the state. This person is appointed as a member of the medical staff and should have considerable specialized training in radiology, either diagnostic or therapeutic or both, and be certified by the American Board of Radiology.

In the larger context, the radiologist, as administrator of the department, is responsible to the administrator of the hospital; as a specialist concerned with the quality of care, the radiologist is responsible to the medical staff. Members of the medical staff send their patients to the department for diagnosis and treatment. The outpatient department sends approximately 50 percent of all the x-ray work, including that from the emergency department. The various inpatient nursing units also send patients down from the unit during the working day.

Location

The x-ray department should be located on the first floor of the hospital and should be conveniently accessible to both outpatients and inpatients. If possible, it is preferable to locate the x-ray department close to elevators and adjoining the outpatient department. It is best to locate the department in a wing of the hospital with the x-ray rooms at the extreme end of the wing. In such a configuration, the traffic pattern through the department will be minimized, and less

shielding from the x-rays will be required due to the exterior walls around the x-ray rooms.

A well-planned x-ray diagnostic department will ensure an efficient flow of service, allowing patients to be scheduled properly and expediently with a minimum of movement for both the x-ray staff and the patients (see Figure 11-2).

Staffing

The basic employee in the radiology department is the radiologic technologist or x-ray technician. These technologists should be trained in x-ray work and should be eligible for membership in the American Society of Radiologic Technologists. Technicians perform their work under the supervision of the radiologist and usually a chief technician. It is estimated that one certified radiologist is needed for every 25 revenue patients per day. The number of technicians required for this workload may vary between two and three.

Radiologic Technologist

(X-ray technician, medical radiographer)

Process radiographs of various portions of the body to assist the physician in the detection of foreign bodies and diagnoses of diseases and trauma. Duties include the following: Prepares patients for radiologic examinations, fluoroscopic studies and other procedures as requested by physician; positions patient, administers contrast media (chemical mixtures designed to radiographically visualize nonopaque organs), practices radiation protection measures; and sets technical exposure factors which result in diagnostic radiographs. Radiologic technologists may also chemically process exposed radiographic film; maintain records or supervise their preparation by clerical staff; maintain equipment in efficient operating condition, including correction of minor problems, and instruct hospital staff regarding radiography and radiologic technology.*

Theft

X-ray does not usually present one of the major theft problems since the only marketable prod-

---

Industry Wage Survey: Hospitals and Nursing Homes, September 1978, Bureau of Labor Statistics, Bulletin 2069, November 1980.

Figure 11-2 Typical 150- to 200-bed hospital diagnostic x-ray suite

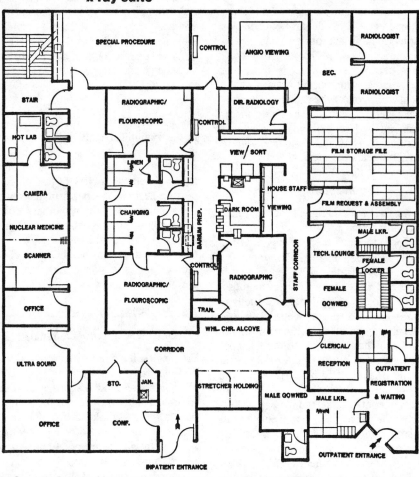

Source: *Project Management—Planning and Design*, Medifac, Inc., Pennsauken, N.J.

uct is the film. There have been incidents where x-ray technicians sold film to x-ray outfits in business for themselves, but these incidents have been sporadic. Film storage requires refrigeration, and good lockup is usually easy to combine with refrigeration. Consequently, quantities of easily accessible x-ray film are usually limited.

A more frequent problem is the fraudulent use of x-ray equipment and film by hospital technicians working in collusion with physicians. This is a practice which is peculiar to inner-city rather than suburban or rural hospitals.

The opportunities for theft vary with work schedules. Where x-ray departments work around the clock, only one or two technicians frequently staff evening, nighttime and weekend shifts. Theft activities are virtually impossible to prevent in these situations.*

Department of Anesthesia**

Most hospitals have a separate department of anesthesiology. Those hospitals that do not have a separate department usually include anesthe-

---

*Source: Walter Nagel, "Health Care Industry's Vulnerability to Theft," *Topics in Health Care Financing*, Winter 1978.

**Source: I. Donald Snook, Jr., *Hospitals: What They Are and How They Work*, Aspen Systems Corporation, 1981.

sia as a function of the department of surgery. Most often, the department of anesthesiology is headed by a physician who is trained in the medical discipline of anesthesia and, hopefully, is board certified. The department may have more than one physician anesthesiologist. It is quite common to have nurse anesthetists, that is, registered nurses who have completed a formalized post-RN anesthesia program or school. Both the physician specialist and the nurse anesthetist administer anesthesia. When a physician anesthesiologist is not available, hospitals use nurse anesthetists exclusively to administer anesthesia. The responsibility for this department is then delegated to either the chief of surgery or to another designated person. In such cases, the operating surgeon is responsible for the professional acts of the nurse anesthetists.

The precise number of physician anesthetists and nurse anesthetists employed in a given hospital will depend upon the number and types of surgical procedures and the number of obstetrical deliveries in the hospital. Personnel in the anesthesia department are required to be on call; this, of course, has an impact on staffing patterns. The nurse anesthetists, depending on the contractual arrangement between the anesthesiologist and the hospital, either work directly for the anesthesiologist or are hospital employees. In any event, the nurse anesthetists function under the technical supervision of the anesthesiologist.

Respiratory Care Department

The Respiratory Care Department embodies the therapeutic value of oxygen and other agents together with, among the newer studies and techniques, pulmonary function studies and blood gas analysis. The department is particularly important in the treatment and diagnosis of patients with pulmonary disease and certain cardiac ailments. The Respiratory Care Department continues to grow, not only in scope of responsibility, but also as a cost and revenue center for the hospital. It has become, in many institutions, a major ancillary department.

The respiratory therapy department is involved in both diagnostic and therapeutic treatment of inpatients and outpatients. All procedures given to the patients are performed either by the physician or by the trained respiratory therapist. These procedures can be administered to the patient only upon the prescribed written orders of a physician.*

Respiratory Therapist**

Administers therapeutic and diagnostic procedures to patients with pulmonary disorders.

Therapeutic procedures include: Setting up and managing mechanical ventilators with respect to flows, volumes, pressures, breathing rates and patterns, and gas composition as prescribed; delivering prescribed therapeutic gases with proper dosing valves, regulators, humidity and prescribed dosages of aerosolized medication to the bronchopulmonary tree; removing bronchopulmonary secretions by means of mechanical suction and bronchopulmonary drainage; assisting patients in deep breathing and coughing with inspiratory positive pressure breathing exercises; performing cardiopulmonary resuscitation and acute airway management procedures including endotracheal intubation; and maintaining artificial airways.

Diagnostic procedures include: Pulmonary function testing (e.g., measuring and interpreting expiratory and inspiratory flows, volumes, and gas composition); obtaining arterial and venous blood to perform blood gas analysis. May also do physiological monitoring and assessment of pulmonary status, i.e., chest auscultation, percussion and observation as appropriate; document and evaluate care in patient's medical records; collaborate and consult with physicians, nurses, and other therapists to coordinate care; instruct residents, interns, nurses, and other staff in the methods and procedures for respiratory therapy; maintain, repair, and decontaminate equipment; and conduct clinical research.

The position normally requires extensive on-the-job training or completion of formal training program and certification or registration by the National Board for Respiratory Therapy.

---

*Source: I. Donald Snook, Jr., *Hospitals: What They Are and How They Work,* Aspen Systems Corporation, 1981.

**Source: *Industry Wage Survey: Hospitals and Nursing Homes, September 1978,* Bureau of Labor Statistics, Bulletin 2069, November 1980.

Electroencephalography*

One of the more specialized ancillary services in hospitals is the electroencephalography or EEG testing service. This is generally part of the neurosurgery or neurology section of the hospital or medical staff. This service is an indispensible tool for solving neurosurgical or neurological problems.

The EEG laboratory does not have a high volume, like laboratory and x-ray. Frequently, however, EEG lab technicians are on 24-hour call for emergency determinations. EEG tests are used in determining both the first signs of life and the last signs of life coming from the brain. Often the EEG test can be the means of determining whether the patient is legally alive or dead.

The field of electroencephalography is concerned with recording and studying the electrical activity of the brain. A machine called an electroencephalograph records this activity and produces a written tracing of the brain's electrical impulses. This record of brain waves is called an electroencephalogram. Neurologists and other qualified medical practitioners use electroencephalograms to help diagnose the extent of injury for patients suspected of having brain tumors, strokes, or epilepsy; to measure the consequences of infectious diseases on the brain; and to determine if there is any organic explanation in cases where individuals suffer from serious adjustment problems or learning difficulties. EEG also may be used prior to vital organ transplant operations, to help determine when the potential donor is "medically" dead.

The people who operate EEG equipment are known as EEG technicians and technologists.

EEG Technician

The main job of an EEG technician is to produce electroencephalograms, under the supervision of an EEG technologist or an electroencephalographer (a physician specializing in electroencephalography). Before doing this job, the technician takes a simplified medical history of the patient and helps the patient relax for the test.

---

*Sources: *Industry Wage Survey: Hospitals and Nursing Homes, September 1978,* Bureau of Labor Statistics, Bulletin 2069, November 1980; and *Occupational Outlook Handbook,* 1982–83 ed., U.S. Department of Labor, 1982.

The technician then applies the electrodes of the electroencephalograph to designated spots on the patient's head and makes sure that the machine is working well. The technician chooses the most appropriate combinations of instrument controls and electrodes to produce the kind of record needed. EEG technicians must be able to recognize and correct any artifacts that appear (an artifact is an electrical or mechanical event that comes from somewhere other than the brain, such as eye movement or interference from electrical lights). If there are any mechanical problems with the electroencephalograph, the technician must advise his or her supervisor, so that the machine can be repaired promptly. EEG technicians must know how to recognize changes in the patient's neurologic, cardiac, and respiratory status. EEG technicians also need a basic understanding of the kinds of medical emergencies that can occur in laboratories to be able to react properly if an emergency arises. For example, if a patient suffers an epileptic seizure, the EEG technician must take the proper action.

Job Duties

Duties include the following: Makes independent judgments concerning the type of electrodes suited to the individual patient; obtains complete wake-sleep tracings to detect epileptic and deep cerebral abnormalities; uses acoustic stimuli during the sleep period to aid in locating a specific abnormality. Must be able to recognize difference between levels of spontaneously varying consciousness, such as alertness, waking, relaxation, drowsiness, and the several levels of sleep. May also make studies requiring the manipulation of a sound or light source, varying its rate of intensity to evoke particular wave patterns; and may use additional electrodes (e.g., basal, nasopharyngeal) when requested. EEG technicians often work with critically ill patients and, therefore, must exercise care in handling such patients, recognize adverse responses, and initiate appropriate emergency procedures, as necessary.

EEG Technologists

EEG technologists usually perform all the duties of EEG technicians but have a broader knowledge of the various aspects of EEG work. They also may use EEG equipment in conjunction with other electrophysiologic monitoring devices, such as tape recorders, computers, and video equipment. They also can repair the equipment if it is not working properly. After producing an EEG recording, the technologist may be asked to write a description of the recording for the use of the electroencephalographer.

Supervising EEG technicians is part of an EEG technologist's job. Besides direct supervision during EEG recordings, this includes such things as arranging work schedules and teaching EEG techniques. Technologists often have administrative responsibilities, such as managing the laboratory, keeping records, scheduling appointments, ordering supplies, and establishing protocol.

Electrocardiography*

Electrocardiograms (EKG's) are graphic heartbeat tracings produced by an instrument called an electrocardiograph. These tracings record the electrical changes that occur during and between heartbeats. Physicians order electrocardiograms to diagnose certain forms of heart disease including irregularities in heart action and to analyze changes in the condition of a patient's heart over a period of time. Some physicians use electrocardiograms as a routine diagnostic procedure for persons who have reached a certain age. In many fields, electrocardiograms are required as part of preemployment physical examinations. Often the test is done for surgery.

Many new cardiac tests are used today, including "invasive" tests such as cardiac catheterization, in which a tube (catheter) is inserted through the patient's blood vessel into the heart. Generally, EKG's are used together with these other cardiac tests.

Throughout the years, the diagnostic tool of electrocardiography has proven to be a necessity in the general community hospital. The EKG is used most frequently on patients having cardiac disease, suspected cardiac disease, or complications of cardiac disease. It is also useful as a chest baseline test prior to surgery. All elec-

---

*Sources: *Industry Wage Survey: Hospitals and Nursing Homes, September 1978,* Bureau of Labor Statistics, Bulletin 2069, November 1980; and *Occupational Outlook Handbook,* 1982–83 ed., U.S. Department of Labor, 1982.

trocardiograph tests are considered diagnostic procedures and must be ordered by a physician. The interpreter of the cardiogram is usually a cardiologist or an internist who is skilled in reading electrocardiogram tracings. The cardiologist or interpreter is usually paid for each electrocardiogram interpreted; however, the payment could be in the form of a fixed salary.

The basic EKG machine is a table-type of apparatus on wheels that is rolled to the inpatient's bedside. It is operated by highly skilled technicians.

The electrocardiograph service is usually a mobile service, in that the technicians frequently must go to the patients' beds while they are inpatients and take tracings while the patients are resting. However, for outpatients and occasional inpatients who can travel to the central cardiograph area, the service is usually located within the department of cardiology.

The Procedure

After explaining the procedure to the patient, the technician attaches from 3 to 12 electrodes—also called "leads"—to the chest, arms, and legs of the patient. Often the technician applies a gel between the electrodes and the patient's skin, to facilitate the passage of the electrical impulses. The patient usually lies down, face up, during this procedure. By manipulating switches on the electrocardiograph and repositioning the electrodes across the chest, the technician produces various tracings of the heart's electrical action. A stylus records the tracings on a long roll of graph paper. The test may be given while the patient is resting, or is doing exercise. The technician must know the anatomy of the chest and heart to properly select the exact locations for the chest electrodes. If the electrodes are placed in the wrong location, an inaccurate reading will result.

After the recording has been completed, the technician prepares the electrocardiogram for analysis by a physician, usually a heart specialist. Technicians must be able to recognize and correct any technical errors, such as crossed wires or electrical interference, that prevent an accurate reading. They also must call the doctor's attention to any significant deviations from the norm.

EKG technicians sometimes conduct other tests such as vectorcardiograms, which are multidimensional traces; stress testing (exercise tests); pulse recordings; and Holter monitoring and scanning, which is a 12- to 24-hour recording of the EKG on magnetic tape. In addition, some technicians schedule appointments, type doctors' diagnoses, maintain patients' EKG files, and care for equipment.

EKG Technician

EKG technicians can be classified into two levels:

Level 1: Operates and monitors equipment in connection with a variety of established examinations or treatment procedures that require a high degree of judgment and skill, adapting techniques to meet special conditions. Duties include: operates and monitors EKG equipment such as echocardiographs and phonocardiographs in specialized cardiac stress tests; recognizes cardiac emergencies, including acute infarction and serious arrythmias, from unmounted tracings, and takes appropriate action, including notifying physician and initiating cardiopulmonary resuscitation. May also operate equipment during difficult special examinations including those using controlled stimuli such as esophageal leads; and autonomic or atropine drug tests; recognizes cardiac arrhythmias and makes long recordings when rhythm is abnormal.

Level 2: Operates and monitors electrocardiograph equipment in connection with standardized examinations in which a series of steps are performed with little deviation from instructions or well established procedures. Duties include: Attaches electrodes to patient's chest and extremities so that proper connections are made to record heart tracings; makes tracings of heart actions before and after treadmill and other exercise tolerance tests. May operate equipment on signal from physician in performing standard controlled stimuli tests (e.g., carotid sinus stimulation). Marks tracings to indicate outside disturbances.

Physical Medicine and Rehabilitation*

The discipline of physical medicine and rehabilitation is a medical specialty concerned with the

_____
*Source: Descriptions of positions from *Industry Wage Survey, Hospitals and Nursing Homes, September 1978,* Bureau of Labor Statistics, Bulletin 2069, November 1980.

diagnosis and treatment of certain musculoskeletal defects and neuromuscular diseases and problems. Physical therapy is commonly prescribed by physicians, and the referred patient is evaluated and treated by the physical therapist. Hospitals may offer occupational therapy services under the direction of a physician. Today, there are only a limited number of hospitals specializing in complete physical medicine and rehabilitation services. However, it is quite common for a community hospital to have a physical therapy section supporting the medical rehabilitation programs of certain patients.*

Supervisor of Physical Therapists

Directs and supervises the physical therapy service in one or more organized physical therapy departments. Duties include: Assigns patient care duties to professional and nonprofessional physical therapy personnel, and supervises and evaluates work performance; interprets responsibilities and hospital policy to physical therapy personnel; periodically visits patients to insure optimal care and to ascertain need for additional or modified services; supervises the execution of doctors' orders and related treatments and the maintenance of physical therapy records (medical, personnel, accounting, billing, etc.); assists in the orientation of new personnel to the department; insures the availability of supplies or equipment; identifies physical therapy service problems and assists in their solution; works on hospital committees and assists in preparing the facility's budget; gives direct physical therapy care in some situations; assists in the in-service education and guidance of physical therapy personnel; researches new procedures and implements and evaluates them; may spend part of the time supervising or instructing student physical therapists, physical therapists' assistants, and physical therapy aides.

Physical Therapist

Treats disabilities, injuries, and diseases through the use of massage, exercise, and effective properties of air, water, heat, cold, radiant energy, and electricity, according to prescrip-

_____
*I. Donald Snook, Jr., *Hospitals: What They Are and How They Work,* Aspen Systems Corporation, 1981.

tion of a physician. May instruct students, interns and nurses in methods and objectives of physical therapy and may supervise physical therapy aides. May consult with other therapists to coordinate therapeutic programs for individual patients. Normally requires training in approved school of physical therapy. Must be licensed in the State in which practicing.

Occupational Therapist

Plans, organizes, implements, and/or directs medically oriented occupational therapy program to facilitate rehabilitation of persons mentally or physically impaired. Identifies and selects activities—utilizing creative and manual arts, recreational and social aids, suited to individual's physical capacity, intelligence level, and interests—to assist patient in developing maximum independence in activities of daily living. Teaches skills and techniques including interpersonal and group process skills, to facilitate and influence patient's participation in program activities and goals. Evaluates progress, attitude, and behavior as related to patient's potential. Consults with other members of rehabilitation team to coordinate therapeutic activities of individual patients. May direct activities of one or more assistants or volunteer workers. May lecture interns, medical, and nursing students on phases of occupational therapy. Normally requires training in an approved school of occupational therapy and registration by the American Occupational Therapy Association.

Speech Therapist

Provides remedial services for speech disorders, including stuttering, voice disorders, and articulatory and speech problems associated with impairments, such as cleft palate, cerebral palsy, and aphasis. Instructs speech handicapped patients in development of desirable speech habits by training in control of articulation and voice. May demonstrate position of lips, jaws, and tongue for forming sounds to produce words. May devise vocal exercises to aid patients in overcoming stuttering and nasal, harsh, or hoarse tones. May teach laryngectomies techniques of speaking with esophageal voice. Prepares patient's progress reports, describing therapy used and progress made. May participate in research to develop diagnostic and remedial techniques. May counsel patients, their families, or teachers concerning social and psychological problems associated with speech disabilities.

Social Services

Social workers in the social service departments are highly trained individuals. Specifically, they must have graduated from a baccalaureate program, and may have taken advanced training at the master's degree level. The social services department provides counselling and assistance to patients to help them deal with social, emotional, and cultural problems. Typically the social service unit offers:*

- Casework services for patients with social and/or emotional problems.
- Referrals to skilled nursing homes.
- Information regarding all health related community resources such as visiting nurse, alcoholics anonymous, and the like.
- Orthopedic and visual rehabilitation centers.
- Assistance in acquiring artificial limbs and appliances.
- Administration of psychological testing.
- Collection of social history.
- Adoption assistance.

Since the American Hospital Association launched its Quality Assurance Program (QAP) and the federal government, through its PSROs, has been pushing for quality assurance programs for hospitals, the social worker has taken on an important role in aiding the process of quality assurance.

As a committee member on the quality assurance program of a hospital, the social worker's most important contribution is in the area of discharge planning. The JCAH recommends that the social service department have a written policy and procedure for discharge planning. Another of the social worker's crucial roles is to find an extended-care bed or a rehabilitation hospital bed for the patient who is unable to go home. In this task, the medical social worker impacts directly not only on the patient's well-being but also on the cost effectiveness and efficiency of the hospital's operations. If the patient is moved into a nursing home bed, the hospital runs a risk of losing reimbursement.

---

*Source: *Orientation to Hospital Operation,* DHEW Pub. No. (HRA) 75-4009, 1975.

Medical Social Worker*

Provides direct service to patients by helping them resolve personal and environmental difficulties that interfere with obtaining maximum benefits from medical care or that predispose toward illness. Performs a variety of services such as counseling on social problems and arranging for posthospital care at home or in institutions, for placement of children in foster homes or adults in nursing homes, and for financial assistance during illness; utilizes resources such as family and community agencies to assist patient to resume life in community or to learn to live with disability. Prepares and keeps current a social case record. Provides attending physician and others with pertinent information to add to understanding of patient. May supervise social work students and beginning case workers.

Psychiatric Social Worker*

Provides psychiatric case work service to patients having problems of social and personal maladjustment. Work involves the following: Studying patient's personal, social, and emotional situation to assist psychiatrists in diagnosis and treatment; assisting patient and family in making mental and emotional adjustment to illness and in developing posthospital plans; and aiding in planning hospital policies related to selection and referral of patients. May also aid in developing community health and welfare programs and engage in research and teaching activities.

---

*Source: *Industry Wage Survey: Hospitals and Nursing Homes, September 1978*, Bureau of Labor Statistics, Bulletin 2069, November 1980.

Chapter 12—The Emergency Department

OVERVIEW*

In the early days of hospitals, an "accident room" was a necessity in the medical institution. The accident room was the place to treat patients who were truly injured with surgical problems, automobile accidents, home accidents, or accidents on the job. At that time, hospital management viewed the accident room as a necessary evil to provide the service necessary for the community. The general practitioners, surgeons, obstetricians, and pediatricians had very little use for the concept of accident rooms. Such rooms were generally staffed by the hospital intern, who was possibly the most inexperienced person to deal with accident situations. Typically, there were registered nurses to support the intern.

By the 1960s the accident room had become a walk-in medical clinic in many communities. Since World War II there has been a continual increase in emergency room visits, making effective emergency department management more difficult. For the last ten years, emergency room visits have increased 175 percent, yet studies show that as high as 60 percent of these visits represent nonemergencies.

On average, emergency room visits show a five to six percent increase each year. In 1972, there were 60.1 million visits; in 1978, the number was 82.8 million. Traditionally, the hospital

---

*Source: I. Donald Snook, Jr., *Hospitals: What They Are and How They Work,* Aspen Systems Corporation, 1981.

has been geared to provide inpatient care, but with the increased demands for emergency and other ambulatory care services, management has had to find ways to integrate the demand for these growing programs into the hospital's future. The emergency room's skyrocketing volume is placing pressure on hospital planners to find appropriate ambulatory care settings to serve their communities. One reason the increased volume is placing pressure on the hospital is that a significant number of the hospital's inpatients are admitted through the emergency room. Some hospitals report as many as one-third of their total admissions come from the emergency room. A hospital's size, location of emergency department, staffing arrangements, and ownership affect the number of inpatients coming from the emergency department.

Who Uses the Emergency Department

As physicians have turned to formal appointment types of practices, emergency rooms have become the place for informal walk-in treatment. A Blue Cross survey in Michigan showed 23 percent of the patients who visited the emergency room came directly to the hospital without calling a physician because they did not believe a physician would be available. Another 12 percent went to the emergency room after they were unable to reach their private physician.

The main reason many people prefer the hospital emergency room for treatment is that they think hospitals have better treatment facilities than physicians' offices. Emergency rooms are being used as afterhours physicians' offices and have become 24-hour outpatient clinics. This places a heavy burden on the facilities, space, staff, and finances of the hospital.

It is important to realize that the emergency department has a significant impact on the hospital's inpatient population. A study by the American Hospital Association indicates that between 16 and 30 percent of the hospital's admissions come through the emergency department. It has been noted that "not only do emergency admission patients generally remain in the hospital for a longer period of time, but also their admissions usually entail greater use of ancillary services than that which occurs with scheduled patients."

Financial Implications

As noted, in an average hospital, a significant portion of the inpatients come through the emergency department. In addition, studies have shown that emergency department patients utilize the ancillary services of the hospital. The high use of the ancillary services by both outpatients and inpatients contributes to the increased charge structure and hopefully an improved cash flow for the hospitals.

Typically, one-third of the bill for a hospital emergency department patient stems from the emergency department; the remaining charges are generated through the utilization of the ancillary services.

The emergency room must be viewed in the sense of total hospital impact rather than as a restricted departmental outpatient center. Emergency departments may increase the hospital's census and cash flow in the inpatient area. Improved physical facilities, competent professional staffing, and the image of high quality patient care in the community all seem to add up to increased volume in the hospital's emergency rooms, which then tends to lower the cost per visit.

Physical Facilities

It is advisable that the emergency department be located on the ground floor with easy access for patients and ambulances. Generally, it is best to have it separated from the main entrance of the hospital. The emergency department should make its entrance easily visible from the street, for example, with proper lighting and signs. It is very important that the ambulance entrance to the emergency department be large enough to admit one or more ambulances negotiating with stretchers. Emergency rooms should have waiting rooms sufficient for patients and their families and friends as well as telephone areas and rest rooms close by. X-ray and laboratory services should be easily accessible to the emergency department. Over 40 percent of emergency patients require x-rays, and over 20 percent need laboratory studies. If emergency rooms handle a patient volume in excess of 1,000 patients per month or handle an unusually high number of fracture cases, they may have their own x-ray facilities. A portable x-ray apparatus is seldom satisfactory. If an x-ray unit is located within the emergency room, provision must be made for the consultation services of radiology technicians and radiologists.

Generally, the emergency department has at least two or three functional areas. Typically, there is the trauma area where the severely injured surgical cases are handled. There should be a medical examining area nearby and a casting area for orthopedic problems. There should be observation beds for patients who need to stay in the emergency room area (for neurological and other medical reasons). These observation beds can be used as a staying area before the patient moves to the inpatient nursing unit.

The National Academy of Sciences identified four categories of emergency care. Type I major emergency facilities include 24-hour specialists in the hospital in addition to other 24-hour backup services. Type II is the basic emergency facility where the emergency room physician is located in the hospital with certain specialists on call. Type III is the hospital that provides standby emergency facilities with perhaps an emergency-room registered nurse and a physician on call. Type IV is a referral emergency room facility that has only an emergency nurse or medical technician in the hospital and that transfers patients to other facilities for life support systems. The JCAH has outlined the requirements of each type's care level needed for accreditation.

ORGANIZATION*

The emergency room is generally considered to be an outpatient nursing unit in the hospital or-

*Source: I. Donald Snook, Jr., *Hospitals: What They Are and How They Work,* Aspen Systems Corporation, 1981.

ganization. However, unlike other hospital nursing units, the medical staff plays a major onsite role in the emergency department and thereby complicates the organization of the emergency room. Typically, the nursing service staffs the emergency room with nursing and auxiliary personnel as they do any other nursing unit. However, since physician coverage is required in the unit (and more recently emergency departments are becoming managed by an emergency department specialist or group), there is a management partnership between physicians and nurses in this unit.

The current organizational trend in emergency rooms is for the unit to be a separate and distinct department under the direction of a full-time physician director. This evolution from a nursing unit within a nursing service to a physician-directed department is more prominent in the larger hospitals that employ full-time physicians to staff the activity. The physicians generally report directly to the medical staff, to the management of the hospital, or through a committee called the emergency department committee of the medical staff.

Typically, the emergency department committee is made up of representatives from the medical staff, nursing staff, and administration. This committee formulates the medical-administrative policies to guide the emergency room operations. It also examines the level and quality of emergency care rendered in the department. More recently, under the PSRO medical care evaluation studies requirement, this committee may be involved in analyzing the flow of patients and the relationship of the emergency department patients to the ancillary services, such as x-ray and laboratory.

With the increased number of emergency visits, the trend has been for full-time emergency room physicians to staff the unit. The simplest model for full-time physicians is one in which the hospital pays one or more physicians a flat salary for attending patients. As a rule, the salaried emergency room physician is a hospital employee. Under these circumstances the hospital bills patients for the use of the emergency room as well as for the physician's services.

Staffing

It is most important that members of any emergency department be highly skilled and competent. In addition, they should be able to work calmly and with self-control. All staff members should receive a thorough orientation and training, including training in how to deal effectively with the public. The staff should be able to communicate well with patients and with family and friends who seek relief from fear and anxiety.

Nursing Staff

Emergency department nurses are almost always employees of the institution, as opposed to emergency room physicians who staff in a variety of ways. The role a nurse plays in an emergency setting is very different from the role played by the traditional nurse on a medical-surgical unit. The emergency nurse at various times must institute life-saving measures, perform triage, begin intravenous solutions, and perform a myriad of other highly skillful nursing tasks—many times under great stress.

Nurses hired as staff members of the emergency department should be highly qualified, intelligent, and flexible. Because the emergency nurse has a broad range of responsibilities, she or he should be given corresponding authority. For example, in emergency departments so small that a physician is not on 24-hour duty, nurses must be given authority to begin life-saving measures.

For the sake of continuity and most efficient patient care, nurses staffing an emergency service should be permanent members of the department and not rotated from other units in the hospital.

The number of nurses staffing the emergency department will vary according to patient load. Peak admissions occur from 8:00 A.M. to 8:00 P.M., so staffing should be planned accordingly. One authority on organization and staffing called for seven to nine nurses per day for each 100 patients seen, when nursing work shifts were tailored to peak load hours.

Medical Staff

In departments with case loads of 20,000 per year or more, the same authority called for a basic physician staff to be on the premises every hour of every day. In high trauma regions, he recommends full staffing as being justified even with a lesser patient load. He then recommends adding one full-time emergency physician for each 7,000 cases seen annually.

MANAGING THE EMERGENCY DEPARTMENT

Policies and Procedures*

Emergency department policies and procedures should be formulated and documented in an emergency department manual that is readily available to all staff members of the department. In order to keep the manual current, it should be revised and updated as needed, at least annually.

The policies must clearly reflect the philosophy of the hospital's administrative, nursing, and medical staff. Therefore, preparation of a policy and procedure manual would necessitate the cooperation of members of each of these three disciplines.

The policy manual, when drafted and adopted, should function as a resource manual for staff members. It should include information on particular problems that arise in the emergency room, including statements released to the press, interaction with law enforcement officers, interaction with other community agencies, and social service needs.

Because emergency room staff deal regularly with such problems as child abuse, injuries that result from criminal activity, and so forth, a number of the policies will have legal implications. Therefore, it is highly advisable to have legal counsel review suggested policies before they are adopted and implemented. It is not important to have a lawyer be a member of the policy-making committee, because many of the procedures and policies do not involve legal questions. Rather, have a lawyer review the entire manual for legal questions. Legal counsel for the hospital would be an appropriate person to perform this crucial task.

Records*

Good medical and administrative practice demands that the hospital initiate medical records on each patient visiting the emergency room department. It is also necessary for the hospital to protect itself legally. Most emergency department medical records are simplified compared to the extensive inpatient records. Generally, they carry administrative and basic statistical data about the patient with a place for appropriate baseline clinical data, such as blood pressure and temperature, plus a space for physicians' and nurses' notes. Generally the emergency room record is limited to one sheet. If a patient is admitted to the hospital, the emergency room record accompanies the patient and is made a part of the patient's inpatient medical chart. If the patient is not admitted, the emergency room record is retained in the emergency department, and another copy is sent to the medical records department for proper storage.

Physician Coverage*

Each hospital, after careful study, must determine which method is most appropriate. As the service grows or shrinks and as there is some change in the availability of physicians for coverage, the method of coverage will have to be reexamined and adjusted.

One acceptable method is the concept of full-time emergency physicians with no other practice. This method, called the *Alexandria Plan,* is an efficient and effective way to organize physician coverage. Introduced in the 1960s, it has proved to be effective where used. The drawback with this plan is that often there were too few physicians able and willing to work as full-time emergency physicians. This resulted in the use of part-time, "moonlighting" physicians or residents, often from other institutions. Thus the continuity this method was designed to achieve was often compromised.

Another method of coverage that has seen wide use involves the rotating of staff members, often called the *Pontiac Plan.* This method has been used on a voluntary and on a compulsory basis. The rationale behind this method is that physicians should be able to give first aid, provide life-saving measures, and make a tentative diagnosis to refer for additional care. However, the drawback of this plan proved to be that there were great disparities in skill as physicians took their turns in rotation.

A newer method is a *variation of the Alexandria Plan.* Full-time physician coverage is pro-

---

*Source: I. Donald Snook, Jr., *Hospitals: What They Are and How They Work,* Aspen Systems Corporation, 1981.

*Source: Marguerite R. Mancini and Alice T. Gale, *Emergency Care and the Law,* Aspen Systems Corporation, 1981.

vided by a partnership or corporation of four or five licensed physicians who sign a contract with the hospital. This method can work well if the contract very clearly delineates the responsibilities as well as the authority of the contracting physicians. With this method, coverage is assured. Furthermore, the liability for acts of negligence would be with the contracting physicians only, as independent contractors, because they are not employees of the institution. Thus respondeat superior would not apply. In this situation patients should be notified that they will be billed separately by the physicians for their services, since the physicians are working as independent contractors. If the contracting physicians maintain a private practice in addition to their contract with the hospital, the practice should be kept separate from coverage of the emergency department.

An even newer method is presently evolving, mainly in large metropolitan areas—*the multihospital emergency physician group.* These groups are large, comprising 50 or 60 physicians. Because emergency medicine is hospital-based, this method offers security to its members. Contracts are established, usually on an annual basis. Thus if one contract is not renewed, the renewal of other contracts compensates. If this method works well for the physicians, it also offers security for the hospital because the emergency physicians do not develop their own private practices. Instead, their work helps build the hospital's emergency department practice.

Still another method used by hospitals involves *using residents and interns* under the direction and supervision of staff physicians. With this method, the lines of authority and chains of command should be clearly delineated and understood. With residents who do not have a good command of English—especially in hospitals with large numbers of patients who do not speak English as their first language—very close supervision should be provided to eliminate problems resulting from language barriers, especially as related to instructions, referral, and consent.

If the hospital chooses to staff its emergency department with house officers, the governing body of the hospital must remember that their skill varies widely. As employees of the hospital they are not independent contractors, and so the hospital's exposure for liability is increased. Their work must be supervised carefully.

The policy manual should delineate the responsibilities of both house and attending staff when both are used. If medical students are used in addition to residents and interns, the policy manual should state clearly who is responsible for their supervision.

Evaluating the Department

Each hospital must study its own situation to determine what kind of emergency department is needed, how to best meet community needs, and how to ensure that quality service is maintained.

By studying facts on past utilization, one can determine what kind of program is needed in the future. Any study of utilization should include data on the number of visits, average length of visits, seasonal variations, variations as to time of day and time of week (to show peak and slack hours), and treatment categories. In studying treatment categories, it would be important to see how many cases seen in an emergency department are not of an emergency nature. It would also be important to study the disposition of patients seen for emergency care. A study of actual costs should be made in order to determine charges for service.

Checklist for an Internal Audit*

1. How closely does the emergency room work with the OPD? Does the emergency room carry a large subacute patient care load that should be handled routinely by the OPD?
2. Are emergency room personnel assigned additional duties when the demand for emergency services is low? If so, with what result?
3. How are charges determined and accumulated? In particular, are all supplies and equipment usages accounted for after emergency care has been delivered?
4. Is the emergency room properly stocked with drugs and supplies and is it well equipped?
5. Where is the emergency room located? Does it provide easy access to unloading facilities for ambulances and walk-in pa-

---

*Source: Seth Allcorn, *Internal Auditing for Hospitals,* Aspen Systems Corporation, 1979.

tients and to other areas of the hospital such as the OPD, diagnostic labs, medical records, and admissions?

6. Are emergency room personnel properly qualified and certified for such service?
7. What is the emergency room policy for extending care outside the hospital for accident victims, disasters, cardiac failure, and maternity cases? Who decides emergency room policy?
8. Does revenue generated by the emergency room support its operation?
9. What are the policies for providing information to journalists and for controlling access to patients and their records?
10. What are the procedures for protecting evidence for victims of crimes such as rape and assault? How are injured criminals handled and, in particular, gunshot wounds?

LEGAL CONCERNS IN THE EMERGENCY ROOM*

Adequate Medical Staffing

A hospital can provide adequate medical staff for its emergency department in a variety of ways: hiring salaried physicians, requiring all members of the hospital medical staff to cover the emergency department under some type of rotation plan, or contracting with an independent group of physicians to serve as medical personnel for the emergency room. In many states statutes or regulations require that the emergency department provide at least a specified minimum amount of physician coverage. A failure to provide appropriate staff and facilities for emergency service, where the hospital is under legal obligation to furnish emergency care, could result in hospital liability if such failure caused harm to a patient. Hospital liability could be predicated on corporate negligence for failure to provide necessary services, or it could be based on the application of respondeat superior for the acts of personnel who sought to provide attention but did so in a negligent fashion.

*Source: Except where noted, this section on "Legal Concerns in the Emergency Room" consists of excerpts from Marguerite R. Mancini and Alice T. Gale, *Emergency Care and the Law,* Aspen Systems Corporation, 1981.

Malpractice

Under respondeat superior, for the hospital to be liable for a physician's malpractice in the emergency room, the hospital must have some control over the work performed; a physician's membership on the hospital's medical staff alone would not be sufficient to lead to the imposition of liability. Thus, where a physician is summoned to the hospital to render care in the emergency room, under a rotation agreement among members of the medical staff, the hospital would ordinarily not be responsible for that doctor's acts. However, some courts may take the position that when the physician has been assigned to the emergency room by the administration, and the appearance of a master-servant relationship is created by the hospital personnel, liability may be imposed on the hospital under respondeat superior for harm suffered by the patient.

A hospital that contracts with a partnership of physicians to provide 24-hour emergency room care, and does not retain the right to direct the specific medical techniques used by physicians, will ordinarily not be liable for negligent treatment rendered by the physicians.

The Right to Treatment*

The Right to Treatment Doctrine historically provided that private hospitals could theoretically pick the patients they wished to treat. The courts, however, have indicated that once treatment is initiated, there is a duty to continue necessary and reasonable care.

Contemporary thinking indicates that if the public is aware that a hospital furnishes emergency services and relies on that knowledge, the hospital has a duty to provide emergency services to those who present themselves for such services. The standards of the Joint Commission on Accreditation of Hospitals, state licensing regulations, and public health department regulations, for example, may be considered by the courts as showing a duty to use due care in hospital emergency rooms.

No matter how trivial a complaint, each patient should be examined. If a patient rejects treatment, he should be requested to sign a release. Transfer of patients should be made only

*Source: George D. Pozgar, *Legal Aspects of Health Care Administration,* Aspen Systems Corporation, 1979.

upon approval of the physician. Appropriate emergency room policies and procedures, medical and administrative, should be developed.

Reporting Laws

In order to promote the detection and appropriate action by public officials in cases involving the safety and health of the community, a number of states have enacted a series of reporting laws. These laws typically require reports to be made to specified officials, provide for the confidential handling of those reports, and protect those who make the reports in good faith from civil and criminal liability. The list of laws will vary from state to state, and some will affect hospitals in differing degrees. Some of the common types of reporting laws relate to child abuse and neglect, elderly abuse and neglect, gunshot and other violent wounds, rape, abortion, poisoning, venereal disease, specified communicable diseases, tuberculosis, cancer, drug abuse, and all suspicious or unattended deaths. It is important for emergency personnel to familiarize themselves with reporting laws and to follow them.

The governing board of each general hospital maintaining an emergency department, together with the emergency department personnel, should address the issue of reportable incidents in the emergency department policy and procedure manual.

Emergency department policies and procedures also must address both the issues of death in the emergency room and coroner or medical examiner cases. These policies and procedures need to cover at least the following:

- reportable deaths
- disposal of bodies
- morgue procedures
- coroner or medical examiner procedures
- police procedures
- next of kin notification procedures
- donation of body and body parts procedures
- identification of the body procedures
- medical record and release form procedures
- autopsy procedures

Death in the Emergency Room

Generally, the issues involving death of emergency patients, the right to possession of the deceased patient, and control of the body for purposes of burial are controlled by state law.

In most states, laws require only that the attending physician complete a death certificate when the patient dies. The next of kin should, of course, be notified immediately or as soon as is reasonably possible. The duty to inform patients extends to the next of kin.

An autopsy should not be performed until the nearest relative grants permission *in writing*. Permission for autopsy can also be obtained from appropriate officials as designated by state laws. Legal authority to perform an autopsy bars objections from relatives.

Dead On Arrival Cases

Patients brought to a hospital emergency department dead on arrival (DOA) must be reported to the coroner or medical examiner of the locality or political subdivision in which the death occurred.

Because such cases come under the jurisdiction of the coroner or medical examiner, the body, clothing, and any other belongings must be turned over to the coroner's office. It is important to not alter the corpse in any way prior to notification of the coroner. It is the responsibility of the coroner or medical examiner to conduct an investigation to determine the possibility of foul play and whether an autopsy or postmortem investigation is advised.

In DOA cases, although pronouncement of death may be made by the emergency room physician, the death certificate must be signed by the medical examiner. When a medical examiner or coroner takes responsibility for the case, by law his or her authority overrides that of the emergency room physician, attending physician, spouse, or other next of kin.

Medical Examiner's or Coroner's Cases

State laws govern when a death comes under the jurisdiction of the medical examiner or coroner. Generally, the following cases are reportable to the office of coroner or medical examiner. The office will determine whether or not to assume jurisdiction.

- All suicides
- All DOAs
- All violent deaths
- All deaths without prior medical care
- All deaths resulting from poisoning
- All deaths resulting from criminal acts

- All deaths wherein patients have been hospitalized for less than 24 hours and a definite diagnosis has not been made
- All deaths for which an attending physician cannot or will not sign the death certificate
- All deaths resulting from an accident
- All deaths wherein the patient has not been seen by the attending physician for 20 days or more prior to death

Anatomical Gifts

The Uniform Anatomical Gift Act, endorsed by the American Bar Association and enacted as state law in many states, details many provisions for the making, acceptance, and use of anatomical gifts.

The donation laws usually permit donors to execute the gift during their lifetimes and preclude liability on the part of surviving relatives for use of the body in conformity with the donation.

The Uniform Anatomical Gift Act provides that the physician who declares the patient dead cannot be a member of the transplant team. This requirement addresses the possible conflict of interest on the part of physicians. It is designed to ensure that the interests of the possible donor will be fully protected by physicians with responsibility for his welfare and not that of the possible recipient.

Under the Uniform Anatomical Gift Act, a donor must be at least 18 years of age and of sound mind. The gift or donation may be made by will or other written instrument and may specify the body parts donated. The act allows donation for purposes of education, therapy, transplantation, or for the advancement of medical or dental science.

The act provides for donation by the next of kin, in a statutory preference order, if consent has not been obtained from the decedent prior to death. If consent is obtained after death from relatives, the statute provides for consent by recorded message. The statute provides that when only a part of the body is donated, custody of the remaining parts of the body is to be transferred to the next of kin promptly following removal of the donated part.

Autopsy

The purpose of conducting an autopsy is to determine the cause of a person's death. The autopsy or post-mortem examination is thus able to determine many legal issues: whether death resulted from criminal acts; whether the cause of death was one for which payment is due under an insurance contract; whether the cause of death is compensable under workmen's compensation and occupational disease acts; or whether death resulted from one specific act or a culmination of several acts. There is a second justification for the performance of autopsies or post-mortem examinations. Autopsies are necessary to hospitals, physicians and nurses, and medical science because they offer a tremendous learning opportunity. Furthermore, the results of autopsies are often used as a check on the medical practice in the hospital. The Joint Commission on Accreditation of Hospitals desires that autopsies be performed on the bodies of at least 20 percent of the persons dying within each hospital, and the American Medical Association requires an autopsy rate of at least 25 percent in facilities and institutions approved for intern training.

Any type of autopsy, whether or not it includes tissue removal, requires consent.

Sometimes the facts are misrepresented to the person possessing the right to consent in order to induce his or her consent. Where a physician or hospital employee states as fact something known to be untrue in order to gain consent, the autopsy would be unauthorized and liability may follow.

In general, the usual priority for consent is as follows: the surviving spouse; surviving children over the age of 18 years; the surviving parents of the deceased; the surviving siblings of majority age of the deceased; other surviving adult relatives in order of closest blood relationship.

If the death is a coroner's or medical examiner's case, the request for the autopsy must be signed by an official of the coroner's or medical examiner's office. A request signed by any other person is ineffective. The autopsy permit must be signed and witnessed and should specify any limitations or restrictions. Any such limitations or restrictions must be adhered to by the pathologist who performs the autopsy.

Approximately half of the autopsy consent statutes provide that the deceased may authorize an autopsy on his or her own body. Such consent should be in writing.

Chapter 13—Ambulatory Care

OVERVIEW

In the past, potentially profitable ambulatory care programs were solely the property of physicians and woe to the hospital administrator who began to talk as if the hospital were more than an economic nonentity. The development of HMOs legitimized the sponsorship of medical care by nonphysician entities, though much resistance still may be encountered.

The chief executive officer has two major questions to decide if the hospital is to sponsor some type of ambulatory care. One is location, either on the hospital grounds or at some distant location. The other is the role and mission of an ambulatory program. Should it be developed to provide primary medical care, or should it be focused on specialty clinics serving needs not met by private practicing physicians? This has appeal where several different specialties are required to diagnose and treat a particular medical problem, such as pain, diabetes, sickle cell, headaches, or back injuries.*

Director of Ambulatory Care: Job Duties**

● Supervises and directs activities of an outpatient clinic and coordinates clinic activities with inpatient facilities to insure adequate and competent outpatient care.

● Establishes clinic policies and procedures in cooperation with inpatient department heads and administrative personnel. Interprets and administers personnel policies established by Board of Governors according to national standards. Reviews clinic activities and makes recommendations for changes in, or better utilization of, facilities, services, and staff. Plans clinic sessions and supervises staff and patient scheduling to meet community needs. Selects personnel and supervises clerical, medical, nutritional, nursing, medical-social, and medical records personnel. Authorizes purchase of supplies and equipment. Prepares department's budget. Prepares statistical data concerning department activities.

● Participates in community activities designed to promote health education. Meets with personnel of other local institutions and organizations (such as public health and public welfare) to establish policies and services for community health problems.

● May administer physical examinations and diagnose and treat ambulatory patients having illnesses which respond quickly to treatment. Refers patients requiring prolonged or specialized treatment to other facilities. May act as consultant to clinic physicians and interns on difficult cases.

Where a physician is required as head of the clinic, he must have an unrestricted State license to practice medicine or osteopathy.

Five to 10 years' hospital supervisory experience may be required, depending upon administrative policies.

---

*Source: Everett A. Johnson and Richard L. Johnson, *Hospitals in Transition*, Aspen Systems Corporation, 1982.

**Source: *Job Descriptions and Organizational Analysis for Hospitals and Related Health Services*, U.S. Training and Employment Service, Department of Labor, 1971.

Organization*

The operations of an ambulatory program should be grouped into three functional areas: nursing staff, business function, and professional staff. Each area should be directed by a working supervisor. For example, the nursing staff should be directed by a designated chief nurse, who in addition to clinical responsibilities, also provides the necessary decision making to keep the nursing staff functioning efficiently and effectively. The two other areas should also have persons appointed to provide the necessary coordination and decision making needed for their activities.

Location

The location of an ambulatory care program is another important factor. A usual rule of thumb is that the patient should travel 20 minutes or three miles for primary medical care. There should be easy parking and public transportation to the site.

Physician Concerns*

There are several potential organizational restraints operating in hospitals that affect ambulatory care programs. When a hospital offers such a program it will usually be seen by physicians as an economic threat. Most physicians become concerned whenever additional providers arrive in their marketplace, even though they always talk about being overworked and having more patients to care for than they can possibly handle. In a similar vein many communities have experienced overt as well as subversive physician activities when a new ambulatory service is planned by nonmedical groups outside of a hospital. If medical staff appointments are needed by physicians in freestanding clinics, difficulty often arises in obtaining medical staff membership.

There are at least two ways an ambulatory care program can appeal to physicians. The first is for the program to provide an opportunity for physicians to develop a specific panel of patients. This means that physicians retain the right to either accept or reject patients for their

*Source: Everett A. Johnson and Richard L. Johnson, *Hospitals in Transition*, Aspen Systems Corporation, 1982.

panel. Since some physicians do not desire to treat certain types of illness, they eventually will leave a practice if forced to provide care in which they are not interested. Staff physicians with the right acceptance can identify more closely with their patients and will have an increased concern for the patients' well-being.

The second way is for ambulatory care physicians to have an opportunity to practice on a fee-for-service basis whenever possible. New physicians are encouraged to settle in a community if they are provided incentives for above average productivity and a guaranteed fee for service. This arrangement places a floor under their income, but does not restrict their total earnings if they exceed the budgeted number of visits for the guarantee.

Because incomes of established physicians in private practice are frequently significantly higher than in ambulatory care programs, physicians recruited may leave after a short tenure if they cannot approach income levels that are available through independent practice.

Direction and supervision of physicians in an ambulatory care program when sponsored by a nonphysician-owned entity is often a sensitive issue and should be handled by a medical director. Whether the physician is fulltime, parttime, or consulting should be based on a recommendation by a medical director, approved by a majority of the fulltime physicians, and appointed by the governing body.

All appointments, both fulltime and parttime, should be made by a written contract in which specific authority, responsibility, and accountability are defined. A desirable contract should include:

- the physician's responsibility for maintaining a practice schedule that has been approved by the medical director;
- participation in limited weekend, evening, and on-call service as determined by the medical director;
- the maintenance of a medical staff appointment at a local hospital;
- the responsibility for providing competent medical care to patients on his or her service;
- participation in the work of physician committees of the ambulatory care program as assigned;
- a grant of a power of attorney to the ambu-

latory care program for billing and collection of patient fees;

- responsibility for visiting hospitalized patients daily, or as frequently as desirable, from his service;
- recognition of the authority of the ambulatory care program for establishing a physician's fee structure;
- referral of patients to the consulting staff of the ambulatory program when additional specialized medical care is required.

The contractual responsibilities of the ambulatory care program should include:

- a definition of the method of payment and productivity level required;
- provision of the same fringe benefits as other employees of the program;
- provision for an annual contract that may be amended with 90-days notice after the first year;
- payment for malpractice insurance at the customary current limits of liability;
- authorization for the purchase of additional fringe benefits through a reduction in the minimum income guarantee of a compensating amount at the direction of the physician;
- the payment of professional and staff dues;
- provision annually for four weeks vacation;
- provision of two weeks of professional leave annually, with expenses paid by the program, for approved educational activities;
- annual review of the physician's medical and administrative performance and providing him with a written evaluation;
- authorization of the physician to accept or reject patients assigned to his service.

The contract provisions outlined apply to both a primary care program and to specialty clinics.

Nursing Activities*

The following list of nursing activities performed in ambulatory care settings is a useful management tool. It can be used in staff selection to assess applicant experience in the responsibilities of ambulatory care nursing. In addition, a

*Source: Joyce A. Verran, "Delineation of Ambulatory Care Nursing Practice," *The Journal of Ambulatory Care Management,* May 1981.

unit orientation guide and skill inventory may be developed from the activity categories. With the addition of behavioral objectives, it is possible to extend the list to an objective clinical evaluation instrument.

Perhaps more valuable is the potential for developing an ambulatory care client classification system from the categories of activities. With further research each of the categories could be scaled in terms of the complexity of the included activities. Clients could be then classified on the basis of the complexity of their nursing care requirements. The final result would be a nursing care complexity index for each clinic setting. Such an index would be useful in determining staffing allocation in terms of numbers required and the ratio of professional to nonprofessional staff.

Patient Counseling

Client advocacy: Protection of client's right to care and attention to complaints regarding care or service.
General support: Attention to concerns and verbalizations regarding health status and reinforcement of positive aspects of health practice.
Clinic procedures: Provision of emotional support before and during clinic procedures.
Terminal/chronic illness: Provision of support and guidance to clients and families of clients who are terminally or chronically ill.

Health Care Maintenance

General assessment: Assessment of client health and knowledge of health maintenance, including socioeconomic status and emotional status.
Follow-up assessment: Assessment of client's status as it relates to compliance with plan of care and progress of a condition or disease.
Provide information: Provision of information regarding general health maintenance and normal body functioning.
Preventive care instruction: Instructions regarding preventive aspects of health care and avoidance of disease development and complications.

Primary Care

Referral: Evaluation of need for and actual referral to other agencies or health care providers.
Triage: Screening of patient problems either in

person or by phone with resolution of that problem either by advice or referral. Involves first patient contact with a health care provider during a specific clinic visit or call.

Protocol care: Provision of medical therapy or the monitoring of that therapy following multiple-decision protocols.

Physical: Performance of a complete physical exam and developmental assessment.

History: Procurement of a complete health and social history.

Patient Education

Health care maintenance program: Provision of a planned educational program related to prevention and health care maintenance.

Illness/condition program: Provision of a planned educational program related to a specific condition or disease state.

Home care: Instructions and demonstrations on procedures for home self-care including:

- General instructions: Instructions that are routine and standardized and do not require the skill of a licensed practitioner.
- Standardized instructions: Instructions designed for a specific patient problem that are unstandardized and nonroutine.
- Individualized instructions: Instructions designed for a specific patient problem that are unstandardized and nonroutine.

Plan of care: Explanation and planned reinforcement of plan of care and physician instructions.

Therapeutic Care

Surgical preparation: Provision of physical care for surgical procedure to be done in clinic or outpatient surgery.

Respiratory treatments: Administration of any therapeutic treatment related to the respiratory tract.

Irrigations: Administration of irrigations, including enemas and removal of impactions.

Applications: Administration of any therapeutic applications to body surface, including dermatology treatments and treatments to reduce fever or injury.

Specimens: Collection of all specimens including cultures.

Measurement: Measurement and recording of physiological and growth indices.

Appliances: Application and removal of casts and other appliances, if performed by a member of the nursing staff.

Recovery: Care given while patient is recovering from surgical or other clinic procedure.

Invasive: Performance of invasive procedures such as catheterizations.

Noninvasive: Performance of noninvasive procedures such as removal of sutures.

Dressings: Application of dressing and wraps.

Medications: Administration of medications by any route except IV.

IV medications: Administration of medications by IV route.

Blood and IV therapy: Administration of blood and blood products as well as IV fluids that contain medication.

Normative Care

Directing: Provision of directions to clients regarding location of other services.

Transporting: Transportation of clients to other services.

Communication: Provision or procurement of special communication assistance.

Chaperoning: Assistance not necessary but physical presence is required for legal reasons.

Assisting: Provision of assistance to physician for procedures including preparation of equipment and clean-up.

Preparation: Preparation of client for physician visit.

Documents: Organization of documents for client's visit.

System: Explanation of ambulatory care system and related services.

Comfort: Attention given to client comfort in regard to hunger, thirst, elimination, and information on reasons for delays, etc.

Coordination: Coordination and timing of client needs with the physician, laboratory, etc.

Nonclient-Centered Care

Maintenance: Maintenance of the clinic and its equipment.

Training: Provision of assistance in the training of students from all disciplines.

Materials: Development of educational materials and standards of care.

Updating: Maintenance of updated knowledge of new care practices and current literature appropriate to service and role.

Internal Audit Checkpoints for Outpatient Departments (OPDs)*

1. Who is responsible for managing the OPD? What is the organization of the business system used by the clinics?
2. Who decides policy for the OPD and what are the policies?
3. Is there an operating manual? If so, is it up to date and complete?
4. How is the OPD staffed? How are the doctors selected? How is the supporting staff selected? Are staffing arrangements planned for flexibility to meet varying patient loads?
5. What reports does the OPD prepare and what is their distribution?
6. What is the fee schedule for the department and the doctors? How were the charges determined?
7. Are patients routinely followed up when they fail to complete prescribed treatments and make return visits? If so, with what effect?
8. How good are the physical facilities? Is there enough modern equipment in good repair? Is there enough space for patients and staff and is the area comfortable?
9. Is there good access to diagnostic labs from the OPD and are patients handled promptly and courteously by the labs? Are test results returned promptly to the OPD?
10. To what extent does the outpatient department earn its way? How are deficits (if any) made up?

MANAGING THE FACILITY

Scheduling System**

Traditionally, a block appointment system has been used, where several patients are given ap-

---

*Source: Seth Allcorn, *Internal Auditing for Hospitals,* Aspen Systems Corporation, 1979.

**Source. Anthony A. Hudgins et al., "Issues in Family Planning Clinic Management," *Family and Community Health,* May 1982.

pointments at the same time, usually at the beginning of the morning or afternoon hours. This type of scheduling system unduly penalizes the patient who must wait an inordinate period of time to see a physician and also creates periods of lower productivity for physicians and program staff during the late morning and afternoon hours.

A preferred method of scheduling for patient convenience is an appointment system. Typically about 80 percent of patient appointments are kept and can be adjusted as operating experience determines a specific rate for a given program.*

Clinic Management

In one large study of clinic management, two overriding problems emerged: First, patients have long waits for services in these clinics, and second, staff do not spend a large portion of their time in patient contact.

Although each clinic studied was unique, with its own mix of problems and causes for these problems, certain fundamental deficiencies existed in many clinics: inadequate patient scheduling; failed appointment rates; patient arrival much earlier than staff; imbalance of staff time available and patient service needs; and improper sequencing of clients through the clinic.

For example, in patient scheduling, five appointment systems were identified—(1) *walk in,* (2) *day only* (i.e., there is a clinic on Friday at 8 AM), (3) *large block* (more than 25% of clients are scheduled at one time), (4) *small block* (fewer than 25% are scheduled at one time), and (5) *individual* appointments. Regardless of the system, however, clients wait. In large day-only clinics, the average client wait is 96 minutes; in those using individual appointments, the wait averages only 29 minutes. With the individual appointment system, the client waits the least amount of time and spends more of the clinic visit with the staff.

In spite of the advantages of a small-block or individual appointment system, only 39% of the time in clinic was actually spent receiving services; the balance was spent waiting. The staff were in contact with clients an average of 43% of

---

*Source: Everett A. Johnson and Robert L. Johnson, *Hospitals in Transition,* Aspen Systems Corporation, 1982.

the time, meaning that only 26 minutes of every hour of clinic time was spent with patients.

Many clinics continue to resist establishing appointment systems. Managers often claim that chronic lateness of patients would be so disruptive in a clinic with a carefully designed appointment system that they prefer to maintain a large-block system. In the clinic studies, however, it was found that 85% of the clients arrived early or on time, and only 16% arrived late. Furthermore, clients of clinics with individual or small-block appointment systems had even better arrival behavior, with only 10% arriving late.

Establishing an Appointment System

In most clinics, clients move through a series of "routing stations"—reception, laboratory, interview, education, physical examination, and possibly others. The station that can handle the least number of patients per hour will determine the ideal number of patients to arrive per hour. If the clinic had an average 20% no-show rate, it would overbook by one patient per hour. An appropriate appointment pattern might be two patients on the hour and one at each 15-minute interval.

Establishing a Patient Sequencing Policy

A clinic should have an established policy for the order in which clients are served, which is known both by the staff and the clients. An example of a policy used to good advantage in some clinics is as follows:

- Patients will be initiated into the clinic as close to their appointment times as possible.
- At all stations within the clinic, patients will be served so that the patient with the earliest appointment is served first.
- At all stations, patients who do not have appointments will be served after those having appointments.
- Patients who are more than 30 minutes late for their appointments will be treated as walk-ins.
- The only deviation from this policy will be that sick patients will always be seen as soon as possible.

A method used for enforcing this policy is to attach a slip of paper to each client's record showing the appointment time and a sequence number reflecting time of arrival of the client. At each station the staff member then selects patients by appointment priority first and by arrival priority second.

Reducing Failed Appointment Rates

A manager should first analyze the factors associated with client no-show, such as type of visit, day of week, time of day, and age of client to see whether certain patterns exist. If it is determined that the no-show rate is generally excessive, there are several methods used by clinics to lower the ratio:

- No-show rates can probably be lowered in most clinics by shortening the interval between making and keeping an appointment.
- Many clinics mail reminders, telephone clients, or even require a client to call in to reconfirm an appointment.
- Clinic sessions should be scheduled at times that clients indicate are most convenient. This information can be learned by administering a simple questionnaire to patients.
- Once the schedule is set, clients should, whenever possible, set their own appointments. In other words, when the client calls, staff do not suggest a time; ask for a time that would be convenient for the client.
- Clinics can simply request that clients call and cancel if they are unable to keep their appointments.

Calculating Personnel Needs

1. Determine the number of patients to be served, by visit type.
2. Define service requirements by visit type.
3. Inventory staff skills.
4. Combine services into tasks.
5. Define task requirements by visit type.
6. Determine average time needed by each patient in each task.
7. Calculate total staff time requirements.
8. Determine personnel needs for clinic session of a given length.
9. Adjust personnel needs by combining tasks and shifting services.

Information System*

Determining Needs

Before designing a management information system, a manager must separate the organization into its component parts and determine what kind of information is needed to manage each one.

1. Patient Care

● Volume

Annual visit volume is the most obvious information needed for facility and staffing purposes. A manager must know the capacity of the physical plant, as well as present, past, and expected future visit volumes. Comparisons of past and present annual volumes may indicate important trends. Of course, exogenous factors affect future volumes. A manager should ask these questions:

- Is there significant in- or out-migration in the facility's catchment areas?
- Are fertility patterns changing in general or in the catchment areas?
- Do census data and vital statistics indicate growth of certain age groups?
- How is consumer awareness affecting health care facilities?
- Will regulatory requirements provide a major impetus for outpatient versus inpatient care delivery? What kinds of outpatient facilities?

● Utilization and Vital Statistics

The number of people who account for total annual visit volume determines utilization (average number of visits per person per year). This figure should be broken down by vital statistics of the population (age and sex) and by service. For instance, population data may indicate that the facility's catchment area will have a high proportion of elderly individuals. Thus a manager must know the historical utilization of this subgroup for facility, staffing, and program planning. Comparison of the facility's utilization

*Source: Alice M. Sapienza, "Managing the Ambulatory Facility: Setting Up the Information System," *The Journal of Ambulatory Care Management*, November 1980.

data with national data may also indicate discrepancies that will be important for future evaluation and marketing efforts.

● Patient Origin

An ambulatory facility's catchment area is not necessarily those neighborhoods contiguous to the physical plant, nor is it the same for each service. The principal catchment area of one service may be distinct from that of another. For example, the internal medicine population may come from surrounding communities whereas the obstetric population may come from an area remote to the facility. Patient origins must also be compared with the expected composition of the catchment areas. If there is a trend toward a high adolescent component of the community using the facility's obstetrical service, a manager must plan staff and program changes to meet expected needs of this population. Fertility and migration trends have an impact on such planning.

● Visit Levels

Most facilities provide several types or levels of visits, even within major services. The internal medicine service may provide annual physicals, short follow-ups, complex treatments, and new appointments. Pediatric service may provide walk-in, acute, and six-month well-child checkups; immunizations; and other kinds of care. The proportion of visits within each level (and service) reflects provider intensity, epidemiology of the population, and revenue sources (assuming that visits are charged according to provider time). This proportion is principally affected by the age and sex of the population and thus will change if the compositions of the catchment areas change. Although visit volume may remain stable, utilization, staffing, and distribution and amount of revenues may change significantly.

● Costs and Revenues

Direct patient care cost includes staff salaries and fringe benefits for time spent in patient care and the cost of supplies consumed in care delivery. Indirect patient care cost includes utilities, insurance, bad debt-free care, and an allocated portion of administrative and other costs. These costs should be broken down by service and matched with revenues by service. Each service should be self-supporting. If this is not possible, because of reimbursement constraints or the financial capacity of certain classes of patients, then an appropriate cross-subsidy should be developed. For example, if most mental health care is provided by social workers to the elderly, then a portion of the internal medicine revenue from this group may be reallocated to mental health activity.

2. Administration Support

Administration support is much simpler in terms of information needs than patient care. Usually, only staff salaries and supply-equipment costs are needed by the manager. Because administration support is non-revenue-producing, its cost must be borne equitably by patient care activities. (For example, administration-support costs could be allocated across services on the basis of gross revenues per service.)

3. Teaching and Research

If these functions are carried out in the ambulatory facility, the manager must know: (1) what proportions of staff time are spent in each activity (and if the stated patient care plus teaching plus research time equals 100 percent of staff time), (2) the corresponding costs (as a percentage of total salary), and (3) supporting revenues (from grants, donations, or other special funds). Under some circumstances, grant funds may support patient care. However, the manager must ensure that there is a clear plan for the eventual elimination of this support.

Data Collection

The next step, and one of the most difficult, is finding appropriate sources of information. Cost data from the facility's billing department are most easily obtained, although they are not likely to be in a format immediately useful to the manager. It may be necessary to break down total salary and other costs by function (for example, patient care versus teaching and research) and then by service. Similarly, revenues may have to be broken down by function and then by service, before they can be matched to costs.

Other data are harder to derive. Total gross billings for the fiscal year should correspond fairly well with total visits, although registration, scheduling, or other logs may be more ac-

curate. For example, volume would be understated if a significant portion of visits were covered by the facility's free-care policy and not reported under gross billings.

Logs of patient appointments by service can be used to determine total volume and utilization. Vital statistics may have to be drawn from medical records, unless the facility collects them in a computerized patient registration file. Patient origins, as well, may have to be drawn from the same source as vital statistics. Given these data, a manager can extract more detailed information such as visit levels by service and visit levels by vital statistics of population within each service.

Implementation

Once these two important steps have been completed—determining what kinds of information are needed and from where—a manager can establish an information system relevant to the ambulatory facility.

Records System

Problems*

The following are potentially significant problems for ambulatory care record management:

1. The fragmented, episodic nature of ambulatory care;
2. The lack of continuity in care by multiple providers, with possible effect on quality of recording;
3. The lack of clearly defined standards for management of facilities and the lack of a centrally accepted accrediting agency;
4. The lack of standardized record format and disagreement as to content qualitatively and quantitatively;
5. The lack of a universal coding system for records, leading to inconsistencies in defining, for example, what constitutes a patient visit, and in obtaining uniform, accurate statistics, lack of utilization of ambulatory care data base;
6. The difficulty of establishing quality assurance systems because of incomplete data,

---

*Source: Judith Weilerstein, "Issues and Problems in Ambulatory Care Medical Record Practice," *Topics in Health Record Management,* March 1981.

lack of follow-up, ill-defined beginning and end points of care, indicating the need for an evaluation system that assesses these and similar problems, nontraditional types of evaluation systems;

7. The difficulty of updating, analyzing, and maintaining availability of highly mobile records due to irregular visits of patients, high volume of service by facility, and use of multiple facilities by patients leading to problems related to record linkage; and

8. The shortage of trained record professionals with experience of or interest in ambulatory care, inadequate administrative support, and lack of interest by many health professionals in records and information handling.

Computerized systems are seen as an answer to many aspects of ambulatory care record management. Certainly the success of the Computer Stored Ambulatory Record (COSTAR) program, a totally computerized ambulatory record system developed by the Harvard Community Health Plan and the Laboratory of Computer Sciences of Massachusetts General Hospital, is evidence that computerization can be accomplished.

Convenience

For large hospitals with active clinics and organized outpatient departments, location of the medical record department should be in excellent relationship to the *outpatient* services with high quality record transport systems to the inpatient zones. Space should be provided for medical record operations in the support zones related to all inpatient and outpatient care areas. If possible medical record clerks should be fulltime staff members of the outpatient departments and should be actively engaged in updating and coordinating the amount of information that goes into the record.

Uniform Ambulatory Medical Care Minimum Data Set*

The National Committee on Vital and Health Statistics recommends that specific items (see

Table 13-1) constitute the minimum data set that should be entered in the records of all ambulatory health care. When so recorded, routinely and uniformly, the value of health records to the patient care process and the potential of health records as an information source are greatly enhanced.

Uses

Minimal ambulatory medical care information may be used for the following:

• To enable physicians to care for their patients;
• To allow professional peer review or self-evaluation;
• To provide the caring professions with a better understanding of the natural history of health, complaints, disorders, and diseases;
• To aid in resource planning, cost allocation, and personnel management in clinics and other settings;
• To serve the data needs of private insurance carriers and federal payment programs; and
• To aid in the development of uniform patient billing forms and insurance claims forms.

Charges and payment data should be recorded as part of the billing process or accounting activity at the time that the fees associated with the specific encounter are determined.

Items of information characterizing a specific encounter may be maintained in a record separate from those describing the patient and provider, with linkage across records achieved by means of the patient and provider identifiers. These items, in conjunction with the data items describing the content of a specific encounter, form the core of the minimum data set. Specific needs of various users can be met by expanding the level of detail within an item or adding additional data items.

An AHA Management Information Service*

The AHA's Hospital Administrative Services for Ambulatory Care (HAS/AC) uses the experi-

---

*Source: *Uniform Ambulatory Medical Care: Minimum Data Set*, National Center for Health Statistics, Pub. No. (PHS) 81-1161, April 1981.

*Source: Bennett McNeal, "New Program for Management Information," *The Journal of Ambulatory Care Management*, April 1978.

Table 13-1   The Uniform Ambulatory Medical Care Data Set

Patient Data Items	Encounter Data Items

1. Personal identification
2. Residence
3. Date of birth
4. Sex
5. Race (American Indian, Alaskan native, Asian, Pacific islander, black, or white) and ethnic background (Hispanic origin or not Hispanic origin)
	10. Data and place of encounter
	  • Private office
	  • Clinic or health center (exclude hospital outpatient department)
	  • Hospital outpatient department
	  • Hospital emergency room
	  • Other (specify)
	11. Reason for encounter
	12. Diagnostic services

Provider Data Items	13. Problem/diagnosis/assessment
6. Provider identification 7. Location/address 8. Type of practice 9. Profession	14. Therapeutic services 15. Preventive services 16. Disposition 17. Expected principal source of payment 18. Total charges

Additional Patient Data Items

A. Highest grade in school completed (persons 18 years of age and over)
B. Current occupation (if student, enter "in school," if "homemaker," record as such)
C. Marital status
	D. Living arrangements
	  1. Family arrangement (spouse and/or children)
	  2. Living with other relative
	  3. Alone
	  4. Other (specify)

Source: Maurice Wood and James D. Lozier, "The Uniform Ambulatory Medical Care Data Set," *Topics in Health Record Management*, March, 1981. [Note: A longer version is available in the *Uniform Ambulatory Medical Care: Minimum Data Set*, National Center for Health Statistics, DHEW Pub. No. (PHS) 81-1161, April 1981.]

ence of the parent HAS program that has provided management information for health care institutions for approximately 18 years.

Through its system of comparative data reporting, the new HAS/AC program presents a subscribing hospital with facts about the staffing, finances and utilization of its ambulatory services, outpatient clinics, emergency departments and outpatient ancillary services. Each month the hospital reports selected financial, statistical and staffing data to the HAS Computer Center in Chicago. The data reported are processed by computer and translated into more than 100 management indicators, such as "nursing manhours per 100 visits," "direct expense per visit," and "x-ray exams per 100 visits."

Comparison of Ancillary Departments/Hospitals

The report contains information on ten hospital ancillary departments where outpatients are provided services, in addition to the outpatient clinics and emergency department. The ancillary departments are hemodialysis, respiratory services, surgical services, lab services, electrocardiography, electroencephalography, diagnostic radiology, therapeutic radiology, nuclear medicine and physical therapy. Revenue, expense and utilization information are provided for these areas. The monthly report to each hospital also includes detailed information on the hospital's emergency department and outpatient clinics. The two major sections of the report, the internal trend data section and the group median data section, enable hospitals to determine where they stand in relation to their own previous performance and in comparison to other participating hospitals (see Tables 13-2 and 13-3).

Although HAS has traditionally stressed the importance of both internal and group median data, some participants in the new HAS/AC program are finding that the format of the internal

Table 13-2   Six-Month Emergency Department Medians
(January to June 1977, HAS/AC Hospitals)

Indicator	Median	Indicator	Median
Visits per month	2,114.00	Percent EMT manhours	15.80%
Average charge per visit	$29.04	Administrative and clerical salaries	
Net revenue per visit	$24.75	per visit	$ 1.64
Deductions—percent of charges	11.02%	Administrative and clerical manhours	
Charges less MD remuneration		per 100 visits	41.23
per visit	$21.54	Other salaries per visit	$ .25
Direct expense per visit	$19.96	Supply costs per visit	$ 2.46
Indirect expense per visit	$11.83	Percent emergency department	
Nonphysician expense per visit	$12.01	patients admitted as inpatients	13.40%
Physician expense per visit	$12.71	Percent inpatients from emergency	
Resident expense per visit	$ 1.66	department	28.05%
Percent visits to hospital-based MD	86.39%	Department square feet per 100 visits	222.68
MD expense—percent total	47.59%	Visits per examination room	228.11
Physician manhours per 100 visits	45.25	Respiratory services per 100 visits	.76
Resident manhours per 100 visits	11.92	Lab units per visit	2.31
Nursing salaries per visit	$ 7.41	ECG examinations per 100 visits	4.21
Nursing manhours per 100 visits	139.26	Diagnostic radiology procedures per	
Percent RN manhours	59.00%	100 visits	52.40
Percent LPN manhours	13.91%		

Source: Bennett McNeal, "New Program for Management Information," *The Journal of Ambulatory Care Management,* April 1978.

trend data section may be of more interest because of the rapid changes that are occurring in many ambulatory service departments.

HAS/AC is intended to enable administrators to evaluate the effects of changes made in the types of services offered, staffing, revenue and expense, and space allocations. Also, the very important area of the generation of revenue by ambulatory service areas can be carefully monitored through continued participation in HAS/AC.

Responding to Consumer Needs

What can organizations do to ensure that they respond to consumer needs? Table 13-4 illustrates what managers should look for and how key elements can be measured in better meeting consumer expectations for ambulatory care.

PLANNING AND DESIGNING THE AMBULATORY CARE FACILITY

For a graphic presentation of the process involved in planning and designing an ambulatory care facility, see Figure 13-1. Layouts of two facilities can be found in Figures 13-2 and 13-3.

AMBULATORY SURGERY CENTERS*

Setting Up a Program

A large number of hospitals have been able to establish a successful program of ambulatory surgery. In virtually every case a committee of some kind has been formed in order to launch the project. Initial support must come from either the administration of the hospital, the board of trustees, or the medical staff, though the motivation can come from more than one source. In any event, hospital administrators should insure that the process is properly managed and that input is obtained from all key areas.

---

*Source: Thomas R. O'Donovan, "The Mechanics of Ambulatory Surgery" and "The Pros and Cons of Ambulatory Surgery," in *Ambulatory Surgical Centers: Development and Management,* ed. Thomas R. O'Donovan, Aspen Systems Corporation, 1976.

Table 13-3   Six-Month Ancillary Service Department Medians
(January to June 1977, HAS/AC Hospitals)

Indicator	Median	Indicator	Median
Hemodialysis:		**Electroencephalography:**	
Percent outpatient treatments	100.00%	Percent outpatient examinations	40.00%
Percent outpatient revenues	81.43%	Percent outpatient revenue	27.85%
Outpatient revenue per treatment	$197.88	Outpatient revenue per examination	$ 58.57
Physician expense per treatment	$ 7.66	Physician expense per examination	$ 16.38
Other direct expense per treatment	$ 97.88	Other direct expense per	
Indirect expense per treatment	$ 35.70	examination	$ 18.60
Respiratory services:		Indirect expense per examination	$ 14.29
Percent outpatient services	.95%		
Percent outpatient revenue	2.02%	**Diagnostic radiology:**	
Percent services of emergency		Percent outpatient procedures	40.00%
department patients	62.00%	Percent outpatient revenue	39.38%
Percent other outpatient services	64.00%	Percent procedures to emergency	
Outpatient revenue per service	$ 20.66	department patients	69.88%
Physician expense per service	$ .84	Percent other outpatient procedures	33.19%
Other direct expense per service	$ 7.98	Outpatient revenue per procedure	$ 27.55
Indirect expense per service	$ 3.07	Physician expense per procedure	$ 6.34
Surgical services:		Other direct expense per procedure	$ 10.55
Percent outpatient visits	11.00%	Indirect expense per procedure	$ 5.94
Percent outpatient revenue	4.94%		
Outpatient revenue per visit	$128.92	**Therapeutic radiology:**	
Physician expense per visit	$ 6.47	Percent outpatient procedures	88.66%
Other direct expense per visit	$ 59.99	Percent outpatient revenue	81.58%
Indirect expense per visit	$ 37.67	Outpatient revenue per procedure	$ 24.08
Lab services:		Physician expense per procedure	$ 7.24
Percent outpatient units	14.02%	Other direct expense per procedure	$ 7.95
Percent outpatient revenue	15.09%	Indirect expense per procedure	$ 3.22
Percent units to emergency			
department patients	24.17%	**Nuclear medicine:**	
Percent other outpatient units	47.50%	Percent outpatient procedures	28.50%
Outpatient revenue per unit	$ 2.98	Percent outpatient revenue	20.36%
Physician expense per unit	$ .20	Outpatient revenue per procedure	$ 65.28
Other direct expense per unit	$ .80	Physician expense per procedure	$ 11.06
Indirect expense per unit	$ .34	Other direct expense per procedure	$ 20.73
Electrocardiography:		Indirect expense per procedure	$ 11.64
Percent outpatient examinations	14.00%		
Percent outpatient revenue	17.06%	**Physical therapy:**	
Percent examinations to emergency		Percent outpatient treatments	33.53%
department patients	93.00%	Percent outpatient revenue	31.99%
Percent other outpatient		Outpatient revenue per treatment	$ 8.72
examinations	55.00%	Physician expense per treatment	$ .97
Outpatient revenue per examination	$ 30.22	Other direct expense per treatment	$ 3.83
Physician expense per examination	$ 7.98	Indirect expense per treatment	$ 2.57
Other direct expense per			
examination	$ 5.89	**Other outpatient services:**	
Indirect expense per examination	$ 6.39	Percent outpatient revenue	6.68%
		Percent outpatient direct expense	.80%

Source: Bennett McNeal, "New Program for Management Information," *The Journal of Ambulatory Care Management,* April 1978.

Figure 13-1 Predesign and program evaluation: Process and schedule

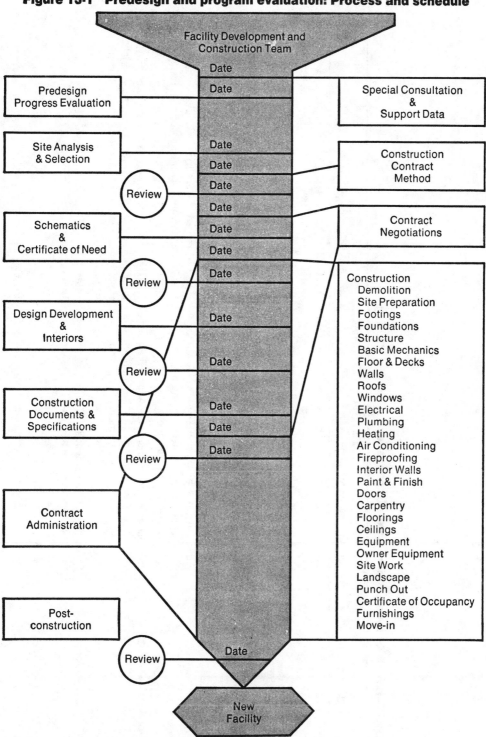

Source: Bruce P. Arneill, "Planning and Design for Ambulatory Care Facilities," *The Journal of Ambulatory Care Management,* January 1978, p. 81.

Table 13-4 Meeting Consumer Expectations of Ambulatory Care

SERVICE ASPECT	BENEFITS OF SERVICE	
	WHAT TO LOOK FOR	HOW TO MEASURE IT
Access	Customers can get into the system when they expect service.	Availability of general physicians for new patients; waiting time for first and subsequent visits.
Humaneness	Staff are polite and warm; they smile and listen.	Satisfaction questionnaires; patient letters of appreciation or criticism; observation on rounds.
Privacy	Privacy of examining facilities (sight and sound); adequate systems for confidentiality of records.	Testing the system by "dummy" patients; observation on rounds.
Continuity	Adequate integrated record system for all parts of the institution, transfer forms between institutions; low staff turnover.	Audit of record system for continuity; requirements for adequate information in transfer records; staff turnover rates.
Quality	All customers receive service which they perceive to be of adequate quality; key staff officials are held accountable for quality.	Satisfaction questionnaires; formal accountability of key officials; focus on key areas which need improvement and periodic measurement of progress.
Information	Customer receives adequate and accurate information on availability and cost of service; providers explain diagnosis and therapy to patients.	Interview with sample of customers; observation of providers by peers.
Input	Growth in demand for services; positive feedback on service delivery.	Interviews with sample of customers; market surveys to improve services; organized advisory groups.

COSTS OF SERVICES

Money	Price charged for the services is competitive with alternative sources of supply; customers understand in advance what services cost and the extent to which insurance covers the fee.	Identification of characteristics of customers served and comparisons of fees with alternate providers; patient satisfaction questionnaires; signs and handouts concerning financial policy; credit arrangements as appropriate.
Time	Amount of time the customer waits prior to receiving service should be no greater than that for other personal services; total time in the facility per diagnosis or treatment should be competitive with alternate providers.	Regular audit of waiting time and of total time in facility for key "package" of services; periodic comparison with other facilities.
Uncertainty	First contact person informs the customer of what he can expect during his first visit to the facility and as desired during subsequent visits; the provider should do likewise during each episode of care.	Interviews with a sample of customers; adequate clerical supervision related to basic standards of behavior; observation of providers by peers.

Source: Anthony R. Kovner and Helen L. Smits, "Point of View: Expectations of Ambulatory Care," *Health Care Management Review,* Winter 1978.

Figure 13-2   Concourse concept of an ambulatory care facility: Sample flow diagram

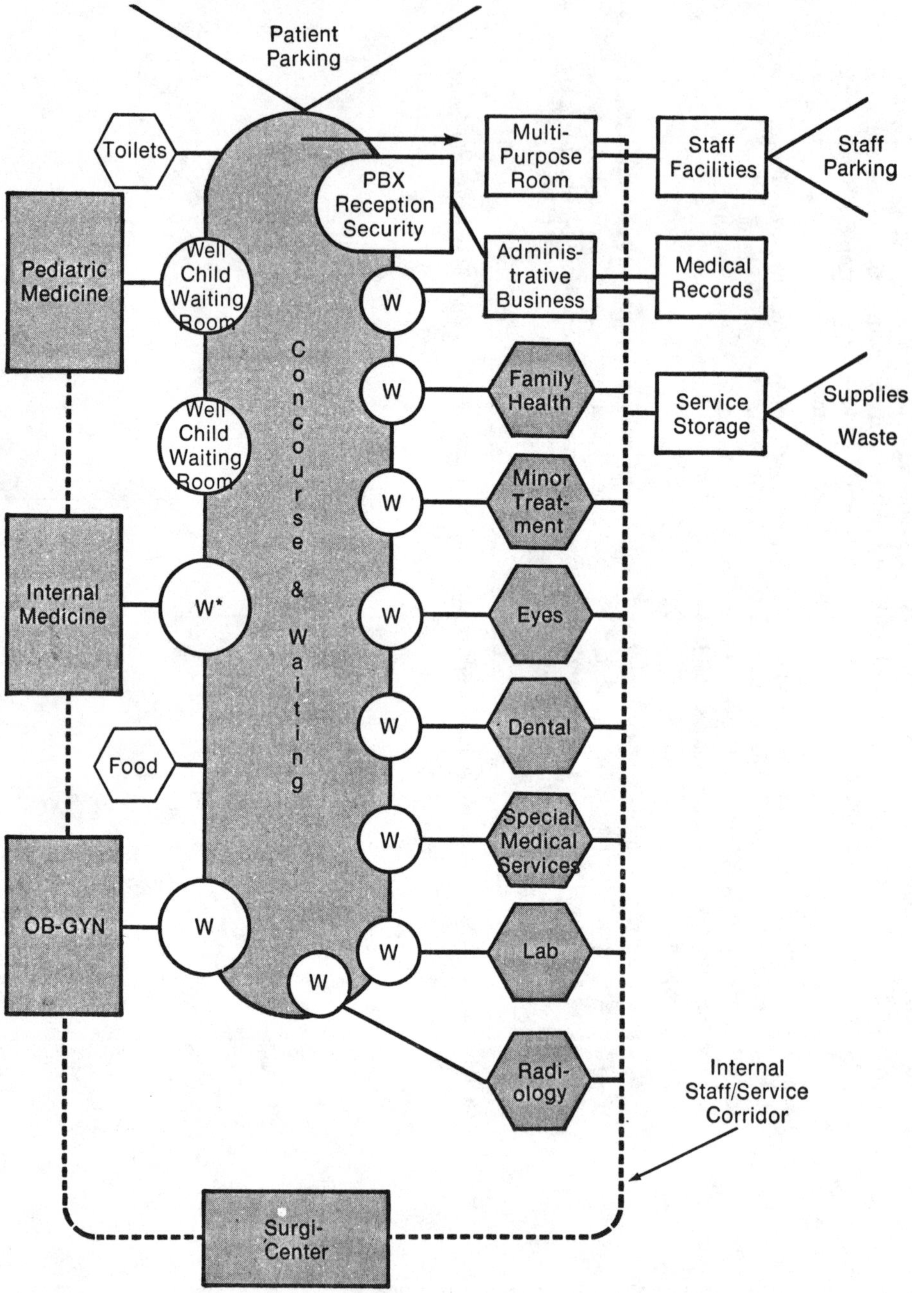

Source: Bruce P. Arneill and Peter H. Nuelsen, "Functional Components of the Ambulatory Care Facility," *The Journal of Ambulatory Care Management,* April 1978, p. 28.

Figure 13-3   Basic layout of a six-provider "pod" ambulatory care facility

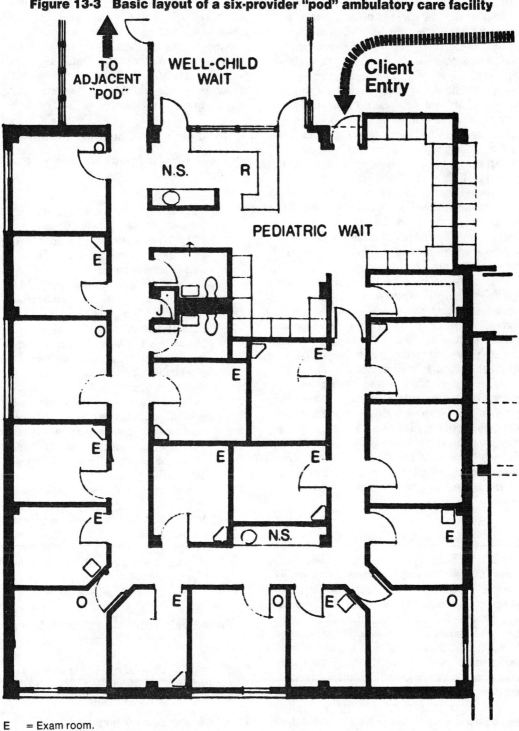

E   = Exam room.
N.S. = Nurse station.
O   = Office.
R   = Reception.

Source: Bruce P. Arneill and Peter H. Nuelsen, "Functional Components of the Ambulatory Care Facility," *The Journal of Ambulatory Care Management,* April 1978, p. 33.

If a committee is charged with the objective of examining the implications of ambulatory surgery with a possible view to establishing a program, it is extremely important to have medical staff representation (particularly anesthesiology, general surgery, and gyn surgery). Of course, plastic surgery and many other surgical subspecialties will eventually be interested in the program, but their membership on the original committee, while valuable, is not necessarily crucial. Other representation should include administration, nursing, and perhaps someone from the office of the controller.

In some hospitals one of the early objectives is an evaluation of whether or not an ambulatory surgery program *should* be created. At other hospitals *that* objective will be assumed, and the approach will be what *steps* should be taken to create such a program.

Once a firm decision has been made to establish an ambulatory surgery program major issues need to be resolved. A subcommittee can be formed to handle the construction and financial details, such as costs and location of the unit (creating a separate tailormade unit or merging it within the existing inpatient system). The physicians will concentrate on the professional aspects. Without the support of the surgeons, the program will die an early death. Anesthesia is a key issue too, because many ambulatory surgery programs have not been able to do an effective job because of the absence of a sufficient number of anesthesiologists. Each situation is different, and approaches must reflect local needs.

Credit Policies

Hospitals are also concerned about credit policies. Since ambulatory surgeries are generally elective procedures, controllers like to have payment assured before the surgery takes place. The same is often true for inpatient elective surgery. The patient's insurance policy information is obtained by the hospital from the patient after the doctor's office "books" the patient. Deposits are usually required if insurance is missing or is in any way inadequate.

To promote financial stability, many hospitals require a 3 to 6 day notice before an ambulatory surgery patient can be operated on. This gives the business office time to verify that financial details are intact. But many doctors may want to book some patients sooner if the operating room time is available. This can serve to limit the utilization of ambulatory surgery.

In most cases two days is enough time for the business office to garner credit information, and both the patient and the surgeon are better served by the availability of reduced waiting time for elective ambulatory surgery.

Problems in Ambulatory Surgery

Some of the problems with ambulatory surgery include:

1. Patient resistance
   a) "My friends always were hospitalized for a D&C, why shouldn't I be?"
   b) "My hospitalization insurance policy pays for inpatient care, and I want all that is coming to me."
   c) "It must be safer to be hospitalized because my doctor never uses the ambulatory surgery program of the hospital."
2. Physician resistance:
   a) Force of habit; lack of general community acceptance; and lack of immediate availability of care in case sudden complications occur.
   b) Possible increased malpractice danger—depends on area practice because court cases lean heavily on what is "considered common usage." In a community with little ambulatory surgery, a physician may tend to take a conservative view of "experimentation."
   c) Reduced physician income in inpatient follow-up care.
      1) Not a strong "con" but some critics may make more of this issue than they should.
3. Potentially reduced hospital income.

Four Basic Models of Ambulatory Surgery Centers

I. Hospital Controlled: Using Existing Inpatient ORs, Admitting, Pre- and Postop Areas

There are also subvariations, e.g., a hospital could use existing ORs but create separate new admitting section, etc. This increases both efficiency *and* cost.

Advantages

a) Enables the hospital to establish a capability for ambulatory surgery, with limited capital investment. It is often possible to create this capability without adding admitting clerks or nurses, although in some cases a small amount of additional personnel may be needed, depending on how busy the unit is. Greater "economies of scale" are provided because the new subunit will be part of the overall system.

b) The capability can be established quicker because the basic inpatient facilities already exist, eliminating construction time.

c) Flexibility: If the medical staff, for whatever reason, does not utilize the ambulatory surgery program, no expensive dollar costs have been wasted. (If a complete new unit were constructed and it was not used sufficiently, serious financial problems would result.)

d) This model allows the surgeon to perform more complex surgical procedures which can result in greater utilization of the ambulatory surgical program. For example, if the pathology report on a breast biopsy shows cancer, more definitive surgery can be performed at that time *rather than* waiting until the patient is transferred to the hospital's inpatient area.

Disadvantages

a) Basically, the hospital is organized and established for inpatient care, and when ambulatory surgery, as well as certain other ambulatory programs, are superimposed upon the existing inpatient system, many problem areas can result. Hospital personnel often regard ambulatory surgery patients as second-class citizens. This can lessen the dignity with which patients are treated. When these problems are not solved, utilization of the unit may not reach its full potential.

b) Longer waits for admission for ambulatory surgery because the inpatient admitting people may be busy with work procedures for their inpatients.

c) Some hospitals treat the ambulatory surgery patients who do not have Blue Cross or Medicare insurance differently than inpatients. For example, they may require

full cash outlay in advance to pay for outpatient surgery if the patient has a commercial insurance policy, whereas that same patient might have had credit extended as an inpatient for his stay.

d) Higher charges than necessary for ambulatory surgery arising from pricing structures modeled after the inpatient pricing system.

e) Outpatients scheduled for surgery may be bumped by emergency cases taken care of in the operating room. In addition, inpatient surgery generally is awarded priority over ambulatory surgery.

f) Since the preop holding areas and recovery rooms are designed for inpatient surgery, ambulatory surgery patients must be merged in the same areas as sometimes critical inpatients. This can result in unnecessary psychological stress.

g) Often proper waiting room areas for ambulatory surgery patients do not exist. When families of inpatients and outpatients are merged, a negative psychological impact on the families of ambulatory surgery patients can result.

h) Since ambulatory surgery patients *awaken earlier* than inpatients, it often occurs that operating room personnel may not be familiar with the special needs of such ambulatory patients.

i) Possibly a greater incidence of nosocomial infections, especially compared to the freestanding centers.

j) An excessively detailed medical record because of the comprehensive nature of inpatient care.

II. Hospital Controlled: Located on Hospital Grounds in a Specially Created, Newly Constructed, or Remodeled Area, Tailormade for Ambulatory Surgery

This includes facilities such as the Santa Barbara Cottage Hospital, in Santa Barbara, Calif.

Advantages

a) The biggest advantage is the tendency to relieve the disadvantages enumerated in Model I above. (Although good management could relieve many of the disadvantages of Model I.)

b) Tailormade area for ambulatory surgery to maximize patient care from a physical facilities standpoint (more than when area is merged with existing systems). If the area is going to be remodeled rather than newly constructed, care should be taken that a suitable area is selected. For example, if a small area of space is chosen, it may be *insufficient* for a sound ambulatory surgery program.

c) Greater satisfaction on the part of personnel, patients, and physicians, because everything is "tailormade."

d) This type of community service may attract a large share of the market because it may appeal to physicians who are not currently members of the hospital's medical staff.

Disadvantages

a) It can cost too much. A degree of flexibility is lost in this approach because if the unit is not successful, it is not likely that the space can be utilized for other hospital services without additional capital investment.

b) Items "c" and "d" under Model I can be disadvantages in Model II as well.

III. Hospital Controlled: The Satellite

Some hospitals have considered opening a satellite health care facility with ambulatory care as the central thrust, with or without ambulatory surgery. Ambulatory surgery, however, could be the main thrust of such a satellite system. Basically, a satellite ambulatory surgery facility is a freestanding facility in which the unit is located some distance from the hospital. It is created specifically for these purposes and is totally controlled by the hospital. Such satellites can be developed by joint hospital efforts as a "shared service."

Advantages

The same as those in Model II; but, in addition, the medical needs of a specific geographic area can be met on a tailormade basis.

Disadvantages

The same as those outlined in "a" in Model II, plus "a" and "b" described in Model IV.

IV. Nonhospital Controlled: The Independently Operated Freestanding Surgery Center

This includes facilities such as the Phoenix Surgicenter® and the Minor Surgery Center® of Wichita.

Advantages

a) If a particular community has an absence of ambulatory surgery facilities, or if existing ambulatory surgery facilities are inadequate, for whatever reason, the freestanding units fill a void by providing ambulatory surgery capability to the community.

b) Lower charges in the freestanding independent units when compared to the hospital charge system.

c) Tendency for increased patient and physician satisfaction. There appears to be an excessive amount of bureaucratic red tape when patients have ambulatory surgery within the hospital setting. The freestanding units have capitalized on this and many perform admirably in terms of patient care and comfort.

Disadvantages

a) Possible increase in net community cost, under certain circumstances. This is an important issue and research is needed in this area.

b) Reduced adjacency to hospital emergency back-up facilities. The independents feel that such back-up is not needed for patient safety; therefore, research in this area would be necessary.

c) As noted in a *Business Week* article recently, Dr. Herbert Notkin is quoted as saying: "Skimming off low-risk, no-overhead surgery from hospitals will simply increase the cost of those operations that must be performed in hospitals." The lead-in to the article states that one-day surgery could improve—or maybe wreck—the health care system. Therefore, independently operated ambulatory surgical facilities can present a challenge to hospital delivery of such care. Such a challenge would exist even if hospitals, alone, dramatically embarked on programs of a high incidence of ambulatory surgery.

WEIGHING THE BENEFITS OF A NEW AMBULATORY SERVICE*

An increasing number of hospitals complete their strategic planning processes with a recommendation to start a satellite ambulatory care center, a health maintenance organization (HMO), or a day surgery program. Before implementing such a program, the hospital administrators must answer yet one more important

---

*Source: Marian C. Jennings, "Financial Modeling: The Impact of Ambulatory Care Services on the Hospital," *The Journal of Ambulatory Care Management,* February 1983.

question: What will be the impact of the program on the overall financial performance of the hospital?

Ultimately, the decision to start or expand ambulatory care programs is an investment decision. Like any investment, these programs should financially benefit the hospital.

A financial model will help determine the impact of the program on the hospital. [See the source below for a detailed description of an eight-step model. Two of the significant steps involve forecasting the demand for the ambulatory care program and determining the ripple or secondary effects on hospital use.]

● **Forecasting demand for the ambulatory care program**

Forecasting the use of the ambulatory care program is accomplished in two steps: (1) forecast of total demand for the specific ambulatory

Figure 13-4 Forecasting use of ambulatory care services

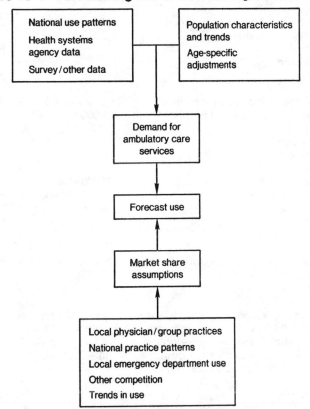

Source: Marian C. Jennings, "Financial Modeling: The Impact of Ambulatory Care Services on the Hospital," *The Journal of Ambulatory Care Management,* February 1983.

care services to be offered and (2) estimation of the market share that the program could reasonably expect to capture, based on the availability of similar services.

Figure 13-4 provides the general methodology for forecasting use of ambulatory care services. Table 13-5 provides a step-by-step approach to forecasting the use of the facility. The first four steps in the table, A through D, result in the development of the two *independent* variables: urgent care visits and visits to the facility's primary care physicians. The last two steps, E and F, result in the forecast of two *dependent* variables: the facility's laboratory services and radiology services. They are called dependent variables because these two services depend on the visits to the facility to generate their volume. Presumably, without the visits, there would be no ancillary use.

The levels of use calculated in this manner often are not achieved in the first year. Indeed, most new programs take 1 to 2 years to achieve their market share objectives. Because of this, a forecast of use for each forecast year is re-

Table 13-5   Forecasting Demand for an Example Satellite Facility

Step	Assumption(s)	Formula	Calculation	Required information
A	Urgent care visits can be estimated based on the service area population.	Population × urgent care use rate	50,000 × 250 visits/ 1,000 = 12,500 visits	Projected population Historical urgent care use rate (age adjusted)
B	Urgent care visits to the satellite can be estimated based on market share data.	Area visits × market share	12,500 × 25% = 3,125 visits	Supply information (see Figure 1) Historical market share data Analysis of competition
C	Primary care physicians' visits can be estimated based on the service area population.	Population × primary care visit use rate	50,000 × 2,900 visits/ 1,000 = 145,000 visits	Projected population Historical primary care use rate
D	Primary care physicians' visits to the satellite can be estimated based on market share data.	Area visits × market share	145,000 visits × 20% = 29,000 visits	Supply information Medical staff analysis Historical practice patterns
E	Laboratory tests are related to the number of visits.	Visits × lab tests per visit	32,125 visits × .75 = 24,094 lab tests	Historical relationship between visits and laboratory use
F	Radiology exams are related to the number of visits; urgent care visits generate more exams than do primary care visits.	(Urgent care visits × x-ray exams per urgent care visit) + (Primary care visits × x-ray exams per primary care visit)	(3,125 × .3 x-rays per visit) + (29,000 × .1 x-rays per visit) = 3,838 x-rays	Historical relationships between visits and outpatient radiology use

Source: Marian C. Jennings, "Financial Modeling: The Impact of Ambulatory Care Services on the Hospital," *The Journal of Ambulatory Care Management*, February 1983.

quired. This allows the hospital to establish realistic objectives for start-up programs.

• Determining secondary effects on hospital use

In addition to forecasting the future use of the ambulatory care program as described, it is critical to evaluate the overall effect on the rest of the hospital.

Patients for a new or expanded ambulatory care program can be drawn from any of three sources:

1. patients who currently receive no care; providing for their unmet needs represents an *expansion of the market;*
2. patients currently receiving care from the hospital or its physicians who now substitute the ambulatory care center's services; this represents *cannibalization* of the physician's or hospital's services; or
3. patients who currently receive care from other area hospitals or their physicians, which represents *market penetration.*

The first group of patients represents a net increase in the ambulatory care, and potentially the inpatient, market. The second group already receives inpatient or outpatient care from the hospital or its physicians. The proposed services may provide more convenience or a more cost-effective alternative for this group, but overall use at the hospital will remain stable or may actually decline. For example, if the hospital were to start an active day surgery program, it might experience significant activity in this new ambulatory service along with a case-for-case decrease in inpatient surgery for all patients in the second group. This would result in fewer admissions, patient days, and perhaps other inpatient ancillary services. The third group of patients represents an increase in market share for the hospital, an increase at the expense of other providers. Overall hospital use would probably increase.

The impact on hospital use can be determined for the example of the free-standing satellite facility. Table 13-6 presents the kind of secondary or ripple effects that should be considered.

As shown, an estimate can be made of the expected decrease in use of the hospital's emergency department because of the opening of the facility (Step G). Based on the emergency de-

Table 13-6   Forecasting the Secondary Effects of the Example Satellite Facility on the Hospital

Step	Assumption(s)	Formula	Calculation	Required information
G	Patients will seek convenience for their urgent care needs; opening of facility will reduce use of hospital ED.	Percentage of population closer to facility than to hospital × ED visits from community	.60 × 2,000 ED visits = 1,200-visit decrease in ED use	Patient origin from ED Population distribution by geographic area Survey data
H	Hospital use will increase based on the increase in hospital urgent care visits.	Hospital admission rate from urgent care services × Incremental urgent care visits	.10 admissions/ visit × (3,125- 1,200) visits = 193 admissions	Admission rate data Incremental urgent care visits (G)
I	Patient days and ancillary use are related to admissions.	Hospital average length of stay × Incremental admissions	9.2 days/ × 193 admissions = 1,776 patient days	Hospital average length of stay

ED = emergency department.
Source: Marian C. Jennings, "Financial Modeling: The Impact of Ambulatory Care Services on the Hospital," *The Journal of Ambulatory Care Management,* February 1983.

partment's patient origin data, the geographic distribution of the population, and the assumption that patients choose the site for urgent care services based on convenience, it is estimated that 60% of the current visits to the hospital's emergency department by area residents would shift to the new ambulatory care facility. In addition, as shown in Steps H and I, estimates can be made of the increases in hospital use because the facility is opened. In addition to the specific examples provided in Table 13-6, assumptions and calculations would also be required for the following: net impact on hospital outpatient ancillary services because of emergency department use changes; net impact on hospital inpatient ancillary services because of changes in admissions and patient days; impact on hospital of changes in admissions, patient days, and ancillary use because primary care physicians are added to the facility; and changes in the hospital's payer class mix because the ambulatory care facility is added.

Chapter 14—Education and Training Department

HOSPITALWIDE EDUCATION

Overview*

Hospitalwide education is directed by a central office with clearly defined accountability for education and training *throughout* the hospital. Responsibility for continuing education, for example, is lodged in the central office rather than within various departments, and the activities of the director of education cross departmental lines. A hospitalwide program may include (but need not be limited to) employee orientation, on-the-job training, inservice continuing education, supervisory and management development, and coordination of training to promote career mobility.

There have been reports from small hospitals as well as from large ones that hospitalwide direction and planning are more efficient means of using resources, of effecting innovations, of improving and upgrading employee performance, and of liaison with other institutions and agencies. Utilization of existing personnel is more efficient; it is easier to arrange for expert personnel to teach in departments other than their own when the need arises, or to participate in team teaching. Purchasing and utilization of educa-

---

*Source: Daniel S. Schechter, *Agenda for Continuing Education: A Challenge to Health Care Institutions,* Chicago: Hospital Research and Educational Trust, 1974, pp. 27–29.

tional materials and equipment are also more efficient and economical when centralized, and unnecessary duplication of purchases may be eliminated.

In many hospitals today, it is the office of the director of nursing inservice education, with long experience in planning continuing nursing education, that is being expanded into a department of hospitalwide training; in others, the training and education function is located as a service area within the personnel department. However, the most prevalent way to organize hospitalwide education today is to make it a separate department of the hospital.

The hospital may [then] employ a director with training and experience in adult education. His role should be that of coordinator, consultant, and trainer of teachers who will help hospital instructors to plan and evaluate their lessons and to use effective methods and materials. The director of a hospitalwide program is in a position to determine needs and recommend educational priorities from an overall point of view, and to evaluate programming by means of a consistent set of standards.

The director of a hospitalwide program is [also] a link between the hospital and these outside resources—the developing network of continuing education directors in other hospitals, in state, regional and national hospital associations, in universities and other educational institutions, and in other professional associations and agencies interested in health care education.

Present Status*

Historically, health care facilities are only beginning to develop education and training departments. In 1970, the American Hospital Association recognized the importance of institutional-based staff development programs when it established ASHET, the American Society for Health Manpower Education & Training. In October 1979, the AHA *Special Survey on Selected Hospital Topics* identified 3,071 hospitalwide education and training departments. In all, 5,663 hospitals responded to the survey. Of those responding, 1,413 or 25.0 percent engaged in some form of preparatory educational activities, 1,211 or 21.4 percent in graduate education, 5,025 or 88.7 percent offered some degree of inservice training, 4,062 or 71.7 percent provided continuing education, and 3,120 or 55.10 percent conducted nonpatient community health education. It should be noted that these statistics frequently represented single-department efforts.

Among the 3,071 institutions with hospitalwide education and training departments, the activities listed in Table 14-1 were identified as the responsibility of the departments named.

Objectives**

The primary objectives of the education and training department are to:

1. Coordinate the total education program for the health care facility.
2. Assess educational needs of the employees and the institution and develop sound education programs to meet those needs.
3. Foster a climate in which staff members identify their own learning needs and seek opportunities to meet them.
4. Design, conduct, and evaluate staff development programs and patient education programs that facilitate the attainment of standards of care established in the agency.
5. Assist staff members to acquire the knowledge and skills necessary to fulfill their role expectations.

---

*Source: Howard S. Rowland, ed., *The Nurse's Almanac,* Aspen Systems Corporation, 1978.

**Source: John E. Baer, "Staff Development," *Handbook of Health Care Human Resources Management,* Norman Metzger, ed., Aspen Systems Corporation, 1981.

Table 14-1   Education and Training Responsibilities

Activity	Percentage of Departments Directing This Activity
Audiovisual services	79.6%
Community health education	46.5
Continuing medical education	45.6
Educational counseling	27.9
Graduate medical education	12.9
Lab, radiology, and other technical staff training	32.1
Management and supervisory development	55.4
Nursing inservice training	89.0
Patient education	68.5
Preparatory allied health education programs	26.1
Support and clerical staff training	44.8
Trustee development	11.2

Source: Reprinted with permission from American Hospital Association *Special Survey on Selected Hospital Topics* by the AHA Hospital Data Center, © 1979.

6. Assist staff personnel to maintain, improve, and update their competency in the provision of health care.
7. Assist in the introduction and orderly adaptation to change in ways that are conducive to the achievement of the institution's goals.
8. Identify, evaluate, and cooperate with internal as well as with outside educational resources to promote and develop programs of basic and continuing education.

Components of a Hospitalwide Education System*

The following options depict the variety of ways that have been used to implement new hospitalwide educational programs. Decisions concerning the components—the framework, content, potential learners, area of responsibility and range of authority—for a hospitalwide education and training program depend upon the unique circumstances of each hospital.

---

*Source: Daniel S. Schechter, *Agenda for Continuing Education: A Challenge to Health Care Institutions,* Chicago: Health Research and Educational Trust, 1974, pp. 27–29.

Framework

A separate department equal to other departments

A subsection within the personnel department

A subsection of community medicine or medical education

A special staff function not attached to any department

An interdisciplinary committee

A department within the organization along with an external consortium (shared)

Content of Program

A broad range of topics that are of general interest

The development of specialized skills

Management development

Potential Learners

All hospital employees

All employees plus patients, prospective patients, and physicians

Any department that can demonstrate the need

Any department except those with their own instructors

Interdepartmental groups

Managerial personnel

Area of Responsibility

To provide all educational services

To coordinate the provision of all educational services

To provide consultative educational services

To provide administrative support to those who provide educational services

To directly provide some educational services and help others provide the balance of them

Range of Authority

Control of all educational resources

Cooperative control of all educational resources

No control of resources but veto power over program

No control over the use of any resources (consultative style)

Control over the way in which programs are developed

Control of a select portion of the educational resources

Control over the use of staff assigned to the function

Personnel

Director of Education and Training: Job Duties*

● Organizes, administers, and conducts training and educational programs in a hospital for purposes of management and promotional development, on-the-job training, and orientation of employees regarding hospital policy and routine.

● Confers with management and line supervision to determine outline and scope of programs. Applies knowledge of hospital procedures, job break-downs, safety rules, supervision techniques, and related information to formulate training curriculum. Makes sure that curriculum for professional trainees adheres to standards established by professional organizations. Organizes lectures, training manuals, examinations, visual aids, reference libraries, and other training implements. Trains instructors and supervisory personnel in proper training methods and techniques and assigns them to specific programs. Coordinates established training courses with technical and professional programs offered in public schools and universities. Prepares budget for training needs and determines allocation of funds for staff, supplies, equipment, and facilities. Maintains records of training activities and evaluates effectiveness and application of programs. Represents institution at vocational and educational meetings. May screen, counsel, test, and recommend employees for inservice educational programs or for promotion or transfer.

● Utilizes a variety of audiovisual aids and training techniques such as case study, role play, and management games.

● Calls upon training personnel of various departments to teach their specialties such as dietitian, clinical instructor, inservice nursing instructor, ancillary nursing instructor, and the general training officer. Also, may have the authority to schedule supervisors and personnel from other departments to give on-the-job or refresher training to recruits.

*Source: *Job Descriptions and Organizational Analysis for Hospitals and Related Health Services,* U.S. Training and Employment Service, Department of Labor, 1971.

Nursing Instructor: Job Duties*

A nursing instructor is a registered professional nurse who instructs student, professional, or practical nurses in theory and practical aspects of nursing art and science. The instructor assists in planning and preparing curriculum and outline for course. Lectures to students and demonstrates accepted methods of nursing service, such as carrying out medical and surgical treatments, observing and recording symptoms, and applying principles of asepsis and antisepsis. Collaborates with nursing supervisors to supplement classroom training assistance wherever needed, and observes performance of students in actual nursing situations. May prepare, administer, and grade examinations to determine student progress and achievement. May make recommendations relative to improving teaching and nursing techniques. May assist in carrying out hospital inservice training program by initiating new procedures and practices and training courses for graduate nurses in theory and practice of general nursing care or clinical specialties. May train auxiliary workers in administration of nonprofessional aspects of nursing care. May teach practical nursing techniques to classes of lay persons.

Department Responsibilities**

If the education system is organized on an institutionwide basis, the needs and resources of the entire organization can be taken into account and activities will not be duplicated or fragmented. Institutionwide education means that all institution-based education is coordinated by a central education and training department with clearly defined responsibility and accountability. The following educational activities would fall under this department.

● Staff Education and Training
Quality control of patient care through educational programming evolves from a process of careful needs assessment, cost identification, se-

---

*Source: *Industry Wage Survey: Hospitals and Nursing Homes, September 1978,* Bureau of Labor Statistics, U.S. Department of Labor, Bulletin 2069, November 1980.

**Source: John E. Baer, "Staff Development: Training and Continuing Education," *Handbook of Health Care Human Resources Management,* ed. Norman Metzger, Aspen Systems Corporation, 1981.

lection of appropriate methodologies and format, and evaluation and documentation of results and costs.

The line manager and the director of education and training share the responsibility for maintaining two-way communication on training needs and job competencies. The line manager should provide input into the education department and seek assistance from it in solving performance problems. The educator can help determine if training is needed and provide learning experiences to eliminate skill deficiencies. However, the line manager, with assistance through training from the education director, is responsible for continued application of on-the-job learning.

● Management and Supervisory Development
The first step in preparing persons to be effective managers and supervisors is to be aware that management is a unique discipline requiring specific skills.

It is being realized more and more that the skills needed for good management have very little to do with the technical function of the specialized area. The higher a person climbs in the management ranks, the greater the shift of priority from technical skills to management skills. Although the supervisor may require a fair amount of technical skills, the ability to manage successfully is more dependent on executive skills.

Health care facilities would be wise to invest both time and money in strengthening their managers' skills in interviewing; employee discipline, development, and motivation; performance appraisal; communications; problem solving; grievance handling; and team building.

Of course, emphasis also should be given to developing management skills in setting objectives, long-range and short-range planning, organizing and controlling work flow, initiating action, and time management.

● Trustee Development
The Joint Commission on Accreditation of Hospitals specifically states that the potential effectiveness of the governing body is influenced in part by a program of orientation and continuing education specifically designed for the board members. Although trustee development remains the primary responsibility of the chief executive officer and the trustees themselves, the education and training department can offer its

resources. As part of this effort, it can assist in planning and organizing programs, arranging for and developing resources, and evaluating effectiveness.

• Educational and Clinical Affiliation
Establishing clinical affiliations with educational institutions should be a function in which the training department participates. Serving as a liaison with those entities, this department can ensure that the benefits derived by the institution are proportionate to the services and facilities it provides.

In addition, by working with the facility's staff, the training department can make recommendations to educational institutions regarding the competencies that will be needed to meet the growing demands of hospital employment.

• Patient and Community Health Education
Although much of the teaching responsibility, especially for specific patient education, rests with the health care team and/or a specially trained health educator, the facility would benefit greatly by having patient and health education activities coordinated by a department that could help identify needs, exchange information, reduce costs through shared resources, ensure quality, and evaluate effectiveness.

• Resource Coordination
All of these activities demand that appropriate teaching aids and educational materials be available to educators, managers, supervisors, professional practitioners, and patients. An education and training department that consistently takes the pulse of the institution's needs is in the best position to determine what resources are required to meet those needs and coordinate with the facility's library services.

Benefits*

The benefits of establishing an education and training department include:

• developing and strengthening internal management skills
• assisting professional staff members to stay abreast of new knowledge and technological advances that impact upon their performance
• promoting high-quality patient care
• maintaining and improving personnel competency in all job categories
• helping to increase productivity

• maintaining high employee morale
• helping reduce staff turnover
• inspiring staff behavioral changes conducive to the achievement of the institution's goals
• assisting administration, through staff education, to overcome operational problems
• providing a convenient resource to assist staff professionals to acquire needed continuing education credits in order to maintain professional licensure
• coordinating programs that satisfy accreditation requirements
• serving as a central depository for staff training and development documents
• serving as a liaison with outside education-affiliated programs
• functioning as a catalyst for staff, patient, and community educational programs

ISSUES*

1. Centralized vs. Decentralized Activities

When determining how to organize an education and training program, the institution must evaluate the benefits of centralizing or decentralizing the function. In general, there appear to be far more advantages to centralization.

The major advantages of a centralized department include:

• a clearly defined accountability for education and training throughout the institution
• a centralized educational budget and its monitoring and control
• cost-effectiveness through more efficient and economical use of staff hours, equipment, and materials by avoiding duplication of programs and purchases, and diversion of instructional personnel time into noneducational activities
• institutionwide needs assessment activities to establish education and training priorities
• central control of educational resources and facilities (class/conference rooms, au-

---

*Source: John E. Baer, "Staff Development: Training and Continuing Education," *Handbook of Health Care Human Resources Management*, ed. Norman Metzger, Aspen Systems Corporation, 1981.

diovisual equipment/materials, training aids) thus providing greater availability and use

- assurance that all educational programs are evaluated consistently with regard to improving/upgrading employee performance
- provision of a centralized system for maintaining training records for each program and each employee in compliance with accreditation requirements
- provision of a coordinating base for community-sponsored programs held at the health care facility
- equal career mobility opportunities for employees in educational reimbursement, scholarships, and grant availability.

2. Organization

For organizations that can afford at least a full-time educator, it is preferable to identify an individual who will be onsite and responsive to the needs of the institution. If the health care facility carefully selects a director of education and training, that individual should be able to design and teach a large number of programs throughout the year. An onsite educator has the advantage of working closely with the line managers and knows the organization structure and climate.

Naturally, many organizational arrangements can be established in an education and training department. The most desirable is to have the department report directly to a senior member of the administration. By establishing this type of relationship, the education and training chief can participate more easily in senior management inner cabinet meetings that allow the director to identify the institution's most pressing needs. An additional advantage of an independent department is that it can better supervise other institutionwide activities such as library, audiovisual services, and medical illustration services and classroom and conference room assignment. This type of organizational arrangement is particularly conducive to the movement toward human resource management being embraced by an increasing number of health care institutions.

3. Assessing Needs

The needs assessment process is to the education and training department as the institutional

budget is to the finance department. It serves as a planning tool and a road map against which to chart its progress.

In determining training needs, a variety of criteria can be used. Real needs are identified through:

1. the specifics of job descriptions
2. information in policy and procedure manuals
3. the results of formal grievances
4. job site observations
5. requirements of quality assurance programs
6. the results of incident/accident reports
7. the mission, goals, and objectives of the institution
8. turnover records
9. attendance records
10. the results of performance evaluations
11. equipment and supply records
12. financial reports

Perceived needs are identified through:

1. formal interviews with staff, patients/families, the community at large, volunteers, physicians, and trustees
2. group discussions
3. questionnaires and surveys
4. suggestion systems
5. informal grievances
6. exit interviews
7. management and/or employee committees

Regardless of what method is used, it is crucial to involve a representative number of persons in the institution in order to achieve a balanced consideration of topics that truly have the highest priority.

4. Evaluation

An evaluation of how good any given program is and how well it accomplishes its objectives must be built into its operation. The evaluation can take several forms:

- employees can be given a pretest and a posttest to determine what they may have learned in terms of skills or knowledge
- the education and training department can work closely with line managers to monitor to what extent classroom concepts have been implemented in the work setting
- employee attitude questionnaires can be

completed to record worker perceptions of the programs

The value of a program is perhaps best determined by measurable results. Consequently, criteria against which to judge its success or failure include such indicators as turnover records, incident/accident reports, performance appraisals, quality assurance results, attendance records, grievances, equipment and supply records, and financial records.

5. Onsite/Outside Programs

On occasion, it may be more cost-effective or desirable to bring in outside resources to supplement the in-house educators. Outside programs tend to be more expensive and may not be as pertinent to the institution's needs. On the other hand outside programs enhance learning by removing personnel from the pressures of the work environment and often give the participants a fresh perspective and new ideas. They also create opportunities for staff members to establish informal relationships with other professional colleagues.

6. Shared Services

Shared services are particularly effective where budgets are tight, educational resources are limited, and where there is a group of health care facilities in reasonably close proximity to take advantage of these services. Increasingly, institutions are sharing educational services via telecommunications. Through a shared service concept, audiovisual equipment and training aids can be used by a number of institutions.

There are, of course, some negatives to consider in a shared service arrangement. Institutions may give up a degree of autonomy, employees may be required to participate in programs outside their facility rather than in the convenience of their own geographic setting, and participating institutions must establish equitable working arrangements.

In one arrangement, participating hospitals contracted to send employees to six one-day workshops at a cost far less than if the same program were not part of this shared service.

7. Costs

Although there is a significant financial investment and an allocation of employee time away from the job in establishing and maintaining an effective education and training program, these expenses will be offset by better management, improved productivity, improved communication and internal systems, lower personnel turnover, and other intangibles.

Cost Effectiveness*

Several factors must be considered in determining the cost effectiveness for any teaching/learning strategy.

- What is the initial cost of the material? (Purchase price vs. rental price)
- How many students will use the material the first time?
- What is the cost per student?
- What is the projected use of the material in terms of semesters, terms, years? (Usually a five-year maximum)
- What number of students would use the material during the projected period? (e.g., 50 students each term for 2 terms each year for five years = 500 students)
- What is the projected cost per student based on expected use? (Cost divided by projected students)
- If the material were rented each time, what would be the total cost over the projected period?
- What is the projected time required to select and prepare the material? (Hours, minutes by faculty, by others)
- What is the projected time *savings* for each future use of the material? (Faculty, others)
- What are the costs related to storage and/or maintenance?
- Are there additional cost factors?
- Is the material more effective than other methods?
- Is the required hardware available and in working order?
- Is special technical assistance required to use the material?

Cost effectiveness can be justified more readily when extended usage is calculated. Costs of rental and postage for repeated uses frequently will equal or exceed purchase costs when con-

*Source: Crystal M. Lange, "Availability and Cost of Media," *Nursing Outlook,* March 1977. © American Journal of Nursing Company.

sidered over a span of several terms. If the material is designed to be part of a self-instructional unit, there may be major savings in time both for instructor and students.

The main consideration, of course, should be the quality of the learning experience in providing the learner with the requirements to meet the objective. If it does not do this, the real cost is then too high.

HOW TO DEVELOP A HOSPITALWIDE EDUCATIONAL PROGRAM*

Generally, four major types of education are offered in hospital settings.

1. *Preservice educational activities* occur before a person assumes work responsibilities and may include general and job-specific orientation, classroom or individualized instruction, and on-the-job training. (A person employed in one job may obtain preservice education for a different job in the organization, as with upward career planning and mobility.)

2. *Orientation educational activities* inform employees of their rights, privileges, and obligations according to the hospital's policies and procedures; attempt to influence employee attitudes and behavior toward compliance with the hospital's philosophy and mission; and instruct new employees in proper techniques and operational procedures necessary for performance of their job duties. (Individual needs are recognized whether the person is new to the health center or to a particular position in the health center.)

3. *Inservice educational activities* are specific to an employee's assigned work responsibilities, and their primary purpose is to meet organizational expectations as defined in job descriptions and policy and procedure manuals.

4. *Continuing educational activities* are designed primarily to improve and/or enrich the individual's knowledge, skills, attitudes, and/or behavior. Their primary purpose is to meet the individual's personal and developmental needs.

---

*Source: Dorothy Lawrence and Robert J. Peoples, "Managers, Educators Collaborate for Hospitalwide Educational Programs," *Hospital Progress*, September 1982, pp. 36ff.

Staff development is defined as educational activities comprising inservice and continuing education.

Because of the increasingly large number of new occupations in the health care field, it is necessary to identify broad categories of persons to be served to ensure their inclusion in educational programs, such as the following eight groups: (1) governance, (2) management/supervisory (administrators, department directors, managers, supervisors), (3) medical staff (attending staff, house staff, medical students), (4) nursing staff (registered nurses, licensed practical nurses, students), (5) allied health staff (medical and radiological technologists, respiratory and physical therapists, social workers, pharmacists, others, students), (6) staff (service/maintenance, secretarial/clerical, technical/analytical, and volunteers), (7) patients (inpatient, outpatient, patient's family), and (8) community.

The institution can sponsor, subsidize, coordinate, or provide fiscal support for educational programs. Which delivery mechanism or combination of mechanisms is used to achieve a particular educational goal depends on the organization's long-range plan, resource availability, and the potential effectiveness and efficiency for ensuring programmatic goal attainment.

A Model Program

At Samaritan Health Center in Detroit a task force, charged with planning a hospitalwide educational program, developed not just a model program but a practical management tool. Any health care facility can replicate the following steps in the development of the model with revisions that allow for institutional autonomy without losing the benefits of the model.

Step 1—Overview of desired educational programs. To obtain an overview of desired educational programs on a hospitalwide basis, the task force independently discussed and reached consensus on the desired types of education that would support the hospital's long-range plans for the various education recipients. For example, the task force members believed that the trustees (governance) should receive all four types of education—preservice, orientation, inservice, and continuing. The delivery mechanisms selected varied for each type. In addition to the institutionally sponsored educational programs for the trustees, the trustees' orientation and continuing education were to be coordinated with the corporate-sponsored orientation program to avoid duplication and gaps. It was further agreed that trustees' continuing education should be supplemented with fiscal support directly to individual trustees who elected to participate in external trustee development programs.

The task force's decisions were recorded on a form (see Table 14-2) which furnished the first overview of the hospital's desired educational programming—a plan for hospitalwide education that was developed in support of the organization's long-range plan. The desired educa-

Table 14-2   Desired Educational Programs and Delivery Strategies for Samaritan Health Center, 1982

Education recipients	Pre-service	Orien-tation	In-service	Contin-uing
			Staff development	
Governance	1*	1,3	1	1,3,4
Management/ supervisory	1,4	1,3	1	1,3,4
Medical staff:				
Attending	—	1	—	1,3
House	—	1	2	—
Students	—	1	2	—
Nursing staff:				
RNs, LPNs	1,2,4	1	1	1,3,4
Students	—	1	—	—
Allied health staff	1,2	1	1,4	1,3,4
Staff (employees and volunteers)	1	1	1,4	1,3,4
Patients	Pread-mission	1	—	1,3
Community	—	1,3	—	1,3

*Key to delivery strategies. *1*, Sponsor: provide educational program (facilities, staff, supplies, programming, evaluation, etc.). *2*, Affiliate: provide an experience or part of a program, the prime responsibility for which belongs to another institution or organization. *3*, Coordinate (with the institution that is sponsoring the program, e.g., in-house college courses): accommodate, integrate, and orchestrate program; ensure communication and harmony with programming, scheduling, etc. *4*, Provide fiscal support: make financial resources available (reimbursement for tuition, fees, and travel expenses). —, None.

Source: Dorothy Lawrence and Robert J. Peoples, "Managers, Educators Collaborate for Hospitalwide Educational Programs," *Hospital Progress*, September 1982.

tional program could now be compared to existing programs to determine needed changes.

Step 2—Identification of persons responsible for education and information required for responsible decision making. Reflecting on the desired educational programs, the task force determined that the next step should involve representative personnel on a hospitalwide basis. This was necessary to obtain accurate data and to elicit ownership and support for any proposed educational plan—key factors for any plan to become operationally successful.

To collect data, the task force needed to identify persons who could provide the desired information—those who were administratively and educationally responsible for each major type of education. It was found that these were not always the same person. The vice-president, professional services, is administratively responsible for the affiliate graduate medical education program, while the director of surgical education is educationally accountable for the clinical education of surgical residents.

The task force determined that the following information should be gathered for each desired educational program: the number of persons to be instructed, instructional time per month, estimated space required, projected use of the space, and special equipment needs.

Step 3—Data collection. Each person administratively or programmatically responsible for education completed a questionnaire like the one shown in Figure 14-1. This format involved representative hospital staff in the specification of current programs and resources as well as in the formulation of future programs and resources.

Step 4—Collation, analysis, and summarization of information in task force report. The format displayed in Figure 14-2 facilitated collation of the information obtained from the questionnaire. The task force analyzed and summarized this information in a final report to management. The projections for educational requirements for the new facility were based on verified information. The report provided information to enable management to make rational decisions for the allocation of personnel, material, and capital resources. Management perspectives were clarified on management activities (planning, program development, and budgeting) needed to accomplish the projected educational programs. Further, the report gave

Figure 14-1 Educational programs planning questionnaire

Type of recipient program: _____

Name of person completing questionnaire: ____

Date: _____

Name of educational program: _____

Type of education (preservice, orientation, inservice, continuing): _____

Delivery strategy (sponsor, subsidize, coordinate, provide financial support): _____

Person(s) administratively responsible for program: _____

Person(s) educationally responsible for program: _____

Primary instructor(s): _____

Current programs and resources

A. Current program:
   1. Frequency of class(es): _____
   2. Classroom hours per month: _____
   3. Recipients per class: _____
   4. Other comments: _____

B. Instructor requirements:
   1. Estimated number of instructor hours per month for programs (planning, preparation, delivery, evaluation): _____
   2. Actual instructor contact hours per month with recipients: _____

C. Facility needs:
   1. Types of space used (classroom, auditorium, laboratory, etc.): _____

2. Special equipment or facility needs (water, mock patient room, storage, A/V equipment, etc.): _____

Future programs and resources (new facility):

A. Briefly describe charges for the programs, i.e., consolidation of current programs: _____

B. Have specific space needs been identified? _____

C. Projected program:
   1. Frequency of class(es): _____
   2. Classroom hours per month: _____
   3. Recipients per class: _____
   4. Other comments: _____

D. Instructor requirements:
   1. Estimated number of instructor hours per month for programs (planning, preparation, delivery, evaluation): _____
   2. Actual instructor contact hours per month with recipients: _____

E. Facility needs:
   1. Types of space used (classroom, auditorium, laboratory, etc.): _____
   2. Special equipment or facility needs (water, mock patient room, storage, A/V equipment, etc.): _____

Source: Dorothy Lawrence and Robert J. Peoples, "Managers, Educators Collaborate for Hospitalwide Educational Programs," *Hospital Progress,* September 1982.

Figure 14-2 Format for summary of future consolidated educational programs

Educational recipients	Number of programs	Instructor needs	Annualized classroom hours			Types of education
			Conference room	Seating for 10–20	Seating for over 20	
Governance						
Management/ supervisory						
Medical staff						
Nursing staff						
Allied health staff						
Staff (employees & volunteers)						
Patients						
Community						

Source: Dorothy Lawrence and Robert J. Peoples, "Managers, Educators Collaborate for Hospitalwide Educational Programs," *Hospital Progress,* September 1982.

a reference point for intelligent discussion of the most effective organization of educational services and the relationship of educational services in the health center so that educational programs would be consistent with and supportive of the organization's long-range plan.

The process described can be used by other hospitals, with revisions to accommodate local differences and preferences, to plan educational programs in alignment with institutional goals. The following merits justify replicating the process, including the use of terms and management tools as a framework:

- No other practical models or management tools are available.

- The planning process solicits input from and support by educators, managers, and staff.

- The model has adaptability, universality, practicality, versatility, and immediate usability and does not require external consultants.

- The model enables planning for educational programs that are consistent with and supportive of the organization's long-range plan.

Development of human resources, each having the knowledge, skills, and willingness to perform in a complex environment, is essential to development of the organization.

GUIDELINES

Guidelines for Initiating Programs*

Before embarking on any new training program or taking advantage of an existing one, ask the following questions.

1. Is there a continuing demand for this skill in your hospital? Could the need be caused by low pay or poor supervision? Could it be remedied more cheaply than through a training program?

2. What benefit will the hospital gain from offering this course?

3. What is the estimated cost per person trained? What is the total cost of the program including space?

4. How long should each training cycle last? When should it be repeated?

5. Does the course already exist elsewhere? Would your present tuition assistance program be less costly?

6. Released time, versus on-the-job training, versus after-hours program—which approach is best?

7. What, if any, academic credit can be given to course graduates? With minor changes, can national accrediting standards be met, if such exist?

8. Will vendors (*e.g.,* telephone company, IBM) help underwrite courses using their equipment?

9. Who will develop the curriculum? What materials are already available and may be bought or borrowed?

10. Who will teach the course? Understanding a subject is one thing, being able to teach it is quite another.

11. Can the course be taught better with audiovisual aids? Have you considered movies, slides, tapes, closed circuit television?

12. Does the course lend itself to individual or small group training as well as to larger classes? Conversely, can you train ten students as cheaply as five?

13. Is your training site conducive to learning? Is it convenient, pleasant, and quiet? Learning is difficult. Do not create additional problems.

14. Are department heads and supervisors supportive? What part did they play in curriculum development? Will they make good teachers?

15. Should course attendance be mandatory?

16. What recognition should be given those completing the course—certificate, promotion, pay increase?

17. What effect will the course have on your employee relations image?

18. Could the program be shared with the employees of neighboring hospitals? Could you reciprocate with other institutions and make training less costly for all?

Guidelines for Inservice Programs*

a. Provision should be made for nurses to participate in the identification of their continu-

*Source: Martin E. Skoler, *Health Care Labor Manual,* Aspen Systems Corporation, January 1981, p. 11:52.

*Source: *Guidelines for Continuing Education,* Veterans Administration, #G-11, M2 Part V, 1977.

ing education needs and in plans for meeting the needs.

b. Programs of continuing and inservice education should be relevant to both the educational needs of professional nurse employees and the needs of the institution.

c. Learning experiences of basic and higher degree programs in nursing should be monitored to determine the appropriateness of selected educational programs or learning activities for continuing education.

d. The staff development program should be consistent with the overall goals and objectives of the institution.

e. Objectives should be defined for each inservice education program and used as a basis for determining content, learning experiences, and evaluation. They should be stated in terms of the terminal overt behaviors which indicate successful achievement of desired outcomes. Plans for continuous and terminal evaluation should be made at the time objectives are identified.

f. An interdisciplinary approach to sponsoring, planning and implementing educational activities is encouraged. Close working relationships should be developed between the nursing service people and the staff development people.

g. Inservice education programs for nurses should be developed under the direction of nurses who are skilled in planning and implementing educational programs, as well as competent nurse practitioners.

h. Faculty expertise in the content to be taught is essential.

i. Maximum opportunity should be provided for participants of continuing education programs to integrate new knowledge and skills into practice, share with others and evaluate the effect on patient care.

j. A variety of formats and teaching methodologies should be utilized, with selection based on the objectives.

k. The time allotted to any inservice education activity should be sufficient to insure achievement of the objectives. Provision should be made for nurses to have time available to devote to these educational activities.

l. Facilities and resources appropriate to the educational program should be provided as follows: Instructional materials, libraries, learning laboratories, conference rooms, secretarial services and consultants if indicated.

m. Adequate funds for planning, conducting, and evaluating the continuing education program should be included in the Nursing Service budget.

n. Programs should be announced well in advance to enable all concerned to make personal and professional plans accordingly.

o. Records of attendance should be recorded and maintained.

p. Counseling and guidance should be offered so that staff will be informed about the range of continuing educational opportunities that may meet their intermediate and long-range career goals.

Guidelines for Selecting Educational Methods*

1. *Effectiveness,* the extent to which an activity achieves the stated goal. An educational method is considered highly effective if it attains the goal. 2. *Efficiency,* the amount of resources used to attain the goal. Efficiency takes into account the variables of manpower, time, materials, and money. 3. *Adequacy,* the degree to which an educational activity can achieve the goal. An activity by itself can be quite inadequate. However, when that activity is combined with another activity, a synergistic effect could occur which would make the contribution highly adequate. 4. *Appropriateness,* the relevancy of the method toward achieving the goal with respect to the culture and environment of the patient.

PATIENT EDUCATION

Decentralized vs. Centralized**

A wide variety of approaches to patient education are described in the professional literature. Most of the methods are individualized to meet the needs and resources of the particular institu-

---

*Source: *A Model for Planning Patient Education,* Bureau of Health Planning Resources Development, DHEW Pub. No. (HRA) 76-4028, 1976.

**Source: Sue Malkin and Pauline Lauteri, "A Community Hospital's Approach: Decentralized Patient Education," *Nursing Administration Quarterly,* Winter 1980.

tion. However, a maximum effect in patient and staff education can be achieved through decentralization, that is, teaching by those professionals currently practicing in the clinical area.

In addition to the differences shown in Table 14-3, two potential advantages of decentralized education are that education is integrated into services already being performed and teaching resources are potentially available at any time. On the other hand, centralized education may be more effective because of specialized personnel training and a possibly better opportunity for posthospitalization follow-up. Both systems, however, are broad, general approaches to patient education and can be molded and modified to meet the needs of an institution.

Use of Instructional Media*

Patient educators need to stay abreast of the rapid changes in the health care delivery system. They must keep in touch with technological advances in the media and communications field and apply the new systems to our instructional methods. Hospitals need to consider computer-assisted instruction; satellite transmission for multihospital, interstate programming; microwave transmission; and for rehabilitation pro-

---

*Source: Wendy D. Squyres, "Using Media in Hospitals," *The Handbook of Health Education,* ed. Peter M. Lazes, Aspen Systems Corporation, 1979.

grams, home video units connected to central terminals in hospitals. (See Table 14-4 for ratings of the various methods and media.)

The CONSICE network in Menlo Park, California, and its prototype, the Health Education TV Network (HETVN) of the Greater Cleveland Hospital Association have developed shared-service approaches to mediated health education in hospital settings. Both projects began by providing staff development television programming to several participating hospitals. (CONSICE has 11 member hospitals; Cleveland has 48.)

Elizabeth Norris, Vice President/Education at HETVN, believes that the economics can't be beat. Their programming costs member hospitals five cents per patient day. They telecast 45 different programs a week to patients' bedside televisions, continuously from 8 A.M. to 8 P.M. each day. Thirteen hospitals receive programming. In between programs, instead of commercials, they feature spot announcements regarding health issues. Each patient receives a TV guide at admission.

Project developers firmly believe that patient education and staff development go hand in hand. HETVN provides regularly scheduled training sessions for hospital staff to ensure appropriate followup to the televised programming.

In addition to these two efforts the literature is full of examples of the use of instructional media in health education. A partial list follows:

Table 14-3 Decentralized vs. Centralized Teaching

Decentralized	Centralized
1. Utilizes all nursing and health personnel for education.	1. Specified individuals responsible for teaching patients and/or coordinating patient teaching activities.
2. Each nurse assumes professional responsibility for patient education.	2. Concentrates responsibilities and accountability on individuals whose specific function is patient education.
3. Provides education to maximum number of patients and families.	3. Number of patients reached may be limited.
4. Educator(s) currently practicing in the clinical area. Possess up-to-date clinical skills and knowledge. Usually less formal training in education.	4. Educator(s) have more formal training in educational approaches. Clinical skills may or may not be in current use.

Source: Sue Malkin and Pauline Lauteri, "A Community Hospital's Approach: Decentralized Patient Education," *Nursing Administration Quarterly,* Winter 1980.

Table 14-4   Ratings for the Various Methods and Media[a,b]

Method, Media/ Materials	Situational/Convenience Factors			Efficiency					Effectiveness											
										Characteristics					Pacing		Teaching Objectives			
	Time Required of Audience	Staff Involvement	Special Space (Sound/ Light) Required	Initial Costs	Labor Costs Initial	Labor Costs Ongoing	Amount of Space	Equipment Repair/ Replacement	Interaction	Light	Color	Motion	Identify	Retention	Repetition	Facts	Procedures	Principles/ Concepts	Attitudes/ Opinions
Visual																			
Still pictures, posters, transparencies, photos	1	1	1	1	2	1	1	1	1	3	3		1	2	1	2	2	2	1
Stills in sequence: bulletin boards, flip charts, exhibits	1	1		1	2		1	1	1	3	3	2	1	2	2	2	2		1
Mobiles					2	3				3	2								
Print: pamphlets, handbills, newspapers	1				1		1		2	3	2		1	1	1	2	2	2	2
Programmed learning	3		1	3	3	3	1	2	2	3	2		1	2	1	2	3	2	2
Audio																			
Tapes and records	2	1		2	3		1		1				1	1	1	2	2	1	2
Radio	1	2		2			1		1				1	1	1	2	2	1	2
Telephone	3	3		1		3		2	3				2	2	2	2	2		2
Audiovisual																			
Filmstrips and slides	2	2-1	3	2	3	1	2	3	2	3	3	2	2	2	3	2	2	2	2
Movies	3	2-1	3	3	2	2	3	3	1	3	3	3	3	1	1	2	3	2	2
TV	1	1	2	3	3	2	2-1	1	2	3	2	3	3	3	1	2	3	3	2
Videotape	1	1	2	3	3	3	2-1	3	2	3	2	3	2	2	2	2	3	3	2
Multimedia	3	1	3	3	3		3	3	3										
Interpersonal																			
Speech	3	3	3	3	3				1	1	1	1	1	1	1	2	2	2	2
Demonstration	3	3	3	3	3				1	1	1	1	1	1	1	1	3	2	2
Play/skit	3	3	3	3	3		2	2	2	2	2	3	2	3	1	2	2	3	3
Role playing	3	3	3	3	3		2	2	2	3	2	3	3	3	1	1	1	3	3
Simulation/games	3	3	3	2	2		2	3	3	3	3	3	3	3	1	2	2	3	3
Small group discussion	3	3	3	1	2									3	2	2	2	3	3
One-to-one counseling, interviewing, consulting	3	3	3	2	3				3	3	1	1	3	2	3	2	2	2	3
Community organization	3	3	3	3	3					2	2	2	2	2	1	2	1		2
Meetings, workshops, conferences	3	3	3	1	3		3	3											

[a]Ratings: 1 = low; 2 = medium; 3 = high.
[b]Ratings assume optimal use of method or medium.

Source: *A Guidebook for Family Planning Education*, U.S. Department of Health, Education and Welfare, DHEW Pub. No. (HSA) 74-16002, December 1973.

- A combination of methods including self-instructional modules, a recording manikin, flip charts, and audio-tapes were successfully used in a heart-lung resuscitation education program.
- A sound-on-slide method was part of a preoperative respiratory teaching program in eleven western state hospitals.
- The American Hospital Association (AHA) 1977 Survey on Hospital Inpatient Education reported that one-to-one teaching is the most prevalent methodology (92 percent of hospitals); the most commonly used media and materials for patient education were brochures, booklets, and pamphlets, followed by filmstrips, films, and flip charts; 23 percent of the responding hospitals used videotapes in the Patient Education Center.
- Six hospitals in Massachusetts used audiocassettes in five languages to convey general health information and orientation to hospital procedures.
- The American Group Practice Association and Core Communications in Health, Inc. developed a planned system of individualized patient education, where a patient receives self-paced programmed instruction via film loop presentations.
- The Santa Clara County Hospital Conference and The Santa Clara County (California) Medical Society sponsor a telephone-access library of recorded messages (over 300 messages in English and Spanish) that operates 24 hours a day. This Tel-Med concept was conceived and developed by the San Bernardino (California) County Medical Society in 1972.
- The Mount Sinai School of Medicine of the City University of New York established a health education program through cable television in an East Harlem high-rise apartment building designed for the elderly.
- Hospitals are sponsoring public service "spots" on 250 radio stations throughout the country featuring one-minute consumer health information announcements.
- A number of patient education programs are being developed for patients with chronic diseases. One program for diabetes combined group instruction and audiovisual techniques.

- A lifelike breast model with variable lumps was used to train patients to do breast self-examinations.
- Many hospitals are cablecasting health information programs through closed-circuit television to patients' bedside television.
- Nurses at the Kansas Medical Center for Health and Sciences Hospital use "teaching baskets," a portable teaching program that can be used by the staff nurse at the patient's bedside. The basket contains teaching material for the nurse educator as well as learning material for the patient and family.
- In addition to the examples cited above, the following strategies for hospital-based programs have been recommended in order to meet educational objectives: individual counseling services, individual behavior modification, meal planning and ordering assistance, videocassettes in waiting areas, and animated programs.

A Model Patient Education System*

(United Hospitals of St. Paul, Minnesota)

The following guidelines suggest how each patient health education program can be integrated into patient care during hospitalization or outpatient visits:

1. Each patient health education program encourages the patient to become as self-sufficient as possible in managing his or her health affairs.
2. Each is multidisciplinary in nature.
3. Team planning and teaching are used.
4. The teachers are the professional health workers already caring for the patients' other health needs.
5. Standard methods are used for:
   a. initiating education for patients and families,
   b. determining the kind of education patients and families need,

---

*Source: Marian Adcock, Tim M. Ettenheim, and Lauren H. D'Altroy, "The Integration of Health Education into Patient Care," in *The Handbook of Health Education,* ed. Peter M. Lazes, Aspen Systems Corporation, 1979.

c. setting reasonable behavioral objectives to be attained through education,

d. delivering the planned educational activities,

e. evaluating the effectiveness of the education,

f. making available to patients and families further guidance in self-care after discharge from the hospital, if this is needed.*

Initiating Patient and Family Health Education

Initially it was found to be more successful to have an attending physician incorporate the patient's health education into routine medical care orders. The physician writes an education order in the same manner as an order for any other form of treatment or care. The education order is then transcribed along with all the other orders. Departments whose services are requested (now including education services) are notified and schedules are set up.

Determining Individual Patient Education Needs

A nurse interviews the patient during the first or second day in the hospital. This is done to assess: (1) what the patient needs to know about the illness and its treatment (and especially what the patient needs to know upon returning home), (2) the patient's normal daily routine so that the necessary changes can be determined, (3) whether the patient intends to follow medical management suggestions or is totally denying the illness and that medical management will help, and (4) whether the patient believes that the illness pattern can be altered if instructions are carried out.

Also during the patient's first or second day in the hospital, other care givers, such as pharmacists and dietitians, visit the patient to discuss current drug-taking and dietary habits.

Once these conversations have taken place, the care givers hold a patient education planning (PEP) conference to pool their information and impressions of the patient, and to formulate educational goals on which they and the patient will work during the remainder of the hospital stay. The priority of goals, teaching methods, and time schedules are agreed upon and recorded in the patient's chart to guide the care givers when they begin their education work with the patient.

Carrying Out the Education Goals

Upon completion of the PEP conference, the individualized education plan becomes a guide for each care giver. As noted previously, the care givers—such as station nurses, pharmacists, or dietitians—assigned to a patient now have education included in their care assignments. Each works with the patient on an individual basis. The care givers use pamphlets, diagrams, actual equipment (like syringes), slide shows, and movies to assist them in the teaching process. The pamphlets contain pertinent information relevant to the patient's disease and treatment and are given to the patient upon leaving the hospital.

Several days before a patient is scheduled to go home, the care givers summarize that patient's progress in achieving the educational goals. Their conclusions are then charted on a summary sheet and used to plan educational assistance to the patient after discharge.

Essentially the same process used for inpatients is used for outpatients. The physician is consulted and agrees to the need. An appointment is made for the patient, who comes to the service and is interviewed by a nurse and a dietitian to further define specific learning needs. Goals are established and appointments are made for the patient to return as often as necessary.

The appointments typically last one hour. Usually a patient is seen once a week for an average of seven weeks, then approximately once every six months. The patient is also encouraged to telephone Outpatient Education Services staff for answers to questions that come up between appointments.

The Organizational System

A multidisciplinary team approach, where direct care givers teach their own patients, requires an organizational framework to function effectively.

The following elements were used by those participating in the education of a patient: (1)

---

*Source: Marian R. Ulrich, "The Hospital As a Center for Health Education," *Health Education Monographs,* no. 31 (1972): 99–108.

procedures that describe in detail what each care giver is responsible for, (2) chart sheets for recording the education plans and patient progress, (3) educational materials (pamphlets, etc.) containing information approved by our medical staff for distribution, and (4) a communication system operating among the departments involved (nursing, health education, pharmacy, etc.) to share information on specific patients, organize the PEP conference, and so on.

The Planning Process

In the development of the educational programs and the organizational system to deliver them, it was important to have one person, preferably a health educator with no patient care responsibilities, working full time to coordinate and lead the planning process.

To develop the specific education programs, this individual relied on planning groups. Eight health care workers (nurses, pharmacists, and others) were chosen to represent their clinical specialties or departments as members of the planning groups. Each of these individuals had direct patient care responsibilities in addition to their planning duties.

These groups met for about one hour each week over several months. During this period the group members conducted a needs analysis of a sample group of patients to be served. Program objectives, content, and program materials were also developed.

During this same time period a second group was formed, the physician advisory council. Its members were appointed by the hospital's medical staff and were expected to serve as medical consultants to members of the planning groups. Members of the physician advisory council also approved the content of the various educational brochures and encouraged other physicians to use the newly developed education programs for their patients.

Program Implementation

A pilot program approach was used to implement each program. After securing the necessary approvals from hospital administration, department heads, and medical staff committees, we decided to use patients from one nursing station to pilot each program over a six-month period.

At the end of this period, the planning group members summarized their findings regarding the effectiveness of the programs. These findings were then presented to the appropriate administrative and medical staff committees with the request to change these programs from pilot status to a regular hospital service. In each case a change in status was granted, and the programs were slowly expanded to serve patients on every nursing station. Outpatients were served through the newly developed Outpatient Education Services Department.

EDUCATION AND TRAINING DEPARTMENT GLOSSARY*

Continuing education: educational activities that are designed primarily to improve and update the knowledge and skills and/or to influence behavior of the individual learner, with the primary purpose of meeting the developmental needs of these individuals.

Continuing medical education: an instructional or training program, generally provided by the employing institution, that is designed to increase the competence or formal education of the medical staff.

Director of Education and Training: a person with a background in adult education, the behavioral sciences, and/or management who directs the activities of the staff of the Education and Training Department.

Education and Training Department: the department providing staff development programs including orientation, preservice and inservice training, continuing education, upgrading and enrichment education, and, in some institutions, patient and community health education, continuing medical education, and development programs for volunteers and trustees.

Enrichment education: educational activities aimed at the personal growth and development of individual employees irrespective of their responsibilities.

Health education: education aimed at specific individuals or groups (patients, families, employ-

---

*Source: John F. Baer, "Staff Development: Training and Continuing Education," in *Handbook of Health Care Human Resource Management,* ed. Norman Metzger, Aspen Systems Corporation, 1981.

ees, community groups) to assist them to maintain or improve their health status.

Inservice education: educational activities that are specific to an employee's assigned responsibility, with the primary purpose of meeting organizational goals outlined in job descriptions, policy and procedure manuals, and so forth.

Orientation: the means by which new staff members are introduced to the philosophy, goals, policies, procedures, role expectations, physical facilities, and special services in a specific work setting.

Preservice education: educational activities that occur prior to an employee's assuming work responsibilities. It may include general or job-specific orientation in the form of classroom or individualized instruction.

Staff development: the total process that includes formal and informal learning opportunities. The focus of the process is on assisting individuals to perform competently in fulfillment of role expectations in an organization. Resources both in and outside the institution are used. The primary goal of a staff development program is to provide opportunities for employed personnel to acquire further knowledge and skills and to learn behavior that will enable them to perform their assigned functions safely and effectively in providing health care for patients and community residents.

Upgrading education: educational activities whose primary aim is to prepare employees for additional and often more difficult work responsibilities.

Chapter 15—Personnel Department

OVERVIEW*

Because a sizable percentage of the health facility's operating expenses is represented by payroll, the personnel department is receiving more attention then ever by health facility management. The fact that there may be as many as 300 different jobs in a large institution also indicates the complexity and importance of this department's functions.

Organization and Scope

The organizational position of the personnel department is usually one of a staff relationship to other departments, and the personnel director reports to the administrator of the institution. (For a typical table of organization for the personnel department of a medium-sized hospital see Figure 15-1). Its role is to develop a framework that assists the various department heads in their line responsibilities with their personnel. Using its experience and resources, the department provides depth in the management and utilization of people. The personnel department is given the responsibility to develop some specific programs within this broad scope. The wage and salary program of the facility, for example, should be designed to help make employment a satisfying experience.

*Source: Robert M. Sloane and Beverly LeBov Sloane, *A Guide to Health Facilities,* 2nd ed., St. Louis, The C.V. Mosby Company, 1977.

Wage and Salary Administration

The approach to a wage and salary program is similar in most institutions. The beginning point is to obtain a complete evaluation of the particular jobs within the facility. The core of such evaluation is the job analysis.

Job Analysis

This is a phase of personnel work in which the employee should actively participate. Pertinent information about the specific nature of the job is gathered and becomes the basis for the analysis. The differences between one job and another, together with the skills and responsibilities necessary to accomplish the tasks successfully, are the required information. This information becomes the job description when documented in a formalized statement (see Figure 15-2, "Chief Engineer").

Although the job description is helpful to the personnel department in selecting a candidate for a job, its purpose covers a much broader range. It gives management the parameters of a particular job.

Job Specifications

To help the personnel department determine exactly which candidate will best fit a particular job, the specifications of that job are compiled and documented (see Figure 15-3). The job specifications include the details from the job de-

Figure 15-1   Personnel department organization structure

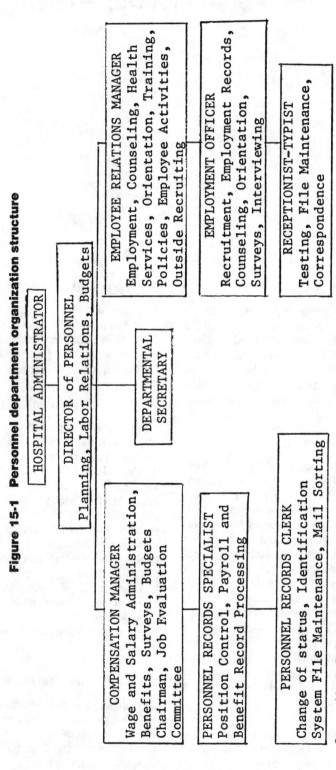

Source: Martin E. Skoler, *Health Care Labor Manual*, Aspen Systems Corporation, January 1981.

scription but also may include facts that are not directly part of the job but that will influence the selection of a particular candidate.

Compensation

Once the personnel department has the relevant data on each job, it uses a systematic method for determining the relative position of each job on the wage and salary scale. A common method is to establish a point scale for the different job factors, that is, skills and education required, responsibility of the job, and working conditions. The higher the total point score of each job, the higher the position is on the salary scale.

Aided by the information on individual jobs in the institution, the personnel department uses community salary surveys, federal and state wage and hours laws, the current labor market, and the cost of living as some of the guidelines to establishing a minimum and maximum wage level for each job classification.

The compiling and constant updating of the facility's total wage and salary program is an ongoing process to be reported annually to the administration and board of directors of the institution along with the other portions of the proposed future expenditures.

Employment, Orientation, and Training Programs

The employment program in the personnel department is designed to secure the best applicants and then select the best person for the job. Although the process of employment is centralized in the personnel office, applicants are only initially screened here. The final judgment should be left to the department requesting an applicant for an approved position.

Orientation programs are designed to help the employee adjust to his new work environment. Each department may have its own formal or informal orientation, although the institution as a whole usually has a program, most often administered by the personnel department. The objectives of the program are to inform the new employee about the conditions of his employment, to get him acquainted with his surroundings, and generally to show an interest in him. The program should be supplemented with an employee's handbook, which explains basic personnel policies, fringe benefits, and other information pertinent to his employment.

Besides providing the orientation program, a health facility may include job training for employees, management development for supervisory personnel, and executive development sessions. The degree of coordination of the personnel department with these programs will vary from institution to institution from providing a clerical function to giving a complete presentation of the program.

As an adjunct to the training programs on the premises, the personnel department may administer tuition reimbursement programs, work-study plans, institution-sponsored off-hour courses, and other continuing educational activities. Some state and national licensing boards are requiring continuing education for professional and vocational recertification, making the institution-sponsored programs an excellent benefit for both the employee and the institution.

Personnel Policies

An important responsibility of a personnel department is the development of written policies and procedures pertaining to all employees. These are approved by the administrator, who in turn must receive approval for major policies from the board of directors. These policies include such items as promotions, transfer, and payroll. The publication of these policies and procedures in a written form tends to provide a uniformity in the relationship between management and the employee. Because of the impact of policies of this nature, it is vital for the personnel department to obtain their information from many sources, including employees themselves.

New Responsibilities

The personnel function is an expanding one. No longer is it concerned solely with traditional matters: wage and salary administration, grievance handling, recruiting and interviewing, benefit administration, and training. In some institutions it has come to include manpower planning, organizational development and community relations. And, where some of the institution's employees have been organized for purposes of collective bargaining, the personnel function may include responsibility for labor relations as well.

One indication that personnel administration has achieved a new level of importance in the

Figure 15-2 A job description (chief engineer)

JOB TITLE: _____ CHIEF ENGINEER _____ CODE: ____ NVRH

DEPARTMENT: _____ DATE: _____

SUMMARY: COORDINATES THE MAINTENANCE, HOUSEKEEPING AND LAUNDRY OPERATIONS. ACTS AS LIAISON WITH OTHER HOSPITAL DEPARTMENTS AND OUTSIDE CONTRACTORS. INSTALLS AND MAINTAINS A PREVENTIVE MAINTENANCE PROGRAM. MAINTAINS RECORDS AS REQUIRED BY REGULATORY AGENCIES.

TYPICAL WORK PERFORMED:

1. COORDINATES DIRECTLY AND THROUGH SUBORDINATES THE OPERATIONS OF THE MAINTENANCE, HOUSEKEEPING AND LAUNDRY DEPARTMENTS (30).

   A. INTERVIEWS PROSPECTIVE EMPLOYEES; MAKES RECOMMENDATIONS RELATIVE TO HIRING.

   B. REVIEWS PERFORMANCE; RECOMMENDS CHANGE IN SALARY AND/OR STATUS.

   C. TRAINS OR PROVIDES FOR ON-THE-JOB TRAINING OF SUBORDINATES.

   D. PROVIDES GUIDANCE, ANSWERS QUESTIONS, RESOLVES PROBLEMS.

   E. ASSURES HOSPITAL POLICIES AND PROCEDURES ARE ADHERED TO.

   F. ASSURES WORK IS PERFORMED ON TIME AND IN ACCORDANCE WITH ESTABLISHED PROCEDURES.

2. PROVIDES A LIAISON WITH OTHER HOSPITAL DEPARTMENTS.

   A. REVIEWS REQUESTS FOR SERVICE, ESTABLISHES PRIORITIES AND SCHEDULES WORK OR CONTACTS MAINTENANCE CONTRACTOR IF BEYOND IN-HOUSE CAPACITIES.

   B. RESOLVES ANY PROBLEMS WITHIN SCOPE OF OWN AUTHORITY.

3. ACTS AS LIAISON WITH OUTSIDE CONTRACTORS.

   A. DESIGNS SPECIFICATIONS FOR SERVICES AS NEEDED, AND PUTS OUT BID; DISCUSSES WITH POTENTIAL CONTRACTORS, OBTAINS REQUIRED INFORMATION AND MAKES RELATED RECOMMENDATIONS TO ADMINISTRATION.

   B. FOLLOWS UP TO RESOLVE PROBLEMS WITH CONTRACTORS.

4. PLANS AND IMPLEMENTS A PROGRAM OF PREVENTIVE MAINTENANCE.

   A. EVALUATES EQUIPMENT BASED UPON COST AND IMPACT IF INOPERATIVE TO ESTABLISH PRIORITIES.

                                              -CONTINUED-

WRITTEN BY: _____ APPROVED BY: _____ APPROVED BY: _____

MANAGEMENT SYSTEMS SERVICES
BEDFORD, NEW HAMPSHIRE

Source: Martin E. Skoler, *Health Care Labor Manual,* Aspen Systems Corporation, January 1981, pp. 16:33–34.

Figure 15-2   continued

JOB TITLE: _____CHIEF ENGINEER_____ _____ CODE: NVRH_____

        B. ESTABLISHES RELATED SCHEDULES AND ESTABLISHES RECORDS TO NOTE WORK PERFORMED.

5.   INSURES HOSPITAL OPERATES BY ALL APPLICABLE CODES AND LICENSING STANDARDS IN AREAS OF BUILDING SERVICES. MAINTAINS RECORDS AS REQUIRED BY THE JOINT COMMISSION ON ACCREDITATION OF HOSPITALS, THE NATIONAL FIRE PROTECTION ASSOCIATION, OSHA, ETC, INCLUDING RESULTS OF TESTS AND INSPECTIONS, PLANS AND SPECIFICATION, LOG OF ACCIDENTS, ETC. ASSURES PROPER RECORDS ARE KEPT OF REQUISITIONS, CONTRACTS, WORK PERFORMED, ETC.

6.   COORDINATES SPECIAL PROJECTS AS REQUIRED.

        A. APPROVES ESTIMATES SUBMITTED ON WORK INVOLVED, EQUIPMENT AND MATERIALS NEEDED, ETC.

        B. OBTAINS APPROVAL.

        C. DETERMINES BEST METHODS AND PREPARES SCHEDULE.

        D. COORDINATES PROJECT WITH DEPARTMENTS AND/OR INDIVIDUALS AND OUTSIDE CONTRACTORS AS NECESSARY.

7.   COORDINATES SAFETY PROGRAM INCLUDING FIRE TRAINING AND FIRE DRILLS.

8.   SERVIES ON VARIOUS COMMITTEES.

9.   ASSISTS WITH MAINTENANCE WORK AS NEEDED.

10.   PERFORMS OTHER ASSIGNED OR REQUIRED TASKS.

Figure 15-3 Constructing job descriptions

Purpose:

This job description questionnaire is designed to assist you in defining the various elements of your job. Such factual information as you provide concerning the duties, responsibilities and other requirements of your job will be used in determining its relative value or ranking in comparison with the other jobs in the hospital. You are requested to complete this form, because you are most familiar with the details of your work.

Completed Job Descriptions, based upon the information you provide, will be reviewed with a representative group of employees and all supervisors to insure that all facts which properly apply have been included.

JOB DESCRIPTION QUESTIONNAIRE

EMPLOYEE:_____ DATE HIRED:_____

DEPARTMENT:_____ LOCATION:_____

PRESENT JOB TITLE:_____ DATE ASSIGNED:_____

PREVIOUS POSITION HELD:_____

NAME & TITLE OF PERSON YOU REPORT TO:_____

OTHERS FROM WHOM YOU
RECEIVE INSTRUCTIONS:_____

1. In a sentence or two summarize the principal functions of your job:
2. What formal educational background is needed to perform the duties of your job?
3. If any specific courses or programs of instruction are needed, what are they?
4. With the above education, what would be the minimum amount and type of prior experience or work background which a new employee would need in order to qualify for your job?
5. What machines and/or equipment do you use, and approximately how much time do you spend on each in a day?
6. Describe briefly the various duties and responsibilities of your job. Describe *what* is done, but not *how*. You may find it convenient to organize your thoughts in terms of work flow, or around types of work (i.e., clerical, patient care, etc.). Provide enough detail so that what you do is clear.
   - Normal daily duties:
   - Weekly, monthly or occasional duties:
7. Give some typical examples of the types of decisions you make or which you share with others:
   - Independent:
   - Shared — decisions made jointly with other personnel:
   - Recommended — decisions which you originate and submit to superior or others:
8. Describe the most complex type of problem that you must solve on your own or give an example:
9. Give some examples of the types of errors that can be made in your job and how these errors are usually discovered and corrected:
10. What work related contacts do you have with employees of other departments and why?
11. What contacts does your work require with persons not employed by the hospital, and how frequent are these? (include patients, patient's families, agencies, etc.):
12. If you have responsibility for the work and time of others draw an organization chart showing the jobs or people you supervise:
13. Do you complete performance appraisals and recommend salary increases for the people under your supervision?   Yes( )   No( )
14. Do you recommend hire, transfer, promotion or termination?   Yes( )   No( )
15. Describe the elements in your job that might cause injury to you, and how frequently these are encountered.
16. What physical aspects of the job or conditions do you consider most disagreeable?

Source: Martin E. Skoler, *Health Care Labor Manual,* Aspen Systems Corporation, January 1981, pp. 16:27–30.

health care field is that an increasing number of institutions have elevated the principal personnel officer to the level of a vice-president or an associate administrator.*

Personnel Director: Job Duties**

● Plans, coordinates, and administers policies relating to all phases of hospital personnel activities:

● Plans and develops a personnel program and establishes methods for its installation and operation. Develops the techniques and procedures for and directs the activities of recruitment, induction, placement, orientation and training. He may also be responsible for the safety and security programs. Interprets hospital policies and regulations to new employees, arranges for their physical examinations, and conducts or advises on training programs. Establishes uniform employment policies and confers with department heads and supervisors to discuss improvement of working relationships and conditions. Assists in development of plans and policies related to personnel and advises supervisors and administrative officials regarding specific personnel problems. Initiates and recommends policies and procedures necessary to achieve objectives of the hospital and insure maximum utilization and stability of personnel. Initiates and directs surveys related to turnover, wages, benefits, morale, and other personnel considerations. Prepares training manuals and directs job analysis program, including preparation of job descriptions and specifications. Acts as liaison between employees and administrative staff. Investigates causes of disputes and grievances and recommends corrective action. Supervises workers engaged in carrying out personnel department functions.

● Plans and sets up system of recordkeeping. Devises forms relative to the personnel functions. Organizes system for maintenance of central personnel files that will provide ready analysis of all personnel management functions.

---

*Source: Martin E. Skoler, *Health Care Labor Manual,* Aspen Systems Corporation, January 1981.

**Source: *Job Descriptions and Organizational Analysis for Hospitals and Related Health Services.* U.S. Training and Employment Service, Department of Labor, 1971.

● Administers benefit services and other employer-employee programs, including recreation, pension and hospitalization plans, credit union, vacation and leave policies, and others. Initiates and implements employee suggestions and performance evaluation systems.

● Informs employees of hospital activities and administrative policies by means of handbooks, house organs, bulletin boards, and other media. Performs research as a basis for recommending changes in procedures and policies. Interviews all terminating employees to determine causes of termination. Represents hospital at conferences relative to personnel activities. Prepares budgets.

PERSONNEL ADMINISTRATION*

Frequently there are danger signals that personnel management is not what it should be. These warnings include the department that somehow becomes overstaffed; the employee who is hired at an excessive (or inadequate) salary, or who is not paid on time; the salary increase that is lost or bears little resemblance to what is expected; or complaints about inequities or lack of responsiveness.

Such problems may be the result of faulty policies or programs, but often they are caused by fragmented administration. They can be the outcome of decentralized interpretation and administration of policy together with inadequate procedures and personnel records which do not insure consistent and efficient policy implementation.

The concept of centralized personnel administration and records management has three primary hospital objectives. They are:

1. to insure the expeditious and consistent application of hospital personnel policies,
2. to develop and provide data for purposes of reference, information and analysis, and
3. to insure compliance with legal recordkeeping and reporting requirements.

Functions

As soon as personnel departments were established in hospitals some centralization of clerical

---

*Source: Martin E. Skoler, *Health Care Labor Manual,* Aspen Systems Corporation, January 1981, pp. 11:41–7.

functions occurred. More recent is the transfer of authority for interpreting personnel policy from the department head to the personnel director, with right of appeal to the hospital administrator.

The administrative section of the personnel department makes no policy decisions. Instead, it processes routine requests according to policy. Unresolved questions are forwarded to the right person. It is the repository for personnel records, and it develops and maintains periodic reports, usually from the computer, for use on a need to know basis. One particularly valuable characteristic of the administrative section is its homogeneous nature. It is concerned with the relationship of all personnel actions to existing hospital policy. Amidst the continuous demand for change and the need to cope with individual problems, the administrative section should be primarily concerned with procedures which efficiently and dependably handle routine matters.

The position control program, employment processing and termination, and salary and benefit administration are duties of the administrative section.

Position Control Administration

Large hospitals with substantial turnover (50 to 60 percent) which have internal mobility and fast changing staffing needs require a position code number assigned for each authorized full or part-time position or an authorization in full-time equivalency for each type of position (*e.g.*, 13.5 RNs in I.C.U.) in an expense center. The staffing is agreed upon at the beginning of the fiscal year and usually retained throughout the year. When the administrative section receives a request to fill a vacancy it verifies the opening, possibly on a computer-produced position control report that compares authorized versus actual current staffing. If there is a vacancy, the request will be forwarded to the employment section for action.

Employment Processing

The employment officer should be made aware promptly of employment decisions and should be a part of those decisions. By the first day of work there should be a folder of information about the new employee sufficient to establish him on both the personnel-payroll computer file and the master employment file. This should be forwarded to the administrative section and should include the employment application and resume, federal, state, and hospital benefit withholding authorization forms (health insurance), benefit declination forms, any reference checks, and a copy of the employment information form. The request form for a new employee should also be returned to the administrative section for its permanent records.

After once again verifying the availability of the opening, the administrative section should prepare and forward the computer payroll input, simultaneously verifying job code, salary grade, and starting salary as being in accord with hospital policy.

Termination Processing

The process of terminating employment has become an imperfect and sometimes costly operation requiring centralized administration. Hospital workers often leave their jobs without giving notice. In addition to the inconvenience to the work schedule, new cost elements are introduced. Where insurance benefits (health, life and disability) are administered on a self-billing basis, the hospital is responsible for reporting additions to and terminations from the plan. Commonly a hospital inadvertently pays for an employee's coverage after he is no longer employed.

Additionally, other operational factors make it important to improve processing of terminations. Not the least of these factors is the accuracy of the payroll file. There is always the possibility of paying a salary to one who is no longer actually working.

Finally, long-range improvement in employee relations and in hospital operations can be suggested by listening carefully to employees during exit interviews. The person who is leaving has a particularly interesting perspective of alterations which might be valuable to hospital policies.

Salary Administration and Salary Planning

The administration section's most important activity is salary administration. No personnel function is more crucial to the hospital or the employee than accurate and prompt management of the salary program.

Most salary programs call for pay increases, either in increments or within a range of increase at appointed review dates. Important to this process is the reminder notice sent to department heads alerting them to salary reviews coming due during the following month. The master file should include the date of last salary increase and the schedule for salary reviews will have to be established by the computer programmer.

The same computer list can be returned with a change form indicating the recommended new salary for the employee. This becomes the change request and computer input.

Whether the response from the department is by computer list or by individual request for salary increase, the administrative section must determine if it is within salary administration policy and approve it. Coincident with this review, the section compels the completion of any performance appraisals expected at the time of increase. A common problem in relating performance and salary review is the surprising number of situations in which they are seemingly unrelated. The correlation should be reviewed by the administrative section and if at all questionable should be brought to the attention of the personnel director.

Benefits Administration

The area of insurance and retirement benefits is growing so rapidly that its administration is becoming a specialty of its own. As a result, some hospitals have established separate benefit administration offices. Whether or not this is done in your hospital, a specialist probably is required to administer enrollments, claims, billing procedures and other procedural matters dealing with such benefits.

This specialist's most common responsibilities are health, life, and long and short-term disability insurance, workmen's compensation, unemployment compensation, and pension and tax-deferred annuity programs.

Personnel Files

As well as being the central administrator of personnel activity, the administrative section is responsible for records relating to hospital-wide personnel management. Though these increasingly involve computerized records, the manual record will remain important.

The master *employee file* is the primary record. It assembles all original documents relating to an employee from his application to his termination. It includes all status changes, salary and otherwise, and is available to back up

any question or challenge to the hospital, legal or otherwise.

The *employee history record* has traditionally been a hand-posted card-type record of employee status changes. There are now alternative approaches to maintaining this manual status record. Current status information is available from computerized reports. Other alternatives are possible if the history is retained in the computer and produced periodically or when a change occurs. The computer can accumulate a chronology of change.

Some hospitals have elected to eliminate the manual card as a continuing record of employee status. If so, it is doubly important to insure the integrity of the computer master file and to provide a standard format for reconstructing a physical record when individual situations require it.

The administrative section has responsibility for other special-purpose files, such as:

Department Salary Plans—indicating when increases of various amounts are planned for individual employees, as estimated in the hospitalwide salary budget policy.
Master Position Control File—indicating the authorized staffing levels for each job and department. Authorized mid-year changes should also be filed here.
Master Personnel Policy Files—including any important backup.
Beneficiary Card Files—for employee life insurance.
A Reminder File—to follow-up on such matters as salary reviews, benefit claims outstanding and deadline-related projects.
Claims Files—including separate files for data relating to disability and workmen's compensation claims.
Termination Information—often keypunched onto IBM cards for periodic analysis using the termination reason codes.
Job Evaluation Files—retained in this section unless there is an authorized person with day-to-day need for the information.

Accessibility of Information

Three general rules are often adopted by personnel departments to protect confidentiality.

1. Information about individual employees is available to managers only on a strict need-to-know basis, with very few having unlim-

ited access (*e.g.*, the administration and personnel director). Thus, managers ordinarily have access only to information on their own employees. Statistical information is available to managers on a need-to-manage basis, with far fewer limitations than personal information;

2. Government agencies may acquire access to information about individuals based on a court order and have access to statistical information to ascertain compliance with laws and regulations with the full cooperation of the hospital, where requests appear reasonable;

3. Other outside parties have access to factual information on individual employees (*e.g.*, salary, length of service) other than management information only with the consent of the employee. Statistical information is available if specifically authorized by the personnel director.

INTERNAL AUDIT CHECKLIST*

Employee Relations: What do employees and prospective employees think of your institution? (Facts are less important than feelings.) What is your turnover rate compared with neighboring hospitals? Does the average employee feel that his needs, opinions, and complaints are given a fair hearing?

Labor Relations: Does the hospital now have union contracts? If not, is unionization or an organizational drive near at hand? (Either of the foregoing can demand enormous amounts of time from the personnel director and his staff.)

Recruitment: Is the recruiting staff sufficiently large and professionally competent to do the job expected of it? Do department heads recruit

*Source: Martin E. Skoler, *Health Care Labor Manual*, Aspen Systems Corporation, January 1981.

through personnel or through sources developed on their own? After spending money to bring in candidates, are the good ones lost in a storage and retrieval system which is inadequate by present day standards?

Personnel Policies: Does a policy manual exist? Is it written clearly and concisely? Are the policies it enunciates fair and defendable by modern standards? Are employees aware of its existence?

Salary Administration: Does a formal plan of any kind exist? Does it reasonably reflect the different requirements of different jobs? Does a sampling of job descriptions show careful analysis of present demands for each position? Are salary levels consistent with those prevailing in the local area for the same work?

Benefits: How do they compare with the community and within the occupational family in which recruitment will take place? Are benefits used as recruiting tools, productivity incentives, employee relations, or have they just accumulated over the years without conscious effort or planning? How much do benefits cost? Are they fairly and effectively administered by the personnel department? Has a profile of workforce by age, sex, or length of employment been undertaken?

Personnel Records: Are they complete, correct, and confidential? Are changes of employee status (insurance beneficiary changes, for example) handled promptly and accurately? Do employees trust the personnel department's record-keeping abilities? Can data processing be more profitably employed in maintaining records and providing a comprehensive data base for future needs?

Training: Are employees adequately trained for their jobs? Where is training done—outside or internally? Are there provisions for continuing programs to keep employee skills up-to-date? How much does training cost? Can economy be realized through cooperative programs among groups of neighboring hospitals?

Chapter 16—Risk Management

ORGANIZATION*

The Risk Management Office

The risk management office will be successful only if a hospital's administration is convinced of the need for such an office. The administrator must assume an interest and a positive role in the development and administration of its program. The administrator's interest in the program almost invariably will be reflected in the attitudes of all members of the supervisory force, and employees' attitudes will reflect those of their supervisors.

The risk management office may be an extension of an existing department or it may be autonomous with full departmental status. It is the logical liability control center and the risk manager is the logical liability control administrator. A central clearinghouse for information is essential, although other functions are equally important to the success of the risk management program.

Some of the basic functions of the office should include:

- receiving, logging, and maintaining incident/accident reports and support information
- maintaining pertinent records and minutes of related committee activities

*Source: Bernard L. Brown, Jr., *Risk Management for Hospitals: A Practical Approach*, Aspen Systems Corporation, 1979.

- preparing appropriate statistical analyses and reviews from gathered information
- coordinating the activities of related committees
- initiating immediate follow-up to risk problem situations
- coordinating and supplementing risk prevention and corrective activities throughout the organization
- performing other related activities as the need arises

The risk management office should not be considered just a receiver of information. A more important function is to initiate and support appropriate action directed toward prevention and correction of risk situations.

Role of the Risk Manager

Most current risk managers' backgrounds and training are in hospital administration, insurance, or safety engineering. The majority were also employed by their hospitals prior to assuming responsibility for risk management activities. Their earlier experience frequently included positions in the area of hospital finance, personnel, research, education, safety, nursing, security, and claims management.

The job description of the risk manager will need to be developed to meet the needs and expectations of the individual hospital. However, certain basic functions should be included, as in the example offered in Table 16-1.

Table 16-1 Job Description—Risk Manager

Title—Director of Safety, Security, and Loss Prevention

Occupational Summary:

- Coordinate all aspects and perform activities related to security, safety, and risk identification, evaluation, and treatment within the hospital.
- Analyze and investigate actual as well as potential risks in the institution.
- Establish operational procedures, programs, and other methods to avoid, reduce, or minimize losses.

Work Performed:

- Develop and maintain a system for the proper reporting, follow-up investigation, analysis, and file of all incidents that occur on hospital property.
- Responsible for aspects of Workmen's Compensation as directed by Occupational Safety and Health Act and Workmen's Compensation laws; work closely with Personnel Department in regard to these activities.
- Serve as Chairman of the Safety and Loss Control Council. Participate in other committees that deal with potential loss situations.
- Select, train, and assign security/safety personnel according to indicated protection requirements.
- Perform fire marshal and disaster coordinator activities related to the hospital; work closely with related committees in regard to these activities.
- Maintain a key control system to meet the hospital's security needs.
- Confer with hospital management and staff to formulate policies and procedures relating to security and loss prevention. Interpret these policies and direct subordinates in their enforcement.
- Direct periodic inspections of the hospital facility to achieve compliance of governing regulatory agencies' requirements. Report discrepancies to the appropriate authority for corrective action.
- Conduct security audits to determine loss vulnerabilities within departmental operations. Consult with the hospital's legal counsel on matters of potential liability. Review loss-prevention methods with management and staff to assure compliance.

Table 16-1 continued

- Assist appropriate departments and committees in periodic review of all release and consent forms and procedures to assure necessary hospital/patient understanding and agreement regarding the treatment or procedural information to be provided.
- Advise and assist the Claims Management Committee in regard to handling of claims, including adjusting.
- Assist in quality assurance activities throughout the hospital as they relate to the risk management function.

Source: Bernard L. Brown, Jr., *Risk Management for Hospitals: A Practical Approach,* Aspen Systems Corporation, 1979.

The Team Approach to Risk Management

The risk management team includes the following: (1) governing body and administration, (2) risk manager, (3) department heads, (4) hospital employees (including volunteers), (5) the Safety and Loss-Control Council and related committees, (6) members of the medical staff, (7) hospital attorney, and (8) outside consultants. Certain functions and responsibilities are assigned to each team member, and each must fulfill these if the program, from an overall standpoint, is to be effective. The following team assignments are suggested:

1. Governing Body and Administration

a. Define overall objectives and establish supportive atmosphere within the organization for the program
b. Commit adequate resources of management, methods, manpower, material, and money to insure its success
c. Require periodic progress reports and analyze the effectiveness of the program

2. Risk Manager

a. Provide management leadership and fulfill the appropriate staff role within the organization
b. Assist other members of the team to fulfill their functions

3. Department Heads

a. Develop written departmental safety guidelines and include same in their departmental procedures manuals
b. Consistently enforce all safety rules and regulations
c. Be constantly alert for unsafe practices and unsafe conditions and be prepared to take appropriate action to correct any irregularities
d. Investigate and complete reports on all incidents/accidents occurring in their area
e. Instruct and train workers in safety, first aid, fire prevention, and disaster planning
f. Provide and enforce the use of required safety devices and protective equipment
g. Cooperate and assist with inspection tours of their departments
h. Appoint employees to serve as members of the Safety and Loss Control Council and related committees
i. Provide for preventive maintenance and repairs of departmental equipment

4. Employees

a. Know and adhere to all safety and fire-prevention rules and regulations
b. Report all unsafe practices and conditions to their supervisors
c. Follow every precaution and safety rule to protect themselves, fellow employees, patients, and visitors
d. Participate in fire and disaster drills as requested
e. Report all injuries to their supervisors immediately

5. The Safety and Loss Control Council and Other Committees

a. See that the hospital facility is maintained in a manner that protects the lives and assures the physical safety of its patients, its personnel, and its visitors
b. See that the hospital is equipped and operated so as to sustain its safe, secure, and sanitary characteristics and to minimize all hazards
c. Conduct periodic inspections of the hospital premises to detect unsafe and unhealthful conditions and practices and recommend appropriate corrective measures
d. Analyze all accident and/or incident reports to determine causes and to suggest such remedial actions as may be appropriate to prevent recurrences
e. Compile and maintain an employee safety manual
f. Act in an advisory capacity to all department heads and supervisors to aid them in their safety responsibilities
g. Assist in periodic rehearsals of fire and disaster plans
h. Promote an ongoing educational program that will involve and inform all levels of hospital management and employees of their primary responsibility for the safety, health, and well-being of all patients, visitors, and hospital staff

6. Medical Staff

Physician identification with risk management can easily be achieved through study of the existing medical staff committee structure.

Some pertinent committee functions include:

- medical staff bylaws, rules, and regulations
- medical care evaluation and audit
- medical records and documentation
- medical diagnosis and treatment standards
- medical staff selection and privilege delineation
- medical staff education
- medical staff and departmental organization
- medical disaster (part of hospital disaster committee)
- patient care/professional liability

Beyond actual formal involvement in such activities as medical committee work, the individual physician can be a valuable source of constructive criticism and evaluation, with resulting improvements in hospital operations and, in the case of risk management, identification of problems.

7. Hospital Attorney

Specific functions fulfilled by the hospital attorney may include:

a. Advisor to the governing body relative to legal implications of bylaws, rules, regulations, policy establishment, and ultimate decisions made by the board; specifically, assists with legal documents, including resolutions, articles of incorporation, trust agreements, and contracts

b. Advisor to the medical staff relative to establishment and enforcement of bylaws, rules, and regulations; assists, when appropriate, medical staff committees dealing with medical evaluation and other related activities with legal implications

c. Assists directly, when needed, the hospital administrator in operational activities having legal implications

d. Advises designated members of the hospital team in operational matters having legal implications (Those designated may include assistant administrators, medical records administrator, director of nursing, admission director, personnel director, and risk manager.)

8. Consultants

Some of the areas in which consultants have been used are:

a. General risk management and loss prevention

b. Risk analysis and evaluation

c. Safety and security programs

d. Self-insurance functions:
   Actuarial services
   Claims surveillance and adjustment
   Trust establishment and management

Using Existing Committees for Risk Management Activities

In developing an effective risk management program, the process of successfully integrating existing activities with new functions is essential but it need not be complicated. In examining current activities, particularly relating to the handling of risk situations, one will find much being performed by existing committees. Therefore, an ideal starting place for structuring the risk management program is the committee organization.

The related committees will generally fall into two basic categories: first, safety and loss control; second, quality assurance. Some of these committee functions currently existing in most hospitals include security, safety, disaster planning, infections control, environmental control, education, patient care evaluation, and others. The risk management program can serve as the means by which related committee efforts are centralized and coordinated.

For example a Safety and Loss Control Council could be composed of multiple committees having specific responsibilities for different aspects of the risk management program. It might include committees such as:

1. *Environment Control and Energy Conservation:* conducts facility inspections and develops policies and procedures relative to the provision of a safe and comfortable environment while attempting to conserve energy resources.

2. *Fire Safety:* coordinates and monitors fire drills and reviews critiques of these drills. Reviews and updates the fire and internal disaster plan and develops policies and procedures relative to fire safety.

3. *Employee Safety:* reviews all accident reports and makes recommendations for appropriate action. Develops policies and procedures relative to employee safety.

4. *Patient and Public Safety:* reviews all incident reports and makes recommendations for appropriate action. Develops policies and procedures relative to patient and public safety.

5. *Disaster:* coordinates and monitors disaster drills and reviews critiques of drills. Reviews and updates disaster plan and develops policies and procedures relative to the handling of an external disaster.

6. *Education:* conducts orientation and training programs to support the hospital's overall safety program. Coordinates these activities with other educational efforts.

7. *Security:* reviews all incident/accident reports that have security implications and makes recommendations for appropriate action. Develops policies and procedures relative to security in and around the hospital.

8. *Infections Control:* reviews and monitors the infection control program and recommends appropriate action. Develops policies and procedures relative to infections control throughout the hospital.

9. *Other:* related committees can be added as needed.

A system of rotating and periodically replacing nonpermanent members may be used to insure broad representation as well as the resulting educational benefits. It is amazing how balanced representation, periodic changes in membership, and broad involvement can vitalize committee functions.

A Risk Management Organization Checklist

__Are existing activities in place which will provide necessary support of a risk management program?

__Is the risk management function located organizationally in a *staff* department or division?

__Have necessary management, manpower, methods, materials, and money been committed to the program?

Risk Manager

__Has a risk manager been designated?

__Does the risk manager have strengths in organizational developments, creativeness, interpersonal relations, and persuasive ability?

__Is the title *risk manager* or other descriptive designation used to establish program identity?

__Has a job description for the risk manager been developed?

Organizational Structure

__Are related committees currently functioning in such areas as safety, environment control, disaster, and education?

__Are the activities of these committees formally coordinated and integrated to improve communication and effectiveness?

__Does an overall risk management coordinating committee exist in some form?

__Does the risk management program involve multiple disciplines, as well as administrative, supervisory, and nonsupervisory levels?

Policies and Procedures

__Is there a general policy established by the governing body relative to risk management or loss prevention?

__Does standard policy and procedure (SPP) include interorganizational policies and procedures related to risk management?

__Does personnel policy and procedure (PPP) include risk management related activities?

__Does departmental policy and procedure (DPP) include each department's activities related to risk management?

The Team

__Does a team approach philosophy exist in the organization?

__Do members of the hospital organization consider themselves involved and responsible in risk management?

__Are team assignments formalized for the governing body, administration, risk manager, department heads, employees, committees, medical staff, hospital attorney, and consultants?

Medical Staff

__Is the working relationship with the medical staff effective as it relates to risk management and problem solving?

__Are pertinent medical staff committees functioning effectively to assure quality medical care in the hospital?

__Is there nonphysician involvement in medical staff committees and physician involvement in risk management committees?

Hospital Attorney

__Does the hospital have a general counsel?

__Is the role of the hospital attorney defined?

__Is the attorney involved in the risk management program?

Consultants

__Are consultants or outside contracts used to enhance the risk management program?

__Are there weaknesses in the program that could be improved with the use of consultants with special expertise?

__Were good principles followed in selecting consultants?

A Risk Management Activities Checklist

Preventive Activities

__Do you have a patient relations program?

__Do you have a patient representative program?

__Do you have a means of immediately handling patient complaints?

__Do you have family support and involvement programs?

__Do you have a patient service questionnaire and are its results distributed?

__Do you have a community or public relations program?

__Is an individual responsible for public relations?

—Do you have an active media relations program?

—Does your hospital have means for community input?

—Does it have public representatives on the governing body?

—Are hospital representatives involved in community activities?

—Do you have an effective volunteer program?

—Do you have a personnel relations program?

—Do you have an effective personnel and employment department?

—Does a healthy family atmosphere exist in the hospital?

—Do you have a hospital slogan, credo, or written purpose?

—Do you have an administrative personnel exchange program?

—Does your hospital have an employee recognition program?

—Do you have an employee newsletter?

—Do you have a medical staff relations program?

—Do physicians serve on the governing body?

—Do effective medical staff-hospital liaison activities exist?

—Does your hospital have a medical director or director of medical affairs?

—Do you have a medical staff secretary?

—Do you have a medical staff newsletter?

—Do you conduct a periodic medical staff opinion poll?

—Are hospital representatives on medical staff committees?

—Do you have an active environmental services program?

—Do you have a preventive maintenance program?

—Do you have an adequate groundskeeping program?

—Do quality control programs for environmental services exist?

—Do you have medical equipment mechanics and/or biomedical engineers on your staff?

—Are zone maintenance and housekeeping programs in operation?

—Do you have ongoing project planning, coordination, and review functions?

—Do you have a formal safety and security program?

—Is a safety and security director on your staff?

—Do you have a surveillance system for facilities and grounds?

—Do you conduct regular safety and security inspection programs?

—Does good liaison with local law enforcement and public safety agencies exist?

Corrective Activities

—Do you encourage problem identification?

—Do programs including rewards and recognition to encourage staff involvement exist?

—Are contests held to identify potential risk problems?

—Do you have area inspection programs?

—Do you have functional inspection programs?

—Are problem situations remedied expeditiously in your hospital?

—Do managers within the organization know how to solve problems?

—Does red tape deter good decision making?

—Are incentives provided to good problem solvers?

—Is there an attitude prevalent of not wanting to get involved?

—Are responsible managers overly defensive to constructive criticism?

—Are problem situations monitored in your hospital?

—Do you have suspense systems to assist in the follow-up?

—Do internal audit functions exist in all areas?

—Are systems of independent audit available?

Documentary Activities

—Are good records a part of ongoing hospital operations?

—Are patient and medical records adequate?

—Are governing body and medical staff records adequate?

—Are personnel records adequate?

—Are administrative and financial records adequate?

—Are policies and procedures recorded?

—Are regulatory reports maintained and referenced?

—Are quality assurance records adequate?

—Are records and reports dealing with potential risk and loss adequately maintained?

Educational Activities

—Are educational activities a part of ongoing hospital operations?

—Are educational functions handled on an intradepartmental basis?

—Do you have an educational services department?

—Are records of educational activities maintained?

—Are personal as well as technical skills included in educational programs?

—Do you have a patient education program?

Administrative Activities

—Has administrative philosophy been formalized in your hospital?

—Is administration a front-office function only?

—Are department heads administrators?

—Is administration an active process in your hospital?

CONVENTIONAL INSURANCE COVERAGE

The primary concern of administrators of hospitals is the protection against losses arising from injuries to patients and those arising from damage to or destruction of physical facilities, equipment and vehicles. Injuries to patients may result from acts of malpractice of professionals as well as the general negligence of the hospital's non-professional employees, and the hospital is subject to the risk of legal action by such patients. The hospital's physical property is subject to risk of fire, theft, and other hazards. Although the hospital should attempt to minimize or eliminate these risks, a program of risk management must include proper insurance coverage against such risks. (See Table 16-2 for a checklist on hospital insurance needs.)

Hospital Professional and General Liability Insurance*

The most critical insurance coverage for a hospital is professional and general liability insurance. Professional liability coverage protects the hospital against loss in those instances in which the hospital is found to be liable for acts of malpractice resulting in injury to a patient.

In most instances, a professional liability insurance policy provides a combination of malpractice and products liability coverage. A typical insuring clause may state that the policy covers liability arising out of the rendering of, or failure to render, professional service, including (1) medical, surgical, dental, or nursing treatment; (2) provision of food or beverages to patients; (3) furnishing or dispensing of drugs or

medical, dental, or surgical supplies or appliances; or (4) performance of autopsies. Under some professional liability policies, the hospital is insured against damages arising from a lawsuit by a physician who is denied staff privileges by a hospital accreditation committee.

To avoid disputes between insurance companies over who is responsible for paying an award, it is best to have the hospital's carrier be the same as the carrier handling the malpractice insurance of individual medical personnel.

Losses from injuries to patients arising out of the negligence of personnel other than professionals are ordinarily covered by a hospital's general liability insurance.

Many hospitals have found it advantageous to buy professional and general liability insurance on a group basis. This practice, in most cases, reduces premium costs. Regardless of the manner in which the hospital purchases liability insurance coverage, a hospital cannot control its premium costs without an effective program of loss control. Each hospital, with the technical assistance of its agent and insurer, should give particular attention to the development and implementation of its own loss control program, including thorough systems for incident reporting and for handling claims.

Other Types of Insurance*

A hospital is involved in many other activities which would not be covered by the professional and general liability insurance, and a hospital should seek separate coverage for these activities.

Directors' and Officers' Liability

Directors' and officers' liability coverage provides protection for directors and officers both as a group and as individuals against personal losses arising out of lawsuits against them for acts done in their official capacities. In many instances, the policy provides funds for the defense of these corporate officials in a class action or shareholder derivative claim. A "company or organization reimbursement clause," present in most policies, protects the hospital corporation for its assumption of the losses or expenses of its

---

*Source: Health Law Center, *Problems in Hospital Law,* Aspen Systems Corporation, 1978.

*Source: Health Law Center, *Problems in Hospital Law,* Aspen Systems Corporation, 1978.

Table 16-2 Checklist for Insurance Needs

	HAVE	NEEDED	NOT NEEDED
LOSS TO REAL PROPERTY			
Fire and lightning			
Extended coverage			
Vandalism and malicious mischief			
Earthquake			
Sprinkler leakage			
Water damage			
Glass			
Replacement cost–building			
Increased cost of construction–building			
Demolition–building			
Improvements and betterments			
All risk			
Optional perils			
LOSS TO CONTENTS (Equipment)			
Fire and lightning			
Extended coverage			
Vandalism and malicious mischief			
Earthquake			
Sprinkler leakage			
Water damage			
Reporting form			
Commercial property coverage			
Industrial property form			
Manufacturers output form			
Auto physical damage			
Aircraft physical damage			
Marine hull			
Electric and neon signs			
Annual transportation floater			
Motor truck cargo floater			
Salesmen samples			
Parcel post			
BOILER AND MACHINERY LOSS			
Boiler and machinery			
Air conditioning			
Business interruption (use and occupancy)			
Outage			
LIABILITY PROTECTION (Premises—Operations)			
Comprehensive general			
Owners, landlords and tenants			
Manufacturers and contractors			
Contractual			
Elevator			
Products–completed operations			
Owners and contractors protective			
Medical payments			
Personal injury			
Occurrence bodily injury and property damage			
Employees as additional insureds			
Water damage legal			
Fire legal			
Aircraft or watercraft liability			
LIABILITY PROTECTION (Automobiles)			
Comprehensive auto			
Owned autos			
Employers nonownership autos			
Hired autos—nonowned			
Drive other cars (limited–broad)			
Medical payments			
HUMAN FAILURE			
Blanket crime bond			
Comprehensive, 3-D bond			
Blanket position bond			
Primary commercial blanket bond			
Fidelity schedule bond			
Depositors forgery bond			
Money and securities broad form			
Open stock burglary			
Open stock theft			
Robbery and safe burglary			
License and permit bond			
EMPLOYEE PROTECTION			
Workmen's compensation			
Group			
Life			
Disability			
Accidental death and dismemberment			
Hospitalization			
Surgical			
Fringe			
Major medical expense			
MANAGEMENT PROTECTION			
Life–keyman			
Personal liability			
Personal auto liability			
Officers and directors			
Umbrella			

Source: Jack C. Wood, "Asset Protection," *Topics in Health Care Financing*, Fall 1974.

officers and directors arising out of any such legal claim. A state corporation law may specifically authorize indemnification and the purchase of insurance to fund these indemnification obligations. For example, the California Nonprofit Corporations Code permits a corporation to indemnify directors, officers, employees, and agents for any suits arising out of their relationships with the corporation.

Medicare and Self-Insurance

Many providers, in an effort to contain costs, are moving towards self-insurance on an individual or, more commonly, on a group basis. A provider is required to meet certain requirements if self-insurance is to be an allowable cost for Medicare reimbursement purposes. The provider must establish a fund with an independent fiduciary, and the fiduciary must have legal title and responsibility for control. Withdrawals are permissible only for malpractice, comprehensive general liability, or unemployment or workers' compensation losses. A provider must submit an annual certified statement from an independent actuary or insurance company that determines the amount necessary for the fund.

Medicare and Adequate Coverage

Damages paid by a provider that should reasonably have been covered by liability insurance are not allowable costs for Medicare reimbursement. If a provider settles or is held liable for an amount in excess of an insurance policy, such an amount is an allowable cost, provided that the intermediary determines the amount of insurance coverage was a prudent management decision. When a provider changes its coverage from commercial insurance to an alternative plan, such as self-insurance, the provider is required to show the intermediary that the new plan meets reasonable cost standards and is consistent with sound management practices.

Automobile Liability

To the extent that a hospital owns and operates motor vehicles, there is considerable exposure to liability, primarily arising out of the negligence of operators. Therefore, a hospital should purchase adequate vehicle insurance, including liability, collision, comprehensive medical payments, and uninsured motorist coverage.

Property Insurance

Fire insurance, the major aspect of property insurance, should be purchased with sufficient coverage amounts to protect all of the hospital's physical assets. In addition to basic fire insurance, coverage against windstorm, hail, explosion, riot, flood, and earthquake is frequently included in property insurance policies. Additional specific types of coverage to be considered include insurance for business interruption, loss or destruction of valuable papers, and loss of amount due from patients as a direct result of

loss of accounts receivable records, all of which may result from a casualty covered by the property insurance policy.

The cost of the property insurance premium will depend, in part, on the size of the deductible feature of the policy. To reduce the cost, the hospital should purchase a higher deductible. The hospital thus, itself, becomes financially responsible to the extent of the deductible, but it avoids the administrative costs of smaller and economically insignificant claims.

Workers' Compensation

Laws in each of the 50 states establish the amount of medical and compensation payments that must be made by an employer to an employee who is injured on the job. Because workers' compensation systems vary considerably among the states, local counsel should be consulted in the preparation of a workers' compensation insurance plan. Generally, the statute specifies the compensation for small claims and provides for a review board, often referred to as the industrial accident review board, to determine compensation for major injuries.

Employers may purchase insurance to cover workers' compensation losses. State regulations often establish the initial premium costs; thereafter, premium costs are based in part on the hospital's own experience. Thus, the hospital's own loss control or employee safety program can markedly reduce, not only direct employee time losses, but also insurance premiums.

Workers' compensation insurance should always include employer's liability coverage to protect the hospital from suits brought by employees who may be injured and who may retain the right to sue the employer in addition to receiving workers' compensation benefits.

Boiler and Machinery

The usual property insurance policy does not cover losses to major pieces of machinery and boilers when the loss is the result of the machinery breaking down or the boiler exploding. Therefore, boiler and machinery insurance should be purchased separately. In addition to the possible physical damage resulting from the breakdown or explosion, the business of the hospital may also be interrupted until the damage is repaired.

Crime

Hospitals frequently self-insure theft losses because of the high premium costs of obtaining such insurance. The major type of crime coverage generally purchased is employee fidelity insurance to cover losses from embezzlement, fraud, and other acts of employee dishonesty.

Providing Patient Data to Insurers*

One of the major problems faced by hospitals and physicians in their dealings with health insurers, and by health insurers in their dealings with hospitals and physicians, centers on the transfer of data concerning the patient to the insurer. From the insurer's standpoint, adequate information is necessary to satisfy the insurer that the claim is, in fact, payable under the provisions of a patient's policy. Furthermore, the insurer needs appropriate information in order to determine the actual amount payable on the claim.

Included in the data set might be such information as a complete itemization of services rendered to the patient, the date on which each service was rendered, the diagnoses and symptoms for which the patient was treated, the date of onset of the illness or symptoms, the charge for each service rendered, the name of the hospital or physician providing the services, and so forth. In addition, if treatment is rendered as a result of an accident, the basic data set might include a brief description of the nature of the accident. Having such information available in the hospital's or physician's insurance department could save having to go back to the medical records department in order to obtain information necessary for the completion of insurance forms. Furthermore, if the insurer requests additional information on the services rendered to an insured patient, having such information readily available in the insurance department could eliminate the necessity of pulling, moving and refiling medical records.

However, it is best to try to avoid creating a situation in which the insurer needs additional information, since such requests for information mean delays in paying claims and are costly for

the hospital and the physician to process. Therefore, the hospital and the physician should be sure to provide all information requested on the insurer's form and provide complete explanations wherever required.

Glossary of Insurance Terms*

Actual Cash Value (ACV). The present-day value of insured real and personal property determined by calculating the present Replacement Cost and deducting an amount representing depreciation caused by physical wear and tear and obsolescense.

Adjustment of Loss. The procedure of determining the cause and amount of the loss and the amount of payment required by the policy conditions.

Agreed Amount Endorsement. An endorsement to a policy indicating an amount of insurance agreed to be sufficient to void the effect of the normal coinsurance condition contained in the contract.

Alienated Premises. Premises previously owned by the insured. Ownership or responsibility for insurance has been transferred to another.

All Risk Insurance. A method of insuring which does not specify the perils to be insured. Coverage is provided against all perils except those specifically excluded by the contractual conditions.

Bailee. An individual or business entity to whom property is given in trust in accordance with a contract, either expressed or implied.

Builder's Risk Insurance. Specific coverage insuring buildings while under construction, resulting in constantly changing values.

Business Interruption Insurance. A specific insurance contract protecting against loss of earnings resulting from the interruption of business caused by damage to real or personal property.

Charitable Immunity. A situation in certain states prohibiting legal suits against charitable institutions.

Claims Made. A liability policy form which covers claims made against the insured during the policy period irrespective of when

---

*Source: J.A. Prussin and J.C. Wood, "Working with the Insurer," *Topics in Health Care Financing*, Fall 1975.

---

*Source: *Topics in Health Care Financing*, Summer 1975.

the event that caused the claim was made. Certain policy forms do not cover claims prior to the issuance date of the policy.

Coinsurance Requirement. A policy provision requiring the purchase of insurance to a specified percentage of the total value of the insured property.

Consequential Damage. Indirect losses resulting from physical damage to insured property. An example would be the thawing of frozen food resulting from fire damage to refrigeration equipment.

Continuity of Construction. Additional building or interior renovations performed to comply with the present quality and type of construction, fire protection and usage.

Deductible Clause. A specific amount to be deducted from each insured loss before the insurance will respond. Generally a deductible clause is provided by the insurance company in return for a reduced premium rate.

Difference In Conditions Policy. A separate policy written in conjunction with a Fire and Extended Coverage policy, providing broader coverage. This policy is normally purchased to provide All Risk insurance.

Dividend. Payments made by a mutual insurer; or payments made by a mutual insurer or a stock insurer because of good loss experience or because of a prior contractual agreement. Normally these payments are made at the expiration of the policy period.

Employers' Liability Insurance. Insures against common-law liability of an employer for accidents to employees, as opposed to the normal liability imposed by a Workmen's Compensation Law.

Experience Rating. A rating procedure by which normal average annual rates are amended depending on the actual losses of the individual insured.

Fidelity Bond. An insurance contract which reimburses the employer for a loss caused by a covered employee resulting from the employee's dishonest act covered by the contract.

First Dollar Defense Cost. Generally in a Liability policy, providing coverage against all legal fees required in defense of insured actions, without any deductible consideration.

First Dollar Insurance. Commercial insurance providing protection against the entire loss covered by the policy, without a deductible provision.

Highly Protected Risk. Usually a building, constructed of generally non-burnable materials, generally including sprinkler protection and other first-aid facilities, and generally close to a superior fire department.

Malpractice Liability Insurance. Insurance against alleged professional misconduct or lack of ordinary skill in the performance of a professional act.

No-Fault. A liability arrangement, such as Workmen's Compensation, whereby liability is determined only as a result of an accident, and not necessarily through courts or other legal activities. In most instances awards are determined in advance based upon the type and severity of the accident, without availability of payment for pain or suffering.

Noninsurance. Generally refers to a minor loss situation, whereby the business entity agrees to absorb its possible financial loss without the purchase of commercial insurance.

Package Plan. A procedure whereby all major insurances are purchased either through a single policy or at least through one insurance company. In this manner the premium income and services are controlled by a minimum of policies and companies.

Personal Injury. Legal liability for injury not involving bodily injury or property damage. Usually applies to slander, false arrest, invasion of privacy, etc.

Personal Property. The contents of a building, specifically separating such insured property from the "building" itself.

Real Property. Specifically defined as the "building" and normally not including excavations, land values, plantings, contents and similar values.

Reinsurance. A common practice of insurance companies involving the protection of themselves against excessive losses by purchasing insurance with other companies that assume a portion of the liability established by the initial insurance contract between the original insurer and its customer.

Replacement Cost Value. An insurance value procedure that will pay the cost of actually replacing the damaged property. The usual Replacement Cost form requires that the property must be replaced before the claim can be collected.

Reporting Form of Insurance. A procedure whereby the amount of insurance is based upon periodic reports. Generally the premium is adjusted on the basis of these reports.

Retrospective Rating. A procedure of rating that adjusts the final premium, normally after the expiration of the policy, in accordance with the actual experience of the insured during the term of the policy for which the premium is paid.

Umbrella Liability Policy. A broad-form liability policy, providing high limits of coverage over primary liability policies, and additional liability coverages, usually in excess of a stated deductible.

Waiver of Subrogation. The standard insurance contract permits the insurer to recover its loss from a guilty third party, if the insured has such right. The insured may waive such right of subrogation *prior* to the happening of any insured occurrence.

RISK MANAGEMENT COVERAGE*

An intelligent insurance decision can be made only if the hospital is cognizant of the various methods of handling risk, is knowledgeable of funding choices available and has an appreciation of the advantages as well as disadvantage of each choice. The viability of each option and the perceived importance of the individual advantages and disadvantages for each option will differ with the hospital's individual set of circumstances. No single option is superior to that of another for all hospitals.

Risk may be managed in five ways. It may be (1) avoided, (2) reduced, (3) assumed, (4) transferred or (5) shared. These five ways of dealing with exposure are not mutually exclusive: an individual hospital in all probability will combine at least three of the above methods in its insurance program. With the exception of avoidance, all methods of dealing with risk require a form of

---

*Source: David H. Schroeder, "The Hospital's Insurance Options," *Health Care Management Review,* Summer 1978.

funding. Methods of funding include (1) no insurance, (2) commercial insurance, (3) self-funding, (4) pooling, and (5) captive (single-owned, multi-owned).

The funding options, again, are not mutually exclusive, and in all probability some combination of the options is likely. Critical to each of the above options for the hospital's evaluation are availability, price, cost reimbursability, claims experience, etc.

Avoiding Risk

To the extent the hospital is successful in avoiding risk, the necessity of funding for possible loss is reduced.

- With due regard for professional, social, geographic, demographic and financial considerations, high-risk procedures and services presently provided by the hospital could be accomplished equally well at another properly equipped and staffed facility. Also, avoidance by shifting would appear to parallel national and local facilities planning objectives in reducing service duplication and cost.
- High-risk services and methods are not limited to the exotic, esoteric and heroic. The hospital may avoid risk by initiation of such programs as self-care, through which the patient and family assume a larger part of the nursing care burden.
- Consider risk exposure for new or expanded services to be offered in the future. If the hospital is self-funding, how does the new service affect previous actuarial projections? An upward revision in the actuarial determination to accommodate a new service is risk exposure cost. If the risk exposure cost is such that the new service cannot be priced competitively, then at least one objective reason for not initiating the service is established.

The individual hospital risk exposure cost is actuarially determined by examining such increments as patient days; admission; units of service by category; surgical procedures; number of employed physicians, surgeons and other professional medical personnel; and number of special care services. Evaluation of risk cost will sensitize the hospital to its risk exposure, permitting risk considerations to become part of decision-making. It may be that exposure cannot be prevented, but it can be avoided.

Reducing Risk

Principles necessary in the development of an effective risk reduction program include:

- Cooperation and Commitment. The development of the program should include the active participation of the hospital trustees, hospital management and hospital medical staff.
- Discriminatory Use of Outside Consultants. The consultant should be only an adjunct to management. Development of the hospital program should not be delegated to the outside consultant.
- Employing or Retaining Legal Counsel. Legal counsel must be well versed in malpractice issues, have a sense of proportion in what lawyers do well and what they do badly, be active in the review of the risk management program and, finally, have the confidence of the physicians.
- Developing a Data Collection Program. Data collection serves as both a detection means and an evaluation means. Data collection may be formal and informal. Formal data gathering may be by way of incident reports, medical care evaluation studies, complaints, suggestions, etc. Informal data collection effort is accomplished by cultivating confidence and applying discretion.
- Recognizing that the Hospital's Exposure to Liability is Growing. Good historical claims experience may be deceptive in dealing with tomorrow's litigation environment.

Assuming Risk

Risk assumption by the hospital is a conscious decision to pay, from hospital assets, potential losses that may occur. Potential losses may be anticipated with appropriate funding provisions or left unfunded. Assumption of risk is often referred to as self-insuring.

Self-insuring should be considered if one of the following four conditions is present.

1. It is impossible to avoid the risk or to prevent the loss from occurring, and it is impossible to transfer the risk.

2. The maximum possible or probable loss is nominal. Should a loss occur, the hospital could absorb it out of current operations with no material adverse effect.
3. The probability of loss is so small that it can be ignored, or the probability of loss is so high that to transfer it would cost as much as the loss occurrence or loss occurrence limits.
4. The hospital can predict fairly well what its loss experience will be.

The hospital has three funding alternatives to consider if it chooses to assume the risk: "going bare," self-retention and single-owned captive insurance company.

Going Bare

"Going bare" may be characterized as a plan that makes no advance provision for loss. It does not fail to recognize the possibility of a loss; rather the plan is to assume the financial consequences of the loss in the period of occurrence. Proponents of this option believe defendants in litigation are selected based on their ability to meet settlement or award demands. As a result, the lack of visible insurance lessens the chances that the hospital will be selected if it is bare. The philosophy is, "You can't get blood out of a stone."

Going bare does not require administrative effort until such time as a claim is filed. Also, no cash demand is made on the organization until the loss is settled.

Principal disadvantages of going bare center largely on cost reimbursability and financial planning. Loss and related expense incurred *are not reimbursable* to the hospital under the principles of reimbursement if the hospital chooses not to maintain adequate protection against likely losses, either through the purchase of commercial insurance, self-funding or other alternatives available.

From an operating standpoint, the losses are unanticipated and, as a result, cannot be budgeted. Not being budgeted, they cannot be built into the product price. Operating statements may vary widely from year to year depending on the loss experience and, as a result, would be unduly influenced by chance results. Hospital equity is fully exposed to settlement demands and jury awards which may destroy the organization.

Self-Retention

Self-retention differs from "going bare" in that the hospital adopts a plan to make an advance funding provision for a possible loss occurrence at some future time.

Self-retention may be advocated for one or more of the following reasons. First, by self-retention, the hospital can save part of the commercial insurer's markup, which ranges between 20 and 45 percent of premium. Certain services such as claims administration, legal and loss control provided by the insurance company for the benefit of the insured would reduce the savings to the extent these services are secured and utilized from alternative sources.

Second, the hospital benefits from the timing difference between funding and loss. Earnings on funded dollars accrue to the benefit of the self-retention fund.

Third, by self-retention, the hospital has a greater incentive to control its losses. It is likely the hospital staff will be more acutely aware of loss prevention and loss reduction measures if the employer is directly and financially responsible and accountable for loss occurrences.

Fourth, by self-retention, the hospital can reduce its annual risk exposure expense. The hospital believes its expected losses will be less than that projected by the insurance company and reflected in the premium quote.

Subject to the extent actually realized, each of these possible advantages must be evaluated in the short-term financial perspective of a possible material loss. Actual loss experience in any single year may vary considerably with actuarially projected loss. In the event of a material loss early in the self-retention program, will the hospital be capable of withstanding the financial strain of the loss—or losses? Is the temperament of the governing board and management such that they can cope with a seriously adverse loss early in the self-retention program? Does the hospital have a bond indenture that permits self-retention, or is it required to insure (transfer the risk) for the comfort of its creditors?

Other immediate considerations include the welfare of hospital trustees and hospital employees. The hospital's directors' and officers' liability coverage may require the hospital to have professional liability insurance; and, in the absence of such insurance, the directors' and officers' policy is void. Hospital employees, including staff physicians, may be uncomfortable in their professional roles if the risk is assumed as opposed to transferred.

No spread of risk is present in the individual hospital self-retention program. The laws of large numbers and probability analysis are of little comfort to the single hospital. Also, the hospital may improperly recognize the risk and underestimate the magnitude of the potential loss.

Single-Owned Captive

The third funding alternative available to the hospital if the risk is to be assumed is the formation of a single-owned captive insurance company. A captive is an incorporated, limited-purpose insurance company established to insure the hospital against malpractice and/or general liability losses that it may have. The single-owned captive serves to insure only the risks of its sole owner. The advantages and disadvantages applicable to self-retention funding also apply to the single-owned captive. The principal reason for forming a single-owned captive is to provide access to insurance markets not available to in-house funding.

Captive insurers may obtain certain covers from reinsurers that the hospital itself cannot obtain. By nature and tradition reinsurers are more flexible, permitting the captive to better tailor its insurance program. The reinsurer is not subject to as many legal restrictions as the insurer dealing with the individual hospital.

Self-retention funding may be considered unsafe or risky for the hospital in the event of a material loss. Obtaining reinsurance transfers part of the risk previously assumed by the hospital to an insurer. (An in-house self-retention fund may accomplish in part the transfer of risk objective by obtaining excess coverage.)

The formation of a captive has some unique problems associated with it. First, the capitalization cost is not reimbursable to the hospital. Second, the Provider Reimbursement Manual requires the captive to meet six additional provisions before premiums are reimbursable. Third, and currently the most serious problem is the possible unavailability of reinsurance in the market; and this, ironically, is the principal reason for forming the captive.

Transferring Risk

Risk transfer is generally accomplished by two-party contract—one party assumes financial responsibility for the other party's risk in consideration of a premium. The hospital pays a certain cost (premium) to avoid responsibility for an uncertain financial loss (contingency insured against). Risk transfer has historically been the most common method of dealing with risk for hospitals.

Transfer of risk by way of insurance appeals to the hospital because it offers the following:

- spread of risk;
- premium reimbursement by third party cost reimbursers;
- fixed and known cost to the hospital;
- loss prevention and claims handling services;
- legal services;
- indemnification up to the insured limits for those who suffer loss; and
- flexible risk-funding tools—primary coverage, excess coverage, quota share.

Disadvantages of risk transfer by way of insurance include the following:

- little immediate reward for good loss experience;
- complex and esoteric pricing methods;
- nonavailability in some cases for primary coverage and an acute lack of excess insurers;
- premium in some cases approaches the insured limits;
- suspicion that present premium pricing may be to cover undercharges of previous years;
- sellers' market; and
- poor anticipatory planning on the part of insurers.

Notwithstanding the recent problems associated with commercial insurance, transfer of risk should continue to be considered a viable option in the insurance program. Commercial insurance can be tailored to the adopted program either in the primary or the excess area. Commercial insurance may be first dollar, limited deductible, quota share participation, quota share with a stop loss, or self-insured retention.

Sharing Risk

Sharing of risk is the process by which uncertainty of loss is reduced. Sharing may or may not involve transfer of risk. Transfer of risk is not present in the shared program that assesses each individual hospital based on its own loss experience. Transfer of risk *is* present if the individual hospitals transfer their individual risks to the shared group. The uncertain financial loss of the individual hospital is exchanged for the more predictable loss experience of the sharing group.

Sharing of risk avails itself of selectivity and the law of larger numbers. The sharing group may make its service available to only those hospitals that meet the group's criteria, such as geographic location, size, claims experience, type of services provided, etc. The law of larger numbers holds that while uncertainty of the amount of loss to the individual hospital is very high, uncertainty of the total amount of loss to a large group is much lower, allowing a fairly accurate estimate of such total loss for the group. The foundation of insurance rests on this law.

Two funding alternatives are available to the hospital if it chooses to share the risk. The first alternative is the formation of a multi-owned captive, which is new to the hospital field though not new to industry in general. The second alternative is the establishment of a pooled trust, which is also new to the hospital field.

Multiowned Captive

Three primary reasons exist for the formation of a multiowned captive. First, it allows the avoidance of existing state insurance commission regulations. Certain state insurance codes do not permit self-insurance (funding), or they force the hospital into a joint underwriting association. Second, a multiowned captive allows the hospital to tailor an insurance plan not available in the market. The hospital may desire broader or more comprehensive coverage than that available in the conventional insurance market. Third, it allows access to the reinsurance market. Reinsurers deal only with insurers, and the captive is an insurer. Other considerations such as spread of risk, timing differences, etc., apply to the multiowned captive but are not unique to this alternative.

Captives are a new concept to the hospital made possible by new regulations which are subject to novel interpretations. (See Transmittal No. 190 updating the *Provider Reimbursement Manual.*)

Pooled Trust

The second alternative available to the hospital that chooses to share the risk is the establishment of a pooled trust. Unlike the captive, assets of the trust are supervised by a third party independent fiduciary.

The pooled trust has all of the advantages of self-retention funding, plus (if so structured) spread of risk. To the extent spread of risk is present, transfer of risk also exists. Transfer of risk may be partial or total depending on the funding structure alternative adopted. Funding alternatives include total risk sharing, risk apportionment by the amount of loss, risk apportionment by fixed percentage participation or risk apportionment on a regional basis.

The pooled trust shares the same problems as that of self-retention funding plus the problems associated with working with a group to establish the structure of the pooled trust. Additionally, some state insurance laws may not allow the establishment of a pooled trust. However, some states, such as Illinois, permit pooled trust for charitable, not-for-profit organizations only.

IDENTIFYING POTENTIAL LIABILITY PROBLEMS*

Overview[1]

An unusual incident is any event that is not consistent with the routine operation of the hospital or the routine care of a particular patient. The purpose of reporting an unusual incident or accident is to alert the institution's risk management program to situations that could lead to claims against the institution and to help in the identification of trends and high risk areas, so that corrective action may be taken.

---

*Sources: Excerpts footnoted "1" in this section are from Ernest J. Crane and Jean M. Reckard, "Hospital Liability Risk Management and the Medical Record," *Topics in Health Record Management,* September 1981; excerpts footnoted "2" are from Bernard L. Brown, Jr., *Risk Management for Hospitals: A Practical Approach,* Aspen Systems Corporation, 1979.

There is general agreement regarding the major components of a successful risk management program with regard to accidents and unusual incidents. These are:

- risk identification
- risk analysis
- risk treatment
- risk evaluation

Risk or exposure identification involves identifying situations that could cause an incident, risk, injury, or financial loss. This process requires a thorough understanding of the organizational and operational characteristics of hospitals in general, and of the particular institution at hand. Risk identification is probably the single most important program element, because until identified, risks cannot be effectively managed.

Risk analysis is the next step in the risk management process. Once loss possibilities have been identified, a determination must be made to ascertain which exposures are significant enough to require some form of intervention. Generally, incidents or risks that are likely to cause financial loss to the institution will demand corrective action. The greater the potential loss, the more urgent is the need for intervention.

Risk treatment is the next step in the process and involves selecting the most appropriate method or methods for managing the risk. Where possible, the exposure should be completely eliminated. This can be accomplished by, for example, correcting defective equipment that has been identified, educating staff concerning hospital procedures they have not followed, and the like. If the risk cannot be eliminated, as is frequently the case, alternative techniques must be employed in an attempt to decrease the potential severity of loss exposures. For example, there are always risks of injury associated with certain treatment equipment, and the risk management program may be able to recommend safety devices or procedures that will reduce the frequency or severity of injury.

Risk evaluation is the final step in the process. It is essentially a continuous process aimed at determining the success of the approach employed in the steps described above. When an approach does not correct the problem, a new strategy must be employed.

Identification of Risks[2]

Defining the cost to the organization of negative situations (for example, risk problems and resulting liability in areas of malpractice, workmen's compensation, small claims adjustment, and legal fees) can be helpful as a first step. Once these negative situations are identified, they may be interpreted to the organization in terms of the dollars which are being paid out for these negative activities rather than for *positive* ones, such as higher salaries, better fringe benefits, and improved working conditions.

Plant and service inspections are excellent methods of problem identification. These usually fall into two basic categories: *area* inspections and *function* inspections. The area inspection approach generally involves a tour and review of a department with the idea of identifying all problem situations, regardless of their origin. Figure 16-1 illustrates such an inspection format. A functional inspection generally is conducted by a specialist seeking to define specific problems. Examples of this type of inspection might be in such areas as electrical hazards, fire prevention, and infections control.

Problem situations generally fall in the following categories:

- patient
- physician
- employee
- environment
- systems
- policy and procedure

Each of these categories should have an appropriate organizational mechanism to encourage identification and documentation of problem situations and referral to appropriate organizational areas for remedial action and monitoring.

Investigative Techniques[2]

When a problem is identified, certain basic steps are suggested.

1. Take care of immediate needs; provide assistance to alleviate critical situations or relieve any pressure that may exist.
2. Gather the facts; fact finding and identification are critical. Facts are differentiated from opinion in this step. This involves examination of physical evidence, obtaining reports from witnesses, establishing time elements, and a basic review of the entire situation.
3. Reconstruct the scene and situation immediately. This might involve the use of such tools as diagrams, sketches, photographs, and detailed descriptions. Log as much descriptive information as possible.
4. Determine whether the problem is part of a pattern; ask certain questions, such as: Have there been other occurrences? Does this mode of operation fit previous situations, or is this an isolated problem? Does the background of those involved relate to this problem situation in any manner? Review circumstantial evidence.
5. Identify responsibility and/or cause. Determine what and/or whom the evidence points to.
6. Build a case from the information and evidence gathered from steps 1–5 and determine an appropriate course of action.
7. Report of investigation should include the who, what, when, where, and how of the case.

Review of Medical Records[1]

Medical record review is an important part of risk management. Medical records requested by patients, their families, attorneys, or those that are subpoenaed should be reviewed by the risk management office. If an initial review indicates a potential liability, the investigator should request a copy of the full medical record to do a thorough review. The hospital attorney also should be apprised of the situation and could recommend a full investigation, including interviews with various hospital personnel.

Legitimate requests for medical records may come from a variety of sources such as physicians, insurance companies, auditors, patients, families, and attorneys. It is essential that personnel in the medical record department know and understand which of these records should be reviewed by risk management staff, and why. This awareness can be readily achieved through inservice education by risk management staff using criteria developed jointly with the hospital's attorney.

Once the medical record practitioner has determined which charts are to be reviewed, the

Figure 16-1 Safety checklist

SAFETY CHECKLIST

SAFETY AND LOSS CONTROL
INSPECTION REPORT

AREA _____
INSPECTED BY _____
DATE _____

Rating   S Satisfactory
Values   U Unsatisfactory

DEPARTMENT

hallways & corridors
stairs & stairways
other traffic patterns
floor surfaces
general housekeeping
waste receptacles
toilet facilities
storage
rodent & insect control
infectious waste control
food preparation & storage
lighting
ventilation
temperature
fire fighting equipment
inspection of extinguishers
fire doors operable
exits (clear & marked)
storage of flammables
storage of medical gases
smoking regulations enforced
fire & disaster manuals
emergency lighting
electrical wiring
electrical panels, labeled
condition of electrical panels
grounding of equipment
condition, use, extension cords
guarding of machinery
use of protective devices
condition of ladders
tools and equipment
handling, radioactive materials
unsafe practices

General Environment: Good | Fair | Poor

Remarks:

Distribution
1. ___ File
2. ___ Follow-up inspection
3. ___ Administration

Note: Report here all unsafe or unsatisfactory conditions. Continue on other side if necessary.

Source: Form used by Kennestone Hospital, Marietta, Ga., 1978, as adapted in Bernard L. Brown, Jr., *Risk Management for Hospitals: A Practical Approach*, Aspen Systems Corporation, 1979.

charts should be turned over to the risk management office.

The next step in the review process is to read the patient's hospital discharge summary, since this report provides a basic outline of the patient's hospital course and may contain clues to problems encountered. Specific attention should be paid to the following:

- unusual incidents;
- bad outcome (e.g., admitted for a diagnostic angiogram, suffered a stroke during the procedure);
- documentation of patient dissatisfaction;
- unplanned return to operating room;
- readmission shortly after previous discharge;
- unexpected or unexplained deaths;
- abnormal laboratory studies with no apparent follow-up or treatment;
- surgical pathology reports that do not correspond to preoperative diagnoses;
- consents not signed or improperly executed;
- documents missing from chart; and
- unexplained corrections in treatment documentation.

Since any of the above findings may indicate possible liability, the risk management staff may complete a formal, written chart review. The situation should be evaluated with the hospital's attorney using this report. If it is determined that there is potential liability, the medical record should be secured in a separate legal file in the medical record department to:

- prevent them from being microfilmed and destroyed;
- allow medical record personnel to alert risk management when these records are requested, and by whom;
- allow the risk management office and the hospital's attorney easy access to the records.

Accidents and Incidents[1]

The use of incident/accident reports should be required and promoted for problem identification purposes. Some may feel that the documentation of problem situations will inflict criticism upon those responsible. This attitude should be emphatically discouraged. Actually, the completion of incident/accident reports demonstrates the conscientiousness and concern of those involved.

In the past, the incident/accident report form was too often used solely to help establish the hospital's defense in a lawsuit resulting from a claim. If used properly, this form can help prevent many claims from being filed in the first place. All appropriate hospital staff should be instructed in the use of the form and encouraged to file their reports immediately after incidents have taken place. For safety's sake, even seemingly inconsequential incidents should be reported.

The method for handling an incident should be a part of the standard policy and procedure (SPP) manual of the hospital (see Figure 16-2).

Accident and Incident Reporting

Incident Reports[2]

Basic information on the incident report (see Figure 16-3) should consist of:

1. Personal data on patient, visitor, or volunteer for identification purposes
2. Designation of category of individual(s) involved in incident and information related to condition(s)
3. Description of incident from those involved and related supporting data
4. Physician's statement and analysis

In most hospitals incident reports are the primary tools used in identifying risk situations. However, other sources of information should be used as well, including the following:

- incidents reported verbally by physicians and employees
- patient complaints to employees, administration, and the business office
- patient ombudsman findings
- letters from attorneys about injuries or other cases of patient dissatisfaction
- malpractice claims
- summaries of past claims experience or the experience of other hospitals
- inspections of the physical plant and audits of policies and procedures, such as relevant positions on the JCAH accreditation report
- the experience of employees and physicians
- findings of the medical audit or other quality assurance committees

Figure 16-2   Flow process in handling potential liability problems

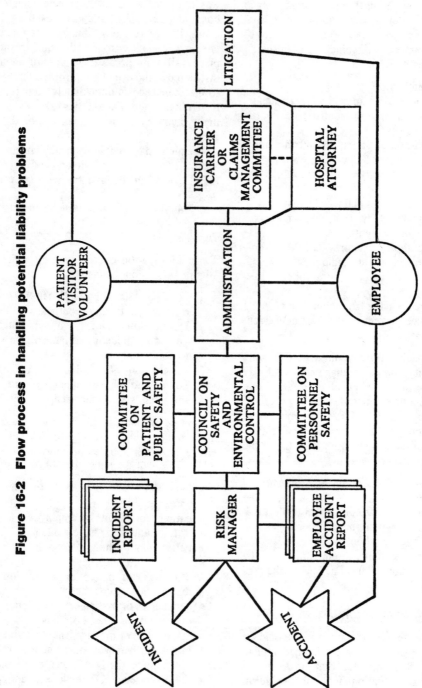

Source: Bernard L. Brown, Jr., *Risk Management for Hospitals: A Practical Approach*, Aspen Systems Corporation, 1979.

Figure 16-3 Incident report form

For Addressograph

Person involved: (Last name)	(First name)	(Middle initial)	Date of report
Age:	Male ( )		Female ( )

	Room no.	State cause for hospitalization
Patient ( )	Patient's condition before incident	
	Normal ( ) Senile ( ) Disoriented ( ) Sedated ( ) Other ( )	
	Were bed rails present Yes ( ) No ( ) Up ( ) Down ( )	Height of bed Up ( ) Down ( )
Visitor ( ) **Other ( )**	Home address	Home phone
	Occupation and place of employment	
	Reason for presence at hospital	

CONFIDENTIAL REPORT OF INCIDENT

Exact location of incident	Date of incident	Time of incident a.m. ( ) p.m. ( )

Employee's account of incident (Describe exactly what happened)

_____

_____

_____

Physical evidence retained (supplies, instruments, etc.)

Statements made by person involved (If possible indicate quotes, note time, and to whom)

_____

_____

_____

Witnesses or persons familiar with incident

Name_____Address_____

Name_____Address_____

Name_____Address_____

Physician notified: Yes ( ) No ( )	Time: a.m. ( ) p.m. ( )	Name of physician
Was person seen by physician Yes ( ) No ( )	Time: a.m. ( ) p.m. ( )	Where

Physician's statement:

Additional comments:

Source: Form used by Kennestone Hospital, Marietta, Ga., 1978, as adapted in Bernard L. Brown, Jr., *Risk Management for Hospitals: A Practical Approach,* Aspen Systems Corporation, 1979.

External data also are available from a wide variety of sources, including:

- the *National Association of Insurance Commissioners Closed Claim Studies* (1975–1977);
- the *California Medical Insurance Feasibility Study* (1977);
- the *Report of the Secretary's Commission on Medical Malpractice* (1973); and
- reports from the local professional standards review organization and health systems agency, the Occupational Safety and Health Administration, state licensure and Joint Commission on the Accreditation of Hospitals surveys, and other agency reports.

Accident Reports[2]

The information contained in the accident report (see Figure 16-4) should consist of:

1. Employee identification data
2. Details of the accident
3. Emergency medical information
4. Pertinent personnel information

Occurrence Screening[1]

Traditional risk management programs generally view the incident report as the cornerstone of their activities. It is usually the means by which the risk management staff learns of the so-called "high frequency-low liability" events. In order to have a truly effective risk management program, some way of also capturing the "low frequency-high liability" events such as complications, death, cardiac or respiratory arrest, and neurological deficit must be developed. One method of accomplishing this is the use of a technique known as *occurrence screening*.

Patient care audits are usually designed using criteria developed for individual medical conditions or diseases and specific procedures or narrowly related processes. Occurrence screening, on the other hand, uses a set of generic criteria like those developed during the California Medical Insurance Feasibility Study in the mid-1970s. The criteria are outcome oriented and basically describe expectations about the course of hospitalization and the consequences of care rendered for a patient.

In occurrence screening, the medical record is reviewed while patients are still in the hospital.

(The more quickly an adverse outcome can be identified and action taken, the lower the potential liability is likely to be.) Since all aspects of patient care are screened regardless of the reason for hospitalization, problems related to both hospital and medical staff are likely to be identified. Nonphysician personnel generally perform the initial record screening, and records with variations from the criteria are flagged and sent to a physician reviewer for a second screening. If this screening confirms the presence of a problem, a report is made to the risk manager, or to the individual responsible for patient safety, for follow-up.

Management Checklist for Health and Safety*

The operational audit should make sure that employees, patients and hospital visitors are provided adequate health protection and freedom from hazards. It should:

1. Ascertain whether there are written policies for the distribution and management of space.
2. Inquire whether definite responsibility for the assignment and utilization of space has been established.
3. Evaluate written policies on health and safety of personnel, patients and visitors.
4. Evaluate the informed-consent policy and determine whether it is being properly administered in diagnostic, treatment and therapy areas.
5. Review waste management policies with special emphasis on areas which produce or come in contact with contaminated or radioactive waste materials.
6. Evaluate the program of insurance coverage with the hospital's insurance agent for completeness and replacement value coverage.
7. Determine whether the hospital is operating in accordance with federal, state and local regulations concerning health, safety and pollution control.
8. Evaluate the security system to ensure that patients, personnel, facilities and other as-

---

*Source: R. Neal Gilbert, "Operational Auditing Checks Effectiveness," *Hospital Financial Management,* August 1977.

Figure 16-4   Accident report form

EMPLOYEE INJURED	Name: (Last) (First) (Middle Initial) — Department:

EMPLOYEE INJURED	Job Title:	Status Full time ( ) Part time ( )	Hours per pay period

DETAILS OF ACCIDENT	Date of accident	Time of accident (a.m.) (p.m.)	Date accident reported by employee
	Date lost time began	Time Lost time began (a.m.) (p.m.)	Employee paid for day of accident Yes ( ) No ( )
	To whom accident reported		Name of supervisor
	Was accident caused by failure to:	Use safety equipment Yes ( ) No ( )	Observe safety rules Yes ( ) No ( )
	Describe how accident occurred and why (Use back if necessary)		
	Name of instrument causing accident, if any		Location of accident
	Was accident due to: Employee's action ( ) Action of others ( ) Equipment failure ( )		
	Name and address of witness:		
	Nature and location of injury (Right or left side, hand or knee, etc.)		
	Has injured returned to work Yes ( ) No ( )	If returned, indicate date and time	
	Signature and title of person preparing report		Date

EMERGENCY MEDICAL INFORMATION	Emergency physician's name:	Date and time seen: (a.m.) (p.m.)	Where examined
	Emergency physician's statement (Use back if necessary)		
	Estimated return to work date		Private physician name, if referred

PERSONNEL DEPARTMENT USE ONLY	Social security number	Address of employee
	Employment date	Marital Status: Single ( ) Married ( ) Divorced ( ) Widowed ( ) Separated ( )
	Sex Male ( ) Female ( )	Birthdate — Home telephone — Rate of pay
	Actual return to work date	Medical charges
	Disposition	

Source: Form used by Kennestone Hospital, Marietta, Ga., 1978, as adapted in Bernard L. Brown, Jr., *Risk Management for Hospitals: A Practical Approach*, Aspen Systems Corporation, 1979.

sets are protected against existing and potential hazards.

RISK MANAGEMENT GLOSSARY*

This glossary includes definitions that relate to risk management in the hospital setting. A glossary such as this cannot provide a short course in such a subject as risk management. Instead, this particular glossary attempts to provide a standard meaning in the context of risk management for those related items that are included. Its object is to enable people to communicate more effectively with each other concerning this timely subject. To a large extent, nontechnical language is used by design in an attempt to increase understanding. It should also be emphasized that these definitions relate to the previous text, which outlines risk management as a hospital function.

Accident: a risk situation or unusual event involving possible harm to employees.

Accident Report: form used to document an accident. Must be completed for all accidents.

Actuarial Study: determination of funding level for self-insurance trust. Must be performed by a recognized actuary.

Administrative Activities: those functions involved in the management and supervision of hospital activities. Should be supportive of the risk management program.

Administrative Personnel Exchange (APE): a formal program established to provide an exchange of ideas between the frontline employees and top administration in the organization.

Claim: demand made against the hospital or its agents; usually precipitated by an incident or accident occurring within the hospital.

Claims Adjustment: settlement of claims resulting from risk situations without litigation; a function usually handled by insurance company, consultant, or claims management committee.

Commercial Insurance: conventional purchased insurance plan obtained through a licensed carrier.

Corrective Activities: those functions that not only remedy existing problem situations, but

---

*Source: Bernard L. Brown, Jr., *Risk Management for Hospitals: A Practical Approach,* Aspen Systems Corporation, 1979.

also seek out and solve hidden or potential risk problems.

Departmental Policy and Procedure (DPP): all intradepartmental policies, procedures, and instructions usually recorded in departmental manuals.

Documentary Activities: formalization of records and reports relative to hospital operations; crucial from a quality as well as a continuity standpoint.

Education Activities: those functions that orient, train, educate, and promote better understanding among all persons working at or served by the hospital.

Employee Recognition: activities designed to recognize and reward employees for excellent service; an excellent motivation tool.

General Liability: includes risk responsibility not specifically included in other types of liabilities; normally included in conjunction with a professional liability insurance program.

General Policy: the policy established by the governing body of an organization based on broad goals and objectives of the institution; serves as a guide for other organizational policies and procedures.

Going Bare: without any type of insurance program or plan. An option some hospitals are choosing because of the unavailability and/or high cost of commercial insurance.

Hospital Attorney: legal counsel and advisor to the hospital. A member of the risk management team.

Hospital Slogan: motto or credo reflecting the hospital purpose, objective, and/or philosophy.

Incident: a risk situation or unusual happening involving patients, visitors, volunteers, and the general public.

Incident Report: form used to document an incident. Must be completed for all incidents.

Liability Control: see **Risk Management.**

Liability Control Center: central clearinghouse for liability information and coordination center for liability related activities.

Line Service: a department or function that usually provides a direct service to the hospital's customers and consumers.

Loss Prevention: see **Risk Management.**

Malpractice: see **Professional Liability.**

Management by Objectives: management technique used to promote efficiency and effectiveness of organizational activities; includes the establishment of functional purpose, accomplishments, objectives, and necessary resources.

Medical Staff Opinion Poll: an opinion survey conducted periodically to determine attitudes of physicians on the medical staff relative to hospital operational activities.

Medical Staff Relations: activities designed to improve physicians' attitudes toward the hospital and involve them in its operations.

Ombudsmen: representatives of the hospital who provide direct liaison with and assistance to patients in addition to regular hospital employees; patient representatives.

Patient Relations: activities designed to improve patient attitudes toward the hospital and the quality of service provided by it.

Patient Service Questionnaire: survey form used to obtain patient evaluation of hospital services. Results should be distributed to those providing such services as well as to the governing body.

Personnel Policy and Procedure (PPP): all interorganizational policies, procedures, and instructions of a personnel and employment nature usually centralized in an institutional manual.

Personnel Relations: activities designed to improve employees' attitudes toward the hospital and their jobs, which hopefully will result in improved patient services.

Policy: basic principles or guidelines that govern and direct an organization's activities and upon which its procedures are founded.

Preventive Activities: activities within the hospital that foster technical as well as personal quality care and seek to accomplish an environment free of risk.

Procedure: operational rules, regulations, and methods based on policies established to provide consistency and direction to organizational activities.

Professional Liability: malpractice occurring in the hospital; usually results from negligence or poor judgment on the part of a hospital employee or physician.

Public Relations: activities designed to improve public attitudes toward the hospital and promote a good hospital image within the community.

Quality Assurance: activities designed to improve and maintain quality service and care;

performed through a formal program with involvement of multiple organizational components and committees.

Risk: the probability that something undesirable will happen; implies the need for avoidance.

Risk Management: the science of the identification, evaluation, and treatment of financial loss. A program that attempts to provide positive avoidance of negative results. Liability control; loss prevention.

Risk Management Office: the physical location or headquarters of the risk management program; the risk manager's home base.

Risk Management Team: includes all those working to reduce risk and problem situations within the hospital: governing body and administration, risk manager, hospital department heads, hospital employees, workers and volunteers, the safety and loss control council/committees, members of the medical staff, hospital attorney, and outside consultants.

Risk Manager: person managing or directing the risk management program; coordinator of the hospital's loss-control efforts.

Risk Retention: the amount of loss due to liability risk that a hospital retains or absorbs; should be limited to an amount that will not impair its financial strength.

Safety: in the purest sense, free from risk or harm; from a practical standpoint, a policy issue that involves the weighing of properly identified risks and benefits.

Safety and Loss Control Council: overall risk management coordinating group. Composed of such committees as environmental control and energy conservation, fire safety, employee safety, patient and public safety, disaster, education, infection control, and others as needed.

Security: protection from harm caused by unlawful activities and the sense of well-being derived therefrom.

Self-Insurance: retaining risk of loss or liability within the organization and providing a funding mechanism to cover cost.

Social Responsibility: an institution's sensitivity to providing quality and safe service.

Staff Service: a department or function generally advisory in nature that supplements and supports line service activities.

Standard Policy and Procedure (SPP): all interorganizational policies, procedures, and instructions of a nonpersonnel nature, usually centralized in an institutional manual.

Trust: a mechanism to fund a self-insurance program; must be restricted and its funding level actuarially determined to receive maximum reimbursement from federal programs.

Workers' Compensation: payment to employees resulting from job-related injury or illness.

Chapter 17—Public Relations Department

OVERVIEW*

The Public Relations Department, unlike many departments, reports directly to the chief executive officer (CEO) in most institutions. This is something of a departure in health care, although it is sine qua non in industry and has been for many years.

The public relations department reports to the CEO for two main reasons. First, the department cuts across organizational lines and is often in the position of having to ask other managers to do things in the interest of the organization that they would rather not do. Public relations must have the support of all departments in the institution and often must get it quickly, as when facts and perhaps an individual are needed to respond to a sensitive press inquiry. In many instances, the authority of the CEO is needed to maintain the effectiveness of the public relations function.

The second, perhaps more important, reason is that there is a pronounced trend toward an expanded public relations role for the CEOs. For example, a 1979 survey revealed that 53.3 percent of all CEOs in hospitals spend more than 10 hours a month on public relations activities, and a third spend over 20 hours a month. These activities include public speaking, lobbying, dealing directly with the media, consumer affairs and meeting with community groups. In

*Source: Lew Riggs, "Organizing the Public Relations Function," *Health Care Planning and Marketing Quarterly*, October 1981.

most cases it is the public relations director who arranges these activities for the CEO, prepares materials for use by the CEO and suggests the most effective ways of carrying out these activities in the best interests of the organization.

The public relations office should be near the administrative offices and the high-traffic area in the institution. Proximity to administration is important because everything of significant consequence that emanates from the public relations office generally requires administrative approval; and since speed is usually required, routing through the mail system is impractical in most instances. In addition, the constant process of planning events, news releases, special programs and the myriad other public relations tasks often must be done in concert with both the CEO and other members of top management.

The Public Relations Director

The key requirements for a public relations director are first and foremost good writing and communications skills, strong administrative abilities and a broad general knowledge of the environment within which the institution functions.

Compensation of the public relations director varies depending on the region. In a survey of health care public relations professionals, it was found that 36 percent of the respondents earned between $20,000 and $30,000 and 6 percent earned over $50,000. A later survey by *PR Reporter* indicated a 1980 median of $23,650, in a range from $13,850 to $57,000. Salaries tend to be higher in the west and northeast and lower in the southern and north central regions.

Reporting Guide for PR Director

Reports should be made to the CEO on a monthly or quarterly basis. The basic rules for effective reports to management should be consistently observed.

The first rule is to *be brief.*

The second is to *describe the action.* What actually happened? When a member of the board of directors asks the CEO what the institution's public relations department has done lately, the CEO should be able to clearly describe the accomplishments of the department in action-oriented terms.

Third, *address the purposes of the department.* If one of the purposes of the public relations department is to produce publicity, then the report should list all placements during the period including the topic, medium and date. If a purpose is to produce publications, then it should list which ones were produced, how frequently and when. If representing the institution at community activities is a priority, then these events should be listed.

The monthly or quarterly progress report should be viewed as a promotional piece for the department as well as an informational device. It should accurately reflect what the department has done on behalf of the institution and the CEO during the reporting period. This is particularly important in larger institutions.

To keep the CEO informed of the specific services being provided by public relations, it is wise to establish a project reporting system for decisions and accomplishments. One system that has proven effective simply summarizes key meetings with clients by stating, in simple narrative form, specific actions taken toward specific objectives. Copies are then circulated to all involved both in the client's organization and the agency's.

In addition to project and monthly or quarterly progress reports, it is important to provide top management with an annual progress report at the end of the calendar or fiscal year. It should succinctly review the accomplishments of the department during the year and, if possible, specify how these accomplishments relate to objectives that were set at the beginning of the year. It should then cite key goals for the coming year.

Policies and Procedures

In concert with top management, the public relations department must establish certain basic policies and determine procedures for their implementation.

It is important that the institution have written policies on at least the following:

- dealings with the media;
- release of information to the media;
- supervision of format and style of publications generated by the institution;
- who may officially speak for the institution;
- institutional advertising; and
- patients' rights.

Procedures should be easy to follow so that employees will not only know what they are but how to carry them out.

Internal Audit Checklist*

Internal auditors may find auditing a function such as public relations strange, and admittedly it is; however, operations auditing can be applied to all functions to some extent and to the degree that this can be done, the unit can benefit. As usual, internal auditors planning to evaluate public relations and communications must prepare by reviewing available literature. They will have to be resourceful when designing audit programs for public relations because the final product is difficult to measure. Below are ten checkpoints for a public relations and communications audit program.

1. How is the function organized and staffed? What policies and procedures have been established, by whom, and are they in writing?
2. Have goals been established and standards set to measure performance where possible? Are the standards in fact measurable?
3. Are the goals of the program compatible with those of the hospital? What provisions are there for reviewing public relations goals and hospital goals to ensure

---

*Source: Seth Allcorn, *Internal Auditing for Hospitals,* Aspen Systems Corporation, 1979.

they will continue to complement each other?

4. What patterns of communication have been established between top management and public relations personnel? Are the patterns adequate? Do they provide for accurate and timely information?

5. Is there overall planning for the public relations program?

6. Have contingency plans been prepared and agreed upon for handling unusual events such as attacks by the media or special interests?

7. What provision has been made for feedback from the public and employees? Is the information acted on?

8. Are files maintained of clippings from newspapers and journals? Are they used to key new ideas on presenting the hospital's health care story?

9. What efforts are made to improve employee attitudes toward patient care and the hospital? How effective are the existing methods of communicating with employees?

10. Does the general atmosphere of the hospital bespeak an effective public relations attitude on the part of the administration?

Internal auditors in hospitals with especially poor track records for public relations and communications may find some assistance by sampling public and employee opinions. If the problem appears serious enough, the internal auditor may want to recommend that consultants analyze the situation.

PROMOTIONAL TOOLS*

[The rest of this chapter is from material originally aimed specifically at professional public relations agency practitioners. However, hospital administrators and their public relations operatives can adapt this to their own situations with very little change since the same basic principles and methods apply to both worlds.]

---

*Source: Robert Rubright and Dan MacDonald, *Marketing Health and Human Services*, Aspen Systems Corporation, 1981.

Promotional tools can be written (brochures, news publications and news releases, annual reports, business and personal letters, signs, posters, and such) or nonwritten (slides, films, videotapes, audiotapes, personal visits, staged events, media appearances). They can: (1) help acquire new business in accordance with the marketing plan; (2) serve as a surrogate agency spokesperson; (3) clarify agency positions, policies, procedures; (4) inform and educate targets; (5) help obtain funds; (6) address competition; (7) recruit staff and volunteers; (8) help form acceptable attitudes and opinions among targets; and (9) reflect the organization's managerial skills.

Characteristics

Most productive promotional tools:

- reflect marketing and organizational objectives and strategies
- are written or prepared for specific targets and communications channels
- carry at least one promotional message
- reflect or suggest service benefits
- reflect organizational purposes
- have a distribution plan
- have an acceptable tone, style, and character
- persuade or inform
- are concisely written, edited
- reflect both reader and management needs
- ask for some action or participation by targets

Tools must direct the targets from unawareness in order to convince a potential client to try the service, repeat its use, and recommend it to others. This flow is called the hierarchy of promotional effects. Specifically, the hierarchy consists of initial awareness, comprehension, a conviction to use the service, and actual service usage.

Basic Types

In its early stages, each tool (see Table 17-1) should undergo a preliminary process resembling that of the marketing plan itself. The process includes steps to:

1. determine the perceived purpose of the tool

2. discuss marketing objectives to be reflected by the tool

Table 17-1 Basic Promotional Tools

Brochure
News releases
Internal newsletter
External newsletter
Public service announcements
Ethical advertising
Factsheets for specific services
Direct mail promotion
Traveling displays
Continuing sampling of user and employee attitudes and opinions
Educational workshops, seminars, special classes, joint projects
Annual social event to raise funds
Videotape capabilities

Source: Robert Rubright and Dan MacDonald, *Marketing Health and Human Services,* Aspen Systems Corporation, 1981.

3. determine the target(s) to be reached
4. devise applicable marketing strategy or strategies
5. agree on methods of distribution
6. designate the tool's writer
7. figure how production (layout, design, typesetting, art, printing, and mailing) will be handled
8. decide who will evaluate the tool as to its conformance to the marketing plan, and when.

Contents

The typical promotional tool also must reflect certain contents if it is to communicate its message to targets.

The Basic Agency Brochure

The basic brochure is a necessity for a good organization. It is a simple confirmation of the agency's existence, it is indicative of an interest to become a part of the greater community, and it is responsive to community and client wants and needs.

The basic brochure should contain much of the following material:

1. What are the purposes of the organization? These purposes should be explained as they are reflected in articles of incorporation or agreement, bylaws, or mission statement.

2. What services are offered? Services should be described according to categories, such as treatment, counseling, outreach, education, or research.

3. What benefits do services provide to targets? This should cite especially benefits suggested by clients and potential clients during the marketing research phase of the market plan, not benefits perceived by agency managers without consulting potential or existing targets.

4. What is the agency's referral network? Can a client self-refer? Is referral restricted to counselors, caseworkers, or professional organizations? How easy is it to refer a new client? Is any extraordinary paperwork involved?

5. How do potential clients make initial contact with the agency?

6. Who do prospective clients first talk with on their initial visit or contact with the agency? What happens after the initial contact?

7. Who uses the agency's services?

8. What is the typical treatment routine for the average user of agency services? How many appointments may be necessary? How long is a typical period of treatment or service? Are services performed in one or more locations? Will there be unusually long waiting periods for services? Which staff members are likely to see clients?

9. How do patients pay for the agency's services? Sliding fee scale, cash only, credit cards, third party payers, charity policy?

10. When are agency services available? What are the hours of business, including after-hours on weekdays, as well as schedules during weekends, holiday? What provisions are made for emergency treatment, counseling, crisis intervention?

11. What happens after the agency's services no longer are appropriate or come to an end? What routine follow-up is practiced by agency staff? Where does the agency normally refer clients who are finished with its services but who require help elsewhere?

12. What constitutes the agency professional staff?

13. How is the agency managed and governed? What is the background of agency managers? Does the board represent a cross section of community interests? Is there a strong voluntary service program?
14. Where is the agency located? Where are branch offices? Is there an advantage in agency location(s) in terms of client traveling time? Do all sites offer full services?
15. What outside organizations are affiliated with the agency? How do such affiliations bring benefits to clients?
16. How does the agency relate to, or share facilities with, other agencies in the community or region?
17. Which organizations certify or accredit the agency?
18. What key memberships does the agency hold? What are organizations with which the targets would be familiar, such as the United Way?

If artwork—photographs or illustrations—is to be used in the brochure, it should depict typical clients (targets) in the process of using agency services (typical service scenes). A cross section of agency staff disciplines should be represented in the art.

The News Release

A news release is mailed or distributed on the agency's letterhead or on a special news release letterhead. Any message or announcement in the release should be of interest to targets identified in the marketing plan. The release, always factual and impersonal, also should modify or reflect a given market strategy as well as the stated marketing objectives. Benefits that will accrue to the target should be stated in some way. If targets, objectives, and strategies can't be identified, the reason for issuing a release, other than for agency ego, should be challenged.

The release can contain information about a current condition of the agency (finances, employee force, staff, board, or volunteers) or its future (a new service, a party or celebration, a long-range plan or policy). Whatever the subject, the copy must relate to a key target of the agency: clients, contributors, legislative supporters, professional staff, employees, volunteers.

The Internal Newsletter

Internal newsletters can be many things: informative, impersonal, personal, instructional, authoritarian, propagandistic, manipulative, inexpensive, direct, informal, formal, intimate, casual. No matter how it is viewed, an effective internal newsletter can be a strong promotional tool, one that should tell much about the organization's integrity.

Employees usually are the primary marketing target for the internal newsletter. Articles should be planned to relate to strategies that can maintain morale, sharpen attitudes, inform, or clarify a situation.

Targeted articles in a hypothetical internal newsletter might be:

1. A discussion of agency-related issues and concerns that may appear in local media in the near future.
2. Announcements of new policies, procedures, and why they were adopted. How will the average employee benefit from such policies or procedures? Were employee opinions and feelings considered when changes were made?
3. A discussion about employee perquisites.
4. Educational opportunities within and outside the agency.
5. Departmental profiles, such as noteworthy things various departments are doing. How do departments respond to agency client needs, expectations?
6. Successful community outreach projects and the clients who have benefited from them.

Secondary Types

When working from a marketing plan, the marketer first ponders the use of the basic promotional tools and the appropriate promotional channels. If the marketed program or service does not mesh realistically with targets and strategies that have been ordained for the agency, auxiliary tools must be considered. For practical purposes, some auxiliary tools are listed, not alphabetically but according to their communications usefulness. By usefulness is meant their ability to transmit a message to a target as rapidly and directly as possible.

- factsheets
- special business letters

- direct mail
- public service announcements
- comment forms from clients
- questionnaires and surveys
- displays, fairs, and exhibits
- information racks
- bulletin boards
- films and audiovisual items
- speakers' bureaus
- feature stories
- inserts and enclosures in mailings
- hotlines (telephone)
- meetings, symposia, seminars, workshops, forums
- handbooks and manuals
- open houses and tours
- videotape programs
- news conferences
- regional and local magazines
- posters
- public address systems
- annual reports
- billboards
- contests
- signs and allied graphics

Guidelines for Selecting Promotional Tools

1. *Design the promotional tool solely for the target or target group you want to reach.* Avoid trying to cover the universe with your message when you are interested mainly in the immediate neighborhood.
2. *Keep tools time-limited.* Don't print 10,000 brochures when your initial main distribution is 2,000. (How many times have stacks of unused printed pieces been removed from agency cupboards?) Times change; so do telephone numbers, addresses, programs, personnel. Think of the short-term and long-term future when budgeting for tools.
3. *Make sure that each tool reflects the aesthetic tastes and cultural background of the target.* A slick, thick, four-color bro-

chure is apt to startle potential contributors who may wonder if their help really is needed. On the other hand, a sloppy, poorly mimeographed report presented to the same people may appear to have been done by a poorly run, unbusinesslike organization.

4. *Establish an order of priority for all tools.* If the budget is important, decide on the one, two, or three tools you cannot do without. Make judgments; will the stickers to be attached to doctor's office telephones be more productive to the agency than renting a booth at the youth job fair? Will 50 personally written letters be more effective than 250 fliers?
5. *Seek quality in the production and use of your tools.* Quality is not synonymous with expense. It means the way in which the tool is written, designed, and distributed. If need be, look outside for volunteer or paid assistance. Quality of tools is one way to distinguish the organization from competitors.
6. *Don't forget marketing's main premise: exchange.* Most tools should convince the target that they can or will receive something from the organization. Exchange should be evident from the benefits listed in the tool.
7. *The tools should provide a return on investment.* Many tools are aimed at bringing in new clients or patients; many others, such as questionnaires to former clients, are intended to yield clues for improvement of services. A tool should not be used as a throwaway item.
8. *Give as much consideration to the deployment of the tool as you did to its production.* Should the beautifully written annual report be mailed to the business offices or to the homes of civic leaders? Should the new ten-minute agency film simply be made available to everyone, or should someone personally get it into every service and civic club in town?

Chapter 18—Volunteer Department*

THE ROLE OF VOLUNTEERS

Hospital volunteers fall into two general groups. One group, usually referred to as hospital volunteers, works primarily in the functional areas of the hospital; the second group works primarily outside the hospital in activities not related to the functions of the hospital. People in this group are referred to as auxiliaries or women's auxiliaries, grey ladies, candy stripers, or guilds. The hospital volunteer provides free services to the hospital. A review of the records shows that there are 37 million volunteers in the United States. Of these, 59 percent are women and 41 percent are men. It is estimated that volunteers give 3.5 billion hours of service per year, an estimated dollar volume of 33.9 billion dollars.

Volunteers have now entered all aspects of the functioning of the hospital. Their mission is to supplement the services provided by the hospital's employees. Volunteers are found operating switchboards, aiding families and friends at the reception desk, and serving as volunteer patient representatives. They may provide nursery service on a day-care basis. They aid the social service department by listening to the terminally ill; they perform puppet shows for the children in the pediatric unit. They may be transportation aides in the x-ray or physical therapy departments. Many of them aid the management of the

*Source: I. Donald Snook, Jr., *Hospitals: What They Are and How They Work,* Aspen Systems Corporation, 1981.

hospital by offering skilled typing services and clerical skills.

The auxiliary services based outside the operating functions of the hospital get involved in gift shop work or snack bar operations, but they also become more directly involved in fund-raising activities. They constitute a strong community-relations arm of the hospital.

ORGANIZATION

The volunteer department in the hospital is usually headed by a director of volunteers who may be a salaried full-time individual. This individual generally reports to the assistant administrator or perhaps to the administrator of the hospital. Frequently, the hospital's auxiliary is a guild affair with its own auxiliary officers. In some instances, the auxiliary is a volunteer department, but it is more common to have a separate auxiliary and inhospital volunteer service.

Director of Volunteers

This individual is responsible for recruiting volunteers, interviewing them, arranging their assignments with various functional department heads in the hospital, providing their orientation, and assisting in training. The director is also responsible for maintaining a strong liaison with the functional department heads with whom the volunteers work and relate. It is the director's job to keep the volunteers informed of pertinent hospital policies and procedures. The volunteer director should recruit based on a reasonable level of hospital need, balancing the recruitment of teenagers and more mature adults against the needs of the hospital.

Specific Job Duties*

• Plans with administrative staff the objectives and scope of the volunteer services program to augment the services of regular hospital staff; recruits and orients new volunteers, arranges for their training and placement, and supervises the program:

• Confers with hospital administrative staff to plan volunteer program consistent with institution's needs. Recommends establishment of policies and procedures for inservice training of volunteers, work hours, types of services to be performed, and assignment of volunteer workers. Meets with department heads to determine volunteer service needs and to interpret service policies and procedures.

• Recruits and interviews applicants to determine their aptitudes, abilities, and other qualifications. Classifies applicants according to qualifications, interests, age, time available for duty, and other characteristics.

• Arranges for formal orientation of new volunteers which should include a description of the institution, its purposes and organization, the place of the volunteer service program within that organization; the policies of the Volunteer Department; and the responsibilities of the volunteer. In cooperation with the staff of the hospital, organizes training courses to instruct volunteers in techniques and procedures of duties to be performed and arranges for or conducts preservice training classes and on-the-job training.

• Receives requests for services of volunteers from various hospital departments and cooperates with department supervisor to define services to be performed by volunteers and to outline duties for each assignment. In cooperation with department supervisors, places volunteers according to their aptitudes and interests. Conducts periodic reorientation for all volunteers.

---

*Source: *Job Descriptions and Organizational Analysis for Hospitals and Related Health Services*, U.S. Training and Employment Service, Department of Labor, 1971.

• Conducts surveys and meets with department heads to evaluate the effectiveness of the volunteer service program. Periodically counsels with and evaluates individual volunteer. Devises methods for improving, modifying, or expanding the program and recommends changes in established policies and procedures. Arranges for appropriate recognition of the volunteer.

• Prepares manuals, handbooks, and guides covering policies, procedures, and programs.

VOLUNTEER'S ORIENTATION

Once volunteers have been selected, it falls to the director of volunteers and the hospital management to place them into a productive position. Volunteers should not feel lost in the environment. They should have the opportunity to understand the mission of the hospital, be acquainted with the functions of the hospital and how it operates, just as any employee would. Volunteers should be assigned tasks in the department in which they are able to perform.

The orientation program sponsored by the director of volunteers can feed upon the employee orientation program. Once volunteers have selected a job and been assigned, they expect some minimal amount of on-the-job training. It is reasonable to expect the employees in the department with whom the volunteer is working to show an interest in the volunteer, just as any fellow employee would be treated. Volunteers should expect to be supervised and treated like all other workers within the department.

ETHICAL AND LEGAL IMPLICATIONS

Caution should be used to make it clear that the volunteer effort is not being used to improve the profits of the institution. In addition, there are certain ethical implications concerning volunteers who might replace paid employees of the hospital. This can become particularly agitating in an area of high unemployment. According to the U.S. Fair Labor Standards Act (Wage and Hour Law), the placing of a volunteer in a position as a typist or in an open employee position establishes a legal employee-employer relationship that violates the spirit of the law and the spirit of volunteerism. The American Hospital

Association seeks to have volunteers perform supplementary tasks that will contribute to the well-being and comfort of hospitalized patients, tasks that are of great importance but that are not normally performed by regular hospital employees, so that employees' jobs will not be in jeopardy.

The hospital is responsible for the volunteer's acts that are performed in the line of duty. Not only is the hospital responsible for the volunteer's actions, it is also responsible for preventing the volunteer from becoming involved in tasks or jobs beyond the volunteer's capacity. A wise hospital manager will ensure protection for the hospital by maintaining a proper insurance policy that covers the volunteers in case of accidental injury on the job or injury to a patient, staff member, or visitor.

Appendix A—Glossaries

LEGAL TERMS GLOSSARY*

Admissibility (of evidence): Worthiness of evidence that meets the legal rules of evidence and will be allowed to go to the jury.

Affidavit: A voluntary sworn statement of facts, or a voluntary declaration in writing of facts, that a person swears to be true before an official authorized to administer an oath.

Agency: The relationship in which one person acts for or represents another; for example, employer and employee.

Allegation: A statement that a person expects to be able to prove.

Appellant: The party who appeals the decision of a lower court to a court of higher jurisdiction.

Appellee: The party against whom an appeal to a higher court is taken.

Assault: An intentional act which is designed to make the victim fearful and which produces reasonable apprehension of harm.

Assignment: Transfer of rights or property.

Attestation: The act of witnessing a document in writing.

Battery: The touching of one person by another without permission.

Best Evidence Rule: A legal doctrine requiring that primary evidence of a fact (such as an original document) be introduced, or at least explained, before a copy can be introduced or testimony given concerning the fact.

Bona Fide: In good faith; openly, honestly, or innocently; without knowledge or intent of fraud.

Borrowed Servant: An employee temporarily under the control of another. The traditional example is that of a nurse employed by a hospital who is "borrowed" by a surgeon in the operating room. The temporary employer of the borrowed servant will be held responsible for the act of the borrowed servant under the doctrine of *respondeat superior*.

Charitable Immunity: A legal doctrine which holds that a charitable hospital cannot be sued by one who has been injured due to the negligence of its employees. The effect of this rule is to force the injured person to sue the hospital employee personally for negligence.

Civil Law: The law of countries such as Germany and France which follow the Roman legal system of jurisprudence in which all law is enacted. It is also the portion of American law which does not deal with crimes.

Common Law: The legal traditions of England and the United States where part of the law is developed by means of court decisions.

Consent: A voluntary act by which one person agrees to allow someone else to do something. For medical liability purposes, consents should be in writing with an explanation of the procedures to be performed.

---

*Source: Adapted from *Nursing and The Law*, 2nd ed., Aspen Systems Corporation, 1975.

426

Coroner's Jury: A special jury called by the coroner to determine whether the evidence concerning the cause of a death indicated that death was brought about by criminal means.

Counterclaim: A defendant's claim against a plaintiff.

Defamation: The injury of a person's reputation or character by willful and malicious statements made to a third person. Defamation includes both libel and slander.

Defendant: In a criminal case, the person accused of committing a crime. In a civil suit, the party against whom suit is brought demanding that he or she pay the other party legal relief.

Deposition: A sworn statement, made out of court, which may be admitted into evidence if it is impossible for a witness to attend in person.

Directed Verdict: When a trial judge decides that the evidence or law is so clearly in favor of one party that it is pointless for the trial to proceed further, the judge directs the jury to return a verdict for that party. The conclusion that one party is negligent or not must be so clear and obvious that reasonable minds could not arrive at a different conclusion.

Discovery: Pretrial activities of attorneys to determine what evidence the opposing side will present if the case comes to trial. Discovery prevents attorneys from being surprised during trial and facilitates out-of-court settlement.

Dissenting Opinion: *See* Opinion of the court.

Emergency: A sudden unexpected occurrence or event causing a threat to life or health. The legal responsibilities of those involved in an emergency situation are measured according to the occurrence.

Expert Witness: One who has special training, experience, skill, and knowledge in a relevant area, and who is allowed to offer an opinion as testimony in court.

Federal Question: Legal question involving the U.S. Constitution or a statute enacted by Congress.

Felony: A crime of a serious nature usually punishable by imprisonment for a period of longer than one year or by death.

Good Samaritan Laws: Laws designed to protect those who stop to render aid in an emergency. These laws generally provide immunity for specified persons from any civil suit arising out of care rendered at the scene of an emergency, provided that the one rendering assistance has not done so in a grossly negligent manner.

Grand Jury: A jury called to determine whether there is sufficient evidence that a crime has been committed to justify bringing a case to trial. It is not the jury before which the case is tried to determine guilt or innocence.

Grand Larceny: Theft of property valued at more than a specified amount (usually fifty dollars), thus constituting a felony instead of a misdemeanor.

Harm or Injury: Any wrong or damage done to another, either to the person, to rights, or to property.

Hearsay Rule: A rule of evidence that restricts the admissibility of evidence which is not the personal knowledge of the witness. Hearsay evidence is admissible only under strict rules.

Holographic Will: A will handwritten by the testator.

In Loco Parentis: A legal doctrine that under certain circumstances the courts may assign a person to stand in the place of parents and possess their legal rights, duties, and responsibilities toward a child.

Independent Contractor: One who agrees to undertake work without being under the direct control or direction of the employer.

Indictment: A formal written accusation of crime brought by a prosecuting attorney against one charged with criminal conduct.

Injunction: A court order requiring one to do or not to do a certain act.

Interrogatories: A list of questions sent from one party in a lawsuit to the other party to be answered.

Judge: An officer who guides court proceedings to ensure impartiality and enforce the rules of evidence. The trial judge determines the applicable law and states it to the jury. The appellate judge hears appeals and renders decisions concerning the correctness of actions of the trial judge, the law of the case, and the sufficiency of the evidence.

Jurisdiction: The right of a court to administer

justice by hearing and deciding controversies.

Jurisprudence: The philosophy or science of law upon which a particular legal system is built.

Jury: A certain number of persons selected and sworn to hear the evidence and determine the facts in a case.

Larceny: Taking another person's property without consent with the intent to deprive the owner of its use and ownership.

Liability: An obligation one has incurred or might incur through any act or failure to act.

Liability Insurance: A contract to have someone else pay for any liability or loss thereby in return for the payment of premiums.

Libel: A false or malicious writing that is intended to defame or dishonor another person and is published so that someone besides the one defamed will observe it.

License: A permit from the state allowing certain acts to be performed, usually for a specific period of time.

Litigation: A trial in court to determine legal issues, rights and duties between the parties to the litigation.

Malpractice: Professional misconduct, improper discharge of professional duties, or failure to meet the standard of care of a professional which resulted in harm to another:

Claims Incurred Policy: Traditional form of malpractice insurance coverage today as contrasted with a claims made policy. In a *claims incurred policy,* the insured is covered for any claims which may arise from an incident that occurred during the policy period. This is true regardless of when the actual claim is made and is limited only by the statute of limitations in the state in which the claim is made.

Claims Made Policy: Alternative form of malpractice insurance coverage to the claims incurred policy. Under this type of insurance arrangement, the insured is covered for any claim made during the policy period, regardless of when the injury may have occurred. Insurance companies contend that a *claims made policy* better enables them to establish more accurate rates. However, there is some transference of risk from the insurer to the insured because many claims for injury will not occur in the policy period.

Limits on Liability: Limits on professional liability that may be imposed by state law. Some states have officially enacted legislation that places limits on the dollar amount of malpractice awards. The constitutionality of these laws is questionable.

Mayhem: The crime of intentionally disfiguring or dismembering another.

Misdemeanor: An unlawful act of a less serious nature than a felony, usually punishable by fine or imprisonment for a term of less than one year.

Negligence: Carelessness, failure to act as an ordinary prudent person, or action contrary to what a reasonable person would have done.

Noncupative Will: Oral statement intended as a last will made in anticipation of death.

Opinion of the Court: In an appellate court decision, the reasons for the decision. One judge writes the opinion for the majority of the court. Judges who agree with the result but for different reasons may write concurring opinions explaining their reasons. Judges who disagree with the majority may write dissenting opinions.

Ordinance: A law passed by a municipal legislative body.

Perjury: The willful act of giving false testimony under oath.

Petit Larceny: Theft of property usually valued below fifty dollars and classed as a misdemeanor.

Plaintiff: The party to a civil suit who brings the suit seeking damages or other legal relief.

Privileged Communication: Statement made to an attorney, physician, spouse, or anyone else in a position of trust. Because of the confidential nature of such information, the law protects it from being revealed, even in court. The term is applied in two distinct situations. First, the communications between certain persons, such as physician and patient, cannot be divulged without consent of the patient. Second, in some situations the law provides an exemption from liability for disclosing information where there is a higher duty to speak, such as statutory reporting requirements.

Probate: The judicial proceeding which determines the existence and validity of a will.

Probate Court: Court with jurisdiction over wills. Its powers range from deciding the validity of a will to distributing property.

Proximate: In immediate relation with something else. In negligence cases, the careless act must be the proximate cause of injury.

Real Evidence: Evidence furnished by tangible things, such as weapons, bullets, and equipment.

Rebuttal: The giving of evidence to contradict the effect of evidence introduced by the opposing party.

Release: A statement signed by one person relinquishing a right or claim against another person, usually for a valuable consideration.

Remand: The referral of a case back to the original court, out of which it came, for the purpose of having a decision made on it there.

Res Gestae: "The thing done." All of the surrounding events which become part of an incident. If statements are made as part of the incident they are admissible in court as *res gestae,* in spite of the hearsay rule.

Res Ipsa Loquitur: "The thing speaks for itself." A doctrine of law applicable to cases where the defendant had exclusive control of the thing which caused the harm and where the harm ordinarily could not have occurred without negligent conduct.

Respondeat Superior: "Let the master answer." The employer is responsible for the legal consequences of the acts of the servant or employee while acting within the scope of employment.

Shop Book Rule: If books are kept in the usual course of business they may be introduced in court so long as they are properly authenticated and held in proper custody.

Slander: An oral statement made with intent to dishonor or defame another person when made in the presence of a third person.

Standard of Care: Those acts performed or omitted that an ordinary prudent person would have performed or omitted. It is a measure against which a defendant's conduct is compared.

Stare Decisis: "Let the decision stand." The legal principle indicating that courts should apply previous decisions to subsequent cases involving similar facts and questions.

Statute of Limitations: A legal limit on the time allowed for filing suit in civil matters, usually measured from the time of the wrong or from the time when a reasonable person would have discovered the wrong.

Subpoena: A court order requiring one to appear in court to give testimony.

Subpoena Duces Tecum: A subpoena that commands a person to come to court and to produce whatever documents are named in the order.

Subrogation: Substitution of one person for another in reference to a lawful claim or right.

Suit: Court proceeding where one person seeks damages or other legal remedies from another. The term is not usually used in criminal cases.

Summons: A court order directed to the sheriff or other appropriate official to notify the defendant in a civil suit that a suit has been filed and when and where to appear.

Testimony: Oral statement of a witness given under oath at a trial.

Tort: A civil wrong. Torts may be intentional or unintentional.

Tort-Feasor: One who commits a tort.

Trial Court: The court in which evidence is presented to a judge or jury for decision.

Waiver: The intentional giving up of a right, such as allowing another person to testify to information that would ordinarily be protected as a privileged communication.

Writ: A written order which is issued to a person or persons, requiring the performance of some specified act or giving authority to have it done.

Written Authorization: Consent given in writing specifically empowering someone to do something.

CAPITAL FINANCING GLOSSARY*

Knowledge of special terminology used in the field of capital financing is necessary for an understanding of health care capital project financing. No attempt has been made to define all accounting and technical terms. The definitions

---

*Source: W. Thomas Berriman, William J. Essick, Jr., and Peter Bentivegna, *Capital Projects for Health Care Facilities,* Aspen Systems Corporation, 1976.

were written to give the reader a working knowledge and are not intended to be legally exact.

Accelerated Depreciation. Term applied to periodic allocations to expense of the cost of fixed assets under a method which provides for a greater allocation during the early portion of their estimated useful lives; generally, the declining balance or sum-of-the-years-digits method.

Accrued Interest. Interest earned on a bond issue from the dated date to the date of delivery. Accrued interest is credited to the issuer at delivery.

Additional Bonds. Parity bonds issued in order to finance additional facilities pursuant to a formula contained in the existing loan documents. Usually the formula is based upon maintaining "coverage" of outstanding and proposed bonds.

After-Acquired Property. All buildings, equipment or furnishings constructed upon the original hospital property (security for loan) after the closing date of the bond sale shall constitute hospital property and therefore be subject to the same mortgage or covenant for protection of bond holders.

Amortization. A process of gradually extinguishing a debt by means of a series of periodic payments. Each payment includes interest and a partial repayment of the principal.

Asked Price. The price at which bonds are offered to potential buyers.

Authority. A municipal or state entity formed through a special legislative act to perform the specific function of distribution of bonds.

Bank Line. The funds that a bank keeps available to a borrower, which can use some or all of its line at any time.

Basis Point. One basis point is equal to one one-hundredth of one percent or .01 percent.

Best Efforts Underwriting. A relationship where the underwriter acts as agent for the issuer and there is no commitment to purchase any of the bonds. If the underwriter has given a Firm Commitment, he is acting as principal and has agreed to buy the entire issue.

Bid. The price buyers offer to pay for bonds; the price at which sellers may dispose of them.

Board Designated Funds. Unrestricted funds set aside by the governing board for specific purposes or projects.

Bond. A certificate of debt of an issuer, paying a stated rate of interest and maturing on a certain date, when a fixed sum of money must be repaid to the holder. Tax-exempt bonds are normally in $5,000 denominations.

Bond Discount (or Debt Discount). Amount by which the selling (or purchase) price is less than the face value of a bond or other form of indebtedness.

Bond Fund. A restricted fund held by the trustee which contains both a principal account and interest account. The hospital under terms of the lease or note deposits money monthly with the trustee sufficient to service interest and principal payments when due on the outstanding bond.

Bond Holder's Risks Section. A portion of the official statement disclosing to bond purchasers that repayment of principal and payment of interest is dependent on future revenues which can be affected by the occurrence of certain events (general and specific) which alone or in combination could affect the borrower's ability to produce such revenue.

Bond Premium (or Debt Premium). Amount by which the selling (or purchase) price exceeds the face value of a bond or other form of indebtedness.

Book Value. Amount at which assets or liabilities are stated on the books; may have no relationship to market value. "Net book value" is generally an asset's cost less any related offsetting amount, e.g., fixed assets less accumulated depreciation. Also applied to shareholder's equity.

Calamity Provision. A bond provision to retire the entire bond issue in the event of destruction or loss of the facility through eminent domain. This provision is sometimes included to permit an early redemption if laws change affecting service to be provided by religiously sponsored institutions.

Capital Asset. Asset having an economic useful life exceeding one year and not acquired primarily for resale, e.g., buildings, machinery, patents.

Capitalization. The capital of a hospital includes the long-term debt (including current portion of long-term debt and capital equipment leases), capitalized leases, and both restricted and unrestricted fund balances. Pro-forma capitalization reflects these categories after giving effect to proposal financing.

Cash Flow. One of the components of "coverage"—defined (although not in the strict accounting sense) as net operating revenue available for debt service, before deduction for depreciation and fixed charges.

Chattel Mortgage. An instrument by which a borrower (mortgagor) gives a lender (mortgagee) a lien on property (other than real estate) as security for payment of an obligation. The borrower continues to use the property; and when the obligation is fully extinguished, the lien is removed.

Commitment Fee. A fee charged by the lender for issuing a loan commitment.

Completion Bonds. A designated amount of parity bonds which can be issued without further approval to complete the original project.

Conditional Sale/Hire Purchase Agreement. A transaction that is recognized in law as providing the seller with security interest in the underlying asset until the buyer has satisfied all the terms and conditions of the contract, at which time the security interest is waived and the buyer owns the asset without lien; or for a nominal sum the buyer acquires the asset. For tax purposes, the transaction is treated in the same manner as a finance lease. CSAs in the United States are about the equivalent of hire purchase or time sales agreements in some markets.

Coupon Rate. The stated annual rate of interest which the borrower promised to pay to the bond holder.

Coverage. Indicates the margin of safety for payment of debt service on the bonds, reflecting the number of times or percentage by which cash flow for a period of time exceeds debt service payable for such period.

Current Yield. The percent relation of the annual interest received to the price of the bond.

Debenture. Debt instrument or security which offers its holder only the general credit of the issuer as protection against nonpayment; as opposed to, for example, a real estate mortgage loan under which the lender is given the additional protection of a

security interest in specified real estate of the debtor.

Debt Service. Required payments for interest on and amortization of the principal amount of outstanding bonds.

Debt Service Coverage Ratio. The ratio of net income available for debt service (net income, depreciation, annual gifts and interest expense) in accordance with GAAP accounting over debt service (equivalent to interest and principal payments due annually under the bond indenture).

Default. Failure to pay debt service when due.

Defeasance. Upon final payment of all principal, interest and premiums, if any, the rights and interests of the bond trustee in the security of the issues for the bondholders is ceased, terminated or defeased. The security provisions or covenants on the issues can also be settled through the creation of a trust (escrow) where sufficient moneys are held for defeasance to occur at a future date (redemption date).

Depreciation. Depreciation accounting is a system of accounting which aims to distribute the cost or other basic value of tangible capital assets, less salvage (if any), over the estimated useful life of the unit (which may be a group of assets) in a systematic and rational manner. It is a process of allocation, not of valuation. Depreciation for the year is the portion of the total charge under such a system that is allocated to the year.

Discount Factor. The factor used to show the present value of dollars due in the future.

Effective Rate of Interest. The percentage determined by dividing the dollar cost to borrow money for one year by the amount borrowed. The effective rate of interest usually differs from the stated interest rate if there is a discount or premium on the debt, a change in required interest payments or lender-required compensating balances.

Endowment Funds. Funds in which a donor has stipulated, as a condition of his gift, that the principal of the fund is to be maintained inviolate and in perpetuity and that only income from investments of the fund may be expended.

Equity. The amount or value of a property above the total value of liens or charges. In hospital mortgage financing, an equity or loan/value ratio is sometimes employed with "value" calculated by representing land at market value, existing facilities at replacement value per appraisal and new construction at cost.

Feasibility Study. A report of an independent recognized firm of accountants or consultants demonstrating that the proceeds from the bonds together with the cash flow generated from the operation of the hospital will be sufficient to complete the project being financed and to pay future annual debt service requirements on the bonds.

Federal National Mortgage Association (FNMA) (Fannie Mae). A federal agency which purchases FHA insured mortgages, to assure a wider secondary market for such securities.

Full Payout Lease. Lease in which the cash flow will return to the lessor (1) the acquisition cost of the asset, (2) the cost of financing, (3) overhead and (4) an acceptable return on the investment. A full payout lease may be either a true lease or a finance lease.

Fund. (1) Cash or other assets held separately for a designated purpose, e.g., a pension fund for the payment of retirement benefits, a sinking fund for the redemption of outstanding debt. (2) To contribute assets to a fund (to fund) or to make other current payments which provide for future obligations.

General Obligation. A bond secured by pledge of the issuer's full faith, credit and taxing power.

Government National Mortgage Association (GNMA) (Ginnie Mae). A federal agency which issues its own securities on the open market, which are backed by the yields on federally insured mortgages.

Gross Pledge of Revenue. All revenues derived from the operation of the hospital and all rights to receive such revenue, whether in the form of accounts receivables or cash, before deduction of any operating expenses, but not including designated gifts, grants or pledges, shall be held first for repayment of the bonds.

Guaranteed Residual. The money a lessor expects to realize at the end of the lease because the lessee or a third party has a contractual obligation to purchase the equipment.

Implicit Interest. Amount of interest on debt determinable by measuring the difference between the total cash payable and the amount of cash borrowed or the fair value of noncash assets received. Often used in leasing.

Indenture. A document that spells out the allocation and disbursement of the funds of a loan.

Investment Banker. Also known as an underwriter, is the middle-man between the issuer and the public market. The investment banker usually functions as principal rather than agent and initially purchases all of the bonds from the issuer.

Issuer. One who borrows money through the sale of bonds. In the case of tax-exempt hospital financing, the issuer is often not the hospital, but a state or local authority who borrows on the hospital's behalf.

Landlord's Waiver. A document signed by the landlord waiving his future rights to leased property affixed to his premises. This is required most often in leasing store fixtures and certain types of office equipment.

Lease. A contract granting possession of land, equipment, machinery, etc. for a fixed or indeterminate period and for a stated consideration, usually known as rent.

Legal Opinion. A written assurance from a recognized firm of approving attorneys to the effect that the issuance of the bonds complies with applicable statutes and court decisions and that the bonds are legally enforcable in accordance with their terms.

Lessee. An individual, company, etc., contracting for the use and possession of property that is owned by another party (the lessor) and paying for that use in the form of rentals.

Lessor. The legal owner of property, who makes it available to a lessee to use in return for rental payments.

Maturity. The date upon which the principal amount of a bond becomes due and payable.

Mortgage Bonds. Bonds secured by a mortgage upon real property. Mortgage revenue bonds have the characteristics of both mortgage bonds and revenue bonds.

Mortgagee's Waiver. A document issued by a mortgagee giving up any present or future rights which he may have (to) equipment located on the premises upon which the mortgage exists.

Municipal Bond. A bond issued by a state or a political subdivision, such as a county, city or village. The term also refers to bonds issued by state agencies and authorities. Generally, interest paid on municipal bonds is exempt from federal income taxes. The term municipal bond is usually synonymous with "tax-exempt bond."

Negative Pledge. A loan agreement condition where the borrower pledges (covenants) not to mortgage its existing property or after-acquired property, except as agreed, unless the bonds or rates outstanding are equally secured.

Negotiated Underwriting. A private sale of the bonds by the issuer as contrasted to the advertisement for public bids. Most hospital bond underwritings are negotiated due to special marketing considerations.

Net Interest Cost (NIC). Also known as the "net effective rate," is the actual borrowing rate—a function of the coupon rate or rates, amortization schedule of the issue and bond discount (or premium).

Obsolescence. Decline in the utility of an asset due to technological or social change rather than physical deterioration.

Operating Lease. A transaction in which the lessor provides specific services, such as insurance and maintenance, as well as financing. The number of services provided by the lessor are negotiable and vary in each transaction. Operating leases are usually non-payout.

Parity Debt. All debt obligations issued or to be issued by the borrower which have the same security provisions and protection and which would share equally in any proceeds resulting from a foreclosure or sale of assets.

Par Value. The face amount of the bond. The amount of money due at maturity—usually $1,000.

Points. The same as "percentage." In the case of a bond, a point means $10 since a bond is quoted as a percentage of $1,000. A bond or bond issue which is discounted two points is quoted at 98 percent of its par value.

Premium. The amount, if any, by which the price of the bond exceeds the par value.

Prepayment Provisions. The provision in the bond or mortgage indenture which specifies at what time and on what terms repayment of principal amount may be made prior to maturity.

Price. Bond prices are generally quoted either in terms of percent of maturity value (premium price = 102, discount price = 99, etc.) or in terms of yield to maturity.

Private Placement. The placement of an issue in the private (i.e., nonpublic) money markets. This private market is composed of different types of financial institutions (banks, life insurance companies, pension funds, REITs, etc.).

Proceeds. The sum of money remaining after the discount has been deducted from the principal amount of the bonds—what the borrower actually receives.

Prospectus. Commonly, a written document conforming to state and federal regulations containing disclosures about a business entity which is seeking additional debt or equity financing, together with information about the terms and purposes of the financing.

Protective Covenants. Restrictive conditions preventing certain action by the borrower which if not waived or corrected could trigger an event of default. Restrictive covenants are usually divided into financial covenants and operating covenants.

Provider. An individual or organization that provides health care services in exchange for reimbursement from a purchaser.

Rate Covenant. A condition in the indenture which requires the hospital to charge rates sufficient to achieve a minimum debt service coverage. In the event debt service falls below this ratio, the hospital is required to retain an independent consultant to analyze operations and make recommendations which the hospital will follow, if feasible.

Redemption Provision. A provision allowing the issuer, at its option, to call the bonds at fixed price after a certain date.

Refunding. New securities are sold by the issuer and the proceeds used to retire outstanding securities. The object may be to save interest cost, extend the maturity of the debt or to relax certain existing restrictive covenants.

Registered Bonds. Bonds which are registered with the bond trustee which designate ownership. Transfer of ownership of the bonds must be registered with the bond trustee in order that new bond holders continue to receive principal and interest.

Reserve Fund. A special fund created under the indenture (usually funded from bond proceeds) to be used only for the payment of debt service on the bonds in the event insufficient funds are deposited in the bond fund.

Revenue Bond. A bond payable solely from the revenue generated from the operation of the project being financed. In the case of hospital revenue bond financing, the bonds are typically payable from the gross receipts of the hospital.

Sale and Leaseback. Transaction in which one party sells real or personal property to another party and concurrently the purchaser leases the property to the seller.

Security Agreement. Written agreement between a debtor and his creditor containing the terms by which a security interest is created in specific assets of the debtor.

Security Interest. Property interest in a debtor's assets which is conveyed to (or retained by) a creditor to secure payment or performance of an obligation that the debtor owes the creditor.

Sensitivity Studies. An analysis of an institution's reputation in its community for the delivery of care, sensitivity to community needs and performance of its functions, often used to determine the community's receptivity to a fund-raising drive.

Serial Bonds. Not a distinct class of bonds but rather an issue of bonds with different maturities, as distinguished from an issue where all of the bonds have identical maturities (term bonds). Serial bonds are usually retired either in equal annual amounts or on a level debt service basis.

Series Bonds. Secured by the same assets or revenue, but issued at intervals with different dates. They may or may not mature at the same time.

Sinking Fund. Separate accumulation of cash or investments (including earnings thereon) in accordance with the terms of a debt or stock security, increased periodically by contributions, generally of cash, from the security's issuer, for the purpose of assuring timely redemption.

"63-20" Financing. A type of tax-exempt hospital financing requiring a special ruling from the Internal Revenue Service based upon a 1963 Ruling (#20). The bonds are issued by the hospital and when fully retired, title is tendered to a municipality or other public body.

Standby Commitment. A promise to make a permanent loan on a construction project upon completion, which contains unusually onerous terms of repayment or interest rate, or both. A standby commitment is not intended to be exercised by the borrower, but does permit the borrower to start construction while awaiting improvement in loan availabilities or market conditions.

Subordinated Debt. Debt that has terms which limit the debtor's assets available to the holder in case of default, usually to those assets remaining after satisfaction of all other creditors' claims, including those of general (unsecured) creditors.

Syndicate. A group of investment bankers usually headed by a manager who underwrites a bond issue and offers it for resale to the public.

Take Out. A permanent loan commitment. When the permanent loan is made, its proceeds are used to pay off or "take out" the construction lender.

Tax-Exempt Bond. A bond upon which the interest is exempt from federal income taxes.

Term Bond. A bond of an issue which has a single maturity. At intervals, a certain percentage of the outstanding bonds are called and retired using the money set aside in a sinking fund. Often, serial bonds and term bonds are combined in one issue.

Third Party Payer. The insurer who pays for the services provided to a patient. The third party payer is particularly one who has a contractual arrangement with the provider to care for a patient under a specific reimbursement arrangement. Includes both private and governmental insurers.

True Lease. A transaction that is recognized both in law and by tax authorities as providing the lessor with the benefits and risks of ownership. A true lease may be either non-payout or full payout. A basic qualification of a true lease is that the lessee may not build an equity position in the asset during the lease term.

Trustee. A bank designated as the custodian of funds and the official representative of the bond holders.

Underwriter. Generally, one or more investment bankers who, for a fee, undertake to market a debt or equity security issue for the issuing entity or, in the case of a secondary offering, for the selling shareholders.

Underwriters Due Diligence. Underwriters are required under provisions of the Securities Act of 1933 to conduct reasonable due diligence (investigation) so as to enable them to determine whether the disclosures contained in the registration statement describe accurately and completely all material facts relating to the issue. This concept is also applied to hospital issues, although the securities are exempt from the requirements of the Securities Act of 1933. Due diligence is required for the preparation of the official statement/loan memorandum.

Underwriting Spread Discount. The difference between the public offering price and the purchase price paid to the issuer by the underwriter. Expenses and selling costs are usually paid from this amount.

Unrestricted Fund. Funds which bear no external restrictions as to use or purpose, i.e., funds which can be used for any legitimate purpose designated by the governing board as distinguished from funds restricted externally for specific operating purposes, for plant replacement and expansion, and for endowment.

Useful Life. Estimated period during which benefits are expected to be derived from the use of an asset by a particular user, generally used in connection with determining depreciation of fixed assets.

Vendor. An equipment manufacturer or distributor who uses equipment financing as a sales tool in selling his merchandise.

Working Capital. Excess of current assets over current liabilities; the net current assets available for the continuing operating needs during the normal operating cycle of the business entity, generally one year.

Wraparound Mortgage. A mortgage loan in which the lender takes a junior lien position, but undertakes to make the payments on the prior lien, usually without assuming any legal obligation to pay it. This device is used to leverage an additional loan by charging a higher rate of interest on both old and new balances, while paying only the lower prior rate.

Yield. The computed percentage of return to the investor. Yield is based upon the cost of the bond, the length of time to its maturity and the coupon rate.

CONSTRUCTION GLOSSARY*

American Institute of Architects (AIA). A society of registered architects which publishes widely accepted copyrighted standard forms of agreements for use in design and construction. Copies of those forms may be obtained at any local office or from 1735 New York Ave., N.W., Washington, DC 20006.

Certificate of Need (CON). A confirmation, usually legal in nature, by an approved agency that a proposal for establishing a program or constructing a facility meets an estimated unmet need in a defined service area.

Cost-Plus Contract. A type of agreement widely used in construction, in which the owner agrees to pay for all costs incurred by the contractor in executing the plans and specifications, "plus" an additional amount (fixed sum, percentage or other arrangement) as fee or profit. Similar to cost reimbursement arrangements with Medicare.

Critical Path. A technique, often computerized, for controlling construction projects so that unwarranted delays are not caused by failures to deliver portions of the work on schedule.

"Fast Track" Construction. The design and bidding of a project in phases or intervals so as to accelerate completion of construction.

Finance Lease. A transaction that is recognized in law as providing the lessor with full proprietary rights in the equipment but is viewed by the tax authorities as a conditional sale agreement.

---

*Source: Adapted from "Capital Financing," ed. Daniel M. Cain and R. Neal Gilbert, *Topics in Health Care Financing,* Fall 1978.

Fixed Equipment. Any major equipment fixed to or any integral part of the building structure (this is realty equipment under HUD-FHA).

Fixed Price Contract. A type of agreement in which a specified service or article is to be delivered in exchange for a specified, certain price.

Preliminary Drawings. Drawings, outline specifications and other material which define in specific detail all the systems, materials and components of a project, sufficiently to establish an accurate cost estimate.

Program. A narrative description of a capital project, expressed in terms of the services to be rendered and the functions which will take place within a department, rather than in terms of partitions and square feet of space.

Program Planning. The development of a service or an activity for a population group. It covers the various steps required to develop, mobilize and coordinate all the resources necessary to carry out the activity. In a real sense, it is the heart of the institutional planning process.

Punch List. A list of construction deficiencies, including omitted matters, usually prepared by the architect as a condition to the release of retainages to the contractor, at or near the end of a construction project.

Schematic Drawings. Drawings indicating the overall scope of the project in broad detail, usually showing only general functional relationships among its elements. Often referred to as "single lines," due to the single-line representation of partitions and walls.

Upset Price. A guaranteed maximum price for a construction project. Usually the person guaranteeing the price must bear full financial responsibility for any excess.

Value Engineering. A continuous process of measurement of costs against values, of services, materials and equipment for the purpose of assuring maximum value is returned for each dollar spent.

Working Drawings. The final plans and specifications from which a project is actually constructed.

EDP (ELECTRONIC DATA PROCESSING) GLOSSARY*

Alphanumeric. A term used to describe data that contain both alphabetic and numeric characters.

Analog Computer. A computer that simulates measurements by electronic means, for example, by varying voltages.

Audit Trail. A means of tracing data back to original source data.

Batch Totals. The sum of a column of input used later to verify data.

Binary System. A numbering system that has only two digits, 0 and 1. The binary system is used by digital computers.

Buffer. That part of a computer system that temporarily stores information until the computer system processes it.

Bug. An error in the program or in the system.

Central Processing Unit. That part of the computer that carries out the instructions and solves the programs given to the computer.

Character. One of the digits, letters, or other symbols that are recognized by a computer.

COBOL. Acronym for Common Business Oriented Language. A computer language widely used in business operations.

Coding. Using symbols and abbreviations to give instructions to the computer. Synonymous with writing the program.

Collating. Combining of data from two or more files into sequence in one file.

Compiler. The program that converts the instructions written by the programmer into instructions that can be interpreted by the computer.

Computer Operator. The person in a computer system who manually controls the operations of the computer.

Control Total. The sum taken on a particular field in a group of records to be used for checking program, machine, or input reliability.

Control Unit. A major part of the computer that directs the step-by-step instructions given to a computer and that oversees the

---

*Source: Donald F. Beck, *Basic Hospital Financial Management,* Aspen Systems Corporation, 1980.

scheduling of the operations called for by the program.

CRT. Acronym for cathode ray tube, which is a television-like device used to display or store data.

Data File. A major unit of information that is stored. Examples of data files include accounts receivable, payroll master file, and general ledger.

Debugging. Identifying and correcting errors in a computer system or program.

Destructive Readin. A process of putting new data into a file in which data previously stored are destroyed in the update.

Digital Computer. A computer that processes data by combinations of digits.

Disk Pack. A device that contains a set of magnetized disks.

Editing. The process of deciding what data to accept, examining them for accuracy, and rejecting those that do not meet predetermined parameters.

Electronic Data Processing. The processing of data and calculating of results by an electronic machine, such as a computer.

Field. A group of consecutive columns of data used for a specific purpose.

File Maintenance. The periodic modification of a file to include changes that have occurred.

First Generation Computer. A class of computers that used vacuum tubes.

Flowchart. A graphic portrayal of a sequence of operations, an accumulation of data, or the steps used to solve a problem.

FORTRAN. Acronym for Formula Translation. A computer language widely used in scientific and engineering applications.

GIGO. Acronym for garbage in, garbage out. A commonly used term meaning that the quality of the computer output cannot be better than the quality of the input.

Hardware. The equipment and other machine devices in a computer system.

Hash Totals. The sum of numbers of a specific field. Used for verifying purposes.

Input. Data entered into a computer system for processing.

Installation. A particular computer system and its overall process.

Machine Language. A system of instructions written in a binary code of electronic impulses that are used to direct the computer.

Magnetic Tape. A tape that has been coded with a magnetizable material. Used to record information in the form of polarized spots.

Memory. A device on which data can be stored for retrieval at a later time.

Mnemonic. A contraction or abbreviation used to represent the full expression.

Nondestructive Readout. A process in which data are read out of storage repeatedly without being destroyed.

Operation Manual. A manual that gives detailed instructions to a computer operator on how to complete a job.

Peripheral Equipment. Equipment that is not under the direct control of the computer, such as a printer, card reader, or cathode ray tube.

Primary Storage. Storage in the main storage area of the computer itself.

Procedure. A predetermined way to accomplish a given task.

Programming. The advance preparation of instructions for use by the computer.

Random Access. A storage device by which access time in retrieval is made to be independent of the location of data or sequence of input.

Real Time. Processing of data instantaneously as they are received, enabling the user to have immediate control.

Second Generation Computer. A computer that uses transistors and operates in millionths of a second.

Secondary Storage. Storage on magnetic tapes, disks, drums, or other devices that are not directly connected to the computer.

Simulation. A representation in a computer program of a real model in order to mirror the effects of changes in the model. Used to determine the probable effects of changes in assumptions.

Software. The programs and documentation of a computer system.

Source Document. Original paper from which information regarding a transaction is recorded.

Subsystem. An identifiable portion of a main system.

Terminals. Devices for input and output that are some distance from the computer. They are often connected to the computer by telephone lines.

Third Generation Computer. A computer characterized by miniaturization and great speed. Operates in billionths of a second.

REIMBURSEMENT GLOSSARY*

(Medicare and Private Health Insurance)

A familiarity with "lingo" (special terminology) used in the health care field is a prerequisite for an understanding of third party reimbursement. This list is not intended to be all-inclusive; it contains selected terms often encountered in the discussion of reimbursement for health care services.

Accrual Accounting: Revenue is reported in the period earned (regardless of when collected) and expenses are reported in the period in which they are incurred (regardless of when paid).

Accumulation: An increase in the amount of benefits provided under a policy, which is used as a reward to the insured for continuous renewal.

Acute Illness: A condition or illness requiring either medical attention or restricted activity and which is expected to last less than three months from the date of onset.

Adjustment Report: A statement by the auditors of their proposed changes in costs claimed by the provider in its cost report.

Allocated Benefits: A situation in which each benefit provided by an insurance policy such as x-ray, drugs, consultations, etc., has a specific maximum stated in the policy, as opposed to an overall maximum for all services rendered.

Allowable Charge: Maximum fee allowable by a third party payer for a covered service.

Allowable Costs: Elements of cost which are reimbursable, usually under a third party

reimbursement formula. Typically, allowable costs under Medicare and Medicaid exclude the costs of such things as luxury accommodations, televisions and telephones.

Allowance: The difference between gross revenue from services rendered and amounts received from patients or third party payers. Allowances are distinguished from uncollectible accounts resulting from credit losses.

Ambulatory Care: Services which are provided on an outpatient basis, in contrast to services provided in the home or to persons who are inpatients.

Ancillary Services: Services other than room and board, physician and nursing care—e.g., laboratory, x-ray, pharmacy, ambulance, equipment, appliances, physical and occupational therapy, etc.—which are related to a patient's care and treatment.

Assignment: Under supplementary medical insurance, if the enrollee and the service provider both agree, the enrollee may assign his rights to benefits to the provider. When this assignment method is used, the provider agrees that his total charge for the covered service will be the reasonable charge approved by the carrier. The provider submits a claim to the carrier, and is reimbursed for the reasonable charge, minus the 20 percent coinsurance and any deductible which remains unmet. The provider may then charge the enrollee only for the coinsurance and any applicable deductible.

Audit: (Medicare) The examination of financial and statistical records of a provider being paid reasonable cost for services rendered to beneficiaries of the program to ascertain that the costs claimed by the provider are in accordance with the Law and the Regulations promulgated by the Secretary.

Automatic Enrollment: Retirement and survivors' insurance beneficiaries are automatically sent Medicare cards three months before the attainment of age 65; those entitled to disability-based benefits are automatically sent Medicare cards three months before the completion of 24 consecutive months of entitlement. These Medicare cards show entitlement to both hospital in-

---

*Source: Adapted from *Topics in Health Care Financing,* Spring 1975 and Fall 1975; William O. Cleverley, *Essentials of Hospital Finance,* Aspen Systems Corporation, 1978; and the *Medicare and Medicaid Data Book, 1981,* Health Care Financing Administration, Pub. No. HCFA-03128, April 1982.

surance and supplementary medical insurance; an enrollee wishing to decline SMI coverage must do so in writing no later than the month prior to the effective date of coverage.

Beneficiary: An individual entitled to have payment made on his behalf or to him under an insurance program (Private or Governmental).

Benefit Period: A benefit period is the time period used to limit Medicare benefits in the health insurance program. A benefit period begins the first day an enrollee is furnished inpatient hospital or extended care services by a qualified provider, and ends when the enrollee has not been an inpatient of a hospital or other facility primarily providing skilled nursing or rehabilitation services for 60 consecutive days. Although there are limits to covered benefits per benefit period, there is no limit to the number of benefit periods an enrollee can have. The enrollee must pay the hospital insurance deductible for each new benefit period.

Benefits: The payment of cash, or provision of services, after the occurrence of specific events, accidents or illness, which are covered by an insurance contract.

Capitation Fee: A per-person charge for services to be provided to individuals or groups for a specified period of time.

Carrier: A carrier is an organization which has contracted with DHHS to process claims and perform other services under Medicare's supplementary medical insurance program.

Catastrophic Insurance Coverage: Insurance coverage for large and unexpected medical expenses. Sometimes such expenses are covered under comprehensive major medical, major medical, or extended benefits coverage provisions.

Categorically Needy: Under Medicaid, categorically needy cases are aged, blind, or disabled individuals or families and children who are otherwise eligible for Medicaid and who meet financial eligibility requirements for AFDC, SSI, or an optional State supplement.

Charity Allowance: The difference between gross-revenue charges at established rates and amounts to be received from an indigent patient or from voluntary agencies or government units on behalf of an indigent patient.

Chronic Illness: Impairments or illnesses which have one or more of the following characteristics: 1) are presumably permanent, 2) leave residual disability, 3) are caused by non-reversible pathological alterations, 4) require special training or rehabilitation of the patient, 5) may be expected to require a long period of medical supervision, and/or care.

Coinsurance: Coinsurance is that portion of reimbursable hospital and medical expenses, after subtraction of any deductible, which Medicare does not cover. Under HI, there is no coinsurance for the first 60 days of inpatient hospital care; from the 61st through the 90th day of inpatient care, the daily coinsurance amount is equal to one-fourth of the inpatient hospital deductible. For each of the 60 lifetime reserve days used, the daily coinsurance amount is equal to one-half of the inpatient hospital deductible. There is no coinsurance for the first 20 days of skilled nursing facility care; from the 21st through the 100th day of SNF care, the daily coinsurance amount is equal to one-eighth of the inpatient hospital deductible. Under supplementary medical insurance, after the annual deductible has been met, Medicare will pay 80 percent of reasonable charges for covered services and supplies; the remaining 20 percent of reasonable charges is the coinsurance payable by the enrollee.

Combination Method: The cost of "routine services" for program beneficiaries is determined on the basis of average cost per diem of these services for all patients; to this is added the cost of ancillary services used by beneficiaries, determined by apportioning the total cost of ancillary services on the basis of the ratio of beneficiary charges for ancillary services to total patient charges for such services.

Community Rating: The practice of basing premiums, in whole or in part, upon the experience of an entire community rather than the particular group insured.

Comprehensive Major Medical Insurance: A policy designed to give the protection offered by both a basic and a major medical health insurance policy. It is generally characterized by a low deductible, a coinsurance feature, and high maximum benefits.

Contestable Clause: The section of an insurance policy which states the conditions under which the insurer can contest the policy. Fraud or material misrepresentation in the application are generally listed as reasons, provided they are discovered during the contestable period, which is usually two years from the effective date of the policy.

Contractual Allowance: The difference between billings at established charges and amounts received or due from third party payers under contract agreements—similar to a trade discount.

Coordination of Benefits: Applied when an insured is covered by more than one policy. It stipulates that the involved insurers will each pay their share of the insured's total covered expenses, but will not pay, in the aggregate, more than those expenses. This eliminates overpayments by insurers, cash windfalls to the policyholder, and excessive premiums for duplicated coverage.

Copayment: Form of cost sharing whereby the insured pays a specific amount per unit of service received. This differs from a coinsurance arrangement under which payment is expressed as a percentage of cost.

Cost-Based Reimbursement: Method of payment used by many third parties based on the actual costs of providing services to the covered patient, not on the charges actually made for those services. There are a variety of cost formulas which specify whether or not a plus factor is allowable and what type of cost apportionment methods may be used. Medicare, Medicaid, most Blue Cross plans and other governmental programs typically reimburse hospitals and other health care facilities on the basis of costs.

"Cost Plus" Factors: An allowance in lieu of specific recognition of other costs not precisely measured or considered in the program cost determination. It is added to reimbursable cost.

Cost Reimbursement: Contractual reimbursement for all reasonable costs of patient care incurred by providers and paid by third party payers (principally Medicare, Medicaid, and Blue Cross), as defined by law, regulation, or contract.

Cost Report: A cost analysis prepared by a provider of health care as a basis for claiming reimbursable costs under third party contract agreements.

Covered Services: Covered services are the specific services and supplies for which Medicare will provide reimbursement. Examples of some covered services are Emergency Services, Skilled Nursing Facility Services, etc. Covered services under the Medicaid program consist of a combination of mandatory and optional services within each State.

Customary Charge: The charge a physician or supplier usually bills his patients for furnishing a particular service or supply is called the customary charge.

Deductible: Deductibles are the amounts payable by the enrollee for covered services before Medicare makes reimbursements. The hospital insurance deductible applies to each new benefit period, is determined each year by using a formula specified by law, and approximates the current cost of a one-day inpatient hospital stay. The supplementary medical insurance deductible is currently fixed by law at the first $60 of covered charges per calendar year.

Departmental Method of Reimbursement: Departmental method of reimbursement is used to apportion the cost of each ancillary department to Medicare patients based on the ratio of beneficiary (Medicare) charges for the specific department to the total patient charges for the specific department.

Desk Review: An examination of the mathematics and logic of a cost report submitted to a third party payer to enable the hospital to receive a tentative payment pending audit and final settlement.

Disabled: For purposes of enrollment under Medicare, individuals under age 65 who have been entitled for not less than 24 months to benefits under the Social Security Act or the railroad retirement system on the basis of disability are considered to be disabled.

Discharge: A discharge is a formal release from a hospital or a skilled nursing facility. Discharges include persons who died during their stay, or were transferred to another facility.

Early and Periodic Screening, Diagnosis, and Treatment (EPSDT): The EPSDT program covers screening and diagnostic services to determine physical or mental defects in recipients under age 21, and health care, treatment, and other measures to correct or ameliorate any defects and chronic conditions discovered.

End-Stage Renal Disease (ESRD): For purposes of enrollment under Medicare, individuals who have chronic kidney disease requiring renal dialysis or kidney transplant are considered to have end-stage renal disease. To qualify for Medicare coverage, the individual must be fully or currently insured under social security or the railroad retirement system, or be the dependent of an insured person. Eligibility for Medicare coverage begins with the 3rd month after the month in which a course of renal dialysis begins. Coverage may begin sooner if the patient participates in a self-care dialysis training program provided by an approved facility; or if a person receives a kidney transplant without starting or receiving dialysis.

Enrollment Period: A Medicare beneficiary may voluntarily enroll for supplementary medical insurance at any time; entitlement begins on the third calendar month following the month of enrollment.

Exclusions: Specific hazards or conditions listed in the policy for which the policy will not provide benefit payments.

Expenditure: Under Medicaid, expenditure refers to an amount paid out by a State agency for the covered medical expenses of eligible participants.

Family Planning Services: Family planning services are any medically approved means, including diagnosis, treatment, drugs, supplies and devices, and related counseling which are furnished or prescribed by or under the supervision of a physician for individuals of child-bearing age for purposes of enabling such individuals freely to determine the number or spacing of their children.

Federal Hospital Insurance Trust Fund: The Federal hospital insurance trust fund is a trust fund of the Treasury of the United States in which are deposited monies collected from taxes on annual earnings of employees, employers, and self-employed persons covered under social security, and other gifts and bequests to the fund. Disbursements from the fund are made to help pay for benefit payments and administrative expenses incurred by the hospital insurance program.

Federal Supplementary Medical Insurance Trust Fund: The Federal supplementary medical insurance trust fund is a trust fund of the Treasury of the United States consisting of gifts and bequests made to the fund, and amounts deposited in or appropriated to the fund as provided by Title XVIII of the Social Security Act including premiums paid in by enrollees under SMI and contributions by the Federal government from general revenues. Disbursements from the fund are made for benefit payments and administrative expenses incurred by the SMI program.

Fee Schedule: A listing of accepted fees or established allowances for specified medical procedures. Usually represents the maximum amounts that a policy will pay for the specified procedures.

Final Cost Settlement: The difference between costs covered by third parties as reflected in the final or audited cost report and any interim payments and/or interim retroactive adjustments.

First Dollar Coverage: Health insurance which pays benefits beginning with the initial services, as opposed to payment after a deductible.

Fiscal Agent: A fiscal agent is a contractor that processes or pays vendor claims on behalf of the Medicaid agency. Under Medicare, fiscal agents are called intermediaries (HI) and carriers (SMI).

Group Practice Prepayment Plan (GPPP): In general, members of group practice prepayment plans pay regular premiums to the plan. In return, the members receive the health services the plan provides, whenever needed, without additional charges. Many prepayment plans have made arrangements with Medicare to receive direct payments for services they furnish which are covered by SMI.

Health Insuring Organization: A health insuring organization is an entity that pays for medical services provided to recipients who pay a premium or subscription charge to the entity, which assumes an underwriting risk with regard to expenses for the services provided.

Health Maintenance Organization (HMO): Some group practice prepayment plans also provide many inpatient services, and therefore have contracts with Medicare as Health Maintenance Organizations which allows them to receive direct payment for services covered by hospital insurance and supplementary medical insurance.

Home Health Agency: A home health agency is a public agency or private organization which is primarily engaged in providing skilled nursing services and other therapeutic services in the patient's home, and which meets certain conditions designed to ensure the health and safety of the individuals who are furnished these services.

Home Health Services: Home health services are services and items furnished to an individual who is under the care of a physician by a home health agency, or by others under arrangements made by such agency. The services are furnished under a plan established and periodically reviewed by a physician. The services are provided on a visiting basis in an individual's home and include: parttime or intermittent skilled nursing care; physical, occupational, or speech therapy; medical social services, medical supplies and appliances (other than drugs and biologicals); home health aide services; and services of interns and residents.

Hospital Insurance: Hospital insurance (also known as Medicare Part A) is an insurance program providing basic protection against the costs of hospital and related post hospital services for individuals who are age 65 or over and are eligible for retirement benefits under the social security or the railroad retirement systems, for individuals under age 65 who have been entitled for not less than 24 months to benefits under the social security or railroad retirement systems on the basis of disability, and for certain other individuals who are medically determined to have end-stage renal disease and are covered by the social security or railroad retirement systems.

Income Ceiling: Refers to the level of family or individual income below which partici-

pating medical practitioners provide services to plan beneficiaries at a charge that does not exceed the amounts listed in the fee schedule. For members with incomes above the ceiling, the practitioner may charge more than the scheduled fee and bill the individual for excesses.

Indemnity Benefits: A policy under which the insured person is paid directly a specified sum of money toward his hospital and medical expenses from which he, in turn, pays the provider of care. In certain circumstances, such benefits may be assigned legally to the provider, removing the patient as the "middle-man."

Independent Laboratory: An independent laboratory is a laboratory certified to perform diagnostic tests independent of a physician's office or hospital and to receive reimbursements from Medicare.

Inpatient Hospital Services: Inpatient hospital services are items and services furnished to an inpatient of a hospital by the hospital, including bed and board, nursing and related services, diagnostic and therapeutic services, and medical or surgical services.

Interim Rate: A negotiated payment made to a hospital for providing services to patients covered by third party insurers subject to final settlement.

Intermediary: An intermediary is an organization selected by providers of health care which has entered into an agreement with DHHS under Medicare's hospital insurance program to process claims and perform other functions.

Intermediate Care Facility: An intermediate care facility is an institution furnishing health-related care and services to individuals who do not require the degree of care provided by hospitals or skilled nursing facilities as defined under Title XIX (Medicaid) of the Social Security Act

Laboratory And Radiological Services: Laboratory and radiological services are professional and technical laboratory and radiological services ordered by a licensed practitioner and provided in an office or similar facility (other than a hospital outpatient department or clinic) or by a qualified laboratory.

Lifetime Reserve: A Medicare hospital insurance enrollee has a non-renewable lifetime reserve of 60 days of inpatient hospital care to draw upon if the 90 covered days per benefit period are exhausted.

Limitations: Exceptions or exclusions to the general coverage. They may be dollar limits of liability, exclusions of specific types of illness, exclusions while performing certain activities, etc.

Major Medical Expense Insurance: Policies designed to help offset the heavy medical expenses resulting from catastrophic or prolonged illness or injury. They generally provide benefit payments for 75%–80% of medical expenses above a deductible paid by the insured person. The maximum amounts provided by such policies are generally quite high.

Medically Needy: Under Medicaid, medically needy cases are aged, blind, or disabled individuals or families and children who are otherwise eligible for Medicaid, and whose income resources are above the limits for eligibility as categorically needy (AFCD or SSI) but are within limits set under the Medicaid State plan.

Miscellaneous Expenses: Hospital charges, other than room and board, such as x-rays, drugs, laboratory fees, and other ancillary charges.

Nursing Salary Cost Differential: Allowance added to Medicare cost to recognize the above average cost of inpatient routine nursing care furnished to aged patients.

Other Practitioners' Services: Other practitioners' services are health care services of licensed practitioners other than physicians and dentists.

Outpatient Hospital Services: Outpatient hospital services are services furnished to outpatients by a participating hospital for diagnosis or treatment of an illness or injury.

Outpatient Services: Outpatient services are medical and other services provided by a hospital or other qualified facility or supplier, such as a mental health clinic, rural health clinic, mobile X-ray unit, or free-standing dialysis unit. Such services include outpatient physical therapy services, diagnostic X-ray and laboratory tests, X-ray and other radiation therapy.

Part A and Part B Services: Medicare benefits are payable from two funds. Part A services, which, in general, are those rendered by institutions, are reimbursed from funds derived from payroll tax. Part B services, generally medical and surgical physicians' services, and outpatient treatment and diagnosis are reimbursed from the fund created by voluntary premium payments and general federal revenues.

Persons Served: Under Medicare, a person served is a Medicare enrollee who uses a covered medical service, incurs expenses greater than the deductible amount, and for whom Medicare paid benefits.

Physicians' Services: Under Medicare and Medicaid, physicians' services are services provided by an individual licensed under State law to practice medicine or osteopathy. Services covered by hospital bills are not included.

Portable X-Ray: A portable x-ray is a radiograph taken with portable equipment, usually in the patient's place of residence, under the general supervision of a physician.

Preexisting Condition: A physical condition of an insured person which existed prior to the issuance of his policy or his enrollment in a plan and which may result in a limitation in the contract on coverage of benefits.

Premium: A premium is a monthly fee paid by enrollees in Medicare. Hospital insurance enrollees who are social security or railroad retirement beneficiaries and who qualify for coverage through age or disability are not required to pay premiums. Aged persons who are not eligible for automatic HI enrollment may pay a monthly premium to obtain HI coverage. Supplementary medical insurance enrollees pay a monthly premium which is updated every July to reflect changes in program costs.

Premium Hospital Insurance: Those persons 65 years and older who are not automatically eligible for hospital insurance may obtain coverage by paying a monthly premium.

Prescribed Drugs: Prescribed drugs are drugs dispensed by a licensed pharmacist on the prescription of a practitioner licensed by law to administer such drugs, and drugs dispensed by a licensed practitioner to his own patients. This item does not include a practitioner's drug charges that are not separable from his other charges, or drugs covered by a hospital's bill.

Prevailing Charge: The prevailing charge is the charge that would cover 75 percent of the customary charges made for similar services in the same locality.

Prior Authorization: Requirement imposed by some third party payers that a provider must justify the need for delivering a service to a patient prior to the actual delivery of that service. Usually prior authorization is limited to the delivery of nonemergency services.

Probationary Period: A specified number of days after the issuance of the policy during which coverage is not afforded for sickness. The purpose of the period is to eliminate sickness actually contracted before the policy went into force.

Professional Component: The services of provider-based physicians (e.g., those on a salary, or percentage arrangement, lessors of departments, etc., whether or not they bill patients directly) include two distinct elements, the professional component and the provider component. The professional component of the provider-based physician's services pertains to that part of the physician's activities which is directly related to the medical care of the individual patient. It represents remuneration for the identifiable medical services by the physician which contribute to the diagnosis of the patient's condition or to his treatment. The portion of the physician's activities representing services which are not directly related to an identifiable part of the medical care of the individual patient is the provider component. Reimbursement for provider component services can be made only to a provider on the basis of its allowable reasonable costs. Provider services include teaching, research conducted in conjunction with and as part of patient care (to the extent that such costs are not met by special research funds), administration, general supervision of professional or technical personnel, laboratory quality control activities, committee work, performance of autopsies, and attending conferences as part of the physician's provider services activities.

Professional Standards Review Organization (PSRO): A PSRO is a physician or other professional medical organization (consisting of physicians and other health professionals with independent admitting hospital privileges) that enters into an agreement with DHHS to assume the responsibility for the review of the quality and appropriateness of services covered by Medicare, Medicaid, and the Maternal and Child Health program. PSROs determine whether services are medically necessary, provided in accordance with professional standards, and, in the case of institutional services, rendered in the appropriate setting.

Proof of Loss: Evidence submitted by the insured to prove that he is entitled to collect benefits due to the occurrence of the event insured against. Such evidence might include: itemized bills, a physician's statement, death certificate, etc.

Proration: The adjustment of benefits paid because of a mistake in the amount of the premiums paid or the existence of other insurance covering the same accident or disability.

Provider: An individual or organization that provides health care services in exchange for reimbursement from a purchaser. The term, as used in the Medicare program, applies only to institutions (e.g., hospitals, skilled nursing facilities or home health agencies) as contrasted to "others" (e.g., physicians).

Provider Component: See Professional Component.

Prudent Buyer Principle: Medicare reimbursement provision that limits reimbursement to a provider for costs in excess of amounts that a prudent and cost conscious buyer would pay.

RCC or RCCAC: *R*atio of *C*harges to *C*harges *A*pplied to *C*ost. Method of determining program reimbursement such as Departmental RCC or Gross RCC.

Reasonable Charge: In processing claims for SMI benefits, carriers use HCFA guidelines to establish the reasonable charge for services rendered. The reasonable charge is the lowest of: the actual charge billed by the physician or supplier; the charge the physician or supplier customarily bills his patients for the same service; and the prevailing charge which most physicians or suppliers in that locality bill for the same service. Increases in the physicians' prevailing charge levels are recognized only to the extent justified by an index reflecting changes in the costs of practice and in general earnings.

Reasonable Cost: In processing claims for HI benefits, intermediaries use HCFA guidelines to determine the reasonable cost incurred by the individual providers in furnishing covered services to enrollees. The reasonable cost is based on the actual cost of providing such services, including direct and indirect costs of providers, and excluding any costs which are unnecessary in the efficient delivery of services covered by the insurance program.

Recipient: A recipient of Medicaid is an individual who has been determined to be eligible for Medicaid and who has used medical services covered under Medicaid.

Recurring Clause: A provision in some health insurance policies which specifies a period of time during which the recurrence of a condition is considered a continuation of a prior period of disability or hospital confinement.

Reimbursement: Under Medicare, the reimbursement amount refers to the dollar amount of medical expenses payable by the Medicare program. (For Medicaid, see Expenditures.)

Reserve: A sum set aside by an insurance company to assure the fulfillment of commitments for future claims.

Rural Health Clinic: A rural health clinic is an outpatient facility which is primarily engaged in furnishing physicians' and other medical and health services, which meets certain other requirements designed to ensure the health and safety of the individuals served by the clinic. The clinic must be located in an area that is not an urbanized area as defined by the Bureau of the Census and that is designated by the Secretary of DHHS either as an area with a shortage of personal health services, or as a health manpower shortage area, and has filed an agreement with the Secretary not to charge any individual or other person for items or services for which such individual is entitled to have payment made by Medicare, except for the amount of any deductible or coinsurance amount applicable.

Self-Insurance: The undertaking by an employer or an employee group to provide coverage directly without contracting with an insurance carrier or service plan.

Senior Citizen Policies: Contracts insuring persons 65 years or older. In most cases, these policies supplement the coverage afforded by the Government under the Medicare program.

Service Benefits: Benefits which are payable directly to the provider of the services.

Spend-Down: Under the Medicaid program, spend-down refers to a method by which an individual establishes Medicaid eligibility by reducing gross income through incurring medical expenses until net income (after medical expenses) meets Medicaid financial requirements.

State Buy-In: State buy-in is the term given to the process by which a State may provide SMI (Medicare Part B) coverage for its needy eligible persons through an agreement with the Federal government under which the State pays the premiums for them.

State Plan: The Medicaid State plan is a comprehensive written commitment by a Medicaid agency to administer or supervise the administration of a Medicaid program in accordance with Federal requirements.

Subscriber: The individual who signs the contract with the health plan. The subscriber is differentiated from the enrollee, who is defined as anyone covered under the contract.

Supplemental Security Income (SSI): SSI is a program of income support for low-income aged, blind, and disabled persons established by Title XVI of the Social Security Act.

Supplementary Medical Insurance (SMI): SMI (also known as Part B) is a voluntary insurance program which provides insurance benefits for physician and other medical services in accordance with the provisions of Title XVIII of the Social Security Act for aged and disabled individuals who elect to enroll under such program. The program is financed from premium payments by enrollees, together with contributions from funds appropriated by the Federal government.

Surgical Expense Insurance: Health insurance policies which provide benefits toward the physician's surgical fees. Benefits usually consist of scheduled amounts for each surgical procedure.

Third Party Liability: Under Medicaid, third-party liability exists if there is any entity (including other government programs or insurance) which is or may be liable to pay all or part of the medical cost or injury, disease, or disability of an applicant or recipient of Medicaid.

Vendor: A medical vendor is an institution, agency, organization, or individual practitioner which provides health or medical services.

Workers' Compensation Programs: Mandatory state social insurance programs that provide cash benefits to workers and their dependents who are disabled as a result of their employment. Medical services are usually covered under these programs.

Appendix B—Licensing and Certification

MEDICAL SPECIALTY BOARDS*

Boards	*Component Certifications*
American Board of Allergy and Immunology (A Conjoint Board of the American Board of Internal Medicine and the American Board of Pediatrics) University City Science Center 3624 Market Street Philadelphia, Pa. 19104 Telephone: (215) 349-9466 Executive Secretary: Herbert C. Mansmann, Jr., M.D.	
The American Board of Anesthesiology 100 Constitution Plaza Hartford, Conn. 06103 Telephone: (203) 522-9851 Secretary-Treasurer: E.S. Siker, M.D.	
The American Board of Colon and Rectal Surgery 615 Griswold, Suite 516 Detroit, Mich. 48226 Telephone: (313) 961-7880 Secretary-Treasurer: Norman D. Nigro, M.D.	
The American Board of Dermatology, Inc. Henry Ford Hospital Detroit, Mich. 48202 Telephone: (313) 871-8739 Executive Director: Clarence S. Livingood, M.D.	

---

*Source: *Directory of Medical Specialties*, U.S. Department of Health, Education, and Welfare, 1979.

Boards	*Component Certifications*

American Board of Family Practice
2228 Young Drive
Lexington, Ky. 40505
  Telephone: (606) 269-5626
  Secretary and Executive Director:
    Nicholas J. Pisacano, M.D.	

American Board of Internal Medicine
200 S.W. Market Street
Portland, Ore. 97201
  Telephone: (503) 228-8880
  President: John A. Benson, Jr., M.D.
	Internal Medicine
	Allergy and Immunology
	Cardiology
	Cardiovascular Disease
	Endocrinology
	Gastroenterology
	Hematology
	Infectious Disease
	Nephrology
	Pulmonary Disease
	Rheumatology

The American Board of Neurological Surgery
LSU Medical Center
1542 Tulane Avenue
New Orleans, La. 70112
  Telephone: (504) 568-5968
  Secretary-Treasurer: David G. Kline, M.D.

The American Board of Nuclear Medicine
(A Conjoint Board of the American Boards of
Internal Medicine, Pathology, and Radiology,
and Sponsored by the Society of Nuclear
Medicine)
475 Park Avenue South
New York, N.Y. 10016
  Telephone: (212) 889-0717
  Secretary: Joseph F. Ross, M.D.

The American Board of Obstetrics and
Gynecology, Inc.
711 Stanton L. Young Blvd.
Oklahoma City, Okla. 73104
  Telephone: (405) 236-0130
  Secretary-Treasurer: James A. Merrill, M.D.

American Board of Ophthalmology
8870 Towanda Street
Philadelphia, Pa. 19118
  Telephone: (215) CH2-1123
  Secretary-Treasurer: Francis H. Adler,
    M.D.

The American Board of Orthopaedic
Surgery, Inc.
444 North Michigan Avenue, Suite 2970
Chicago, Ill. 60611
  Telephone: (312) 822-9572
  Executive-Secretary
    William A. Larmon, M.D.

Boards	*Component Certifications*

American Board of Otolaryngology
220 Collingwood, Suite 130
Ann Arbor, Mich. 48103
  Telephone: (313) 761-7185
  Secretary-Treasurer: Walter P. Work, M.D.	

The American Board of Pathology
112 Lincoln Center
5401 W. Kennedy Blvd. P.O. Box 24695
Tampa, Fla. 33623
  Telephone: (813) 879-4864
  Executive Director: Murray R. Abell, M.D.
	Clinical Pathology and Pathologic Anatomy
	Blood Banking
	Clinical Bacteriology
	Clinical Chemistry
	Clinical Microbiology
	Clinical Pathology
	Forensic Pathology
	Hematology
	Medical Chemistry
	Medical Microbiology
	Neuropathology
	Pathologic Anatomy

The American Board of Pediatrics, Inc.
Suite 402 NCNB Plaza
136 E. Rosemary Street
Chapel Hill, N.C. 27514
  Telephone: (919) 929-0461
  Executive Secretary:
    Robert C. Brownlee, M.D.
	Pediatrics
	Pediatric Allergy
	Pediatric Cardiology

American Board of Physical Medicine and Rehabilitation
Suite J, 1A Kahler East
Rochester, Minn. 55901
  Telephone: (507) 282-1776
  Executive Secretary-Treasurer:
    Gordon M. Martin, M.D.	

The American Board of Plastic Surgery, Inc.
Room S-2221 Vanderbilt University Hospital
Nashville, Tenn. 37232
  Telephone: (615) 322-6404
  Secretary-Treasurer: John B. Lynch, M.D.	

The American Board of Preventive Medicine, Inc.
Graduate School of Public Health
University of Pittsburgh
Pittsburgh, Pa. 15261
  Telephone: (412) 624-2089
  Secretary-Treasurer:
    Herschel E. Griffin, M.D.
	Preventive Medicine
	Aerospace Medicine
	General Preventive Medicine
	Occupational Medicine
	Public Health

Boards	*Component Certifications*

American Board of Psychiatry and Neurology, Inc.
One American Plaza, Suite 808
Evanston, Ill. 60201
  Telephone: (312) 864-0830
  Executive Director:
    Lester H. Rudy, M.D.
	Child Psychiatry
	Neurology
	Neurology with Special Competence in Child
	  Neurology
	Psychiatry
	Psychiatry and Neurology

The American Board of Radiology
Kahler East
Rochester, Minn. 55901
  Telephone: (507) 282-7838
  Secretary: C. Allen Good, M.D.
	Radiology
	Diagnostic Radiology
	Diagnostic Roentgenology
	Roentgenology
	Radium Therapy
	Therapeutic Radiology

The American Board of Surgery, Inc.
1617 John F. Kennedy Blvd.
Philadelphia, Pa. 19103
  Telephone: (215) 568-4000
  Secretary-Treasurer:
    J.W. Humphreys, Jr., M.D.

The American Board of Thoracic Surgery, Inc.
14640 East Seven Mile Road
Detroit, Mich. 48205
  Telephone: (313) 372-2632
  Executive Director/Secretary-Treasurer:
    Herbert Sloan, M.D.

The American Board of Urology, Inc.
4121 West 83rd Street, Suite 124
Prairie Village, Kan. 66208
  Telephone: (913) 341-6321
  Secretary-Treasurer:
    William L. Valk, M.D.

HOSPITAL LICENSING FOR ANCILLARY AND OTHER SERVICES

Although the length and specificity of health facility regulations varies from state to state, almost all state regulations detail special program requirements for facility subparts and services. Table B-1 identifies the most common of these services and subparts that receive special attention in state health facility licensure regulations. Each of the services and subparts listed in the table has special requirements for licensure.

Table B-1 Hospital Services with Special Licensing Requirements

NAME OF STATES	Maternity and Newborn	Surgical Services	Laboratory	Radiology	Pharmacy	Medical Records	Physical Therapy	Occupational Therapy	Medical Services	Outpatient Services	Emergency Services	Dental Services	Psychiatric Services	Communicable Disease Services	Pediatrics	Social Services	Patient Activities	Patient Rights
Alabama	X	X	X	X	X	X	X			X							X	
Alaska	X	X				X							X		X			
Arizona	X	X	X	X		X					X		X	X				
Arkansas	X	X	X	X	X	X	X				X	X	X	X				
California	X	X				X		X	X							X		
Colorado	X	X		X	X	X	X	X		X	X	X		X	X	X	X	X
Connecticut	X	X		X		X	X				X	X		X				X
Delaware				X	X								X					X
District of Columbia	X	X	X	X	X	X			X	X	X		X	X	X	X		
Florida	X	X	X	X	X	X	X	X			X	X	X					X
Georgia	X	X	X	X	X	X	X			X	X	X	X			X	X	
Hawaii	X	X	X	X	X	X				X	X				X			
Idaho	X	X	X	X	X	X	X	X	X		X		X		X	X	X	
Illinois	X		X	X	X	X	X				X	X		X				
Indiana	X		X	X	X	X	X	X		X	X		X				X	X
Iowa	X	X	X	X	X	X	X	X		X	X		X		X			
Kansas	X	X	X	X	X	X	X	X	X	X	X	X	X	X	X	X	X	
Kentucky	X		X	X	X	X				X	X	X		X	X			
Louisiana	X	X	X	X	X					X	X	X	X			X		
Maine			X	X	X	X	X	X	X	X	X	X	X			X		X
Maryland	X	X	X	X	X	X	X	X		X			X	X		X	X	X
Massachusetts	X	X		X	X					X	X							
Michigan	X					X									X	X	X	
Minnesota	X	X	X	X	X	X				X								
Mississippi	X	X	X	X	X	X	X	X		X	X				X	X		
Missouri	X	X	X	X	X	X	X	X		X	X							
Montana	X	X	X	X	X	X	X	X		X	X	X	X			X	X	X
Nebraska	X	X	X	X	X	X					X	X						X
Nevada	X	X	X	X	X	X	X	X		X	X	X	X			X		
New Hampshire	X	X	X	X	X	X								X				
New Jersey	X					X	X		X	X			X			X	X	X
New Mexico	— none —																	
New York	— unknown —																	
North Carolina	X	X	X	X	X	X	X	X		X	X	X		X	X	X	X	
North Dakota	X	X	X	X	X	X	X			X				X		X	X	X

Table B-1   continued

SERVICES

NAME OF STATES	Maternity and Newborn	Surgical Services	Laboratory	Radiology	Pharmacy	Medical Records	Physical Therapy	Occupational Therapy	Medical Services	Outpatient Services	Emergency Services	Dental Services	Psychiatric Services	Communicable Disease Services	Pediatrics	Social Services	Patient Activities	Patient Rights
Ohio	X		X	X	X	X	X	X						X				
Oklahoma	X	X	X	X	X						X							
Oregon	X	X	X	X	X	X								X	X			
Pennsylvania	X	X	X	X	X	X				X	X	X	X		X	X	X	X
Rhode Island		X	X	X	X							X				X	X	X
South Carolina	X	X	X			X	X	X		X	X	X			X	X		
South Dakota	X	X	X	X	X	X				X	X						X	X
Tennessee	X	X	X	X	X	X				X	X	X	X					
Texas	X	X	X	X	X	X	X	X			X				X	X	X	X
Utah	X	X	X	X	X	X	X		X	X	X		X		X		X	
Vermont	X	X	X	X	X	X	X							X				
Virginia		X	X	X			X			X	X							
Washington	X	X	X	X	X	X	X			X	X							
West Virginia	X	X	X	X	X	X				X	X	X			X	X		
Wisconsin		X	X	X	X	X				X	X	X				X	X	
Wyoming				X	X	X							X			X	X	
American Samoa					— no licensure agency —													
Guam					— unknown —													
Puerto Rico	X	X	X	X	X	X	X			X	X	X			X	X	X	X
Trust Territories					— unknown —													
Virgin Islands					— unknown —													

Source: Kirschner Associates, *Characteristics of State Health Facility Licensing Practices: A Comparative Review,* Bureau of Health Planning and Resources Development, DHEW, Pub. No. (HRA) 78-14016, 1978.

INDEX